OXFORD MEDICAL PUBLICATIONS

Oncology

Oxford Core Texts

Clinical Dermatology
Endocrinology
Human Physiology
Paediatrics
Psychiatry
Medical Imaging
Neurology
Oncology

ONCOLOGY

Edited by

Roy A. J. Spence OBE JP MA MD FRCS
Consultant Surgeon, Belfast City Hospital; Honorary Professor,
The Queen's University of Belfast and
Honorary Professor, University of Ulster

and

Patrick G. Johnston MD PhD FRCP FRCPI
Professor of Oncology, The Queen's University of Belfast
and Belfast City Hospital

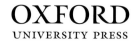

OXFORD
UNIVERSITY PRESS

OXFORD

UNIVERSITY PRESS

Great Clarendon Street, Oxford OX2 6DP

Oxford University Press is a department of the University of Oxford.
If furthers the University's objective of excellence in research, scholarship,
and education by publishing worldwide in

Oxford New York

Athens Auckland Bangkok Bogota Buenos Aires Calcutta
Cape Town Chennai Dar es Salaam Delhi Florence Hong Kong Istanbul
Karachi Kuala Lumpur Madrid Melbourne Mexico City Mumbai
Nairobi Paris São Paolo Singapore Taipei Tokyo Toronto Warsaw Shanghai

with associated companies in
Berlin Ibadan

Oxford is a registered trade mark of Oxford University Press
in the UK and in certain other countries

Published in the United States
by Oxford University Press Inc., New York

A catalogue record for this title is available from the British Library.

Library of Congress Cataloging in Publication Data
(Data available)

1 3 5 7 9 10 8 6 4 2

ISBN 0 19 262982 4

Typeset by EXPO Holdings, Malaysia

Printed in Italy
by Vincenzo Bona s.r.l., Turin.

Contents

Contributors   xi

Preface   xiii

Acknowledgements   xvii

1 The principles and practice of oncology – Patrick G. Johnston and Ultan McDermott   3

2 The aetiology of cancer – Hilary Russell   15

3 The epidemiology of cancer – Frank Kee   27

4 The molecular biology of cancer – D. Paul Harkin   37

5 The pathology of cancer – Damian T. McManus   47

6 Cancer prevention and screening – Richard D. Kennedy   61

7 The radiology of cancer – William Torreggiani and Michael J. Lee   81

8 The psychology of cancer – Robin Davidson   93

9 The principles of cancer surgery – Roy A. J. Spence   105

10 The principles of chemotherapy – Patrick. G. Johnston   119

11 The principles of radiotherapy – Frank Sullivan   133

12 Palliative care in cancer – Sheila Kelly   143

13 Skin cancer – Ronnie J. Atkinson   171

14 Head and neck cancer – Ruth Eakin   191

15 Gynaecological malignancy – John H. Price   209

16 Gastrointestinal cancer – James J. A. McAleer   231

17 Genitourinary Malignancy – Patrick F. Keane, John D. Kelly, and James J. A. McAleer   257

18 Thoracic tumours – Kieran McManus   283

19 Haematological and lymphoid tumours – T. C. M. (Curly) Morris   317

20 Bone and soft tissue tumours – Angus J. Patterson and
David C. Harmon   355

21 Paediatric tumours – Peter C. Adamson and
Brigitte C. Widemann   383

22 Breast cancer – William Odling-Smee   413

23 Central nervous system malignancies – Brian Orr   443

24 Endocrine tumours – Patrick M. Bell and
A. Brew Atkinson   463

25 Oncological emergencies – Sarah McKenna   489

Index   513

Dedication

To Iseult, Seamus, Eoghan, Niall, Ruairi
P. G. J.

To Di, Robert, Andrew, Katherine
R. A. J. S.

Contributors

Peter C. Adamson MD
Associate Professor of Paediatrics, Chief, Division of Clinical Pharmacology and Therapeutics, Children's Hospital of Philadelphia

A. Brew Atkinson DSc MD FRCP FRCPI
Consultant Physician, Honorary Professor of Endocrinology, Royal Victoria Hospital, The Queen's University of Belfast

R. J. Atkinson MD FRCS FRCOG
Senior Lecturer/Consultant in Medical Oncology, Royal Victoria Hospital, The Queen's University of Belfast/Belfast City Hospital

Patrick M. Bell MD FRCP
Consultant Physician Honorary Senior Lecturer, Royal Victorian Hospital, The Queen's University of Belfast

Robin Davidson BSc(Hons) MSc MSc(Clin Psych) DPhil ABPS
Consultant Clinical Psychologist, Honorary Lecturer, Belvoir Park Hospital/ The Queen's University of Belfast

Ruth Eakin MRCPI FRCR
Consultant in Clinical Oncology, Northern Ireland Cancer Centre

D. Paul Harkin BSc PhD
Lecturer in Oncology, The Queen's University of Belfast

David C. Harmon MD
Associate Physician, Massachusetts General Hospital; Assistant Professor, Harvard Medical School, Boston

P.G. Johnston MD PhD FRCP FRCPI
Professor of Oncology, The Queen's University of Belfast; Consultant Oncologist, Belfast City Hospital

Patrick F. Keane MCh FRCS(Urol)
Consultant Urologist, Belfast City Hospital

Frank Kee MB BCh BAO(Hons) MSc MD FRCP(Edin) FFPHM
Consultant in Public Health Medicine, Northern Health and Social Services Board, County Hall, Ballymena, Co Antrim

John D. Kelly MD FRCS(Urol)
Specialist Registrar, Belfast City Hospital

Sheila Kelly MB FRCSI
Consultant in Palliative Medicine, Belfast City Hospital/The Queen's University
of Belfast; Medical Director, Marie Curie Centre, Belfast

Richard D. Kennedy MB BSc(Hons) MRCP
Macmillan Specialist Registrar in Medical Oncology, Belfast City Hospital

Michael J. Lee MSc FRCPI FRCR FFR(RCSI)
Professor of Radiology, Beaumont Hospital Dublin and Royal College of
Surgeons in Ireland

James J. A. McAleer MD FRCP FRCR
Senior Lecturer and Consultant in Clinical Oncology, Belfast City Hospital/The
Queen's University of Belfast

Ultan McDermott MB MedSci MRCP
Specialist Registrar, Belfast City Hospital

Sarah McKenna MB BCh BAO MRCP
Research Registrar, Medical Oncology, Belfast City Hospital

Damian T. McManus BSc MD MRCPath
Consultant Histo/Cytopathologist, Belfast City Hospital

Kieran McManus BMedSc MB BS, FRCS(I)
Consultant Thoracic Surgeon, Royal Victoria Hospital, Belfast

T. C. M. Morris MD FRCPath FRCPI FFPath RCPI FRCP
Consultant Haematologist, Head of Service, Belfast City Hospital

William Odling-Smee MB FRCS
Senior Lecturer in Surgery, The Queen's University of Belfast; Director of the
Breast Clinic, Belfast City Hospital

Brian Orr MA MSc MRCP FRCP
Consultant in Clinical Oncology, Belvoir Park Hospital, Belfast

Angus J. Patterson MB BCh MRCP(UK) FRCR
Consultant Clinical Oncologist, Belfast City Hospital

John H. Price MD FRCOG
Consultant Gynaecologist and Obstetrician, Belfast City Hospital; Honorary
Senior Lecturer, The Queen's University of Belfast

Hilary Russell BSc PhD
Senior Lecturer, The Queen's University of Belfast

R. A. J. Spence OBE JP MA MD FRCS
Consultant Surgeon, Belfast City Hospital/Honorary Professor, The Queen's
University of Belfast, Honorary Professor, University of Ulster

Frank Sullivan MB BCh BAO MRCPI
Medical Director, Maryland Regional Cancer Care; Adjunct Scientist, Radiation
Oncology Branch, National Cancer Institute

William Torreggiani MB, BCh, BAO, CRCP, MRCPI, FRCR
Specialist Registrar, Beaumont Hospital, Dublin

Brigitte C. Widemann MD
Attending Physician, Pharmacology and Experimental Therapeutics Section,
Paediatric Oncology Branch, National Cancer Institute

Preface

Cancer is second only to cardiovascular diseases as the cause of death in the Western world.

It is anticipated that in the next 5–10 years deaths from cancer will overtake cardiovascular disease. Against this background, cancer studies have become an increasingly important part of the undergraduate medical curriculum in universities. Virtually all doctors will have contact with cancer patients in their practice. The principles of cancer therapy and the presentation, investigation, and management of the common cancers should be familiar to all doctors. This has been emphasized by the government, following the publication of the Calman Report on the reorganization of Cancer Services.

This book has arisen out of a need for a comprehensive textbook for undergraduate medical students that is written in the modern educational style. We were encouraged to write this book by our own students, because they had difficulty obtaining information within one volume on the principles of cancer and details on the common specific cancers, in a language and depth that they could comprehend. Postgraduate nurses have also approached us to write a text, along a similar theme. This book covers the principles and practices of oncology and is aimed primarily at undergraduate students.

The book is divided into two sections, the first being the general principles of cancer, including chapters on the aetiology, epidemiology, biology, and pathology of cancer. Other chapters include cancer prevention, staging, and psychology. The principles of cancer surgery, chemotherapy, and radiotherapy are described. There is a detailed chapter on modern palliative care of cancer.

The second half of the textbook gives information on each of the common cancers and discusses the aetiology, clinical presentation, examination findings, investigation, and management of each cancer. Each chapter includes up to 10 articles to which the reader can refer, for further information. Chapters are liberally illustrated and have bullet points, outlining core principles, for ease of reference for the reader. Finally, most chapters are illustrated with a number of case histories, in line with modern educational practice.

While the primary focus of the book is undergraduate students, the book will be of interest to junior postgraduate hospital doctors and doctors in family practice and postgraduate nurses.

The book will also be of interest to trainees in oncology, nursing, and to colleagues in specialities allied to medicine such as physiotherapy and occupational therapy. Doctors involved in palliative care will also find this book to be of interest, as will doctors involved in pain management.

We trust the reader will find this text to be an important educational resource and ultimately of benefit to their approach and clinical management of the cancer patient.

R. A. J. S.
P. G. J.
2001

Acknowledgements

The authors are pleased to acknowledge the enormous help received from Oxford University Press, initially by Mrs Esther Browning at the early stages of the book and latterly by Ms Catherine Barnes, both of whom gave us much encouragement, help and advice with the text.

We would also like to acknowledge the work of our respective secretaries, Miss Anne Wilkie (P. G. J.) and Mrs Ethel Archer (R. A. J. S.) in the preparation and typing of parts of the manuscript.

We are grateful to our colleagues, who are busy clinicians from the United Kingdom, Ireland and the United States, who have given of their time to write chapters in their respective expert areas.

We would also like to acknowledge feedback from our students, for whom this text is primarily written, and our many colleagues who gave advice.

Specifically we gratefully acknowledge help with the following chapters, by Drs Houston and Moore (Chapter 14), Dr Mirakhur for illustrations in histopathology and Dr Arthur Grey for radiological illustrations (Chapter 23), advice and support from Dr Eli Glatstein (Chapter 11), Dr Andrew Rosenberg and Ms Simonne Longerich for supplying photographs and graphic advice (Chapter 20). We acknowledge the help of Dr Seamus McAleer and Dr John Foster for help with the text and illustrations (Chapter 25). We acknowledge the inspiration of Dr Robert Twycross for Chapter 12 and Dr Paul Rice for provision of radiological figures for Chapter 16. We also acknowledge the assistance of Dr Geraldine Markey (Chapter 19).

Above all we acknowledge the support, patience, and forbearance of our respective families, who tolerated much burning of the midnight oil.

We dedicate this book to our respective wives and children.

R. A. J. S.
P. G. J.
2001

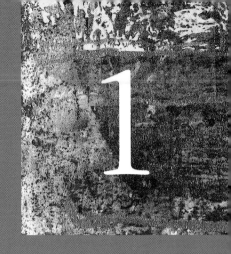

The principles and practice
of oncology *Patrick G. Johnston*
and Ultan McDermott

- Introduction

- International comparison

- Aetiology

- Screening procedures

- Clinical detection of cancer

- Cancer detection, diagnosis and staging

- Cancer staging and histological classification

- Tumour markers

- Principles of cancer treatment

- The cancer multidisciplinary team

The principles and practice of oncology

Introduction

In the UK cancer is a major problem today. Approximately a quarter of a million people are diagnosed with cancer and 120 000 die each year. While improvements in cardiovascular disease have resulted in a decline in mortality from heart disease, cancer mortality continues to rise and is expected to be the major cause of death across the next decade. Currently one person in three living in the UK will develop cancer during their lifetime and one in five will die from the disease. Over 60% of all cancers will occur in the over-65 age group and as our populations get older clinicians will be faced with increasing numbers of patients at risk or presenting with malignant disease. An individual's risk of developing cancer depends on many factors such as genetic inheritance, background, smoking behaviour, and diet. However, it is now clear that the cause of cancer is not due to one single event, but is multifactorial. Several major cancers account for over 50% of all new cases and include cancers such as lung cancer, which accounts for 16% of all cancers, non-melanoma skin cancers, which account for 12%, and breast and colorectal cancer, each of which account for approximately 14% of cancers, whilst 8% of cancers are due to prostate cancer (Fig. 1.1, Table 1.1). In females, the most common cancers are those of breast, lung, colon, and skin, and in males the commonest cancers are those of the lung, prostate, gastrointestinal, and skin. The annual cost of diagnosing and treating cancer is currently £1.5 billion for the National Health Service.

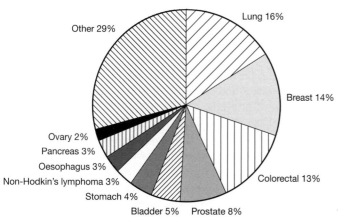

Total cancers excluding non-melanoma skin cancer = 245, 950

Fig. 1.1 Ten commonest cancers in people living in the UK, 1995. CRC Incidence Factsheet 1.1, 1998.

Table 1.1 Estimates of the percentage of the population who will develop cancer over a lifetime and the lifetime risk

Site	%	Risk
Males		
Lung	9.1	1 in 11
Skin (non-melanoma)	5.7	1 in 18
Prostate	4.4	1 in 23
Bladder	2.8	1 in 35
Colon	2.6	1 in 38
Stomach	2.4	1 in 42
Rectum	2.0	1 in 50
Non-Hodgkin's lymphoma	1.1	1 in 93
Pancreas	1.1	1 in 95
Oesophagus	1.0	1 in 96
Females		
Breast	8.6	1 in 12
Skin (non- melanoma)	5.0	1 in 20
Lung	3.8	1 in 26
Colon	3.1	1 in 33
Ovary	1.8	1 in 55
Rectum	1.5	1 in 67
Cervix	1.4	1 in 72
Stomach	1.4	1 in 72
Uterus	1.3	1 in 75
Bladder	1.1	1 in 93

The survival rates for all cancers have risen steadily over the last 20 years. Overall survival is generally higher for women than men. The current 5-year relative survival rates for all cancers rose from 18% to 29% for men and 33% to 43% for women between 1970 and 1990 (Fig. 1.2). In females the leading causes of death due to cancer are lung, breast, and colorectal, whilst in males the leading causes of death are lung, prostate, and colorectal. Together these cancers represent over half of all cancer cases and deaths (Cancer Research Campaign Factsheet, 1998; CRC CancerStats, 1999a). For the same time period, the outlook for childhood cancers has improved dramatically with overall 5-year relative survival rates of over 50%. Amongst adults, relative survival is lower for elderly patients than for younger patients for almost all cancers, even when the generally higher mortality amongst the elderly is taken into account. Cancer survival is also heavily influenced by material deprivation with a lower survival among patients from more deprived areas than those from more affluent groups. For children however there is no significant difference in survival between these groups.

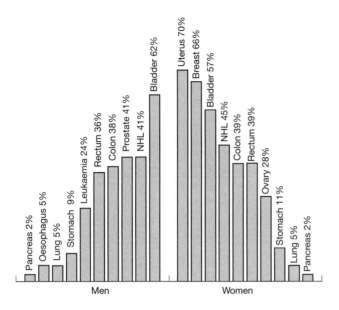

Fig. 1.2 Five-year age standardized relative survival %. Adults diagnosed during 1986–90, England and Wales. NHL, non-Hodgkin's lymphoma.

International comparison

There have been many recent advances in the treatment and outcome for patients with cancer over the last 20 years. Improvements such as the use of more specialized surgical techniques, the advent of chemotherapy, and improvements in radiotherapy techniques have led to the combined modality or multidisciplinary

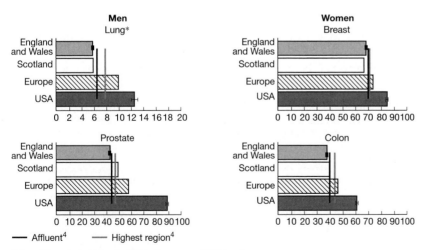

* Note different horizontal scale: 20% for lung cancer, 100% for others
1 Average survival rate for England and Wales, with 95% confidence interval
2 Average survival rate for European countries (incl Scotland) and regions (incl parts of England and Wales) covered by EUROCARE II study
3 Average survival rate for US states covered by SEER programme, with 95% confidence interval
4 Survival rate for affluent group (England and Wales); and highest survival rate among NHS Regions (all deprivation groups combined)

Fig. 1.3 International comparison of 5-year relative survival (%), selected cancers: England and Wales[1] (adults diagnosed 1986–90), Europe[2] (1985–89), and USA[3] (1986–90).

approach to the treatment of cancer patients. Despite these improvements, outcomes for cancer patients in the UK vary widely. Five-year relative survival rates for men and women diagnosed in England, Wales, and Scotland have been compared with the average survival rate for the European countries participating in the Second Eurocare Study (1985–89), and with areas of the USA covered by the Surveillance, Epidemiology and End Results (SEER Programme 1986–1990) (Fig. 1.3) The relative survival rates for England and Wales are similar to Scotland, but are much lower than the average for Europe and the USA (Berrino *et al.*, 1995; CRC CancerStats, 1999b). Moreover, the differences in survival between the UK and other western European countries for diseases such as colon and breast cancer arose primarily in the first 6 months after diagnosis, suggesting international differences in our early management and staging of the disease and/or access to optimal treatment. For diseases such as testicular cancer, Hodgkin's disease and leukaemia, survival rates in England and Wales were similar to those in Europe and the USA.

Political concern was expressed when it was clear that the survival of patients with certain cancers in the UK was much lower than in most European countries.

As a result of the Eurocare study, further concern was expressed when it appeared that some specialists seemed to do cancer surgery better than generalists, although the data in many cancers apart from breast are somewhat conflicting (Berrino *et al.*, 1995). Generally, surgeons treating larger numbers of patients produce better results. Data to support this has arisen in cancers such as ovary, breast, oesophagus, stomach, testis, and sarcoma. It also appears that children with cancer have better survival when treated in specialized centres. Several studies have shown that patients with colon and rectal cancer have great variability in their mortality, morbidity and long-term survival between different surgeons. It has been shown that patients who have cancer of the testis have better survival when treated in specialized centres, with defined treatment protocols, when managed with a multidisciplinary approach and when treated in centres with large case numbers.

When cancer of the breast was studied, it seemed that surgeons who specialize in the condition could obtain 17% better survival. It has been shown that there is great variation in treatment geographically in the UK, in breast cancer, with respect to patients who obtain breast conservation, those patients who are offered breast reconstruction, and those patients who are given postoperative chemotherapy and radiotherapy. There also seems to be a survival difference, depending upon where the breast cancer patient lives in the UK.

It seems, therefore, that patients with cancer do better in specialized centres, in the following areas: breast, ovary, oesophagus, pancreas, stomach, and lung. It has also been shown that patients who are in clinical trials do better than patients who are treated outwith trials.

Subsequent to the emergence of these data the **Calman–Hine Report** was published in April 1995. To correct the deficiencies noted above, this report proposed the creation of cancer centres and units with experts in cancer working together in a multidisciplinary fashion. The cancer units would be based in a district hospital and would have arrangements for close integration of primary and secondary care. The cancer unit would be an integral part of the hospital and within the unit there would be surgical sub-specialization. The cancer unit would look after the more common cancers and would not have radiotherapy services. Multidisciplinary management of patients would be core to the working practices of the unit. Palliative medicine, access to counselling, and psychological help would be central to the function of the unit, with other supportive care, including prosthetics, stoma care, and complementary therapies available. Other services such as physiotherapy, dietetics, speech therapy, occupational therapy, and social services would all be readily available.

The cancer centre would be part of a large general hospital, providing services for patients with common cancers, as well as additional specialized services, in the same way as the cancer unit. The cancer centre would deliver the full range of cancer treatment, encompassing treatment programmes for less common and rare cancers. The cancer centre specialization would be further developed for both diagnosis and treatment, with surgeons and physicians specializing to develop their skills. Multidisciplinary consultation for all patients with cancer would be central to the management to the patient. The cancer centre would serve a population of at least one million. Specialist clinical nurse skills would include intravenous chemotherapy, palliative care, breast care, rehabilitation, psychological support, stoma care, and lymphoedema management. The cancer centre would provide radiotherapy for the region. It would also provide a specialist surgical service, including plastic and reconstructive surgery, intensive chemotherapy, bone marrow transplantation, and peripheral blood cell support. There would be sophisticated diagnostic imaging such as magnetic resonance imaging (MRI) and computerized tomographic (CT) scanning.

These recommendations have now been accepted by the UK government and currently cancer units and centres are being developed throughout the UK.

Table 1.2 The aetiological causes of cancer

Viruses (papilloma, Epstein–Barr, hepatitis B, retroviruses)
Radiation exposure
Environmental industrial carcinogens
Tobacco and alcohol consumption
• Asbestos
• Aromatic amines
• Bischloromethyl ethers
• Beta-naphthalene and benzedrine
• Polycyclic hydrocarbons
• Drug-induced cancers (alkylators such as melphalan and cyclophosphamide)
• Nickel
• Vinyl chloride
• Isopropyl alcohol
• Diet and nutrition
Immunodeficiency syndromes
Genetic susceptibility syndromes

Aetiology

The cause of cancer is multifactorial and includes lifestyle, environmental factors and inherited genetic susceptibility. It is thought that as many as 80–90% of all cancers may be due to environmental or lifestyle factors. Smoking is the single major cause of cancer accounting for 30–40% of all cancer deaths. The major known causes of cancer are shown in Table 1.2 and discussed in more detail in Chapter 2.

In addition to environmental and occupational agents that have been identified, diet, nutrition and immunosuppressive states (inherited or induced) may also lead to the development of cancer. There are also many genetic susceptibility syndromes such as Li–Fraumeni syndrome and hereditary non-polyposis coli syndrome, which are associated with a higher prevalence of cancer (Table 1.3). These causal factors may act together or in sequence to initiate or promote carcinogenesis.

Screening procedures

In the absence of practical preventive measures for cancer, the control of cancer can in some instances be achieved through early detection and treatment. In an attempt to detect cancer at an early stage, it is important to focus on the occult

Table 1.3 Syndromes of inherited predisposition to cancer

Inherited cancer syndrome	Principal tumours	Lifetime risk of cancer in gene carrier	Cancer cases/year in UK	Gene
Retinoblastoma	Retina	90%+	100?	RB1
Familial adenomatous polyposis (FAP)	Colorectal	90%	< 100	APC
Multiple endocrine neoplasia type 1	Parathyroid Pituitary Endocrine Pancreas	> 70%	< 100	MEN1
Multiple endocrine neoplasia type 2 Adrenal	Thyroid	70%	< 50	RET
Neurofibromatosis type 1	Brain Sarcoma	5–10%	< 100	NF1
Neurofibromatosis type 2	Acoustic nerve Schwannoma Meningioma	90%	< 50	NF2
Li–Fraumeni	Breast, sarcoma Brain	90%	< 100	TP53
von Hippel–Lindau	Renal, CNS Angiomas Phaeochromocytoma	90%	< 50	VHL

phase when the lesion is asymptomatic. Currently, there are some diseases where effective screening is possible. These include cervical and breast cancer screening, and evidence is now emerging for the efficacy of large bowel screening. Screening for cancers of prostate and lung do not as yet have proven efficacy. Screening is addressed in more detail in Chapter 6.

Clinical detection of cancer

Early clinical detection

Early detection of cancer is very critical as any delay in cancer detection may be detrimental to the patient. Therefore, screening patients for early lesions of the skin, uterus, breast, colon, and rectum is extremely important. Early clinical detection means that the cancer may be detected when it is localized and has not developed regional or distant spread to nodes or other viscera. It is at this early stage that most cancer patients will have the greatest chance of cure.

Important clinical tools in early clinical detection include:

- complete physical examination
- regular Pap smear
- regular mammography and breast self examination
- haemoccult for occult blood in faeces, in particular over the age of 40 years
- urinalysis and blood count
- a complete clinical history
- an in-depth family medical history.

Clinical symptoms or signs of cancer

Cancer normally presents with signs or symptoms due to changes in normal physiological function. These include:

- alteration in eating habit
- loss of appetite
- problems in swallowing
- change in bowel habit
- the presence of a lump at any site
- the appearance of bleeding
- unexplained recurrent pain
- recurrent fevers
- unexplained weight loss
- repeated infections which do not clear with treatment.

Cancer detection, diagnosis and staging

Once cancer is suspected, a careful work-up is essential (Fig. 1.4). The clinical findings may require periodic follow-up or surgical intervention to establish or exclude the diagnosis. Fine needle biopsy, surgical biopsy and/or excision of the

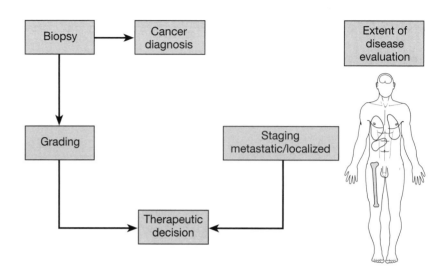

Fig. 1.4 The management of patients presenting with symptoms and signs suggestive of cancer.

mass is the single most important procedure in establishing the diagnosis. Once the diagnosis is made other tests will be necessary in order to determine the extent of the disease.

Radiological imaging

An increasing number of medical imaging procedures exist to detect cancer, as described in Chapter 7. New diagnostic imaging procedures have largely replaced exploratory surgery for cancer patients. These include:

- plain film radiography
- arteriography
- radioisotope scanning
- ultrasound and computerized tomography
- magnetic resonance imaging
- positron emission tomography.

MRI and CT techniques are two non-invasive techniques which can produce cross-sectional pictures of the body to show the shape, size, and location of the tumour. These imaging modalities are important in staging patients and in assessing response to treatments. Another advance has been the development of three-dimensional images using several imaging procedures. This technology now permits better staging and planning for surgery and radiation therapy treatment.

Cancer staging and histological classification

Clinical decisions regarding the treatment of a particular cancer are based upon the anatomical stage and the histological diagnosis of cancer.

The objectives of cancer staging and histological classification are:

- to aid the clinician in planning of treatment
- to give some indication of prognosis
- to evaluate the efficiency of treatment

- to facilitate exchange of information
- to assist in continuing clinical studies of cancer.

Through prospective studies the relationship between stage and clinical outcome has been defined for the majority of cancers. From these studies it is possible to provide more accurate prognostic information to patients with specific malignancies (CRC CancerStats, 1999b).

Histopathological staging and classification

Histopathological classification is extremely important in defining the tumour type and it is crucial for decisions on treatment planning and predicting outcome. There is an important need to define the histopathological type, grade, and degree of differentiation of the tumours. This is highlighted in Chapter 5.

Histopathological classifications of tumour include:

- adenocarcinoma
- squamous carcinomas
- small cell carcinomas
- large cell carcinomas
- sarcomas
- lymphomas
- leukaemias (myeloid and lymphocytic)
- gliomas
- seminomas
- teratomas.

Staging depends on measuring and defining the extent of the disease (Fig. 1.4). The tumour stage is a reflection of the tumour burden and is determined by three major criteria which are:

- T – primary tumour
- N – regional lymph node
- M – metastases.

The TNM classification defines the primary site as T1–T4 with increasing size of the primary lesion, advancing nodal disease N0–N3, and the presence or absence of metastases is M0 or M1. The exact criteria for staging depend on the individual primary organ sites.

A typical type of stage grouping is the following:

Stage 1 – $T_1N_0M_0$

Clinical examination revealing a tumour confined to the primary organ. This lesion tends to be operable and completely resectable.

Stage 2 – $T_2N_1M_0$

Clinical examination shows evidence of local spread into surrounding tissue and first draining lymph nodes. The lesion is also operable and resectable but there is a higher risk of further spread of the disease.

Stage 3 – $T_3N_2M_0$

Clinical examination reveals an extensive primary tumour with fixation to deeper structures and local invasion. This lesion may not be operable and may require a combination of treatment modalities.

Stage 4 – $T_4N_3M_1$

Evidence of distant metastases beyond the site of origin. The primary site may be surgically inoperable.

The degree of differentiation is classified as:

• well differentiated
• moderately differentiated
• poorly differentiated.

Tumour grade is classified as:

• low grade
• high grade.

High grade poorly differentiated tumours tend to have a much worse outcome.

Tumour markers

Biological markers may also be useful as an adjunct to staging and histological classification of tumours. Tumour markers such as CEA, β-HCG, ACTH, alpha-fetoprotein (AFP), prostate specific antigen (PSA), and CA-125 help further define the histopathological classification of tumours. Markers such as epithelial membrane antigen and common leucocyte antigen help differentiate between epithelial and lymphoid malignancies. Some of these markers such as CA-125, β-HCG and AFP may also be useful in monitoring a patient's response to treatment (Fig. 1.5).

Principles of cancer treatment

The major principle governing the initial approach to treatment for a cancer patient is initially to define the goals of clinical management. For those patients

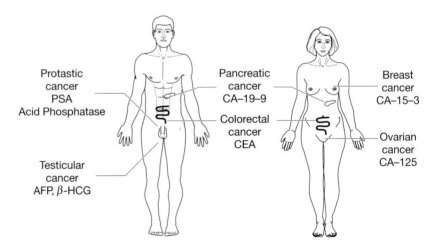

Fig. 1.5 Tumour markers used in the diagnosis and evaluation of cancer.

with curable disease, the goal is to cure the patient using proven single or combined modality treatments. However, if the cancer patient is not curable, then the goals of treatment are to improve the quality of the patient's life and possibly prolong life (with good quality).

Treatment principles are based upon:

- the biological behaviour of the cancer
- the mortality and morbidity of the therapeutic procedure
- the efficacy of the therapeutic procedure under consideration
- the performance status of the patient

In the treatment of cancer it is important to realize that:

- patients with localized cancers are curable
- patients presenting with positive lymph nodes tend to have poorer prognosis
- patients with distant metastases are rarely curable but in some cases may survive 5 years with multimodality treatments
- standard treatments for cancer patients are based upon large clinical studies that have shown improved disease-free and overall survival
- the most commonly chosen parameter to measure survival and benefit of treatment is 5-year disease-free and overall survival rates.

The cancer multidisciplinary team

Treatment of the cancer patient has become increasingly complex and requires a multidisciplinary team of professionals, including:

- surgical oncologists
- radiation oncologists
- medical oncologists
- palliative care specialists
- psychologists
- social workers
- nurses
- chaplains.

Cancer treatment includes three major treatment modalities:

- surgical treatment
- radiation treatment
- chemotherapy treatment.

These therapies should only be undertaken by people who are properly trained and skilled in the proper delivery of these treatments for patients.

Current advances in treatment have come from prospective randomized trials that have shown major benefits in survival for patients. Future advances in cancer treatment will only come from the performance of multi-centre randomized clinical trials. Therefore the enrolment of patients into these trials is an essential part of patient treatment.

Further reading

Berrino, F., Sant, M., Verdecelina, A., Capocaccia, R., Hakulinen, T., and Esteve, J. (eds) (1995) *Survival of cancer patients in Europe: The Eurocare Study*. IARC Scientific Publications No. 132.

Berrino, F., Capocaccia, R., Esleve, J., Gatta, G., Hakulinen, T., Micheli, A., Sant, M., Verdecelina, A., (1999) *Survival of cancer patients in Europe: The Eurocare Study*. IARC Scientific Publications No. 151.

Cancer Research Campaign Factsheet 1.1 (1998) – Figure One. Ten Commonest Cancers, persons, UK, 1988.

CRC CancerStats (1999a) Survival. England and Wales 1971–1995: April 1999. Figure One: Five-year age-standardized relative survival % – adults diagnosed during 1986–90, England and Wales.

CRC CancerStats (1999b) Survival. England and Wales 1971–1995. April 1999. Figure Ten: International comparison of five-year relative survival (%), selected cancers: England and Wales (adults diagnosed 1986–90), Europe (1985–89) and the USA (1986–90).

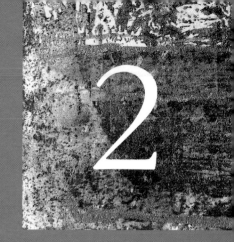

2

The aetiology of cancer
Hilary Russell

- Introduction
- Chemical carcinogens
- Radiation
- Viruses

The aetiology of cancer

Introduction

It is now accepted that cancer arises within a single cell as a result of an accumulation of abnormalities (mutations) within the DNA of that cell. When these mutations occur within key genes, e.g. those involved in control of the cell cycle, apoptosis, DNA repair, etc., it can lead to uncontrolled cell growth and eventually, perhaps, to a cell type that has acquired the ability to metastasize. A large number of aetiological agents have been recognized that cause genetic damage and lead to neoplastic transformation. They fall into three general categories:

- chemical carcinogens
- radiation
- viruses.

Although each of these groups will be considered separately, it should be remembered that members of one group may interact with another and perhaps synergize the effects of others.

Chemical carcinogens

The role of chemicals in tumour development is widespread and was recognized because of some obvious occupational diseases. It is estimated that 80–90% of human tumours are due to a chemical aetiology.

A variety of experiments in animal models have confirmed the multistep nature of carcinogenesis and identified two main stages in the overall process as **initiation** and **promotion**. The initiation step occurs when a cell is exposed to an appropriate dose of a carcinogenic agent (the initiator) and is altered in such a way that it is

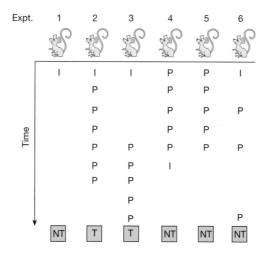

Fig. 2.1 The role of tumour initiators and promoters during carcinogenesis. Experiment: 1, initiator only; 2, initiator followed by promoter at twice weekly intervals over several months; 3, initiator and then delay before promoter at twice weekly intervals over several months; 4, promoter and then initiator; 5, promoter only; 6, initiator followed by promoter at suboptimal intervals. I, Application of initiator (polycyclic hydrocarbon); P, application of promoter (croton oil); T, tumours, NT, no tumours.

Table 2.1 **Historical observations of chemical carcinogens**

Date	Observation	Carcinogen
1761	Excessive use of snuff leads to the development of nasal 'polypusses' or polyps	Nitrosamines
1775	High incidence of scrotal cancer in chimney sweeps	Soot
1860s	High incidence of bladder cancer in workers preparing fuchsin dyes from aniline	Aromatic amines
1915	Rabbit ears painted with tar developed papillomas	Benzpyrene

likely to give rise to a tumour. The initiation step is usually rapid and irreversible and due to DNA damage (i.e. mutations). Promotion describes the step in which there is proliferation and clonal expansion of initiated cells. However, in contrast to initiators, promoters do not affect the DNA directly and their effects are reversible. The initiator must be applied before the promoter; there may be a long delay before application of the promoter, but this must be applied repeatedly and at regular intervals. The experiments which gave rise to these general principles of initiation/promotion are summarized in Fig. 2.1.

Initiation

A variety of natural and synthetic compounds that initiate carcinogenesis have been identified. They fall into two groups (Table 2.2):

- direct-acting compounds, which are themselves carcinogenic;
- indirect-acting compounds or procarcinogens which are metabolically converted *in vivo* to the ultimate carcinogen.

Table 2.2 **Major chemical carcinogens**

Direct-acting carcinogens	Indirect-acting carcinogens
β-Propiolactone	Benzypyrene
Ethyl methanesulfonate (EMS)	Dimethylnitrosamine
Dimethyl sulphate (DMS)	Vinyl chloride
Nitrogen mustard	2-Naphthylamine
Methylnitrosourea (MNU)	Sassafras
Diepoxybutane	Aflatoxin B_1
Anticancer drugs, e.g. cyclophosphamide, chlorambucil	Benzidine

However, all chemicals that are capable of transforming a cell are highly reactive electrophiles, i.e. they have electron-deficient atoms that can react with nucleophilic (electron-rich) sites within the cell. Although the primary target within the cell for these electrophilic reactions is DNA, other electron-rich sites such as RNA and proteins will also be attacked. This will sometimes cause lethal damage but if this does not occur, the DNA damage will be transmitted to daughter cells and perpetuated in subsequent generations of cells. In an effort to prevent this, the cellular DNA repair mechanisms will attempt to reconstitute the DNA before cell division.

A major class of enzyme involved in the metabolic activation of inactive procarcinogens to the active ultimate carcinogen is the family of cytochrome P-450-dependent mono-oxygenase isoenzymes. Within the general population, the activity and inducibility of these enzymes shows considerable variation. For example, one of the P-450 enzymes, CYP1A1, is responsible for the metabolism of polycyclic aromatic hydrocarbons such as benzpyrene. Within the population, approximately 10% of individuals carry a highly inducible form of this enzyme and this is associated with an increased risk of lung cancer in smokers. Therefore, individual susceptibility to a particular carcinogen will be influenced by polymorphisms in the genes that encode these enzymes. A further example of how response to a carcinogen is genetically influenced is seen with the various polymorphic forms of enzymes which inactivate or detoxify the procarcinogen. The enzyme glutathione-*S*-transferase is involved in the detoxification of polycyclic aromatic hydrocarbons. In approximately 50% of the population, this locus is deleted completely. This is associated with a high risk of lung cancer in such individuals when exposed to tobacco smoke.

Therefore the ability of a compound to initiate carcinogenesis is influenced not only by the reactivity of the compound *per se*, but also by a balance of mechanisms that activate and detoxify.

Promotion

The process of promotion, in contrast to initiation, is gradual, partially reversible and requires prolonged exposure to the promoting agent. Promoters do not need to be metabolized to the active compound; they have no tendency to react as electrophiles and they rarely induce tumours themselves. When a cell that has undergone initiation is exposed to a promoter, that cell is stimulated to divide and the number of genetically damaged cells increases. With continued cell division there is selection for those cells that have an increased growth rate and enhanced invasive properties as a result of genetic mutation. Promotion can therefore be regarded as the proliferation of preneoplastic cells, malignant conversion, and tumour progression. At each step of this multistep process, additional mutations are acquired by the initiated cell, resulting in the formation of a malignant tumour.

Promoters are non-mutagenic and contribute to tumourigenesis by induction of cell proliferation mechanisms. The mode of action of promoters is typified by the compound tissue plasminogen activator (TPA), a member of the phorbol esters found in croton oil derived from the seeds of the tropical plant, *Croton tiglium*. TPA activates protein kinase C, a component of the phosphoinositide signalling pathway normally controlled by the second messenger, diacylglycerol. The activation of protein kinase C leads to the phosphorylation of a variety of target proteins and ultimately stimulates cell proliferation. Thus TPA stimulates cell proliferation by its ability to substitute for diacylglycerol in normal cellular mechanisms.

Radiation

Radiant energy, whether as ultraviolet rays or ionizing radiation, will transform cells *in vitro* and induce tumours *in vivo* in both humans and animals. There are many similarities in the basic mode of action of chemical and radiation-induced carcinogenesis. As with most chemical carcinogens, radiation is mutagenic and thought to cause malignant transformation by DNA damage. There are usually many years between exposure to the initiating dose of radiation and the appearance of malignancy. This would suggest that exposure to promoting agents is involved in proliferation of radiation-damaged cells and ultimate tumour development.

Ultraviolet radiation

Ultraviolet radiation of the appropriate wavelength can be absorbed by DNA bases and generate changes in them. The UV portion of the solar spectrum can be divided into three wavelength ranges: UVA (320–400 nm), UVB (280–320 nm) and UVC (200–280 nm). UVB is thought to be responsible for the induction of cutaneous cancers. The most common damage is the generation of dimers between adjacent pyrimidine residues in one DNA strand. These dimers subsequently interfere with the transcription and replication of DNA. This type of DNA damage is repaired by the nucleotide excision repair pathway. The five steps in this pathway are:

- recognition of the DNA lesion;
- incision of the DNA strand on both sides of the lesion;
- removal of the damage;
- synthesis of a nucleotide patch;
- ligation of the patch to adjacent nucleotides.

The products of at least 20 genes are thought to be required for excision repair. It is postulated that with excessive sun exposure, the excision repair mechanism is overwhelmed and some DNA damage remains unrepaired. The importance of the excision repair pathway is observed in patients with the autosomal recessive disorder xeroderma pigmentosum, in whom there is an inherited inability to repair UV-induced DNA damage. Such patients demonstrate extreme photosensitivity and have a 2000-fold increased risk of skin cancer in sun-exposed skin. Xeroderma pigmentosum is genetically heterogeneous, with at least seven different variants, each of which is caused by a mutation in one of several genes involved in the excision repair pathway.

Ionizing radiation

Ionizing radiation includes electromagnetic (x-rays and γ-rays) and particulate (α-particles, β-particles, protons, neutrons) radiation. All of these are carcinogenic and are a part of the natural environment. The main source of ionizing radiation is

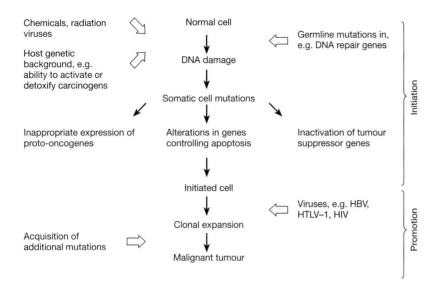

Fig. 2.2 General scheme for carcinogenesis in which promoters cause clonal expansion of the initiated cell. Further proliferation leads to an accumulation of additional mutations and eventually a malignant tumour.

the radiation background, i.e. cosmic rays, radon and terrestial radiation; however, approximately 18% is due to medical and industrial sources. Ionizing radiations have been called universal carcinogens because of their ability to induce cancers in almost all tissues of all species at all ages, including the fetus. Unlike UV radiation, a single exposure to ionizing radiation is sufficient for tumour formation as demonstrated by survivors of the Nagasaki and Hiroshima atomic bombs. In such individuals, leukaemias (principally acute and chronic myelocytic leukaemia) appeared after about 6 years and solid tumours after approximately 20 years. Even therapeutic radiation has been shown to be carcinogenic. Thyroid cancers have developed in approximately 10% of those exposed during infancy to head and neck irradiation. Another human disease that is due to defects in DNA repair and results in a highly elevated cancer risk is the recessive disorder ataxia telangiectasia (AT). Homozygotes often die from malignant disease before the age of 25 and even individuals who are heterozygous for the condition are thought to have an increased risk of malignancy. Patients with AT are sensitive to x-rays but not to UV radiation and the excision repair pathway is intact. Cells cultured from AT patients show chromosome instability, with numerous breaks and translocations.

Viruses

Evidence for the role of viruses in tumour aetiology stems mainly from observations in animals and was first proposed as early as the 1900s. However, a number of DNA and RNA viruses have now been implicated in human tumours. These tumour viruses cause transformation as a consequence of their ability to integrate their genome into the host cell DNA. Usually the virus is responsible for the production of a *transforming protein*, coded for by an oncogene, which maintains the transformed state within the cell. For the DNA tumour viruses, the oncogene is an integral part of the viral genome, whereas for the RNA viruses, it may be of viral origin or may be a host gene that is inappropriately expressed following viral infection.

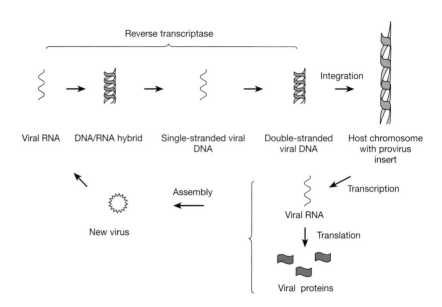

Viral RNA — DNA/RNA hybrid — Single-stranded viral DNA — Double-stranded viral DNA — Host chromosome with provirus insert

Fig. 2.3 Retroviral life cycle.

There is also another fundamental difference in the life cycle of the DNA and RNA tumour viruses. For the DNA viruses, entry into the host cell is followed by transcription of viral DNA into viral mRNA and translation into viral proteins. Both cellular and viral DNA are replicated prior to cell division and eventually one or more copies of the viral genome becomes integrated into the host genome. As such, it is then replicated along with the host genome and no new mature virus particles are produced. For the RNA viruses, direct integration into the host genome is not possible since their genome is RNA. Initially, viral RNA is converted into a DNA copy, the provirus, using the RNA as template and the viral-encoded enzyme, reverse transcriptase. The provirus is then integrated into the host genome and replicated with it. Single-strand RNA viruses which use this pathway are called retroviruses (Fig. 2.3).

Oncogenic DNA viruses
Epstein–Barr virus (EBV)

Epstein–Barr virus (EBV) is a herpesvirus and is implicated in two major types of cancer: Burkitt's lymphoma and nasopharyngeal carcinoma. Approximately 98% of cases of Burkitt's lymphoma in Africa are thought to be due to an EBV infection whilst outside Africa, the virus is only detected in 15–20% of cases. In developed countries, where EBV infection is common, the virus causes infectious mononucleosis, which is a self-limiting infection of B cells, and therefore additional factors must be involved in the development of Burkitt's lymphoma. A feature of Burkitt's lymphoma cells is a translocation involving chromosomes 8 and 14 in which the region of the *myc* oncogene on chromosome 8 comes under the influence of the immunoglobulin loci (chromsome 14 or occasionally chromosomes 2 and 22) (Fig. 2.4). One role for the virus in the development of Burkitt's lymphoma has been the demonstration that the viral-encoded protein EBNA-1

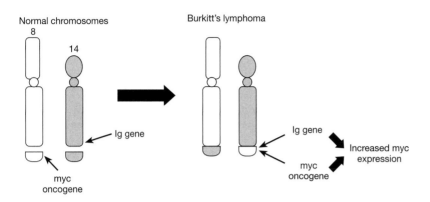

Fig. 2.4 The chromosomal translocation and genes involved in Burkitt's lymphoma.

activates the machinery for rearrangement of immunoglobulin genes, increasing the likelihood of a t(8;14) translocation and activation of *myc*. The other tumour type associated with EBV is nasopharyngeal carcinoma. This tumour is endemic in southern China and some parts of Africa and 100% of nasopharyngeal carcinomas have EBV DNA. This suggests that the virus plays a role in the genesis of these tumours but the restricted geographical distribution would indicate that genetic and/or environmental factors are also important.

Papillomaviruses

The papillomaviruses are small DNA viruses and members of the papovavirus family. They are responsible for warts and other benign tumours as well as malignancies. Currently over 30 distinct human papillomaviruses (HPV) have been recognized, some of which are associated with benign lesions whilst others are associated with malignancy. Thus, HPV 16 and 18 are associated with squamous cell carcinoma of the uterine cervix and also their presumed precursors (dysplasia and carcinoma in situ), whilst HPV 6 and 11 ('low-risk types') are common in benign cervical lesions. A further difference between the carcinomas and benign lesions is the observation that in benign lesions the HPV genome remains in a non-integrated form whilst in the carcinomas, the viral genome is integrated into that of the host cell. The site of integration into the host genome is random. The region of the viral genome at which the viral DNA is disrupted at integration is always at the E1/E2 open reading frame. The E2 region normally represses transcription of the viral E6 and E7 genes and thus viral integration causes overexpression of these two gene products. The E6 and E7 proteins are able to inactivate two important tumour suppressor genes, p53 and Rb, respectively, which regulate important cellular processes such as the cell cycle and apoptosis. It is interesting to note that the E6 and E7 of HPV 16 and 18 ('high-risk' viruses) show high affinity for p53 and Rb, whereas E6 and E7 of HPV 6 and 11 ('low-risk' viruses) have a much lower affinity. Although HPV is clearly implicated in the development of cervical tumours, it is most likely that the viral infection acts as an initiating event and that additional somatic mutations are necessary for the development of malignancy. Such changes are probably achieved by cofactors such as smoking, coexisting microbial infections, dietary deficiencies and hormonal changes.

Hepatitis B virus (HBV)

Hepatitis B virus (HBV) is associated with chronic hepatitis, cirrhosis and carcinoma of the liver. In areas of Africa and south-east Asia, infection with HBV is endemic and the virus is transmitted vertically from mother to child. Such children have a high incidence of hepatocellular carcinoma (HCC) at a very early age, typically 20–30 years. In virtually all cases of HBV-related HCC, viral DNA is integrated into the host cell genome but no consistent pattern of integration has been recognized. The viral genome does not include an oncogene; however, one viral gene product, the HBx protein, acts as a transcriptional activator of several growth-promoting genes as well as inactivating the p53 tumour supressor gene. It therefore appears that the role of HBV in the development of HCC is indirect and that the virus is perhaps responsible for hyperproliferation. In these mitotically active cells, mutations in key growth control genes may arise spontaneously or through insult by environmental agents such as the dietary aflatoxins, which are toxic metabolites of the fungus *Aspergillus flavus*.

Oncogenic RNA viruses

Human T-cell leukaemia virus (HTLV-1)

Human T-cell leukaemia virus (HTLV-1) is one of few examples of a retrovirus causing a human cancer. The virus is implicated in adult T-cell leukaemia/lymphoma (ATLL). Viral infection is common in southern Japan, South America, and parts of Africa and precedes the development of malignancy by several decades. The virus dislays a tropism for CD4+ cells and viral infection is by transmission of infected T cells by sexual intercourse, blood products or breast-feeding. HTLV-1 is an example of a retrovirus that does not carry its own oncogene in the viral genome, nor has a consistent site for viral integration been observed. As with other retroviruses, it contains three genes – *gag*, *pol*, and *env* – which code for the viral structural proteins (*gag* and *env*) and the reverse transcriptase (*pol*). In addition, the viral genome contains another region, *tat*, which is apparently responsible for the transforming activity. The *tat* gene product has a number of roles:

- it stimulates transcription of viral mRNA and host IL-2 (a T-cell growth factor) and its receptor;
- it prevents formation of the complex between CDK4 and its inhibitor p16^{INK}, leading to dysregulation of the cell cycle.

Viral infection, therefore, leads to uncontrolled proliferation of T cells through autocrine stimulation and a monoclonal T-cell leukaemia/lymphoma results when one of these proliferating cells acquires additional mutations.

Human immunodeficiency virus (HIV)

The human immunodeficiency virus (HIV) or acquired immunodeficiency syndrome (AIDS) virus is another retroviral-induced condition that leads to a variety of different tumours. These are of two main types:

- those which are related to immunosupression, e.g. following Epstein–Barr infection in which the virus is released from its normal immune control. This loss of immune function also makes AIDS patients prone to 'opportunistic' infections, which are often the cause of the patient's death;

- Kaposi's sarcoma in which plaques or nodules appear on skin and mucosa. These probably develop as a result of growth factors released from HIV-infected cells and multiple lesions are regarded as being independent in origin rather than as a result of metastasis. In addition to the *gag*, *pol*, and *env* genes, common to the retroviruses, the HIV genome has at least six additional genes. Multiple small mRNAs are produced from these genes by virtue of spliced mRNAs, all of which allow the virus to grow much more vigorously than other retroviruses. The precise role of many of the HIV genes is unclear but is thought to involve the activation of transcription and alternate splicing and/or transport of mRNAs. The HIV virus does, in fact, cause cell death rather than cellular transformation and in this way leads to a profound immunodeficiency.

Further reading

Ames, B. N., and Gold, L. S. (1998) The causes and prevention of cancer: the role of environment. *Biotherapy* 11, 205–20.

Balmain, A., and Harris, C. C. (2000) Carcinogenesis in mouse and human cells: parallels and paradoxes. *Carcinogenesis* 21, 371–7.

Bishop, P .C., Rao, V. K., and Wilson, W. H. (2000) Burkitt's lymphoma: molecular pathogenesis and treatment. *Cancer Invest* 18, 574–83.

Brechot, C., Gozuacik, D., Murakami, Y., Paterlini-Brechot, P. (2000) Molecular bases for the development of hepatitis B virus (HBV)-related hepatocellular carcinoma (HCC). *Semin Cancer Biol* 10, 211–31.

Cantelli-Forti, G., Hrelia, P., and Paolini, M. (1998) The pitfall of detoxifying enzymes. *Mutat Res* 18, 179–83.

de Boer, J., and Hoeijmakers, J. H. (2000) Nucleotide excision repair and human syndromes. *Carcinogenesis* 21, 453–60.

de Gruijl, F. R. (1999) Skin cancer and solar UV radiation. *Eur J Cancer* 35, 2003–9.

Goodman, A. (2000) Role of routine human papillomavirus subtyping in cervical screening. *Curr Opin Obstet Gynecol* 12, 11–14.

Hidalgo, J. A., MacArthur, R. D., Crane, L. R. (2000) An overview of HIV infection and AIDS: etiology, pathogenesis, diagnosis, epidemiology, and occupational exposure. *Semin Thorac Cardiovasc Surg* 12, 130–9.

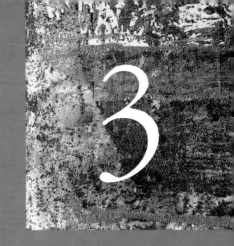

The epidemiology of cancer
Frank Kee

- Introduction

- What causes cancer? What causes a cause?

The epidemiology of cancer

Introduction

The World Health Organization established a subcommittee on the registration of cancer which provided the initial spur for the establishment of the International Union Against Cancer (UICC) in 1950 and ultimately the International Agency for Research on Cancer (IARC).

Since that time, data collection and quality assurance systems have been established that ensure that national and international comparisons of cancer rates can be made.

Some common principles underpin an effective registration system and two of the most important are that it be population based (rather than practitioner- or hospital-based) and that a uniform data set is collected in a uniform way. A population-based registry must use multiple sources for case ascertainment and this increasingly relies on methods of electronic data capture. Several regions of the UK now routinely receive data files from Hospital Patient Administration Systems, Pathology and Haematology Laboratories, from Screening Programme Administration Systems and from the Office of the Registrar General. Whilst such a wide net can help maximize completeness, data-cleaning and data-validation routines are now rigorously codified to avoid duplication and to ensure key pieces of information, such as the data of diagnosis and gender of the patient, are consistently reported for individual cases. The advent of such electronic data capture facilitates the compilation of basic quality assurance data such as the proportion of cases with documented histological verification, the proportion of death certificate only registrations, and the mortality to incidence ratio (Jensen *et al.*, 1995). Eventually this should become more straightforward, if the principle of the Unique Patient Identifier becomes a practical reality, as has been the case for some decades in Scandinavian countries whose cancer registration systems are well developed.

A major challenge to all registers is the consistent recording of a uniform data set and to ensure comparability coding schemes have been internationally agreed for various key pieces of information such as tumour grade, behaviour, and stage, and other more basic data such as date of onset and place of residence. Without such agreement, there is little potential for a register to fulfil its *raison d'être* and achieve it goals:

- to measure the incidence and distribution of cancer in a population;
- to measure survival from the disease; and
- to provide information of relevance to the planning and evaluation of preventive screening and therapeutic services.

The effect of data collection systems and quality on these goals can be illustrated if one were to consider an assessment of time trends. For incidence data, time series may partially reflect progressive improvements in registration rate whether resulting from the development and refinement of diagnostic techniques or improved reporting systems for the registry. For example, in the Connecticut tumour registry, from 1935 to the 1980 the percentage of histologically confirmed cases increased from 73% to 93% of cases. The problem of imprecise data is accentuated by the differences in the evolution of precision between regions or age groups. Errors in diagnosis are generally more serious in older people and improvements in precision can therefore have a fundamental effect on incidence rates in this age group. The phenomenon is probably a partial explanation for the recent increase in myeloma in the elderly. Detection of tumours at an earlier stage and the refinement of staging techniques can also artefactually affect survival trends. For example, many more prostatic cancers are being detected as an incidental finding at surgery. This will tend to inflate the stage I tumours with cases that may never have caused symptoms during life and consequently may suggest an improvement in survival for the disease. A variant of this, the so-called Will Rogers' phenomenon[1] – which may manifest if more refined detection of spread leads to an apparent stage shift of a certain proportion of cases – may also produce a purely artefactual improvement in survival (Feinstein *et al.*, 1985).

Thus when confronted by claims of an unforeseen trend in or distribution of cancer, it is sensible first to test the robustness of the data before attempting to answer any aetiological question. Methods of evaluating putative aetiological risks are considered below.

What causes cancer? What causes a cause?

Susceptibility bias

This can be problematic if the subjects who become 'exposed' are prognostically more likely to develop the outcome event than those who are not exposed. The classical clinical example of susceptibility bias occurs in the therapy of cancer. Surgical treatment is generally reserved for 'operable' patients with more localized cancer and no major co-morbid disease whilst the inoperable patients with metastatic disease or major co-morbidity may be preferentially referred for radiotherapy or chemotherapy. Survival rates are often rather superficially compared for the two groups without regard to the confounding distortion of susceptibility bias.

Detection bias

This may arise when the outcome event is sought and identified with different rigour or methods in the exposed and the unexposed groups. Feinstein has recently decried as scandalous the fears and suspicions evoked by so-called risks from electric power lines, microwave ovens and cellular phones when no account is taken of any greater propensity for worried users to seek out medical attention or a CAT scan (Feinstein, 1995).

---

1 The American humorist Will Rogers once observed that when the Okies left Oklahoma and moved to California, the average intelligence in both states rose (Feinstein, A. R., Sosin, D., and Wells C., 1985).

Exposure bias

Biases in exposure measurement arise if systematic errors or distortions are made when obtaining (e.g. interviewer bias) or when reporting information on exposure (e.g. recall bias). The former can occur if the interviewers are aware of the study hypotheses and employ different interviewing strategies for diseased and non-diseased whilst the latter may arise if study subjects, aware of the putative association sought, systematically inflate or deflate their recalled exposure.

Confounding

Confounding, on the other hand, arises when associations between a putative risk factor and disease actually arise from the correlation between both and a third factor. For example, if a randomly selected group of healthy men, who happened to be carrying a box of matches in their pockets, were followed up for 20 years and their incidence of lung cancer then compared with the general population, then the real effect on risk is more likely to be due to a smoking habit than to carriage of matches.

When the effects of chance, bias and confounding have been examined, the investigator must still apply judgement about the likelihood of a causative association. The panel below is an adaptation of factors identified by Bradford Hill (1965) to assess the likely role of cause in an association:

Association or causation?

- Strength
- Dose–response
- Temporality
- Consistency
- Specificity
- Plausibility
- Reversibility

Sir Richard Doll compiled a monograph in the early 1980s detailing the proportion of cancer incidence attributable to various known or suspected causes (Doll and Peto, 1981). The Harvard Report on Cancer Prevention has recently updated this and its findings still bear witness to the fact that what we are dealing with is largely a preventable disease (Harvard Report on Cancer Prevention, 1996). Table 3.1 illustrates this.

Whilst the figures in Table 3.1 present an overall pattern for a developed nation, clearly the attributable risks would vary several-fold according to the cancer and the country. For example, a high proportion of nasopharyngeal cancer in Asia is likely to be attributable to viral infection. In an era when billions of dollars are invested in chemotherapy by drug companies and health care systems, figures like those in the table should remind us of the enormous opportunity for saving lives through better prevention programmes. The following Table (Table 3.1) illustrates this potential

Table 3.1 Estimated percentage of total cancer deaths attributable to established causes of cancer

Risk factor	Percentage
Tobacco	30%
Adult diet/obesity	30
Sedentary lifestyle	5
Occupational factors	5
Family history of cancer	5
Viruses/other biologic agents	5
Perinatal factors/growth	5
Reproductive factors	3
Alcohol	3
Socioeconomic status	3
Environmental pollution	2
Ionizing/ultraviolet radiation	2
Prescription drugs/medical procedures	1
Salt/other food additives/contaminants	1

Tobacco

In 1993, the US Environmental Protection Agency designated tobacco smoke as a group A carcinogen, for which there is no known safe level of exposure. The risk of cancer is not only determined by the number of pack years but also by the age at commencing smoking. The UK Government in December 1988 released a special White Paper – Smoking Kills – with the following specific aims:

- reduction and eventual banning of tobacco advertising;
- protection of young people by tougher enforcement of under-age sales legislation;
- reduction in tobacco smuggling and fraud;
- promotion of Approved Codes of Practice on smoking at work, including new and improved signage identifying non-smoking areas;
- reduction of smoking prevalence from 28% to 24% in adults and from 13% to 9% in children by the year 2010.

Diet and alcohol

The role of diet in cancer causation is complex and difficult to unravel. However, probably 30% of cancers are associated with poor diet and obesity (Willett, 1994). Specifically, the population intake of fruits, vegetables, legumes and grains should increase, paralleled by a reduction in consumption of red meat, salt and saturated fats.

Lifestyle

The evidence is now considered overwhelming that physical exercise helps protect against colon cancer (Pate *et al.*, 1995), though the picture is a little less clear for breast cancer. Sedentary lifestyle probably doubles the risk of colon cancer. Whereas the mean age at diagnosis is around 70 years, the protective effect can be manifest with only moderate activity such as vigorous walking, so few should exempt themselves from the simple health-promotion message.

Occupation

In 1970 the first comprehensive list of exposures judged to cause human cancer was published by the International Agency for Research on Cancer (1979). Body surfaces that have direct contact with carcinogenic agents in the workplace are at highest risk for developing cancer. These surfaces are the skin (e.g. after exposure to coal tar and soots), nasal passages (e.g. after nickel or formaldehyde exposure) and lung (e.g. after exposure to a variety of heavy metals). The primary internal body surface that has contact with carcinogens is the bladder. The risk obviously depends on the dose and the duration of exposure but with modern occupational hygiene practice it is hoped that no worker in a developed country will succumb to an occupationally acquired cancer. This goal will only be attainable through a sustained commitment to vigilance and surveillance, perhaps in future based on monitoring of physiological or genetic damage at a cellular level.

Infectious agents

It is now generally accepted that both HTLV-1 (human T-cell lymphoma virus type-1) and Epstein–Barr virus are causal factors for several lymphomas, whereas hepatitis B and C are linked, especially in Asia, to the occurrence of liver carcinoma. These infections are quite common but the risk of malignancy is probably linked to latent infection and secondary genetic damage to target tissues. Whilst most carriers will have no serious sequelae, there are some simple prevention messages which can mitigate the risk in the population:

- avoid blood and body fluid exposures – for example, by sharing or re-use of needles or through sexually transmitted infections;
- mothers positive for hepatitis B should have their infants given HBV immunoglobulin followed by vaccination. Those positive for HTLV-1 should bottle feed.

Genetic epidemiology

Molecular epidemiology has gained a prominent place in medical science (McDade and Anderson, 1996; Risch and Merikangas, 1996). What has become clear is that while gene 'detection' through linkage tests can uncover effects of moderate size, the 'lesser' effects of the more frequent genes involved in polygenic disease. For complex diseases, as for rare single-gene defects, statistical analysis of family data can provide clues to the existence of a basic metabolic defect. However, the demonstration that a familial pattern of disease is consistent with Mendelian segregation ratios is considerably more difficult for a disease with a complex aetiology than for a simple autosomal dominant or recessive disorder. Although susceptibility to thrombosis may be determined by numerous genetic loci, most may have only a minor effect. There may be one or a few which independently or in combination have a major effect. In addition, complex diseases such as coronary heart disease may exhibit aetiological heterogeneity with one locus having a major impact in some families and another locus or an environmental variable having a bearing in others. Because of these complications, statistical analysis of family patterns of such diseases may sometimes yield ambiguous results.

The frequency of association between a gene marker and a 'disease' gene will depend on variations in the frequency of the marker in different populations. If controls have a different ethnic background from cases, and if marker allele frequencies differ between ethnic backgrounds, spurious associations may emerge that are unrelated to a disease susceptibility gene. In addition, it is important to remember that these studies are based on a concept of statistical association rather than physical proximity of the relevant loci.

Another issue often not addressed in studies of genetic marker–disease associations is that of biological interaction between the genetic marker and other genetic and environmental factors. In the presence of gene–environment interaction, a truly causal association between a marker and disease may be diluted by the proportion of the population that are or are not exposed to environmental factors which interact with the susceptible genotype (Sing and Moll, 1989).

Not surprisingly, analysis of data from different populations sometimes yields discrepant results. Disease susceptibility loci detectable in one population may not be discerned in another due to differences in environmental risk or other genetic or racial factors or because of differing methods of ascertainment. A further problem resides in the fact that many genetic diseases exhibit aetiological heterogeneity. Whilst these potential shortcomings must always be borne in mind, more advanced statistical approaches beyond the scope of this section are continually being developed, which can at least partially take account of such factors.

Evidence synthesis

The Canadian epidemiologist David Naylor is of the view that the Cochrane Collaboration is an endeavour which will rival the Human Genome Project in its potential significance to clinical medicine. Set up originally in honour of the British epidemiologist Archie Cochrane, this is a worldwide network of biostatisticians, epidemiologists, and clinicians, whose primary purpose is to provide an unbiased synthesis of evidence on the efficacy of treatments or the aetiology of diseases. A host of statistical issues in meta-analysis remain as much a matter of judgement as of science (Spitzer, 1995), as does the older debates between the traditional frequentist and Bayesian views of statistics. Frequentists deduce the probability of observing an outcome given the true underlying state whereas Bayesians induce the probability of the existence of the true, but as yet unknown, underlying state given the data. Probabilities of different states of nature can be combined with pre-specified benefits and costs that would result from taking a certain decision in the face of those 'givens'. The Bayesian approach would then be to choose the decision that maximizes the expected benefit. For example, such an approach, it is claimed, would have demonstrated that although it looks fairly likely that venous thromboembolism occurs somewhat more frequently with third-generation oral contraceptive pills (OCPs), there is considerable doubt about which preparation is safer overall (Lilford and Braunholtz, 1996). Faced with data presented in Bayesian terms, one would more readily appreciate how the probabilities attached to alternative states of nature vary according to different interpretations of the 'starting' information and that the final decision (to initiate contraception) should take account of all the relevant personal trade-offs. A Bayesian approach can thus do justice to the disparate evidence that may have an impact on prior beliefs and will allow for assumptions to be handled openly and explicitly. The reality is that degrees of belief are often continuous, not dichotomous, varying from person to person or situation to situation, in the face of inconclusive evidence. The Bayesian approach seems certain to gain ground in the policy-making arena (Freedman, 1996).

Further reading

Doll, R. and Peto, R. (1981) *The causes of cancer*. Oxford University Press, Oxford.

Feinstein, A. R., Sosin, D., and Wells, C. (1985) The Will Rogers phenomenon. Stage migration and new diagnostic techniques as a source of misleading statistics for survival in cancer. *N Engl J Med* 312, 1604–8.

Feinstein, A. R. (1995) Biases introduced by confounding and imperfect retrospective and prospective exposure assessments. In Graham, J. D. (ed.), *The role of epidemiology in regulatory risk assessment*. Elsevier, Amsterdam.

Freedman, L. (1996) Bayesian statistical methods. A natural way to assess clinical evidence. *BMJ* 311, 569–70.

Harvard Report on Cancer Prevention (1996) In: *Cancer Causes and Control* 7 (Suppl. 1). Rapid Science Publishers, London.

International Agency for Research on Cancer (1979) *Chemicals and industrial processes associated with cancer in humans*. IARC Monographs, vols 1–20. Lyon, France.

Jensen, O. M., Parkin, D. M., MacLennan, R., Muir, C. S., and Skeet, R. G. (eds) (1995) *Cancer registration: principles and methods*. IARC Scientific Publications No. 95, Lyon.

Lilford, R. J. and Braunholtz, D. (1996) The statistical basis of public policy: a paradigm shift is overdue. *BMJ* 313, 603–7.

McDade, J. E. and Anderson, B. E. (1996) Molecular epidemiology: applications of nucleic acid amplification and sequence analysis. *Am J Epidemiol* 18, 90–7.

Pate, R. R., Pratt, M., Blair, S. N. *et al.* (1995) Physical activity and public health. A recommendation from the Centers for Disease Control and American College of Sports Medicine. *JAMA* 273, 402–7.

Risch, N. and Merikangas, K. (1996) The future of genetic studies of complex human diseases. *Science* 273, 1516–17.

Sing, C. F. and Moll, P. M. (1989) Genetics of variability of CHD risk. *Int J Epidemiol* 18, S183–94.

Spitzer, W. O. (ed.) (1995) The Potsdam International Consultation on Meta-analysis. *J Clin Epidemiol* 48, 1–172.

Willett, W. (1994) Diet and health. What should we eat? *Science* 14, 393–418.

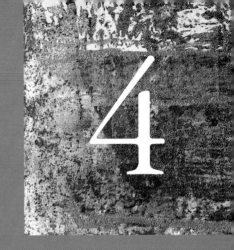

The molecular biology of cancer
D. Paul Harkin

- Introduction

- Oncogenes

- Tumour suppressor genes

- DNA repair genes

- Multistep nature of cancer

The molecular biology of cancer

Introduction

Cellular growth and division is a carefully regulated process that depends on the precise interaction of multiple regulatory factors. Cancer represents a deregulation of this process, in which some of the normal constraints on cell growth and division have been lost. How this deregulation occurs has been the focus of intense interest over the last three decades. However, it is now generally accepted that tumours arise through the accumulation of several genetic changes affecting the control of cellular growth. Recent advances in molecular biology have made it possible to define some of the molecular changes that regulate the mechanisms by which certain tumours arise.

The following three major classes of genes have now been implicated in the development of cancer:

- Oncogenes
- Tumour suppressor genes
- DNA repair genes

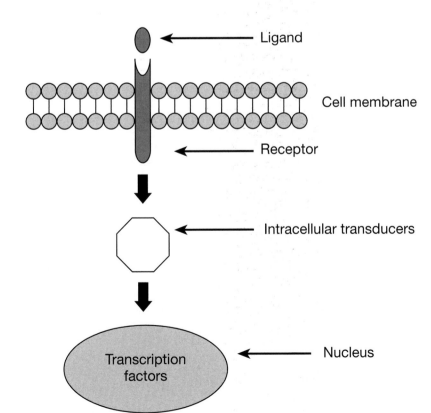

Fig. 4.1 Cellular proliferation is regulated by both positive and negative growth signals. These signals are relayed to the nucleus via receptor–ligand interactions which activate intracellular transduction pathways. These intracellular transducers transmit this signal to the nucleus where the appropriate transcription factor is activated.

Oncogenes

The first class, termed oncogenes, are mutated forms of normal cellular genes called proto-oncogenes and tend to function as positive regulators of cell growth. Oncogenes were first discovered in transducing RNA tumour viruses, which acquired cellular genes, by transduction. When these cellular genes are incorporated into the viral genome they become activated oncogenes. Oncogene activation has also been shown to occur by retroviral insertion near a proto-oncogene, resulting in abnormal expression of the gene. A number of other mechanisms such as translocations, point mutations, and gene amplification have also been shown to result in activated oncogenes. The signalling pathways by which a cell divides or remains quiescent involves a complex array of growth factors, growth factor receptors, intracellular transducers, and transcription factors (Fig. 4.1). Tumourigenesis reflects a malfunction in one or more of these pathways, caused in part by the action of oncogenes. To gain an overall insight as to how oncogenes disrupt normal cellular controls, it is necessary to examine oncogene function in the context of these signalling pathways. Signalling molecules can be loosely grouped according to their cellular location and function as follows:

- growth factors
- growth factor receptors
- intracellular transducers
- transcription factors.

Growth factors

In recent years a large variety of growth factors have been identified, including platelet-derived growth factor (PDGF), insulin-like growth factors (IGFs), epidermal growth factor (EGF), and its structural and functional homologue, transforming growth factor-α (TGF-α), to name but a few. Growth factors mediate their mitogenic effect by binding to specific receptors on the cell surface. This results in the upregulation of a cascade of genes, termed immediate early genes, such as *fos, myc*, and *jun*. Some of these genes are themselves pleiotrophic regulators of growth. A characteristic of tumour cells is their ability to grow in an autonomous fashion and lacking dependence on one or more growth factors whose presence is required for growth of their normal counterparts.

Growth factor receptors

One of the best-studied growth factor receptors, the EGF receptor (EGFR), was initially characterized as a ligand-stimulated protein tyrosine kinase. The receptor was subsequently shown to consist of an extracellular EGF binding domain, a transmembrane region of 23 amino acids, and a cytoplasmic domain with tyrosine-specific protein kinase activity. Mutations within the protein tyrosine kinase domain of EGFR were shown to abrogate its transforming potential, indicating that receptor tyrosine kinase activity was necessary for neoplastic transformation. The importance of protein tyrosine kinases (PTK) in normal signalling pathways is highlighted by a number of other studies. For example, the oncogenic effect of c-*erb* B-2, a transmembrane glycoprotein homologous to the EGFR, is mediated by increased PTK activity caused by gene amplification or by a point mutation in the transmembrane region (Bargmann *et al.*, 1986).

Intracellular transducers

The discovery of cyclic adenosine-3′,5-monophosphate (cAMP) more than 30 years ago gave rise to the idea that hormones can regulate cells by initiating the production of intracellular second messengers. Since then a number of other intracellular molecules, including calcium and the products of phosphoinositide metabolism, have been discovered. In most cases these second messengers are stimulated via a family of small heterotrimeric G-proteins (called G-proteins because they bind GTP). The specificity with which a receptor can bind a particular G-protein defines the range of responses a cell is capable of making in response to a particular stimulus. The *ras* family of proto-oncogenes encodes a group of closely related 21 kDa proteins that control regulatory pathways critical for normal proliferation and differentiation. The discovery that Ras proteins could bind GTP and GDP and were localized to the inner surface of the plasma membrane led to the suggestion that Ras proteins and G-proteins may have functional similarities.

Nuclear oncogenes (transcription factors)

A number of proto-oncogene products are located in the nucleus where it has been suggested that they provide the final stage in the signalling pathway governing cellular proliferation. The best-described nuclear oncogene is c-*myc*, which was initially identified as the homologue of the transforming sequence of the avian myelocytomatosis virus MC29 (Donner *et al.*, 1982). It has subsequently been shown to be amplified in a variety of cancer types including colon carcinoma, small cell lung carcinoma and breast cancer. A number of related genes have been discovered based on their homology to c-*myc*. The two best-described family members are n-*myc* and l-*myc*, both of which are amplified in certain types of tumours.

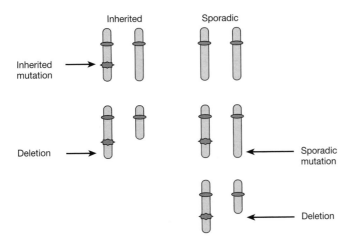

Fig. 4.2 Both copies of a TSG must be lost or inactivated in order to promote tumour progression. In this figure, inactivation is represented by mutation in the first allele, followed by loss through deletion of the remaining wild-type allele. (a) In familial forms of cancer, the first mutation is inherited through the germline, followed by a second sporadic mutation. This tends to result in an early age of onset of the disease. (b) in sporadic forms of cancer, both mutational events are somatic, with the result that the age of onset tends to occur later in life.

Tumour suppressor genes

The second class of genes, termed tumour suppressor genes (TSG), act as negative regulators of cell growth. Loss or inactivation of a TSG results in loss of growth inhibition and results in a selective growth advantage for the cell. The observed recessive nature of TSGs means that both copies of a TSG must be lost or inactivated in order that the malignant phenotype may be expressed (Knudson, 1971) (Fig. 4.2). In the case of hereditary forms of cancer such as retinoblastoma one of these mutations is inherited through the germline, usually resulting in an earlier age of onset of the disease. A number of mechanisms by which TSGs are lost or inactivated have been identified. These include deletions, resulting in complete loss; translocations, which interrupt the coding sequence; point mutations, which inhibit gene function or result in protein truncation; and imprinting, which may result in abnormal gene expression.

Somatic and microcell genetic studies

The first suggestion that cancer may occur as a recessive event came from the fusion of malignant and non-malignant mouse cells. The resultant hybrid clones exhibited a reduction in tumourigenicity, indicating that malignancy acts as a recessive trait (Harris *et al.*, 1969).

Familial cancers as indicators of tumour suppressor genes (TSGs)

Knudson and others have stressed the importance of genetic inheritance in the search for cancer-related genes. The observation of specific chromosomal abnormalities associated at high frequency with particular hereditary conditions has proved invaluable in this search. In the absence of detectable cytogenetic abnormalities, localization of a particular disease gene will usually rely on linkage analysis, which allows the ordering of inherited markers relative to each other.

Loss of heterozygosity studies

Using a combination of these approaches, an increasing number of genes have been isolated which fall into this category. These novel tumour suppressor genes carry out a diverse series of functions within the cell, ranging from cell cycle checkpoint to cell migration (Table 4.1).

The RB paradigm

Retinoblastoma (RB), which has an incidence of approximately 1:20 000, occurs in cells of the embryonal neural retina in young children up to age 5 years and exhibits both sporadic and familial forms. The observation that as many as one-third of retinoblastomas appear to arise from a genetic predisposition with a dominant mode of inheritance led Knudson to postulate the now classical 'two-hit' theory. He suggested that retinoblastoma is caused by two mutational events. In the dominantly inherited form, one mutation is inherited through the germline and the second mutation is somatic. In the sporadic form of the disease both mutations are somatic. It was subsequently shown that in retinoblastoma the target of these mutational events was the RB tumour suppresser gene (Cavenee *et al.*, 1985).

Table 4.1

Gene	Tumour	Localization	Function
RB	Retinoblastoma, osteosarcoma	13q14	Cell cycle checkpoint
p53	Majority of tumour types	17p13.1	DNA damage responsive gene, cell cycle arrest & apoptosis
WT1	Kidney tumours	11p13.3	Nuclear transcription factor
NF1	Neurofibromas, Schwannomas	17q11.2	GTPase-activating protein
NF2	Schwannomas, meningiomas	22q	Cytoskeletal reorganization
VHL	Kidney tumours	3p25	Component of the cellular ubiquitination machinery
APC	Colon carcinomas	5q21	Cellular adhesion and signal transduction
BRCA1	Breast and ovarian	17q21	Cellular response to DNA damage & regulation of transcription tumours
BRCA2	Breast cancer, pancreatic cancer	13q12-13	DNA repair
p16INK4	Melanomas	9p21	Cell cycle checkpoint
p19ARF	Melanomas	9p21p	Cell cycle checkpoint, regulation of p53 protein levels
PTEN	Hamartomas, breast tumours thyroid tumours	10q23	Cell migration

The p53 tumour suppressor genes (TSG)

The p53 gene was initially identified by the ability of its encoded protein to complex with the SV40 large T antigen in SV40-transformed cells. It has been described as the guardian of the genome, due to its role in the cellular response to DNA damage. It is now estimated that approximately 50% of all tumours carry a p53 gene mutation, making this gene the most frequently mutated in human cancers. In most tumours where p53 is mutated, one allele contains a missense mutation and the second allele is lost by deletion, thereby fulfilling the essential criteria for its classification as a TSG, originally proposed by Knudson.

DNA repair genes

A third class of genes, termed DNA repair genes have more recently been implicated in the genesis of cancer. The initial observation that an association may exist between DNA repair deficiencies and cancer came approximately 20 years ago with the report of an elevated risk of skin cancer in the human disease xeroderma pigmentosum. However, the major breakthrough in this field was the cloning of a human mismatch repair gene, *hMSH2*, identified based on its homology to the *Saccharomyces cerevisiae, MSH2* gene. It was subsequently shown that this gene was mutated in families with hereditary non-polyposis colorectal cancer (HNPCC), resulting in what has been described as a mutator phenotype (Cleaver, 1994). Conceptually, inactivation of DNA repair genes can be considered as an initiation events in tumour development but is not rate limiting. Mutations within DNA repair genes tend to result in an intrinsic genetic instability, which subsequently leads to additional mutational events such as inactivation of tumour suppressor genes.

Mammalian cells have evolved a highly regulated mechanism for dealing with DNA damage incurred through spontaneous mutation, nucleotide mismatch during DNA synthesis, exposure to ultraviolet or gamma radiation or exposure to reactive metabolites that cause oxidation and alkylation of DNA.

Nucleotide excision repair

Nucleotide excision repair (NER) is the process whereby DNA damage is removed and replaced with new DNA using the intact wild-type strand as a template. It is one of the most extensively studied and complicated of the excision-repair processes, involving up to 30 gene products. The NER machinery has broad specificity and is able to recognize a wide variety of chemical alterations to DNA, which result in distortion of the DNA structure. A typical lesion repaired by this mechanism is the pyrimidine dimer which, is induced by the photochemical fusion of two adjacent pyrimidines in response to ultraviolet radiation. It is estimated that skin cells would acquire thousands of pyrimidine dimers each day in response to sunlight exposure, if they were not removed by excision repair. A large number of the genes implicated in NER have been shown to be involved in transcription regulation, and mutations affecting different domains of these multifunctional proteins can lead to widely differing clinical phenotypes (Lehmann, 1998). The best described cancer syndrome caused by mutation of genes involved in excision repair is the human skin disease xeroderma pigmentosum (XP), which is characterized by hypersensitivity to sun (UV) light and predisposition to skin cancer.

Mismatch repair

It has been known for some time that mismatch repair (MMR) plays an essential role in the correction of replicative mismatches that escape proof-reading polymerases, and in the processing of recombination intermediates. MMR, therefore acts as an important fail-safe mechanism to ensure the fidelity of DNA replication. Studies in *Escherichia coli* have provided much of the fundamental information on how the MMR system works.

Interest in this field received a considerable boost with the observation that the underlying genetic defect in hereditary non-polyposis colorectal cancer (HNPCC) could be attributed to mutations within various members of the mismatch repair genes, particularly *hMSH2* and *hMLH1* (Fishel *et al.*, 1993). Phenotypically patients with mutations of mismatch repair genes exhibit a mutator phenotype, which manifests itself as instability within simple repeat sequences. In addition to HNPCC, mutations within mismatch repair genes have also been observed in numerous forms of sporadic cancer, including endometrial, pancreatic, gastric, ovarian and breast cancer to name but a few.

Multistep nature of cancer

There is now compelling evidence to suggest that cancers arise via a multistep process resulting in an accumulation of genetic changes in a single cell. Molecular analyses of human cancers, which are typically clonal, exhibit multiple genetic lesions including the activation of oncogenes and the inactivation of TSG. The net effect of this accumulated genetic damage is a deregulation of the normal controls on proliferation with the result that cells continually enter the cell cycle and divide (Fig. 4.3). Colorectal cancer has provided an ideal model for the study of this multistep process. Colorectal tumours progress through easily recognizable clinical stages in which tumourigenesis is preceded by widespread cellular hyper-proliferation from which foci of benign adenomas arise. The adenomas increase in size and dysplasia and may invade through the basement membrane to become by definition a carcinoma. Further progression may result in metastasis to distant sites. The genetic changes underlying this clinical progression have, to a large extent, been defined and involve the inactivation of key TSG and the activation of specific oncogenes, which combine or co-operate to induce the malignant state (Vogelstein *et al.*, 1988) (Fig. 4.4). This stepwise selection within the tumour population results in an increased growth rate in those cells that have acquired the necessary number of genetic hits to allow a selective advantage over their neighbours. The net effect of this process of selection is an increase in the malignant potential of the tumour, which eventually manifests itself as an ability to spread from the primary site and metastasize to other regions of the body.

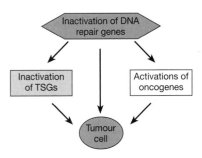

Fig. 4.3 Tumourigenesis reflects the underlying genetic changes that occur over time in a specific cell. These alterations include inactivation of TSGs and DNA repair genes, in addition to the activation of specific oncogenes. The combined effect of these changes results in deregulation of the normal constraints on cell growth, the net effect of which is the ability to proliferate in an uncontrolled manner.

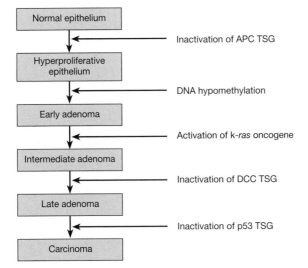

Fig. 4.4 The molecular changes underlying the phenotypic progression observed in colorectal cancer have to a large extent been described. Although the exact order of the molecular changes may vary, a consistent pattern has emerged. This involves as an early event the inactivation of a critical TSG, APC (adenomatous polyposis coli) followed by a series of other genetic alterations detailed in the text.

Further reading

Bargmann, C. J., Hung, M. C., and Weinberg, R. A. (1986) Multiple independent activations of the *neu* oncogene by a point mutation altering the transmembrane domain. *Cell* 45, 649–57.

Cavenee, W. K., Hansen, M. F., Nordenskjold, M., Kock, E., and Maumenee, I. (1985) Genetic origin of mutations predisposing to retinoblastoma. *Science* 228, 501–3.

Cleaver, J. E. (1994) It was a very good year for DNA repair. *Cell* 76, 1–4.

Donner, P., Greiser-Wilke, I., and Moelling, K. (1982) Nuclear localization and DNA binding of the transforming gene product of the avian myelocytomatosis virus. *Nature* 296, 262–5.

El-Deiry, W. S., Tokino, T., Velculescu, V. E., *et al.* (1993) WAF1, a potential mediator of p53 tumour suppression. *Cell* 75, 817–25.

Fishel, R., Lescoe, M. K., Rao, M. R. S., *et al.* (1993) The human mutator gene homologue MSH2 and its association with hereditary nonpolyposis colon cancer. *Cell* 75, 1027–38.

Hansen, M. F. and Cavenee, W. K. (1987) Genetics of cancer predisposition. *Cancer Res* 47, 5518.

Harris, H., Miller, O. J., Klein, G., Worst, P., and Tachibana, T. (1969) Suppression of malignancy by cell fusion. *Nature* 223, 363–8.

Hermeking, H., Longauer, C., Polyak, K., *et al.* (1997) 14-3-3σ is a p53-regulated inhibitor of G2/M progression. *Molecular Cell* 1, 3–11.

Knudson Jr, A. G. (1971) Mutation and cancer: statistical study of retinoblastoma. *Proc Natl Acad Sci U S A* 68, 820–82.

Lehmann, A. R. (1998) Dual functions of DNA repair genes: molecular, cellular, and clinical implications. *Bioessays* 20(2), 146–55.

Polyak, K., Xia, Y., Zweier, J. L., Kinzler, K. W., and Vogelstein B. (1997). A model for p53-induced apoptosis. *Nature* 389, 300–5.

Vogelstein, B., Fearon, E. R., Hamilton, S. R., *et al.* (1988) Genetic alterations during colorectal tumour development. *N Engl J Med* 319, 525–32.

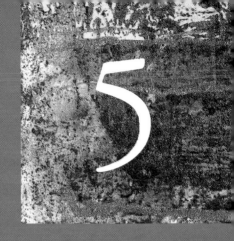

The pathology of cancer
Damian T. McManus

- Introduction, definitions, and classifications
- Carcinogenesis
- Spread and effects of malignant tumours
- The role of tissue diagnosis in malignant disease

The pathology of cancer

Introduction, definitions, and classifications

Neoplasia

Neoplasia (literally 'new growth') has been defined by Willis in functional terms as a disorder of cell growth in which there is a permanent and inherited change in cells resulting in a pathological proliferation of tissue which is excessive, purposeless, and autonomous, continuing indefinitely regardless of stimuli or effects of the expanding neoplasm on the surrounding tissues. It is a disorder which is characterized by the irreversible disruption of the normal homeostatic mechanisms that regulate:

- cell proliferation,
- differentiation, and
- apoptosis,

resulting in a caricature of normal tissue growth. Key features of the caricature include uncontrolled cellular proliferation of relatively undifferentiated cells with defective senescence and cell death programmes.

Neoplasms may be categorized as benign or malignant. Not all neoplastic growths form tumours or swellings: acute leukaemia, for example, represents malignant transformation of pluripotent white cell precursors (blasts) within the bone marrow and only very rarely forms tumours or mass lesions. The hallmark of malignant tumours is their ability to destructively **invade** locally and to spread to distant parts of the body by **metastasis**. Invasion and metastasis are the cardinal behavioural characteristics that distinguish benign and malignant tumours. Some benign tumours, e.g. adenomatous polyps of the colon, may be precursors of malignant tumours, although this is not always the case.

Benign tumours may still result in clinically significant and life-threatening complications for a number of reasons:

- patient anxiety, e.g. a fibroadenoma of the breast;
- anatomical location, e.g. obstruction of cerebrospinal fluid drainage by a posterior fossa ependymoma or choroid plexus papilloma;
- compression of adjacent anatomical structures, e.g. compression of the optic chiasma by an expanding adenoma of the anterior pituitary;
- secretion of biologically active substances, e.g. Cushing's disease, where a pituitary adenoma secretes ACTH which causes the adrenal glands to release excess glucocorticoids.

Benign tumours are often well circumscribed and may be encapsulated. They are not fixed to surrounding structures. They may have been present for some time and grow slowly. Their surface is generally not ulcerated and they may show an exophytic or polypoid growth pattern. By contrast, malignant tumours often have diffusely infiltrative margins and may be fixed to surrounding structures. They may grow rapidly and there may be a history of recent change, e.g. itch or change in shape in a skin lesion. Their surface may ulcerate and on removal the cut surface may be variegated with areas of haemorrhage and necrosis. There may be an endophytic invasive growth pattern in addition to an exophytic non-infiltrative component.

Tumours may be classified histogenetically or perhaps more accurately according to the differentiation patterns displayed by the tumours. Histologically, benign tumours are usually well differentiated, closely resembling their tissue of origin. Malignant tumours may also show an obvious line of differentiation or may be so poorly differentiated or anaplastic that their histogenetic origins are not apparent. Certain histological and cytological features are often associated with malignancy:

- an infiltrative unencapsulated margin;
- invasion of basement membrane or surrounding structures such as muscle or nerve;
- evidence of invasion of blood vessels or lymphatics or metastases to lymph nodes;
- tumour necrosis;
- architectural abnormalities such as an increased gland to stroma ratio and increased gland complexity;
- cytological abnormalities including increased nuclear to cytoplasmic ratio, nuclear hyperchromasia with coarsening of the chromatin pattern, and pleomorphism;
- numerous mitotic figures and abnormal mitoses.

Some examples of benign and malignant tumours are given in Table 5.1.

Carcinogenesis

Morphologically recognizable precancerous changes occur in many tissues prior to the development of a frankly malignant tumour. The term **dysplasia** is used to describe a reversible disorder of cell growth characterized by architectural and

Table 5.1 Nomenclature of malignant tumours

Name of tumour	Tissue of origin	Examples
Carcinoma	Epithelium	Adenocarcinoma
Sarcoma	Mesenchymal	Liposarcoma
Malignant lymphoma	Lymphocytes	Follicular lymphoma
Malignant melanoma	Melanocytes	Superficial spreading malignant melanoma
Malignant mesothelioma	Mesothelium	Pleural malignant mesothelioma
Teratoma	Germ cells	Testicular teratoma
Choriocarcinoma	Trophoblast	Uterine choriocarcinoma

cytological changes similar to those seen in malignant neoplasms but of less severe degree. The maturation or differentiation of tissues may also be impaired. Although such changes occur most often in epithelia, they are increasingly recognized in other tissues, e.g. bone marrow where certain myelodysplastic syndromes may be associated with subsequent leukaemic transformation.

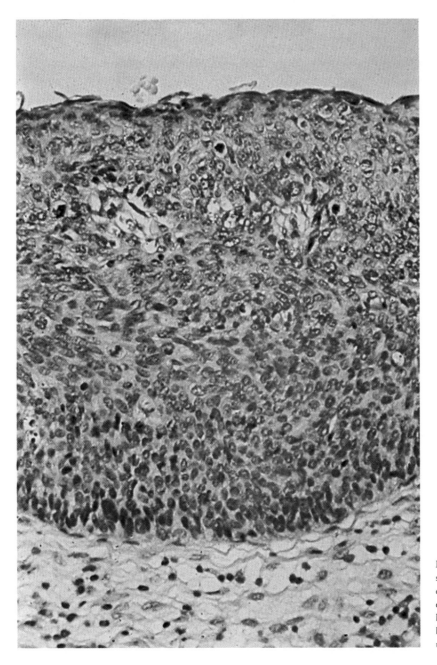

Fig. 5.1 Severe dysplasia or CIN III of the stratified squamous epithelium of the uterine cervix. Note the lack of maturation with extension of abnormal mitotically active basaloid cells onto the surface and intact basement membrane at the interface with underlying stroma. H&E staining.

The maturation disturbances and architectural disturbances that are seen depend to a large extent on the specific tissues involved. Dysplasia of glandular mucosa is characterized architecturally by an increased gland density with a reduction in intervening stroma. The complexity of individual glands is increased and there are abnormalities of polarization of the cells lining the glands. Dysplastic stratified squamous epithelium is characterized by relatively increased layers of basaloid cells in comparison to mature superficial cells (Fig. 5.1). Cytological abnormalities such as nuclear hyperchromasia and pleomorphism similar to those seen in malignant tumours are also seen in dysplastic tissues.

Metaplasia describes the replacement of one fully differentiated tissue by another. Metaplasia may coexist with dysplasia and metaplastic epithelia may also develop dysplastic change. Thus the metaplastic columnar mucosa of Barrett's oesophagus and metaplastic stratified squamous epithelium of the transformation zone of the cervix are both susceptible to malignant change.

Disordered epithelial growth often shows a continuous spectrum of change in response to persistent injury. Regenerative changes as a reaction to ulceration and inflammation can show similarities to, and be difficult to distinguish from, mild or low-grade dysplasia; at the other end of the scale, severe dysplasia merges imperceptibly with **carcinoma in situ**. Carcinoma in situ is a term used in the context of epithelial premalignancy when the histological abnormalities are sufficiently severe to suggest carcinoma but in the absence of basement membrane invasion (Fig. 5.1).

Low-grade dysplasia may spontaneously regress and can often be managed conservatively by continued surveillance. High-grade dysplasia or carcinoma in situ is unlikely to regress and may progress rapidly to or be accompanied by invasive squamous carcinoma. Metastatic potential is heralded by the destruction of basal lamina and invasion of underlying stromal tissues by the malignant epithelium.

Whereas squamous carcinoma is often preceded by dysplastic changes, some common types of adenocarcinoma, e.g. endometrial adenocarcinoma of the uterine corpus, may instead be preceded by **hyperplastic** change. Hyperplasia is traditionally viewed as a reversible growth disturbance occurring, for example, secondarily to stimulation of a tissue by hormones. **Atypical hyperplasia** is a term which has been introduced to describe precancerous morphological changes in endometrium and in the breast, showing a range of hyperplastic morphological features overlapping with dysplasia.

The process of neoplastic transformation is also referred to as **carcinogenesis**. The incidence of many types of cancer, particularly carcinoma, increases with age; statistical analysis of age/incidence curves for such tumours suggests that carcinogenesis is often a multistep process requiring perhaps six to eight steps. Carcinomas are derived from epithelial tissues, which are generally continuously renewing cell populations and often exposed to a variety of environmental carcinogens. Multiple redundant negative regulatory systems in such tissues prevent uncontrolled cell proliferation and must be progressively degraded before an uncontrolled, autonomous malignant cell population emerges. Cancer arises as a result of cumulative non-lethal damage to DNA. The development of genetic models for colorectal and other carcinomas has confirmed the multistep model and illuminated its molecular and cellular basis. Each step represents a somatic mutation that provides a growth advantage for the affected cell, progressively overcoming negative regulatory controls and permitting clonal expansion. The eventual outcome of this somatic evolutionary process is the emergence of a clone of malignant cells refractory to normal homeostatic controls that continues to evolve in the process of **progression**.

Many carcinomas show gross numerical and structural chromosomal abnormalities with allelic imbalance at multiple loci reflecting tumour suppressor gene inactivation and oncogene amplification. By contrast, certain lymphomas, sarcomas, and other small, round, blue cell tumours are commoner in young adults and children. Sarcomas and lymphomas often show fewer cytogenetic abnormalities and frequently contain specific, clonal karyotypic abnormalities such as reciprocal translocations involving transcription factors important in regulating development and differentiation. It is likely that fewer steps are needed for the malignant transformation of such tissues, which lack the multiple redundant negative regulatory systems characteristic of epithelial tissues.

Mutations may either be inherited in the germline or acquired as somatic mutations. Mutations may behave in a dominant or recessive manner at the level of a cell, depending both on the gene target and the type of mutation. Inherited germline mutations that increase susceptibility to cancer affect three main categories of genes:

- inheritance of allelic polymorphisms indirectly increasing susceptibility to cancer: polymorphisms within MHC type II antigens may predispose to the development of cervical carcinoma by reducing the effectiveness of the immune response to human papilloma virus infection. Polymorphisms affecting the activity of enzymes responsible for the metabolism and detoxification of xenobiotic chemical carcinogens constitute another example.

- inheritance of faulty DNA repair mechanisms: e.g. mismatch repair enzyme defects *hMSH1* and *hMSH2* in hereditary non-polyposis colorectal cancer. This is an example of a so-called **caretaker** gene where inactivation promotes genomic instability manifest as **microsatellite instability**.

- inheritance of a faulty tumour suppressor gene: statistical analysis of the age incidence data for hereditary and sporadic retinoblastoma led Knudson to a two-hit model of retinoblastoma carcinogenesis. This and cell fusion studies led to the notion of recessive **tumour suppressor** genes whose inactivation is associated with carcinogenesis.

Inactivation of a classical tumour suppressor gene is rate limiting for the initiation of specific tumours. Such genes are also known as **gatekeeper** genes. These directly regulate cell proliferation or cell death in specific tissues. In inherited tumours, a germline missense or non-sense mutation disables one allele but the full oncogenic effects are not manifest whilst the remaining allele continues to function. Only a single somatic mutational event is then needed to initiate a cancer. Sporadic tumours develop when both copies of the gene are disabled by somatic mutations. The risk of acquiring a single mutation is exponentially greater than acquiring two mutations in a single cell or a clone of cells and there-

Table 5.2 Familial cancer syndromes and associated genes

Entity	Gene	Locus
Retinoblastoma	*RB1*	13q14
Wilm's tumour	*WT1*	11p13
Li–Fraumeni syndrome	*TP53*	17p13
Familial adenomatous polyposis	*APC*	5q12
Neurofibromatosis type 1	*NF1*	17q11
Neurofibromatosis type 2	*NF2*	22q12
von Hippel Lindau syndrome	*VHL*	3p25
Hereditary breast/ovarian carcinoma	*BRCA1*	17q
Hereditary breast/ovarian carcinoma	*BRCA2*	13q12-13
Multiple endocrine neoplasia type IIa	*RET*	10q11

fore patients with hereditary mutations are at greatly increased risk of developing specific tumours. Moreover, inherited tumours in such kindreds usually present at an earlier age and are often multifocal and bilateral.

Hereditary cancer kindreds due to germline mutations in gatekeeper tumour suppressor genes behave as Mendelian autosomal dominant with incomplete penetrance but behave in a recessive fashion at a cellular level. The application of **linkage analysis** and **positional cloning** to such kindreds has led to the identification of tumour suppressor gene loci with the subsequent isolation and characterization of the affected genes. Some examples of such familial cancer syndromes are given in Table 5.2.

The second allele is often inactivated by physical deletion, or loss and reduplication, during somatic mitotic recombination events in both sporadic and hereditary tumours. Analysis of **polymorphisms** close to or within such tumour suppressor gene loci will show **loss of heterozygosity** in tumour DNA in comparison to the constitutional genotype.

Somatic genetic abnormalities may inactivate recessive tumour suppressor genes as discussed above or activate **oncogenes**, which generally have dominant effects. Oncogenes may be activated by a variety of mechanisms:

- **gene amplification:** increased copy numbers of the gene in homogenously staining regions (e.g. the *erbB2* oncogene) or as extra-chromosomal double minutes (the n-*myc* oncogene) result in increased expression of the oncogene protein product. The *erbB2* oncogene is frequently amplified in breast carcinoma with concomitant over-expression of the protein at the cell membrane.
- **reciprocal translocation:** translocations between chromosomes can result in a gene coming under the influence of a new promoter or enhancer sequence, resulting in dysregulated or increased transcription. In Burkitt's lymphoma, the c-*myc* oncogene from chromosome 8 is translocated to 14q32 near the immunoglobulin heavy chain locus, resulting in constitutive expression of

c-*myc* without reference to the cell cycle. Translocations can also result in fusion of one part of a gene to another, giving rise to novel chimaeric mRNA species. The Philadelphia chromosome was the first specific cytogenetic abnormality to be detected in cancer. It is highly specific for chronic myeloid leukaemia and is characterized by a reciprocal translocation with fusion of the *abl* proto-oncogene to *bcr*.

- **point mutations** causing amino-acid substitutions: point mutations at codon 12 in the *ras* oncogene causing substitutions for glycine can result in major conformational changes affecting GTPase activity and locking the Ras protein into an active conformation.

- **viruses:** the introduction of mutated oncogene sequences by retroviruses into cells is very unusual. However, integration of DNA or retroviruses into host DNA may result in dysregulated transcription of oncogenes nearby due to proximity of viral enhancer sequences, e.g. c-*myc* and the human papilloma virus.

In contrast to the activating mutations detected in oncogenes, tumour suppressor genes are inactivated by a variety of mechanisms including missense or nonsense mutation and loss of all or part of a chromosome.

The cell cycle describes how the process of cell proliferation or mitosis is coupled to DNA synthesis (Fig. 5.2). It is regulated by numerous influences, including the protein products of several tumour suppressor genes and oncogenes. The retinoblastoma gene protein product serves as a critical regulator at a restriction point in G1 of the cell cycle just before the cell commits itself to divide.

Apoptosis is a morphologically and biochemically distinctive form of programmed cell death that occurs physiologically in many normal tissue. It is now clear that the accumulation of abnormal cells that constitutes a cancer doesn't only arise from uncontrolled cell proliferation, but is often at least partly due to dysregulated apoptosis. Apoptosis is regulated by several genes, important in carcinogenesis, including *TP53*, *bcl2*, and c-*myc*.

The TP53 gene has been described as the guardian of the genome and is frequently mutated in a variety of cancers. It is thought that in some normal tissues, DNA damage such as strand breaks causes induction of p53 protein. This stalls the cell cycle and offers an opportunity for DNA repair to supervene. If this is unsuccessful, then the apoptosis programme is activated, destroying the cell and preventing transmission of the genetic damage to daughter cells in proliferating tissues. Inactivation of p53 prevents the selective destruction of genetically damaged cells, allowing the accumulation of such cells within cancers.

When cells are grown in tissue culture, they do not divide indefinitely but rather they eventually stop dividing and become senescent. As cells divide, the **telomeres** (repeat sequences at the ends of chromosomes) progressively shorten due to incomplete replication of one end of each DNA strand. It is thought that the phenomenon of progressive telomere truncation acts as a lifespan-limiting clock. The enzyme **telomerase** catalyses telomere extension and is expressed by germ cells and stem cells. Biochemical analysis of homogenates of many different cancer types shows increased telomerase activity. Derepression and expression of

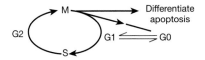

Fig. 5.2 The cell cycle. G0 represents the resting state. Diploid cells are recruited into G1 of the cell cycle. During S phase, DNA synthesis occurs, culminating in reduplication of the genome and tetraploid DNA content, G2. During mitosis (M) the chromosomes are equally divided between the two daughter cells. Cells may leave the cycle by a process of differentiation to mature specialized post-mitotic cells or by programmed cell death or apoptosis.

telomerase during carcinogenesis immortalizes cells, allowing them to continue to divide indefinitely and to accumulate further mutations.

Neovascularization of the growing mass of cells allows proliferation and eventually metastasis and is regulated by the balance between angiogenic and anti-angiogenic polypeptide factors secreted by the tumour.

Normal tissues have a specific architecture where the spatial relationships between cells depend on adhesive interactions between cells and between cells and the extracellular matrix. Alterations in the expression of **cell adhesion molecules** on the surface of tumour cells are often associated with invasive behaviour and metastasis. E-cadherin expression may be reduced in signet-ring type gastric adenocarcinomas and lobular carcinoma of the breast, both tumours classically showing diffuse infiltrative behaviour.

Adhesive interactions between tumour cells and the extracellular matrix are also important in invasion and metastasis. Certain types of integrins mediate attachments to the extracellular matrix through fibronectin. Basement membranes represent specialized extracellular matrix at the interface between epithelia and underlying connective tissue stroma. They are rich in laminin and collagen IV. Tumour cells often secrete metalloproteinase enzymes with proteolytic activity that degrade such basement membrane components, permitting invasion and metastasis. Some tumours provoke an intense fibrous scarring reaction (**desmoplasia**), which makes the tumour hard or scirrhous.

Spread and effects of malignant tumours

The local effects of a malignant tumour mainly depend on the anatomical relations to surrounding structures:

- Tumours arising within a hollow viscus such as the distal colon or common bile duct may lead to obstruction and intestinal obstruction or obstructive jaundice, respectively. For example, bronchogenic carcinoma frequently arises in the proximal portion of a major bronchus. The intraluminal exophytic tumour growth may obstruct the bronchial lumen and result in atelectasis and retention of secretions in the distal lung.
- The surface of malignant tumours frequently ulcerates and this and/or invasion of blood vessels may lead to haemorrhage. Bronchogenic carcinoma may invade major branches of pulmonary vessels and lead to haemoptysis, which can be dramatic. Carcinoma within the caecum may ulcerate and bleed silently into the bowel lumen, resulting in an iron deficiency anaemia, or may present as melaena. Invasion of nerves may be painful or produce other symptoms or signs. Apically located lung cancers may invade the stellate ganglion around the dome of the pleura and cause ipsilateral Horner's syndrome. Involvement of the recurrent laryngeal branch of the vagus nerve can cause vocal cord paralysis. Ulceration of the visceral pleura may lead to the accumulation of a pleural effusion containing malignant cells and extension to involve the pericardium may precipitate supraventricular arrhythmias.

Tumours may metastasize by three main routes:

- lymphatic system to local lymph nodes, e.g. breast carcinoma;

- bloodstream to distant organs, often the liver, lungs, brain or bones;
- across body cavities, e.g. ovarian carcinoma and the peritoneal cavity.

In general, carcinomas often spread initially to regional lymph nodes and then to distant sites. By contrast, sarcomas may disseminate via the bloodstream to distant organs without regional lymph node involvement. Many tumours show characteristic patterns of spread or a predilection for metastasis to particular organs. These depend both on anatomical patterns of lymphatic or venous drainage and on the ability of micrometastases to colonize and proliferate in a particular micro-environment. The latter ability may depend on variable expression of **cell adhesion molecules** on the surface of the cancer cells.

Some of the characteristic complications of advanced cancer are not readily explained by the effects of local invasion or metastatic spread. Such **para-neoplastic** syndromes are frequently explained by the secretion of biologically active substances by the tumour:

- Small cell carcinomas frequently secrete polypeptides with ACTH activity, causing adrenal hyperfunction and Cushing's syndrome, or ADH, resulting in hyponatraemia.
- Renal carcinomas may secrete erythropoietin, leading to polycythaemia.
- Mucin-secreting adenocarcinomas are particularly prone to increasing the coagulability of the blood, resulting in thromboembolism.

Lung cancers may also be associated with various neurological syndromes such as Eaton–Lambert syndrome, a condition closely related to myasthenia gravis. Finger clubbing may be seen in a variety of conditions and is not specific for cancer, but could also be regarded as a paraneoplastic phenomenon. Acanthosis nigrans – pigmentation and thickening of the skin in the axilla – is sometimes associated with malignancy as is intractable pruritus.

Many patients with advanced or metastatic carcinoma show marked weight loss and muscle wasting (**cachexia**). This is not only due to reduced nutrition or the parasitic demands of the tumour but rather reflects disordered metabolism with increased catabolism due to biologically active substances secreted by the tumour such as tumour necrosis factor.

Tissue diagnosis in cancer

Histological typing of a tumour is fundamental to cancer diagnosis. The current classification system is based on tissue **differentiation** and, by inference, histogenesis. Whilst the classification of well-differentiated tumours is generally achieved by inspection, typing of poorly differentiated or **anaplastic** tumours can be problematic and the pathologist may be forced to rely on ancillary methods of diagnosis such as **immunohistochemistry** or **electron microscopy**. The judicious use of antibodies to intermediate filaments and other markers allows differentiation between the main subtypes of cancer such as sarcoma, carcinoma, and lymphoma.

Even when a specific type of cancer has been diagnosed, histopathology may be able to provide further information affecting the prognosis and/or management by **typing** or **grading** the tumour. Grading and typing systems exist for many different cancer types. These attempt to predict the likely behaviour of the cancer by standardized evaluation of features such as mitotic indices. The Nottingham Prognostic Index in breast cancer is derived from tumour size, histological grade, and axillary lymph node status, and can be used to predict outcome and assist in the selection of patients for adjuvant chemotherapy.

The prognosis of many cancer types is dependent on **staging**; the stage describes the extent to which the tumour has invaded surrounding normal anatomical structures and sites of distant metastasis. Whilst the staging of tumours such as soft tissue sarcomas depends largely on radiological investigation, the staging of tumours such as colorectal adenocarcinoma or transitional carcinoma of the urinary bladder depends largely on histopathological examination of resection specimens.

Tissue diagnosis of cancer is based on histological or cytological evaluation of specimens. For histology, specimens are fixed, processed to paraffin wax and thin slices or sections are stained and examined under the microscope. Histological diagnosis of cancer is the gold standard against which other modalities are compared. Small **endoscopic** biopsy specimens may be obtained during examination of the respiratory or gastrointestinal tract. **Core** or **needle** biopsies may be obtained from superficial lesions such as breast lumps, from the prostate, or under radiological control from more deep-seated lesions.

It is important to appreciate that small biopsies may not always be representative of a lesion. Many malignant tumours will show **heterogeneity** with respect to differentiation between different areas; the heterologous elements such as malignant cartilage which characterizes a carcinosarcoma of the endometrium may not be represented in an endometrial curettage. A small biopsy may give a false-negative diagnosis for invasive cancer. Adenocarcinoma of the oesophagus often coexists with extensive areas of metaplastic and dysplastic mucosa; adequate sampling is essential to ensure that the full range of pathological changes present are represented.

Cancer may also be diagnosed by excision biopsy or resection, where the tumour and surrounding normal tissue are removed. The purpose of histopathological evaluation in such circumstances is to provide prognostically relevant information as well as confirmation of malignancy. Other features that may be commented on include a statement indicating if the surgical excision margins are free of tumour.

Cancer may also be diagnosed by cytological techniques. This is achieved by microscopic examination of stained cells. A variety of approaches are used to obtain samples and stain the cells:

- fine needle aspiration (FNA) cytology. A fine (21 or 22 gauge) needle and syringe is used to aspirate a cell sample from superficial or palpable masses such as a breast lump. The sample may be stained and examined within minutes. This has led to its adoption as an out-patient procedure with immediate reporting in one-stop breast clinics. FNA is also useful in the management of solitary thyroid nodules, salivary gland masses and palpable lymph nodes. Radiologically guided FNA may be used to sample impalpable breast lesions or deep-seated masses in, for example, the lung or liver.

- exfoliative cytology. Cervical smears are obtained by scraping the transformation zone of the uterine cervix with a wooden spatula and smearing the cellular material onto a glass slide. Brushing techniques may be used in association with endoscopy to obtain cytological specimens, e.g. bronchial brushings. The combination of such approaches with conventional biopsy often results in increased sensitivity of cancer diagnosis.

Malignant cells in urine or body cavity effusions may be concentrated by cytocentrifugation and examined microscopically.

Whilst tissue diagnosis of cancer has previously been dominated by purely morphological and anatomical consideration, two trends have emerged in recent years:

- the development of assays/tests yielding information relating to the functional properties of a tumour;
- the development of a multidisciplinary team approach in Cancer units and Cancer Centres.

It is now possible to phenotype and genotype formalin-fixed tumour material very precisely by immunohistochemistry, polymerase chain reaction based nucleic acid analysis and *in situ* hybridization. Techniques such as flow cytometry can detect abnormal DNA content and provide a measurement of proliferation index. Some of these approaches have already found limited roles in diagnostic practice. The immunohistochemical detection of oestrogen receptors in tumour sections is routinely used to assist in the rational selection of adjuvant therapy for patients with breast cancer. Polymerase chain reaction detection of clonal immunoglobulin gene rearrangements or T-cell receptor gene rearrangements may be of help in subclassification of certain types of lymphoma. The detection of specific diagnostic molecular abnormalities in certain sarcomas, lymphomas, and childhood tumours has led to the development of classification systems for these tumours, which are heavily dependent on immunophenotyping and genotyping. The introduction of novel therapies such as monoclonal antibodies to *HER2/neu* or *erbB2* may also lead to a demand for immunohistochemical assays to detect overexpression of this protein product of the *erbB2* gene in breast cancers.

Regular multidisciplinary clinicopathological meetings in Cancer Centres and Units improve communication between histopathologists, clinicians, and radiologists, reduces the risks of misinterpretation of histological or cytological abnormalities, and also assists in tailoring treatment to the individual patient. The triple approach of synthesizing clinical, radiological, and cytological findings used in the assessment of women with breast lumps is a model for good practice in other branches of surgical oncology.

Further reading

Bodmer, W. F. (1994) Cancer genetics. *Br Med Bull* 50, 517–26.

Bodmer, W. F. (1997) The somatic evolution of cancer. *J R Coll Physicians Lond* 31, 82–9.

Jones, D. and Fletcher, C. D. M. (1999) How shall we apply the new biology to diagnostics in surgical pathology. *J Pathol* 187, 147–54.

Karp, J. E. and Broder, S. (1995) Molecular foundations of cancer: new targets for intervention. *Nature Med* 1, 309–20.

Kinzler, K. W. and Vogelstein, B. (1997) Gatekeepers and caretakers. *Nature* **386**, 761–2.

Knudson, A. G. (1993) All in the (cancer) family. *Nature Genet* **5**, 103–4.

Kumar, V., Cotran, R. S., and Robbins, S. L. (1997) *Basic pathology*, 6th edn. WB Saunders, Philadelphia.

Lakhani, S. R., Dilly, S. A., and Finlayson, C. J. (1998) Cell growth and its disorders. *Basic pathology, an introduction to the mechanisms of disease*, 2nd edn, 217–80. Arnold, London.

Ruoslathi, E. (1996) How cancer spreads. *Scientific American September Review Issue: What you need to know about cancer*, 42–7.

Underwood, J. C. E. (1996) Carcinogenesis and neoplasia. *General and systemic pathology*, 2nd edn. Churchill Livingstone, Edinburgh.

Weinberg, R. (1996) How cancer arises. Scientific American September Review Issue: What you need to know about cancer, 32–40.

Internet sites

• http://www-medlib.med.utah.edu.webPath/webpath.html: This site has numerous archived images illustrating gross and microscopic pathological findings and also includes mini-tutorials.

• http://cancer.med.upenn.edu:

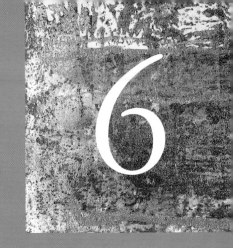

Cancer prevention and screening *Richard D. Kennedy*

- Primary prevention of cancer

- Secondary prevention of cancer

Cancer prevention and screening

Cancer prevention can be divided into two areas:

- primary prevention: this is an attempt to modify factors that promote or protect against carcinogenesis. Examples include dietary modification, smoking cessation, reducing sun exposure, reduction of carcinogens in the workplace, prophylactic surgery, and the use of chemopreventative drugs.
- secondary prevention: this is the early identification and treatment of premalignant or early malignant disease. Examples include population screening, surveillance of high-risk groups, and genetic susceptibility testing.

Primary prevention of cancer

Epidemiological studies have demonstrated that migrants tend to display cancer rates specific to their adopted country rather than their place of origin. An example of this is the increased incidence of breast cancer in Japanese migrants to the USA. These trends suggest that factors other than genetic predisposition must be involved in the development of cancer and opens the possibility to cancer prevention. Table 6.1 lists possible causes of cancer that may be modified.

Diet and cancer

Carcinogens in the diet

Epidemiological studies suggest that up to one-third of cancer deaths are related to dietary carcinogens (see Table 6.2). The relationship between certain food types and carcinogenesis is difficult to prove. Less than 1% of carcinogens so far identified in the diet are attributable to food additives or pesticides. The majority of potential cancer-causing agents are a natural part of foodstuffs. Others are produced by microbial contamination or during cooking, such as the following:

Table 6.1 Cancer mortality due to behavioural/environmental factors

Factor	Percentage of cancer deaths (%)
Smoking	30
Diet (includes obesity)	30
Infectious agents	5
Alcohol	3
Sedentary lifestyle	3
Ultraviolet and ionizing radiation	2
Air pollution	2

Table 6.2 Dietary carcinogens

Carcinogen	Food
Naturally occurring	
Caffeic acid	Apples, pears, cherries, carrots, celery, grapes, lettuce, potatoes, coffee, beans
Allyl isothiocyanate	Cabbage, cauliflower, Brussels sprouts
Furocoumarins	Lime, carrots, celery, parsley, parsnips
Hydrazines	Mushrooms
Mycotoxins	
Aflatoxins	Corn, peanuts
Deoxynivalenol	Wheat, maize
Nivalenol.	Wheat, maize, barley
Produced by cooking	
Heterocyclic aromatic amines	Barbecued chicken, fish, pork, bacon, beef, lamb
Polynuclear aromatic hydrcarbons	Charcoaled beef, chicken, pork, bacon, fish
N-Nitroso compounds pickled vegetables	Cured meats, cured fish, salami, beer, whiskey,

- aflatoxins – metabolites produced by *Aspergillus* moulds found on the surface of crops such as groundnuts, maize, and cottonseed. These toxins are implicated in the development of hepatocellular cancer, especially in the developing world. Improved food storage conditions have been introduced in many countries to try to reduce the risk from these moulds.
- aromatic compounds – heterocyclic and polynuclear aromatic compounds are produced on the surface of fish, chicken, and red meat products when cooked at high temperatures. Methods such as frying, grilling, or barbecuing particularly generate these compounds. Aromatic amines and hydrocarbons have been found to be strongly carcinogenic in animal models, causing cancers of the breast, colon, liver, and skin. Boiling, poaching or microwaving methods do not produce these toxins and may be safer methods of cooking.
- *N*-nitroso compounds – these chemicals are found in salted, smoked or pickled fish or meat. They are consistently carcinogenic in animal models and epidemiological studies have found a positive correlation to human stomach, oesophageal, nasopharyngeal, urinary bladder, and hepatocellular cancer.

Dietary fibre

Dietary fibre is defined as the components of fruit, vegetables, and grain that human digestive enzymes cannot degrade. It can be classified as:

- **non-soluble fibre**, including cellulose and lignin that add bulk to food. This reduces gut transit time and decreases intestinal exposure to potential carcinogens.

- **soluble fibre**, such as pectin or gum, which increases microbial fermentation, leading to a fall in colon pH that may reduce carcinogenesis.

Cancer incidence is lower in populations where a high-fibre diet is consumed. A number of studies on human populations suggest that a high-fibre diet helps prevent colonic cancer and possibly breast cancer. As high-fibre foods often contain important vitamins and minerals, it is difficult to be sure of the exact contribution of the fibre to cancer prevention.

Current evidence suggests that the average person should take 20–30 g of fibre daily to reduce the risk of cancer.

Dietary fat

Animals receiving high-saturated-fat diets have an increased incidence of cancer. Human colorectal cancer is associated with an increased intake of saturated animal fat but red meat may actually be a more important risk factor.

Prostatic cancer has the strongest association with saturated animal fat, although, like colorectal cancer, this may also be confounded by red meat ingestion.

Obesity and a sedentary lifestyle are well-recognized risk factors for several cancers including:

- breast cancer
- colorectal cancer
- renal cancer
- endometrial cancer.

The high calorific value of fat may be its most important reason for being a risk factor in cancer.

Mono- and polyunsaturated fat found in plant oils and fish have been found to be beneficial in preventing atherosclerosis and, importantly, have not been demonstrated to cause cancer.

Exercise and control of body weight, along with a low-saturated, increased mono- and polyunsaturated fat diet should reduce the risk of both cancer and cardiovascular disease.

Fruit and vegetables

These foods are plentiful sources of vitamins, minerals, biologically active compounds, and fibre. They are also relatively low in calorific content, which reduces the risk of obesity (an independent risk factor for cancer). The protective effect of fruit and vegetables against cancer has been consistently demonstrated in human studies. To date it has been difficult to identify which components of these foods are active in preventing cancer and it is likely that they contain many active chemicals. Possible anticarcinogenic agents identified in fruit and vegetables include:

- vitamin A
- vitamin C
- folate
- β-carotene
- retinol

- selenium
- zinc
- calcium.

The cruciferous vegetables (broccoli, cauliflower, and Brussels sprouts) contain isothiocyanates, indoles, and selenium, which seem particularly protective against most cancers. Garlic has been associated with a reduction in gastric cancer in Italy and China.

Current recommendations are to eat at least five portions of varied fruit or vegetables per day.

Alcohol

In the UK, 39% of men and 21% of women aged over 16 drink more than 14 units of alcohol per week. Alcohol is associated with cancers of the:

- oral cavity
- pharynx
- oesophagus
- liver
- breast.

The exact mechanism of carcinogenesis is unclear and the frequent association between smoking and alcohol consumption complicates population studies. Currently alcohol contributes to 1 in 30 cancer deaths, although this figure may be higher. In the case of breast cancer, it appears to have its largest cancer-promoting effect in people who are folate deficient.

The advice for cardiac and liver disease prevention is to limit alcohol consumption to a maximum of 14 units per week for a female and 21 units per week for a male. It is probable that these limits should be lower for cancer prevention.

Obesity

Obesity is almost invariable in developed countries. A body weight 20% over that in a standard height–weight table is considered as obesity. It is an established risk factor for endometrial and postmenopausal breast cancer, explained by the production of oestrogens by adipose tissue. Increasing evidence suggests a link between the development of colorectal cancer and obesity, although the mecha-

---

Information box 6.1 Recommendations for healthy diet

- Exercise regularly and avoid overeating to maintain ideal body weight.
- Eat 20–30 g of fibre daily.
- Reduce saturated fat in the diet.
- Eat red meat at most once weekly.
- Eat five varied portions of fruit and vegetable daily.
- Avoid charring food. Boiling, steaming or microwaving is preferable.

nism is unclear. In line with cardiovascular disease prevention, current recommendations are to maintain an ideal body weight by a combination of reduced calorific intake and increased exercise.

Information box 6.1 summarizes current advice on a healthy diet.

Smoking and cancer prevention

Tobacco was introduced to Europe from the American continent at the end of the fifteenth century. Initially regarded as medicinal, it was not until the 1950s that the dangers of smoking were established. In 1956 an epidemiological study by Doll and Hill found a positive correlation between smoking and lung cancer in British doctors. Now more that 3000 chemicals have been identified in tobacco smoke of which the aromatic hydrocarbons have been found to be the most carcinogenic.

Within the UK, because of public awareness of the health risks along with government taxation and healthcare policies, smoking has declined in the adult population (see Table 6.3). In 1998, 13% of children between the age of 11 and 15 years smoked regularly.

Smoking cigarettes causes each year 120 000 deaths in the UK (1 in 5 of all deaths). The main causes of death due to smoking are cancer and cardiovascular disease.

From the cancer perspective, smoking causes 30% of all cancer deaths. It is the main factor in 80–90% of all lung cancer deaths. Tobacco consumption is also a major factor in several other malignancies (see information box 6.2). Tobacco and

Table 6.3 Percentages of UK adult population who smoked regularly in 1972 and 1998

Population group	1972	1998
Adult male smokers	52%	28%
Adult female smokers	41%	27%

Information box 6.2 Smoking-related cancers

- Lung cancer
- Oropharyngeal cancer
- Stomach cancer
- Cervical cancer
- Pancreatic cancer
- Renal cancer
- Bladder cancer
- Liver cancer
- Leukaemia

Information box 6.3 'Smoking Kills – a white paper on tobacco'

1. Protection of children
- Parliamentary measures to stop billboard advertising.
- New criminal offences for repeated sales of tobacco to children.
- Plans for industry-led proof of age card to protect shopkeepers and children.
- Increased restrictions on siting of vending machines.

2. Promoting clean air
- A new charter to ensure consumers are better able to choose whether to eat, drink, or socialize in smoky atmospheres.
- Increased smoke-free provision in public places.
- Industry-led scheme of symbols available outside restaurants, pubs, and bars to indicate smoking policy inside.
- New code of practice on smoking in the workplace which will need to be adhered to in line with Health and Safety at Work Act 1974.

3. Support for adults wishing to stop
- The first ever national NHS smoking cessation programme will be introduced.
- GPs will be able to refer to special smoking cessation counsellors.
- Counsellors will be able to offer 1 weeks' supply of nicotine replacement therapy.
- Health improvement programmes will contain local strategies to tackle smoking.
- Pregnant women will be a particular focus for NHS help.

4. International action on tobacco
- An extra £35 million will fund action against tobacco smuggling.
- International development aid will not be used for any purpose which supports the tobacco sector in the recipient country.
- Guidelines to diplomats not to be involved in advertising or promotion of tobacco.
- Support of World Health Organization's antitobacco work.
- Take part in European Union proposals to control tobacco labelling, constituents, and additives.

5. Tough new targets
- New targets to reduce smoking in England. Separate targets will be set in Scotland, Wales, and Northern Ireland.
- Reduce smoking in children from 13% to 9% or less by 2010.
- Reduce adult smoking in all social classes so that overall rate falls form 28% to 24%.
- Reduce percentage of women who smoke during pregnancy from 23% to 15%.

Department of Health, UK, 1998

alcohol act synergistically in the case of oral and pharyngeal cancers where there is a 35-fold increased risk in people who smoke two or more packs per day and take 4 or more units of alcohol per day.

Smokers who smoke 1–14 cigarettes per day have eight times the risk of dying from lung cancer compared with a non-smoker. If greater than 25 cigarettes are smoked daily, then the risk is increased to 25-fold. The risk of lung cancer falls by 50% after 10 years and by 90% after 15 years of abstention from smoking.

A recent meta-analysis of 37 epidemiological studies has found a 24% excess risk of lung cancer in lifelong non-smokers who live with smokers. Specific cigarette-related carcinogens have been identified in the urine and blood of passive smokers. This evidence, along with concerns about continued high levels of smoking in adults and children, persuaded the UK government to release a white paper in December 1998 (information box 6.3).

Air pollution

This is now in decline in most developed countries. Epidemiological studies have suggested a higher incidence of lung cancer in urban areas compared to rural areas. Socioeconomic differences between urban and rural dwellers may confound these studies. For example, town-dwellers are statistically more likely to smoke (or passively smoke) and have poorer diets than country-dwellers. Atmospheric pollution, however, does have an effect on lung cancer and current measures to reduce fume emissions (usually for asthmatic control) are also likely to help to reduce the incidence of cancer.

Occupational carcinogens

In 1775, Sir Percival Pott, a London surgeon, identified chimney soot as the cause for squamous cell carcinoma of the scrotum in chimney sweeps. Encouraging the sweeps to wash off soot markedly reduced the incidence of this cancer. This was the first report of occupational carcinogen exposure. Numerous other agents have since been identified as carcinogens in the workplace (see Table 6.4).

Asbestos is an infamous example of a modern occupational chemical that has become recognized as a carcinogen and a serious health risk.

Asbestos and cancer

Asbestos is a mixture of silicates of iron, magnesium, aluminium, cadmium, and nickel. It has been used for its heat-resistant properties as a thermal insulator and fire retardant, particularly in the ship-building industry. There are two major, commercially important forms:

- chrysotile (white asbestos)
- crocidolite (blue asbestos).

Both forms of asbestos are carcinogenic. Crocidolite is two to four times more potent than chrysotile in causing mesothelioma, although both are equally potent in the development of lung cancer.

Mesothelioma typically occurs up to 40 years post-exposure and often can occur in those with relatively light contact with asbestos. Asbestos alone can cause lung cancer but it also has a synergistic effect with smoking (×5 risk).

Table 6.4 **WHO recognized carcinogens in workplace**

Substance or process	Site of cancer
Aluminium production	Lung
Asbestos	Pleura, peritoneum, lung
Benzene	Haematological system
Beryllium	Lung
Cadmium	Lung
Coal tars	Skin
Diesel exhaust fumes	Lung
Formaldehyde	Nose and nasopharynx
Glass manufacturing	Lung
Hairdressing	Bladder
Iron founding	Lung
Mineral oils	Skin
2-Naphthylamine	Bladder
Nickel	Nose
Painting	Lung
Petrol refining	Skin, haematological system
Radon	Lung
Rubber industry	Bladder, haematological system
Silica	Lung
Soots	Skin
Vinyl chloride	Liver
Wood dust	Nasal cavity

Skin cancer and ultraviolet light

Skin cancer is the most common malignancy seen in Western civilizations and, when advanced, accounts for 2% of cancer deaths. This type of cancer is increasing in incidence, which may partly reflect a fashion for suntans. A 1% decrease in the ozone layer over the past 20 years has resulted in an increase in ultraviolet B levels at the Earth's surface by 2%, which may also be contributing to the rise in incidence of skin tumours. The lifetime risk for developing melanoma in the 1930s was 1 in 1500, whereas current figures suggest a risk of 1 in 75. The majority of skin cancer deaths are due to malignant melanoma.

Most evidence for the role of ultraviolet sunlight in skin cancer comes from epidemiological studies, although laboratory work has confirmed its ability to cause direct DNA damage. It appears that squamous cell and basal cell carcinomas are associated with cumulative exposure to ultraviolet sunlight, whereas malignant melanoma is associated with episodes of acute ultraviolet damage. The shorter wavelengths (ultraviolet B and C) are the most damaging to DNA but ultraviolet A (often used in sunbeds) has also been shown to cause damage. Currently, health

Information box 6.4 The British Cancer Research Campaign recommendations regarding sun exposure

- Avoid the midday sun.
- Seek natural shade when in sunlight, e.g. trees.
- Wear cover-up clothing, including T-shirts and hats.
- Use a broad-spectrum sunscreen of sun protection factor 15 or higher. (Sun protection factor is a guide to how much longer it is possible to stay in the sun before becoming burned.)
- Re-apply sunscreen frequently.
- Especially protect children from sun exposure.

education programmes reinforce that deliberate ultraviolet exposure for tanning purposes is to be strongly discouraged (see information box 4).

It is important not to forget the role of secondary prevention in skin cancer. Individuals should be encouraged to monitor their moles and report any:

- itching
- bleeding
- change in pigment
- increased size
- altered shape
- appearance of new moles.

Early excision of malignant melanoma is usually curative.

Prevention of viral-related cancer

Table 6.5 lists some of the viruses associated with certain cancers. Each year at least 850 000 international cases of cancer are attributable to infection. Vaccination programmes against hepatitis B would have a major impact on hepatocellular cancer in the developing world. Education on safe sexual practice would be expected to reduce the risk of human papilloma and immunodeficiency virus-associated malignancies.

Table 6.5 Viruses associated with cancer

Virus	Cancer
Hepatitis B,C	Hepatocellular cancer
HIV	Kaposi's sarcoma, lymphoma
Epstein–Barr virus	Nasopharyngeal cancer, Burkitt's lymphoma
Human papilloma virus	Cervical cancer

Chemoprevention of cancer

Identification of chemopreventative agents arises from epidemiological studies, laboratory experiments, or from drugs used to treat established tumours. An ideal chemopreventative agent would be:

- highly effective
- non-toxic
- inexpensive
- easy to administer
- easy to comply
- widely available.

Antioxidants and lung cancer

The carotenoids are a group of plant pigments found widely in nature. Their role is to 'mop up' free radicals formed as a byproduct of photosynthesis in plants. It has been suggested that β-carotene (a carotenoid found in human tissues) may act as an antioxidant, preventing damage to DNA by reactive molecules. Epidemiological studies have suggested that a high intake of food containing β-carotene is protective against several types of cancer, especially lung tumours. Disappointingly, trials of β-carotene as a lone food supplement have not been found to reduce the risk of lung cancer and may actually promote the growth of established tumours.

Retinoids and head and neck cancer

Retinoids are natural and synthetic analogues of vitamin A. They act on specific cell receptors that are involved in cellular differentiation. 13-*cis*-Retinoic acid (isotretinoin) has been demonstrated to reverse oral leukoplakia (a premalignant phase of oral cancer), but this effect only lasts for as long as the drug is taken. Isotretinoin has been demonstrated to reduce the risk of second tumours following treatment for primary cancers of the oral cavity and lung. This drug has also been used to prevent skin tumours in xeroderma pigmentosum and basal cell naevus syndrome.

Isotretinoin can only be recommended in patients at particularly high risk of cancer as it is associated with significant side-effects such as drying of mucous membranes, abnormal liver function, and raised serum lipids.

Colorectal cancer and the non-steroidal anti-inflammatory drugs (NSAIDs)

Numerous human epidemiological studies have confirmed that 15 years of non-steroidal anti-inflammatory drugs (NSAIDs) can reduce the risk of bowel cancer in the general population by as much as 50%. Bowel tumour cells over-express cyclo-oxygenase 2 (an enzyme involved in prostaglandin production) in the adenomatous phase of tumour development. This enzyme seems to be important in tumour growth and resistance to apoptosis. NSAIDs are known to inhibit cyclo-oxygenase enzymes 1 and 2 and therefore may have an antiproliferative action on the premalignant phase of bowel cancer. In support of this theory, the NSAID sulindac has been found to cause regression of polyps in patients suffering from familial adenomatous polyposis coli.

Breast cancer and tamoxifen

Tamoxifen is a well-established treatment for oestrogen-sensitive breast cancer. It also has a known benefit in reducing osteoporosis and improving serum lipid levels, making it a particularly favourable drug for chemoprevention. The Breast Cancer Prevention Trial studied the effects of tamoxifen on reduction of breast cancer in American females with no previous cancer history. Tamoxifen was seen to reduce the risk of breast cancer by almost 50%. The initial enthusiasm generated by this trial was tempered when early results from two European trials failed to find the same benefit. As with the other chemopreventative drugs discussed above, the side-effects of tamoxifen must be considered. A rise in endometrial cancer, venous thromboembolism, and possibly stroke were seen in the treatment groups of the trials, along with troublesome sweats and facial flushing. Tamoxifen's role in chemoprevention may eventually apply only to high-risk females such as those with *BRCA1* or *BRCA2* mutations rather than the population at large.

Prophylactic surgery

Certain congenital or genetic abnormalities are associated with a high risk of cancer development. Sometimes prophylactic surgical excision of a possible cancer site can be offered. Examples include:

- orchiopexy to prevent testicular cancer following cryptorchism;
- colectomy to avoid tumours in patients with hereditary colorectal cancer or ulcerative colitis;
- thyroidectomy to prevent medullary cancer of thyroid in patients with multiple endocrine neoplasia type II;
- mastectomy in patients with familial breast cancer;
- oophorectomy in patients with familial ovarian cancer.

Information box 6.5 Basic requirements of a screening test

- The test must be highly sensitive.
- The test must be highly specific.
- There must be a high predictive value.
- Screening should be applicable to large number of individuals.
- The test should be easily and quickly accomplished.
- The test must not be harmful.
- The test must be acceptable to the patient to promote compliance.
- The test should be cheap.
- The natural history of the disease must be known.
- There must be a proven beneficial outcome from early detection of the disease in question.

Secondary prevention of cancer

This is the detection of premalignant or early malignant lesions at a time when treatment is potentially curative. For a screening test to become acceptable it must meet certain criteria (see information box 5).

Screening test validity

The validity of a screening test can be defined as its ability to correctly identify individuals who have a disease and those who do not. It consists of three components (see information box 6).

Sensitivity

This is the test's ability to correctly identify those individuals with disease. If the test is not sufficiently sensitive, then many individuals who have cancer will be wrongly reassured by a false-negative result.

Specificity

This is the test's ability to correctly identify those individuals who do not have disease. The screening test must be sufficiently specific to prevent undue anxiety in a large number of individuals who are given a false-positive result but do not have cancer.

Positive predictive value

This is a measure of the reliability of a positive test result indicating true disease. Screening tests with a high positive predictive value lead to less unnecessary follow-up investigations.

Screening for breast cancer

Mammography is the only breast cancer screening method that has been demonstrated to reduce mortality. It is highly specific (90%) and sensitive (90%) in the detection of breast cancer in postmenopausal women. The combined estimate from all randomized trials using mammographic screening demonstrates an overall reduction in mortality by 25% in women aged over 50. In women aged under

---

Information box 6.6 Screening

Diagnosis

Test result	Disease	No disease
Positive	a	b
Negative	c	d

Sensitivity (%) = a/(a+c) × 100

Specificity (%) = d/(b+d) × 100

Positive predictive value (%) = a/(a+b) × 100

50, no benefit has been demonstrated. This is mostly due to the difficulty of interpreting mammograms of the relatively dense premenopausal breast.

Currently, routine screening with 3-yearly mammography is offered to all women in the UK between the ages of 50 and 65. A positive result is followed by a fine needle aspiration or core biopsy of the suspect lesion. The breast-screening programme in the UK is believed to prevent 1250 deaths per year.

Although the results from the breast-screening programme are impressive there are still some problems:

- 80% of women find the procedure uncomfortable, which may reduce compliance.
- False-positive results occur in 1% of tests, causing unnecessary anxiety.
- Breast tumours can still occur in the time interval between visits (16 per 10 000 women screened).

The risk of causing malignancy due to mammography appears to be negligible.

Breast self-examination

At present there is no compelling evidence that formal self-examination is effective in reducing morbidity or mortality from breast cancer. The majority of breast lumps identified are benign, causing undue anxiety. Instead of teaching ritualistic examination technique, it is probably more useful to inform women of the changes in their breasts that should be brought to a doctor's attention.

Cervical screening

Cancer of the uterine cervix is the second most common cancer in middle-aged women (after breast cancer) and the detection and treatment of its precancerous state can modify its outcome. Cervical screening has been shown to be successful in reducing cancer deaths retrospectively in several countries. It has never undergone a prospective, randomized clinical trial.

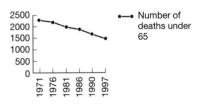

Fig. 6.1 Trends in cervical cancer incidence in the UK.

Around 1500 women died in the year 2000 from invasive cervical cancer. This has decreased from over 2000 per year in 1971 (Fig. 6.1).

In 1964, a cervical screening programme, using pap smears, was launched in the UK. Screening is carried out 5-yearly for females from the ages of 20 to 64. At present, 85% of women in the target group comply with screening. Unfortunately, women in lower socioeconomic groups, who are at the highest risk of developing cancer, often do not comply. The UK government's aim is to reduce the incidence of cervical cancer by at least 20%. In order to increase uptake of cervical screening, general practitioners are financially rewarded for reaching certain screening goals.

Abnormal smear tests are reported as a grade of cellular abnormality (dyskaryosis). Follow-up depends on the severity of the abnormality:

- borderline or mild dyskaryosis: repeat smear 6 months later and if still abnormal colposcopy is performed. A minimum of two consecutive negative smears 6 months apart are needed after a borderline or mildly dyskaryotic result before standard screening can be resumed.
- moderate and severe dyskaryosis : refer for colposcopy immediately.

Colposcopy allows direct identification and biopsy of carcinoma in situ (CIN):

- if grade 1 CIN is present, this can be kept under surveillance, as a proportion of these will revert to normal.
- if grade II or grade III CIN is identified, then immediate local treatment is required.

The human papillomavirus (HPV) is a cofactor in cervical cancer development. A strong association with HPV types 16 and 18 has been noted. HPV viral identification in smears is currently being evaluated as an adjunct to the standard pap screening test to see if this will improve its sensitivity and specificity.

A possible primary preventative measure for the future may be HPV vaccination. This, however, will not prevent all cervical cancers, as some do not appear to be associated with viral infection.

Screening for colorectal cancer

There is good evidence from clinical trials that faecal occult blood testing every 2 years will allow the early detection of colorectal cancer. This has the potential to reduce mortality by 20%, which is comparable to the UK breast cancer screening programme. With a compliance rate of 60%, screening of 50–69-year-olds would be expected to prevent 1200 deaths per year in the UK.

Faecal occult blood testing has a positive predictive value of 50%. This means for every 10 people who test positive, five will have significant findings on further investigation. A positive faecal occult blood test should be followed by endoscopy. At present two methods are being considered:

- **flexible sigmoidoscopy** followed by a **double contrast barium enema** with an 80% sensitivity for detection of tumours;
- **full colonoscopy**, also with a sensitivity of 80%, although some experts have reported tumour detection rates of 90–100%.

In the future, virtual colonoscopy may be the method of choice to follow-up faecal positive occult bloods. In this method, a CT scan of the abdomen is carried out and a computer reconstructs the bowel wall. The procedure takes less than 1 minute but interpretation may take longer.

Before faecal occult blood analysis can be carried out the patient must be taking a special diet. This, along with a false-positive result of 10%, may reduce patient compliance.

In summary, colorectal screening has proven benefit in cancer prevention but the financial and manpower issues, along with concerns about patient compliance, have to be resolved prior to its introduction.

Prostatic cancer screening

In the UK, 10 000 men each year die from prostatic cancer and this figure is rising annually. This death rate is considerably more than that for cervical cancer for which there is a well-established screening programme. Efforts to develop a screening test for middle-aged men have been attempted but results have been disappointing. Screening modalities used to date include the following:

- **digital rectal examination** – this was traditionally used prior to 1990. Unfortunately, despite annual tests, only 20% of those men having an abnormal rectal examination had localized disease. Of men with metastatic disease, 25% had a normal prostatic examination. This method was therefore of low sensitivity and specificity.
- **transrectal ultrasound** – when this was evaluated as a screening test it proved to be insensitive and non-specific. It is, however, used in the work-up of proven prostatic cancer.
- **prostatic specific antigen** – an elevated prostatic specific antigen (PSA) of over 4 ng/ml predicts subsequent prostatic cancer with a sensitivity of 71% and a specificity of 91%. This makes PSA a potential screening modality.

One of the criteria for a screening test is that there must be a proven beneficial outcome from early detection of the disease. A meta-analysis of six studies, which involved the long-term follow-up of patients with low-grade disease, demonstrated prolonged survival with no therapy. Also the frequency of prostatic cancers found at autopsy steadily increases for each decade over 50 years and most of these tumours are clinically silent. By detecting early prostatic cancers we may cause unnecessary anxiety along with the significant morbidity and mortality associated with surgery of unknown benefit. It is apparent that some prostatic cancers have a favourable outcome and others are rapidly fatal. Current research is focusing on identifying factors that may predict patients requiring treatment and those who can be safely watched.

Until such times as we have a better understanding of this disease's natural history and its optimum treatment in the early stages, prostatic cancer screening should only be undertaken within the context of a clinical trial.

Surveillance

Surveillance is secondary cancer prevention offered to individuals known to be at high risk of malignancy. It must be distinguished from screening that is applied to a population at large. An example of surveillance is regular colonoscopy in patients suffering ulcerative colitis or familial colorectal cancer. Patients with a strong family history of breast cancer are recommended to have regular surveillance mammography. This starts 5 years before the age of onset of cancer in the youngest affected family member.

Genetic susceptibility testing

In families with hereditary cancer syndromes, an increasing number of associated genetic abnormalities are being recognized. Testing for these genetic mutations allows the physician to identify individuals in a family at high risk of developing cancer.

'Susceptibility testing' differs from screening in that:
- it is only applied to a small, high-risk group rather than the population at large;
- it is only performed once;
- it is usually expensive.

When a positive result is obtained, the physician may then offer primary cancer prevention (such as chemoprevention or surgery), or may recommend secondary

Table 6.6 **Genetic susceptibility tests in use**

Hereditary cancer syndrome	Gene mutations identifiable
Breast and ovarian cancer	BRCA1, BRCA2
Hereditary nonpolyposis coli	MSH2, MLH2, PMS2, PMS1, MSH6
Familial adenomatous polyposis coli	APC
Multiple endocrine neoplasia type 1	MEN1
Multiple endocrine neoplasia type 2	RET
Von Hippel–Lindau disease	VHL
Retinoblastoma	RB1
Li–Fraumeni syndrome.	P53
Melanoma	P16, CDK4

prevention in the form of regular surveillance (such as colonoscopy in hereditary colorectal tumours or mammography in *BRCA* mutations). Genetic susceptibility tests currently used are listed in Table 6.6.

BRCA1 and *BRCA2* testing is being used increasingly within the UK.

BRCA1 and BRCA2 testing

Genetic testing for *BRCA1* and *BRCA2* gene abnormalities has become available in the last 5 years. A women with a *BRCA1* or *BRCA2* mutation faces about a 60–85% lifetime risk of breast cancer and a 20–60% risk of ovarian cancer. Genetic testing in families with a strong family history of breast or ovarian cancer may allow prevention of some of these malignancies.

The current difficulty is that there are no recognized primary interventions in *BRCA1* or *BRCA2* mutation. Possible measures include:

- **prophylactic surgery** – bilateral mastectomies and oophorectomies have been suggested to reduce the risk of breast and ovarian cancer but have not been proven in large randomized trials. Unfortunately, prophylactic surgery cannot guarantee elimination of cancer risk and may be associated with considerable psychological morbidity.

- **chemoprevention** – tamoxifen for prevention of breast cancer or low-dose oestrogen for reducing risk of ovarian cancer are possible measures under investigation but, again, these are as yet unproven.

At present, *BRCA1* and *BRCA2* testing in high-risk individuals may be of value in guiding secondary rather than primary prevention in the form of regular mammography, transvaginal ultrasound and CA-125 levels.

Legal issues regarding the disclosure of *BRCA1* or *BRCA2* status to financial or insurance companies may become important. As there are possible long-term implications to the individual plus her relatives, counselling and informed consent are essential prior to genetic testing.

Further reading

Annas, G. J. (1997) Tobacco litigation as cancer prevention: dealing with the devil. *N Engl J Med* **336**(4), 304–8.

A look at how legislation may be used to stop tobacco promotion.

Atkin, W. (1999) Implementing screening for colorectal cancer. *BMJ* **319**, 1212–13.

A review of the evidence for colorectal screening along with the problems of implementation.

DeVita, V. T. Jr, Hellman, S., and Rosenberg, S. A. (eds) (1997) Dietary carcinogens. In *Cancer: principles and practice of oncology*, 5th edn, Chapter 22.4. Lippincott-Raven, Philadelphia.

A review of the carcinogens recognized in the diet.

Hill, D. (1999) Efficacy of sunscreens in protection against skin cancer. *Lancet* **354**, 699–700.

Discusses the evidence for the effectiveness of sunscreens.

Landrigan, P. J. (1998) Asbestos – still a carcinogen. *N Engl J Med* **338**(22), 1618–19.

A useful overview of some of the issues still relevant to asbestos exposure.

Lane, D. (1998) The promise of molecular oncology. *Lancet* **351** (Suppl. 2), SII17–20.

Discusses the future application of molecular oncology to cancer prevention.

Olopade, O. I. (1996) Genetics in clinical cancer care – the future is now. *N Engl J Med* **335**(19), 1455–6.

A review of the advantages and disadvantages of genetic susceptibility tests.

Osborne, M., Boyle, P., and Lipkin, M. (1997) Cancer prevention. *Lancet* **349** (Suppl. 2), SII27–30.

A brief review of primary cancer prevention, especially focused on chemoprevention.

Potter, J. D. (1999) Fiber and colorectal cancer – Where to now? *N Engl J Med* **340**(3), 223–4.

Does fibre protect against cancer? This editorial reviews the evidence.

Sox, H. C. (1998) Benefit and harm associated with screening for breast cancer. *N Engl J Med* **338**(16), 1145–6.

A review of the benefits and risks associated in breast screening, especially when applied to women under 50 years.

Websites

Action on smoking and health (ASH) website: http://www.ash.org.uk
Cancernet from the national cancer institute PDQ statements on cancer prevention and screening: http://www.oncolink.upenn.edu/pdq

Department of Health screening information: http://www.doh.gov.uk/publich.htm

Cancer Research Campaign 'Reducing the risk': http://www.crc.org.uk

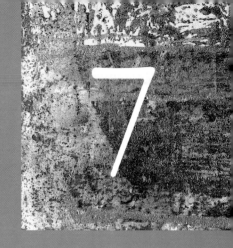

7

The radiology of cancer William Toreggiani and Michael J. Lee

- Imaging modalities

- Ultrasound

- Computerized tomography (CT)

- Magnetic resonance imaging (MRI)

- Nuclear medicine (radioisotope imaging)

- Positron emission tomography (PET)

- Interventional radiology including angiography

- Conclusion

Modern radiological imaging plays a major role in the diagnosis, staging, and follow-up of cancer. The choice of which imaging modality to use depends on several factors, namely, the information being sought, the most appropriate imaging modality to detect the cancer being sought, and the local availability of various imaging modalities.

Whilst the radiological detection of cancer is generally based on the suspicion that a cancer is present, it is not uncommon for cancer detection to be incidental. For example, in an elderly patient referred for assessment of abdominal pain, the incidental detection of a liver or renal tumour is not uncommon. However, the widespread use of imaging as a screening tool for cancer detection has not happened. At present, mammography is the only diagnostic imaging modality currently used in both the UK and the USA as a screening tool for the detection of breast cancer.

Table 7.1 Advantages and disadvantages of imaging modalities

Advantages	Disadvantages
Ultrasound	
No ionizing radiation	Difficult in fat people
Cheap	Overlying bowel may make visualization difficult
Almost universally available	Operator dependent
Good patient acceptance	Hardware variability
Little preparation in most cases	Limited use in the thorax
CT	
Anatomical detail well shown	Exposes patients to ionizing radiation
Overlying bowel not generally a problem	Time consuming
Almost completely operator independent	Some patients experience claustrophobia
Obese patients easy to scan	Relatively expensive
Bone and calcifications well seen	Metal hardware in-patients causes artefact
MRI	
No ionizing radiation	Expensive
Excellent multiplanar capabilities	Not universally available
Brain and spinal cord well demonstrated.	Claustrophobia common
Good tissue characterization	Prone to movement artefacts
Nuclear medicine	
No preparation generally required.	Poor spatial resolution
Functional information may be obtained	Exposes patient to ionizing radiation
PET allows quantitative data analysis	PET imaging is very expensive
Few contraindications	Not universally available

Imaging modalities

Table 7.1 summarizes the advantages and disadvantages of the main imaging modalities.

Plain radiographs play an important but somewhat limited preliminary role in the radiological assessment of cancer. The only exception to this is the plain chest radiograph (Fig. 7.1) and bone radiographs for lung cancer and primary bone cancer, respectively. A chest radiograph may reveal a typical lung cancer (Fig. 7.1) in a patient with haemoptysis who is a known smoker. Associated fea-

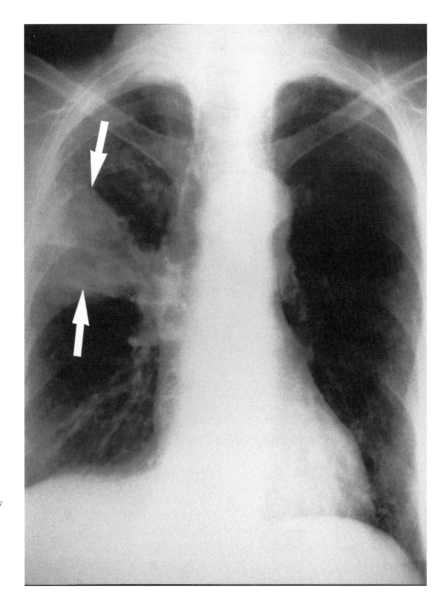

Fig. 7.1 Frontal chest radiograph of an elderly patient who presented with haemoptysis. The patient was a known heavy smoker. The radiograph shows a large mass (arrows) extending from the right hilum to the periphery of the lung. The mass was biopsied percutaneously by a radiologist and was shown to represent a primary lung cancer.

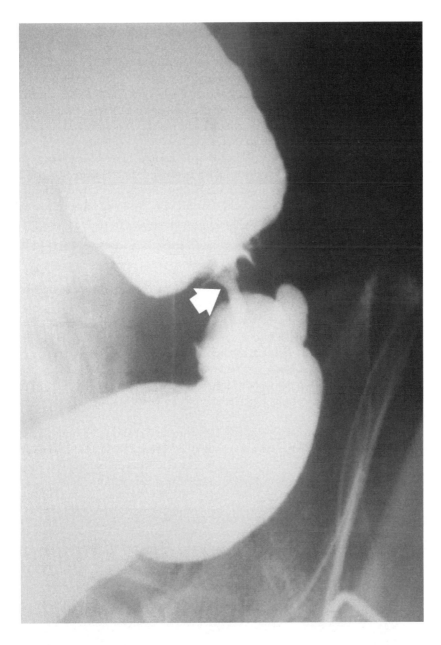

Fig. 7.2 A spot view from a barium enema in another patient with a history of rectal bleeding shows the typical appearance of a cancer involving the descending colon. There is marked concentric narrowing of the bowel lumen with associated shouldering of the edges, giving the typical apple-core appearance of a bowel cancer (arrow).

tures such as pleural effusions, lung collapse, and bony metastases may be identified and in these cases the diagnosis of lung cancer may be made with some certainty. However, in many cases the diagnosis is not so clear-cut and further imaging with other modalities such as computerized tomography (CT) is required. This may give more definitive proof and also allow for staging of the neoplastic process.

In many cases, plain radiographs show secondary signs of cancer rather than the primary cancer itself. For example, a colonic carcinoma may present with plain abdominal radiographic findings of large bowel obstruction. The actual diagnosis of colonic cancer may then be made with a barium enema (Fig. 7.2) or colonoscopy.

Barium studies of the oesophagus, stomach, small bowel, and colon are a useful adjunct to endoscopy in the investigation of gastrointestinal tract tumours. Both endoscopy and barium studies have their inherent advantages and disadvantages. Unlike endoscopy, barium studies expose the patient to ionizing radiation. In addition to this, biopsies are not feasible with barium studies. Endoscopy, on the other hand, allows for direct biopsy of any visualized abnormality. Cancers of the stomach causing linitis plastica (leather bottle stomach) are easily detected on a barium meal but can be missed during gastroscopy. The small bowel is also an area that is not amenable to endoscopy and barium studies play an important part in the evaluation of disease processes in the small bowel.

Ultrasound

Ultrasound is the imaging modality of choice in the investigation of abdominal and pelvic malignancies.

In the abdomen most of the solid organs are generally well visualized. The kidneys, spleen, liver and gallbladder are well seen (Fig. 7.3). Visualization of the pancreas can be difficult as overlying bowel gas can obscure detail. The retroperitoneum is variably assessed with imaging of this area being both operator and patient dependent, being particularly difficult in obese patients.

Table 7.2 lists some of the more common organ related cancers visualized on ultrasound.

Assessment of the female pelvis with ultrasound has traditionally been via the transabdominal route. This gives a good overall delineation of the bladder, uterus, and ovaries. However, there is now an increasing acceptance of transvaginal scanning which allows a clearer visualization of the uterus and ovaries.

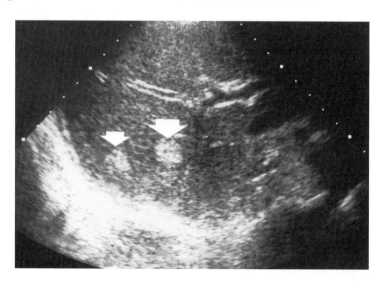

Fig. 7.3 Ultrasound of the liver in a patient who had a previous colonic resection for colon cancer and who now presents 2 years later with weight loss and abdominal pain. The ultrasound shows two bright echogenic lesions in the liver, suggestive of metastases (white arrows). These were biopsied percutaneously by a radiologist and confirmed to represent colonic metastases.

Table 7.2 Organ related cancers commonly visualized on ultrasound

Liver	
Primary tumours	Hepatoma, fibrolamellar carcinoma and cholangiocarcinoma (biliary tree origin)
Secondary tumours	Metastases (most common liver malignancy)
Kidney	
Adults	Renal cell carcinoma, lymphoma and metastases
	Transitional cell tumours (often difficult to visualize)
Children	Nephroblastoma (Wilms' tumour)
Pancreas	Ductal adenocarcinoma, cystadenocarcinoma (cystic tumour) and islet cell tumour
Lymph nodes	
Primary disease	Hodgkin's lymphoma, non-Hodgkin's lymphoma
Secondary disease	Metastases
Small organs	
Testes	Seminoma, teratoma and lymphoma
Thyroid	Thyroid carcinoma and metastases
Adrenal gland	
Adults	Adrenal carcinoma, metastases (commonest malignancy of adrenals)
Children	Neuroblastoma

In the male pelvis, the bladder again is well assessed using the trans-abdominal route. The prostate, however, is more suitably evaluated by transrectal ultrasound in which anatomy is better demonstrated and smaller lesions are more clearly delineated.

Computerized tomography (CT)

CT now plays an increasingly important role in the detection, staging, and follow-up of cancer. In the thorax, lung cancer is particularly well evaluated by CT. As well as the size and characteristics of the primary lesion, CT can detect mediastinal invasion, the presence of lymphadenopathy, and pleural involvement with a high degree of accuracy. Suitability for resection can also be assessed.

CT is the most sensitive imaging modality for detecting lung metastases. By altering the computer software settings of the CT image, the lungs may be optimally imaged and even small parenchymal abnormalities (< 5 mm) can be seen. The number, size, and distribution of metastases can be evaluated and where therapy is instigated the response to therapy can be assessed by performing follow-up CT scans of the thorax.

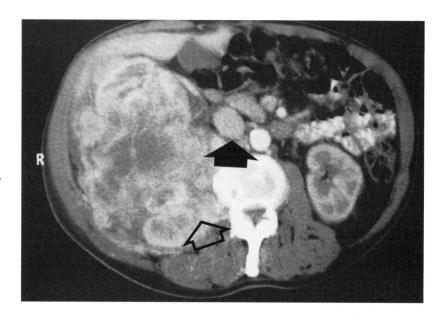

Fig. 7.4 Axial CT scan of a middle-aged man who presented with haematuria. The scans were performed through the level of the kidneys following the injection of intravenous contrast material. There is a large mass involving the right kidney. There is marked enhancement of the mass, indicating hypervascularity. The right psoas muscle is directly invaded by the tumour (open arrow). The inferior vena cava is displaced anteriorly by the mass (closed arrow). The mass was confirmed histologically to represent a renal cell cancer. The presence of local muscle invasion carries a poor prognosis.

In the abdomen, CT plays a major role in the detection, staging, and follow-up of many intra-abdominal malignancies. In general, oral contrast should be given to patients prior to scanning as this helps label loops of bowel that otherwise could be mistaken for lymphadenopathy or other pathology. Intravenous contrast material is also commonly given, as many cancers are much easier to detect after intravenous contrast. Indeed, a sizeable percentage of tumours will be missed without intravenous contrast.

CT has largely replaced staging laparotomy in the assessment of patients with lymphoma. In a well prepared patient, enlarged lymph nodes are well demonstrated with nodes greater than 1 cm in size generally being considered abnormal as in other parts of the human body.

In the liver, both primary and secondary liver tumours are generally well visualized on CT. Helical CT has an approximate 75–85% detection rate for hepatic metastases. Intravenous contrast is essential to visualize these lesions to maximum effect.

CT is excellent for evaluating tumours of the kidneys, pancreas, and retroperitoneum. Again, intravenous contrast usually helps not only in visualizing the tumour mass but also in identifying spread into adjacent vascular structures. For example, it is not uncommon for renal cell carcinoma to spread into the adjacent renal vein and inferior vena cava and without the use of intravenous contrast such spread may be difficult to detect (Fig. 7.4).

CT is the preferred imaging modality in the initial evaluation of brain tumours and metastases. Intravenous contrast aids detection and may help in distinguishing benign from malignant lesions of the brain by the type of enhancement they demonstrate. Tumours often demonstrate ring enhancement (rim of high density at the periphery of lesions). However, some other pathologies such as brain abscesses may also show ring enhancement, making distinction difficult. In such cases, correlation with clinical symptoms and findings may help. Alternatively, magnetic resonance imaging (MRI), which is more accurate for imaging the cranial cavity, may also help to resolve the problem.

Magnetic resonance imaging (MRI)

The major two advantages of MRI over other imaging modalities are its lack of ionizing radiation and the ability to view anatomy and pathology in multiple planes. Most examinations with MRI involve an evaluation of both T1- and T2-weighted images. (T1 and T2 refer to the type of sequences used in MRI imaging.) T1-weighted images best demonstrate anatomy. T2-weighted images best demonstrate pathological conditions because most inflammatory and neoplastic processes appear bright in signal as a result of their increased water content.

As described above, MRI is superior to CT in assessing space-occupying lesions of the brain. When a focal space-occupying lesion is detected within the brain, the multiplanar capability of MRI often helps to determine its position as intra-axial (within the brain parenchyma) or extra-axial (outside of the brain, distorting the brain's contour). This information is key in formulating a differential diagnosis.

MRI plays a primary role in the diagnosis of spinal cord tumours. Previous techniques such as myelography are now seldom used where MRI is available to identify cord tumours. Both primary and metastatic disease may be identified.

Whilst the major role of MRI in cancer detection involves the brain and spinal cord, its role is now expanding to include the evaluation of the thorax and, in particular, the mediastinum. The multiplanar capability of MRI makes the detection of mediastinal invasion by tumour or encasement of the pulmonary artery by tumour straightforward to detect, particularly if the relationship of the tumour to the mediastinum is not clear on CT.

Whilst CT is generally considered superior to MRI in the evaluation of abdominal cancer, certain anatomical structures such as the liver are well assessed by MRI. Hepatomas and metastases may be identified and their size, number, and distribution noted. MRI may in addition demonstrate portal vein involvement, which is typical of a hepatoma. Perhaps the primary role of MR in liver imaging lies in the differentiation of benign cavernous haemangiomas from metastases. Cavernous haemangiomas occur in approximately 17% of people and can be confused with liver metastases. MRI is highly accurate in differentiating haemangiomas from metastases (> 95%).

In patients with renal disease, CT is generally considered superior because of its high sensitivity in detecting calcification and perinephric disease. Calcification is not well seen on MRI and many renal tumours, as well as stone disease and inflammatory conditions of the kidney such as tuberculosis, demonstrate calcification. However, in patients in whom CT findings are equivocal, MRI is an excellent adjunct with its multiplanar imaging capabilities being useful in determining the organ of origin of large masses projecting into the renal fossa.

MRI of the pelvis

The high sensitivity of MRI in the pelvis makes it the most accurate imaging modality for evaluating pelvic cancer. Because respiratory motion is minimal in the pelvis, high quality, artefact-free images can be obtained. In the female, uterine and, in particular, cervical cancer can be assessed. Whilst the diagnosis of cervical cancer is primarily made clinically with histological confirmation, MRI is the method of choice for tumour staging.

Nuclear medicine (radioisotope imaging)

Radioisotope imaging differs from other radiological techniques in providing regional biochemical or physiological, rather than anatomical, data. It is often necessary to correlate these data with anatomical information. Radioisotope imaging involves the labelling of a compound with a radioactive tracer. In most cases the radioactive tracer is technetium-99m (^{99m}Tc), as this is easily available and can be tagged on to many compounds. The compound to be tagged depends on the organ to be imaged. For bone imaging, there are a number of phosphate or phosphonate derivatives available in kit form ready for labelling with ^{99m}Tc. Following *in vitro* labelling, the radiolabelled compound is injected intravenously.

Other uses of radioisotope scanning include assessment of the thyroid gland. In cases where a nodule has been detected clinically, thyroid scanning is often performed to see if the nodule is hot or cold, single or multiple. In general, a single cold nodule in the thyroid gland is more likely to be malignant. However, sensitivity and specificity are poor, and correlation with other imaging modalities such as ultrasound is essential. For example, a simple cyst will show up as a cold nodule, but should be easily confirmed as being a cyst on ultrasound.

Positron emission tomography (PET)

PET is proving useful in certain aspects of tumour localization and follow-up. PET scanning uses positron-emitting isotopes of oxygen, nitrogen, carbon, fluorine, and rubidium. Positrons are particles identical to electrons except that they are positively charged. Positrons travel a short distance, giving up kinetic energy by coulomb interactions, and finally colliding with a free electron, resulting in total annihilation. It is the photons from the total annihilation of the positron and electron that are detected by PET scanning. A ring of detectors is placed around the area to be imaged and this picks up the energy released from the annihilation process. Since each annihilation originates from a specific point in space, an image is generated which contains spatial information.

One of the commonest agents used in PET scanning is 5-FDG (a fluorinated deoxyglucose). Because glucose is such an important cellular molecule and avidly taken up by actively dividing cells such as cancer cells, 5-FDG tends to collect in cancer cells so that tumours are portrayed as bright spots. PET provides information about the metabolic activity of tumours and may therefore help to distinguish some benign from malignant lesions. It can also be helpful in deciding whether a residual mass after cancer therapy is a sterile mass or residual cancer.

Interventional radiology including angiography

The role of angiography in the diagnosis of cancer has reduced substantially since the advent of modern imaging modalities such as ultrasound, CT, and MRI. However, angiography still plays a role in difficult cases. The demonstration of

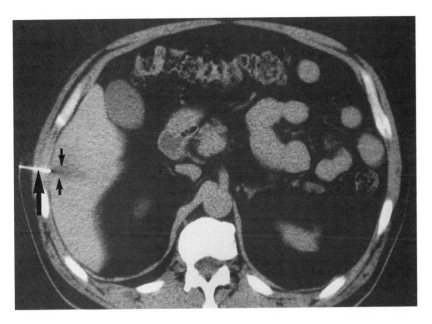

Fig. 7.5 Patient with colorectal cancer who had a liver lesion detected on follow-up CT scanning. The lesion (small arrows) was biopsied under CT guidance with a 20 gauge needle (large arrow). The lesion proved to be a metastasis.

neovascularization (small abnormal tortuous blood vessels) in a suspect mass is suggestive of malignancy. As well as helping to diagnose cancer, angiography sometimes plays a role in mapping out the vascular supply to a tumour prior to surgery. In addition, targeted chemotherapy and embolization play a limited but important role in cancer treatment for certain liver cancers.

The modern interventional radiologist plays a major part in the diagnosis of cancer. Many tumours or suspected tumours seen on plain film, ultrasound, or CT are amenable to biopsy. Peripheral lung lesions, hepatic lesions, and many abdominal masses may all be selectively localized and biopsied (Fig. 7.5). Both primary and secondary tumours can be biopsied. In some cases biopsy may help to decide if residual tissue post-chemotherapy represents sterile tissue or residual cancer. There are two broad categories of biopsy. The first is called a fine needle aspirate biopsy (FNAB) in which a thin needle (20 or 22 gauge needle) is introduced into the lesion and manual syringe aspiration removes cells. The second type of biopsy is termed a core biopsy requiring a needle of larger calibre (16–20 gauge) with which a tissue sample is obtained. Biopsies may be performed under ultrasound, CT, or fluoroscopy.

Some tumours such as hepatocellular carcinoma may be treated and often cured by trans-arterial chemo-embolization (TACE). In the Far East this technique is almost solely used in the treatment of small hepatocellular carcinomas. The technique involves selective catheterization of the hepatic arterial branch supplying the tumour and injecting a combination of lipiodol, which is taken up by hepatocytes and therefore acts as a carrier, and daunorubicin, the active chemotherapeutic agent. Another method of treatment of these tumours is the direct injection of alcohol into the lesion under CT or ultrasound guidance. This causes direct tissue death and tumour ablation.

Conclusion

The radiological assessment of cancer involves a diverse range of imaging modalities and investigations. The key in maximizing the yield from these various imaging modalities lies in having good clinical information and having the results of appropriate biochemical tests available. Availability and expense both need to be considered. The modern imaging department has a key role to play in the diagnosis, staging, follow-up, and, in some instances, treatment, of many different cancers.

Further reading

Blamey, R. W. (1998) The role of the radiologist in breast diagnosis: a surgeon's personal view. *Clin Radiol* 53, 393–5.

Cardoza, J. D. and Herfkens, R. J. (1994) *MRI survival guide*, Chapter 3, pp. 77–101. Raven Press, New York.

Chapman, S. and Nakielny, R. (1995) *Aids to radiological differential diagnosis*, 3rd edn, Chapter 13, pp. 456–79. W. B. Saunders, Philadelphia & London.

Gedgaudas-McClees, R. K. and Torres, W. E. (1990) *Essentials of body computed tomography*. W. B. Saunders, Philadelphia & London.

Grainger, R. G. and Allison, D. J. (1986) *Diagnostic radiology, an Anglo-American textbook of imaging*, 2nd edn, Chapter 50, pp. 947–65. Churchill Livingstone, Edinburgh.

Peters, M. E. and Voegeli, D. R. (1989) *Breast imaging, handbooks of diagnostic imaging*. Churchill Livingstone, Edinburgh.

Sutton, D. (1992) *A textbook of radiology and imaging*, 5th edn, Chapter 14, pp. 391–412. Churchill Livingstone, Edinburgh.

Watkinson, A. and Adam, A. (1996) *Interventional radiology, a practical guide*, Chapter 5, pp. 36–58. Radcliffe Medical Press, Oxford.

Whitehouse, G. H. and Worthington, B. S. (1990) *Techniques in diagnostic imaging*, 2nd edn, Chapter 26, pp. 427–37. Blackwell Scientific Publications, Oxford.

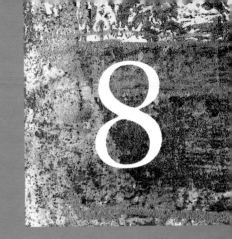

8

The psychology of cancer
Robin Davidson

- Introduction

- Psychological risk factors

- The psychological impact of cancer

- Psychotherapy for cancer patients

- Overview

The psychology of cancer

Introduction

This chapter summarizes the scientific literature from the following areas:

- psychological carcinogenic risk factors;
- adjustment and coping strategies after diagnosis;
- psychological morbidity associated with cancer;
- the impact of psychotherapy on quality of life and disease course.

Psychological risk factors

Behaviour and cognitions

Behavioural, lifestyle factors contribute to almost half of cancer mortality, whilst smoking behaviour alone accounts for almost 30% of all cancer deaths. Models, which include the Health Belief Model and the Theory of Planned Behaviour, enable us to understand how people reduce carcinogenic behaviours like smoking, alcohol use, or exposure to ultraviolet light, and how they permanently acquire positive behaviours like breast and testicular self-examination, physical exercise, or healthy eating habits. Most of these health behaviour models focus on a person's beliefs about the impact of current behaviour on their future health. There are a number of key beliefs that predict health behaviour change and, more important-ly, its maintenance over the lifespan. These are illustrated in Table 8.1.

Strong outcome and normative beliefs predict the **initiation** of new positive health behaviour, whereas strong self-efficacy beliefs are better predictors of **long-term maintenance**. By way of example, these theoretical principles are translated into a number of practical steps in Table 8.2, which should be incorporated into any typical quit-smoking programme.

Table 8.1 Key predictors of health behaviour change

- Self-efficacy beliefs: this is perceived behavioural control, the expectation that one has the intrinsic ability to implement and persist with a new behaviour

  Can I succeed?

- Outcome beliefs: the expectations that change will increase positive reinforcing effects or decrease negative reinforcing effects

  Is change worthwhile?

- Normative beliefs: the importance which significant others attach to particular behavioural change

  Do other people really want me to change?

Table 8.2 Essential components of all quit-smoking programmes

- Bolster outcome expectations by personalizing the costs of continuing and benefits of stopping
- Increase efficacy by debriefing after relapse
- About a month before the stop day, initiate coping skills training and begin to cut down by using behavioural strategies like nicotine fading or scheduled reduced smoking
- Stopping with other people can help motivation and increase normative expectations
- After stopping, promote efficacy by nicotine replacement (transdermal patch or gum) and continue to practise coping strategies for high-risk situations

Personality

As well as behavioural factors, there is now some support for the view that personality variables may be aetiologically significant in the development of some cancers although research findings are inconsistent. There are a number of components of the so-called cancer-prone or type C personality, including:

- a need to nurture;
- lack of awareness of one's own emotional needs;
- feelings of powerlessness/helplessness;
- conventional, passive, and appeasing in relationships with other people.

It has been suggested in a small number of studies that this personality type may have greater predictive validity for cancers that are aetiologically linked to hormonal or immunological factors. However, it is, as yet, too early to draw any definitive conclusions on the general aetiological and prognostic significance of a cancer-prone personality.

It is more likely that people who develop cancer do not have a discrete personality type, but rather possess certain personality traits. Most of the good prospective studies in this area have been carried out on samples of women who later develop breast cancer. Breast cancer patients are more likely, premorbidly, to demonstrate emotional suppression. In other words, they will hide their feelings and tend to suppress negative emotions more than women who do not develop breast cancer. It does seem that when other important predictor variables like age and family history are statistically controlled, the aetiological relationship between emotional suppression and breast cancer remains.

It used to be thought that stressful life events are associated with the development of cancer. However, important recent evidence suggests it is almost certainly not adverse life events *per se*, but rather the perceived personal control attributed to these events which is important (Petticrew *et al.*, 1999). People with internal locus of control feel that they are responsible for their own destiny, whilst those high on external locus of control believe events in their life mostly occur by chance, accident, or fate. The interaction between locus of control and life events is currently the subject of a number of research trials. If there is a psychological vulnerability towards the development of cancer, this may facilitate more appropriate targeting of primary intervention strategies.

The psychological impact of cancer

The psychological sequelae of cancer wax and wane throughout the disease trajectory from symptom appearance, diagnosis, early stage, recurrence, long-term adaption, or death. The psychological impact is also predicted from perceived disease severity.

The way in which information is given to the patient at the point of diagnosis is important and there is considerable literature on the relationship between breaking bad news and future psychological distress. At this time, **all** clinicians should relate to patients using three basic counselling principles:

- **unconditional positive regard**: genuinely caring and accepting the patient as a person;
- **empathy**: an ability and willingness to view the world through the patient's eyes;
- **congruence**: a consistency between the way the doctor feels and the way he or she behaves.

Table 8.3 illustrates the key findings on how bad news should best be broken.

After the individual deals with the initial trauma of diagnosis, psychological morbidity may become manifest, particularly in the presentation of depression or anxiety. Among newly diagnosed cancer patients, the prevalence of serious depressive illness is 5–6% and therefore not significantly higher than the general population. However, the prevalence of clinically significant adjustment disorder with depressed mood (DSM IV) is much higher, with estimates ranging from 16 to 25% (Sellick and Crooks, 1999). The predisposing factors associated with

Table 8.3 Breaking bad news: key steps

a	See patient in a private setting
b	Introduce yourself if you are not already known
c	Find out what the patient knows and wants to know
d	Start from the patient's starting point (aligning)
e	Give information in small chunks
f	Use warning shot, e.g. 'I am afraid things are not as straightforward as we thought'
g	Use plain English
h	Frequently monitor and acknowledge the patient's reaction: clarify accordingly
i	If diagnosis is asked for, start vaguely: move to more accurate predictions if the patient is able
j	Warn that the interview is soon to close, e.g. 'I am afraid I am going to go in a minute, is there anything else you would like to know?'
k	Offer to speak to relatives

Adapted from Buckman, R. (1992)

Table 8.4 Factors associated with increased psychological morbidity among cancer patients

- History of mood disorder
- History of alcohol/drug abuse
- Cancer treatment associated with visible deformity
- Younger age
- An aversive experience of cancer in the family
- Poor social support
- Low expectation of effective treatment outcome
- The presence of distressing side-effects
- Associated and concurrent stressful life events

depressed mood, which is underdiagnosed in oncology, are not surprising and are summarized in Table 8.4. Key symptoms, like loss of appetite, lack of energy, low libido, loss of weight, poor self-esteem, anhedonia, insomnia, or suicidal ideation, may at times be attributed to malignant disease or treatment when they are in fact due to a depressive condition. Only one-third of cancer patients who may potentially benefit from antidepressants actually received them.

The features of anxiety are easier to recognize and generalized anxiety disorder would normally be expected in up to 10% of the cancer population. According to DSM IV, as well as demonstrating excessive worry, people with this disorder should also manifest at least three of the following behavioural or somatic symptoms:

- restlessness
- fatigue
- difficulty concentrating
- irritability
- palpitations
- muscle tension
- sleep disturbance.

Some account should be taken of the relationship between the disease process, treatment, and psychopathology. Biological complications of the illness, for example, cerebral metastases or hypercalcaemia, will clearly influence a patient's mental state. Certain cytotoxic agents and steroids can in themselves cause depression, and the psychological impact of side-effects such as nausea, alopecia, or fatigue must be monitored. Disturbance of body image and psychosexual functioning is well documented after mutilating surgery. For example, psychosocial morbidity after breast surgery is three times more likely than matched samples in the general population. However, a consistent, if somewhat counter-intuitive finding, is that there is little difference in the prevalence of long-term psychological problems between women who have undergone mastectomy and those who have had a breast-conserving local excision. This highlights the general view among patients

Table 8.5 Psychosocial interventions

Information and education

A didactic approach which provides information on the disease, medical treatment, coping issues and self-care measures

Support counselling

Support and encouragement in a caring environment in which the emotional consequences of the disease and its treatment can be expressed

Therapeutic counselling

Patient-centred process of exploration, clarification and problem-solving using procedures such as active listening, reflection, and empathic responding

Psychoanalytical psychotherapy

This class of interventions is based on specific psychological theories of human functioning, e.g. Freudian theory, and focuses primarily on interpretation of largely unconscious conflicts and tensions

Cognitive behavioural psychotherapy

An approach in which emphasis is placed on the influence of conscious thought and behaviour on feeling and emotion. It can include techniques like visualization, anxiety management, problem-solving, behaviour modification, and cognitive appraisal and reframing

that it is the cancer itself which is the primary source of most psychological distress.

Psychotherapy for cancer patients

Psychotherapy and psychosocial outcome

Psychosocial interventions employed with cancer patients are outlined in Table 8.5.

A number of well conducted meta-analyses and treatment reviews on the impact of psychotherapy on the adult cancer patient have come to the following broad conclusions:

- Psychological interventions have a very positive effect on psychological morbidity, functional adjustment, disease-related symptoms and overall quality of life.
- Psychological interventions may convey survival advantage for particular illnesses, notably melanoma and breast carcinoma. However, the effect size in the Meyer and Mark (1995) meta-analysis of 45 treatment trials falls just short of statistical significance.
- While all psychological interventions have a beneficial effect on most outcome measures, cognitive behavioural psychotherapy is emerging as the most therapeutic and cost-effective approach.

Because of the burgeoning interest in the use of psychotherapy, the NHS commissioned a wide-ranging review of psychotherapeutic interventions (NHS

Executive, 1996). The review concluded that there is currently an absence of sound evidence to support the effectiveness of client-centred counselling and psycho-analytic therapy for most psychological disorders (see Table 8.5). On the other hand, cognitive behavioural psychotherapy for a range of psychological problems, including depression and anxiety, was regarded as sound, evidence-based practice. In line with this trend, Moorey *et al.* (1994) developed a cognitive behavioural intervention specifically tailored to the needs of cancer patients. This so-called **adjuvant psychological therapy** is a brief, problem-focused approach which aims to improve adjustment and enhance mood. Components include:

- **the promotion of emotional expression**: this is the acknowledgement of negative emotions to help adjustment.
- **activity scheduling**: activities and daily structures are planned to promote mastery over one's personal environment, thereby promoting self-efficacy.
- **relaxation and visualization**: this helps patients deal with anxiety. Guided imagery of the host defences destroying cancer cells can be used in conjunction with hypnosis or relaxation.
- **cognitive restructuring**: monitoring thoughts and training in distraction, reality testing or re-attribution of their meaning.

Current evidence clearly indicates that psychological intervention, particularly cognitive behavioural strategies, can improve quality of life and reduce psycho-logical morbidity in cancer patients. This effect is independent of the severity of illness and primary tumour site.

Psychotherapy and survival

Psychological therapies are said to enhance survival by promoting a better adjust-ment to the illness. A number of common adjustment styles have emerged in factor analytic studies and these are summarized in Table 8.6. Factor analysis allows researchers to identify clusters of psychological test items which tap a common attribute.

Some studies have shown that patients who adopt **fighting-spirit** and **denial** coping styles live longer. The adjustment and attitude towards cancer may have immunological correlates that mediate apparent survival affects. In this area of psychoneuroimmunology there are a growing number of reports which demon-strate a relationship between mental state and immunological parameters such as natural killer cell activity.

Table 8.6 Adjustment styles to a diagnosis of cancer

Fighting spirit: 'I am not going to let this disease beat me'
Denial: 'I don't really think that this is cancer'
Stoic acceptance/fatalism: 'I'm just going to have to learn to live with this'
Helplessness/hopelessness: 'This is the end. There is nothing I can do'
Anxious preoccupation: 'I can't get the thought of this tumour out of my mind'

There are some frequently cited, methodologically sound, randomized, controlled trials that seem to demonstrate survival advantage resulting from psychological intervention. Fawzy *et al.* (1993) combined psychological, immunological, and disease end point data and showed significantly greater immune upregulation and better survival rates among malignant melanoma patients who participated in a 6-week group psychotherapy programme. The most widely cited trial is that of Spiegel (1992), who demonstrated a striking survival difference between a control group and an experimental group of women with metastatic breast cancer. The experimental group intervention consisted of weekly group psychotherapy for a period of 1 year. The group therapy was cognitive behavioural in orientation in that emotional expression was encouraged and strategies like problem-solving, life-priority recording, cognitive restructuring, anxiety management and self-hypnosis were employed. A number of other studies have also demonstrated a relationship between survival rate and psychological intervention following diagnoses of colorectal and lung cancers.

These results, however, should at the moment be treated with caution for a number of reasons:

- Some well-conducted trials have supported the null hypothesis.
- Biological processes may be mediated indirectly by behavioural variables. There may, for example, be better treatment compliance, healthier dietary habits, less smoking and alcohol use, and more appropriate use of exercise arising indirectly from psychotherapy. In other words, psychological treatments may empower individuals to engage more actively in health behaviour.
- These longitudinal studies present very real methodological problems. The power of the study should be sufficient to allow a range of illness variables, like site and stage of tumour, as well as psychological and demographic variables to be statistically or experimentally controlled.

Treatment provision

There are two important considerations in the provision of psychological therapy for cancer sufferers; **when** is the optimum time to intervene, and **how** should the intervention be structured. It is emerging in the post-traumatic stress literature that formal psychological therapy has greater long-term benefit if it is given some months after the traumatic event, rather than immediately. This finding is mirrored in cancer studies. Initial diagnosis can be regarded as a discrete trauma, and in the first few months people may be too overwhelmed to benefit from psychotherapy. At this stage they need good and empathic social support to individually process the meaning of their illness. Edgar *et al.* (1992) elegantly demonstrated that a general group of cancer sufferers whose psychotherapy began several months after initial diagnosis showed significantly less psychological morbidity, reported a greater sense of self-control, and experienced less intrusive thoughts than an early intervention group at 1 year follow-up.

In most published trials, cancer patients have received psychotherapy in a group rather than a one-to-one setting. Whilst both modalities are important, there is now some evidence to suggest that individual therapy, particularly for women with gynaecological and breast cancers, can be more effective than group therapy in the longer term. These important issues on the optimum timing and modality of psychological interventions for cancer patients require further research.

Overview

There is a growing body of literature which illustrates the central importance of the mind–body interaction in the aetiology, prognosis, and management of cancer. Contemporary, comprehensive approaches to the care of the cancer patient and their family emphasize the needs of the whole person. Because of this, clinical psychologists play the central role in the multidisciplinary cancer team. Oncologists will prescribe the medical treatment whilst psychologists can help promote better adjustment and psychological health, thereby influencing adherence to these medical treatments. Medical and psychological intervention can work together to improve quality of life and possibly disease course. The psychologist has also a role to play in the provision of a staff support programme for the cancer team. Burn-out among clinical staff will clearly have a significant and adverse effect on patient care. In this field it is important that the mental health of professionals as well as of patients is considered.

Case history Alison

Alison is a nurse in her mid-forties. A local excision of a breast lump was followed by an axillary node clearance and adjuvant CMF chemotherapy. The initial shock and trauma of diagnosis was replaced by a very positive attitude towards her illness. 'I was like *a* patient rather than *the* patient.' However, towards the end of her chemotherapy she began to worry how she could cope without the security and protection offered by treatment and frequent hospital contact. She reported a sense of helplessness and that her illness had become a personal reality. Alison described a deterioration in mood, she ruminated constantly about her future, and more particularly that of her teenage children. Every ache and pain was construed as recurrence. She also reported very distressing emotions about the death of her mother some 11 years ago, which she had hitherto repressed. She became tearful, withdrawn from the family, and experienced terminal insomnia, and some diurnal variation in mood. After being prescribed antidepressants, she requested a referral from her oncologist for psychotherapy.

Alison attended conscientiously and was initially given space to discuss her apprehensions regarding the future. She was unable to talk to family and friends as 'I did not want to burden them with my troubles'. These sessions were followed by some work in helping her monitor and challenge negative thoughts, and activity scheduling to replace the helplessness with a sense of mastery and control. Relaxation and visualization also promoted self-efficacy: 'I feel more in control of my recovery.' Therapy concluded with bereavement counselling to help her begin to deal with unresolved issues, triggered by her own illness regarding the death of her mother.

Alison's mood slowly improved and after 3 months she reported a greater sense of control and what she called 'a different set of priorities'. It was probably a combination of the psychotrophic medication, psychotherapy, and time that led to the improvement in Alison's mental state.

Further reading

American Psychiatric Association (1994) *Diagnostic and statistical manual of mental disorders*, 4th edn. APA, Washington, DC.

Anderson, P. (1998). Cancer. In Bellack, A. and Hersen, M. (eds), *Comprehensive clinical psychology*, Vol. 8. Pergamon, New York.

Barraclough, J. (1994) *Cancer and emotion*. Wiley, Chichester.

Buckman, R. (1992) *How to break bad news: a guide for healthcare professionals*. London, Pan Books.

Cwikel, J., Behar, L., and Zabora, J. (1997) Psychosocial factors that affect the survival of adult cancer patients: a review of research. *J. Psychosoc Oncol* 15(3), 1–34.

Edgar, L., Rosberger, Z. and Nowlis, D. (1992) Coping with cancer during the first year after diagnosis. *Cancer* 69(3), 817–28.

Fawzy, F., Fawzy, N., Hyun, L., *et al.* (1993) Malignant melanoma: effects of an early structured psychiatric intervention, coping and affective state on recurrence and survival six years later. *Arch Gen Psychiatry* 50, 681–9.

Guex, P. (1994) *An introduction to psycho-oncology*. Routledge, London.

Hughes, J., (1991) Anxiety and depression: psychotrophic medication. In Watson, M. (ed.), *Cancer patient care*. BPS Books, Cambridge, 111–25.

Meyer, T. and Mark, M. (1995) Effects of psychosocial interventions with adult cancer patients: a meta-analysis of randomized experiments. *Health Psychol* 14, 101–8.

Moorey, S., Greer, S., Watson, M., *et al.* (1994) Adjuvant psychological therapy for patients with cancer: outcome at one year. *Psychooncology* 3, 39–46.

NHS Executive (1996) *Psychotherapy services in England, review of strategic policy*. Department of Health, London.

Petticrew, M., Fraser, J. M., and Regan, M. F. (1999) Adverse life-events and risk of breast cancer: a meta-analysis. *Br J Health Psychol* 4(**Part 1**), February, 1–18.

Seligman, L. (1996) Promoting a fighting spirit. *Psychotherapy for cancer patients, survivors and their families*. Jossey-Bass, San Francisco.

Sellick, S. M. and Crooks, D. L. (1999) Depression and cancer: an appraisal of the literature for prevalence, detection and practice guideline development for psychological interventions. *Psychooncology* 8(4), 315–33.

Spiegel, D. (1992) Affects of psychosocial support on patients with metastatic breast cancer. *J Psychosoc Oncol* 10(2), 113–20.

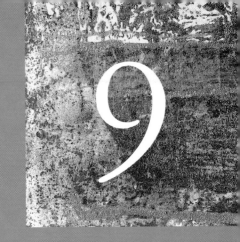

9

The principles of cancer surgery Roy A. J. Spence

- The surgeon as part of the oncology team

- Ethics of surgical oncology

- Surgical oncology

- Complications of treatment

- Surgical emergencies in oncology

The principles of cancer surgery

The surgeon as part of the oncology team

With the current emphasis on a multidisciplinary approach to cancer management, the surgeon is one member of a closely knit team who can all be involved at various stages of the treatment of the patient's disease. All should be involved in the discussion of the patient's management in the initial stages. The team may include an oncologist, cancer surgeon, radiologist, pathologist, nurse counsellor, geneticist, plastic surgeon, nursing staff, dietetics, pain team, social worker, and psychologist.

Ethics of surgical oncology

It is good medical practice to avoid unnecessary surgery. A huge resection operation in a terminal patient is clearly inappropriate. Discussion with the family is important, but the patient's wishes are paramount, provided he or she is competent and can give fully informed consent, including full knowledge of the consequences of not having surgery.

Avoidance of unnecessary surgery

One of the major changes over the past two decades is the avoidance of unnecessary surgery in cancer patients. Twenty years ago the procedure of laparotomy was not uncommon and a number of patients were opened and closed for no significant benefit. Whilst some patients still occasionally require the procedure of laparoto-

Oncology
multidisciplinary
team
- Oncologist
- Surgeon
- Oncology nurse
- Radiologist
- Pathologist
- Nurse counsellor
- Geneticist
- Plastic surgeon
- Pain team
- Social worker
- Dietitian
- Psychologist
- Palliative care team
- Chaplaincy

Key points
- Ethics
- Patient's wishes
- Autonomy
- Competence
- Resources
- Trials

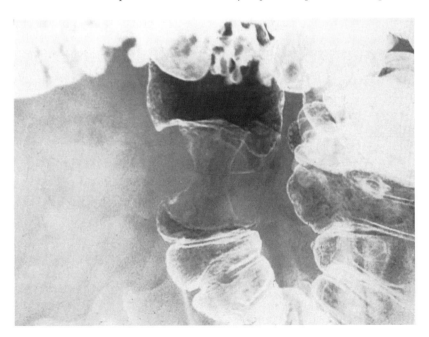

Fig. 9.1 Radiograph of a cancer of the colon on barium enema.

my for diagnostic or trial resection purposes, this is increasingly uncommon. Modern preoperative investigations including fine needle biopsy, ultrasound, CT, and MRI scanning have helped to avoid this potentially unnecessary procedure. Over the past decade, the procedure of laparoscopy has been increasingly used, particularly in gastrointestinal cancer.

An additional helpful investigation is intraoperative ultrasound. This is particularly useful for liver and pancreas cancer where ultrasound picks up other tumours that have not been seen on preoperative CT, ultrasound, or MRI scanning, and which are not palpable at operation. Inappropriate liver resection and pancreatectomy are hence avoided.

Diagnosis

Much preoperative diagnosis is performed by the radiologists with MRI, ultrasound, CT scanning, and scan-guided fine needle biopsy. The surgeon may still be required to obtain pre-resection tissue with procedures such as endoscopic, laparoscopic, and occasionally open surgical biopsy.

Surgical staging

Staging may not be complete until surgery is performed. For example, some liver secondaries may be small and not picked up with preoperative imaging. Similarly, some secondaries may not be picked up even at laparoscopy (peripancreatic nodes are difficult to see and biopsy at laparoscopy). However, the most important aspect of the surgeon's role in terms of staging is the final pathology specimen that is produced. The definitive guide to the extent of spread of the tumour is the resected specimen. Of considerable importance is invasion of the adjacent lymph nodes, blood vessels, and lymphatics, which hold the key to future treatment and prognosis.

Key points

- Staging
- Clinical
- Imaging – preoperative
- Fine needle aspiration – preoperative
- Intraoperative imaging
- Intraoperative pathology
- Resection specimen

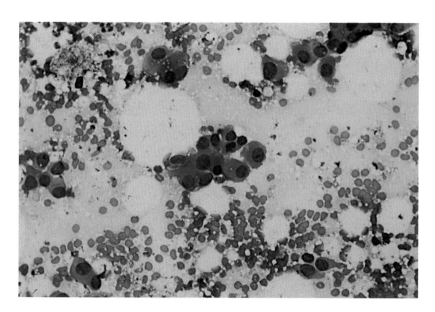

Fig. 9.2 Fine needle aspirate of cancer of the breast.

Surgical oncology
Anatomy and pathology

The anatomy of the organ which contains the tumour is extremely important; for example, a knowledge of the spread of rectal tumours to the mesorectum is important. It has been shown that excision of the mesorectum is important in the widespread clearance of rectal cancers to decrease the incidence of local recurrence in the pelvis. Similarly, resection of the colon tumour, along with its potentially involved lymph nodes, is important. A clearance procedure is now the preferred method of dealing with axillary lymph nodes in patients with breast cancer. However, biopsy of the sentinel node may make axillary clearance a more selective procedure. A knowledge of the blood spread of tumours is equally important, e.g. cancer of the colon tends to spread to the liver and therefore a very full assessment of the liver is important both pre- and intraoperatively.

Combined treatment modalities

Most cancers can be treated by a number of different modalities. These include surgery, chemotherapy, radiotherapy, hormonal manipulation, immunotherapy, and other modalities such as embolization of tumours.

Many tumours are suitable for a combination of treatments. The rationale is that some solid tumours have micrometastases at the time of diagnosis. The purpose of adjuvant chemotherapy is to destroy those cells that have already spread at the time of diagnosis and surgery.

Either before or after the primary surgery it is appropriate for many tumours to offer the patient either pre- or postoperative management with other treatment modalities. Examples include preoperative radiotherapy for patients with a large

> ### *Key points*
> - Combined treatment modalities
> - Preoperative chemotherapy – breast osteogenic sarcoma
> - Postoperative chemotherapy – breast, colon
> - Preoperative radiotherapy – rectum
> - Postoperative radiotherapy – lung, breast, rectum

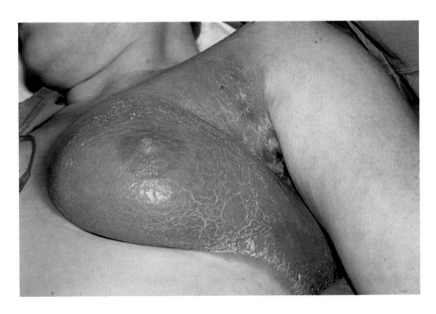

Fig. 9.3 Clinical photograph of a patient with breast cancer.

fixed rectal cancer or those with a large apparently unresectable breast cancer that is fungating. This can sometimes shrink the tumour to allow surgery to take place. Preoperative chemotherapy is appropriate in some young patients with large breast cancers. It is also helpful, occasionally, in stomach cancer.

Postoperative adjuvant treatment with either radiotherapy or chemotherapy is given to many patients with tumours including lung, breast, and colon. Finally, the timing of primary surgery may be important in those patients who have tumours that are, at least partially, hormone dependent. This applies to the timing of surgery with respect to the menstrual cycle in patients with breast cancer.

Conservative and radical surgery

Surgical procedures in cancer can be subdivided into conservative or radical. Conservative surgery aims to preserve as much function and cosmesis as possible. Conservative surgery, for example, includes partial mastectomy for breast cancer where most of the breast is preserved while still doing an adequate cancer operation with a 1 cm clearance margin. These patients usually require postoperative radiotherapy to decrease the chance of local recurrence. Conservative cancer surgery is now available to young patients with bone tumours around the knee. Such a patient with an osteosarcoma around the knee may be offered replacement of the femur by a prosthesis (endoprosthesis) instead of an amputation. Clearly the functional results are much better.

Similarly, in patients with lung and liver cancer, it may be possible to perform less radical surgery, provided the margins are clear. The caveat is that the patient may require a further operation to perform a wider resection if the margins are not sufficiently clear of tumour. Surgery can then range up to the massive cluster transplants offered by one or two centres in the USA.

Radical surgery includes hemihepatectomy for hepatoma and simple mastectomy for large breast cancers. Occasionally, liver transplantation is performed for primary liver cancer or secondary endocrine tumours in the liver, but the benefits of such a transplant are debatable.

Reconstruction

In an effort to return patients to a reasonable quality of life after their cancer surgery, reconstruction after the initial cancer procedure is offered where possible. The breast can be reconstructed using various techniques, e.g. implants, tissue expanders, TRAM and latissimus dorsi flaps. After major head and neck resections, plastic surgeons use free vascularized flaps to replace skin, muscle, and bone; examples include free radical forearm and free fibular flaps. Although there has been one forearm and hand transplant in the world, it is unlikely that transplants for sarcoma amputees will be available for the foreseeable future.

Palliative surgery

There is a role for palliative surgery in patients who are not amenable to curative surgery. For example, jaundice caused by cancer of the head of the pancreas or bile duct can be relieved, either by the insertion of a stent or by an operative bypass. Patients who have gastric outlet obstruction may be helped by an operative bypass using either open surgery or laparoscopic techniques. In those patients who have no gastric outlet obstruction, endoscopic retrograde cholangiopancreatography (ERCP) and stent insertion is more appropriate. Similarly, in some patients who have colon cancer at an advanced stage (and who may have liver secondaries), it may still be reasonable to proceed to surgery (if they are sufficiently fit and fully informed) to remove the primary tumour to prevent intestinal obstruction. Although rare nowadays, surgery may still be appropriate in an occasional patient to relieve severe pain from cancer (see later).

Some patients who have intestinal obstruction due to tumour may be helped with a bypass procedure, but if the patient has widespread secondary disease throughout the peritoneal cavity such procedures are rarely of benefit.

It should be borne in mind that even in advanced cancer a proportion of patients will have a non-malignant cause for their obstruction. Therefore, each patient needs to be assessed individually and some symptoms of intestinal obstruction can be controlled with medication.

Bleeding from an oesophageal, bronchial, or bladder tumour can be controlled with either laser or diathermy. Even if local resection is incomplete, fulguration may still be valuable for a locally advanced tumour that is odorous and necrotic. For example, a toilet mastectomy is still appropriate even for advanced disease, provided the patient's general condition permits.

A surgeon may be involved in the management of malignant ascites where the ascites is re-accumulating at a rapid rate despite frequent aspiration and when other treatments such as chemotherapy have failed. Although a peritoneal–venous shunt from the peritoneal cavity to the internal jugular vein (Denver shunt) carries a small risk of disseminated intravascular coagulopathy, it does give excellent palliation from the unpleasant symptom of gross ascites.

Generally, the modern management of pain is excellent in oncology units, with a combination of various drugs, radiotherapy to control bone metastases, and occasionally nerve blocks. These are generally given by the pain team who have trained in anaesthesia. In a small subgroup, neurosurgery is helpful for the management of pain which is not amenable to control by other means. Neurosurgical techniques include anterior-lateral cordotomy, medial thalmotomy, and hypophysectomy. These techniques are rarely required nowadays but are useful in a small group of patents with unilateral pain. Side-effects limit their usefulness.

Minimally invasive surgery

Over the past decade minimally invasive surgery has become very popular for procedures such as laparoscopic cholecystectomy and hiatus hernia repair. There is controversy regarding its use in surgical oncology. Whereas it may give less morbidity and there is a shorter stay in hospital, it may not give a sufficiently wide clearance of the tumour and survival may, therefore, be compromised. The data are currently not available to be dogmatic but there has been concern over the past few years that laparoscopic port recurrences are a significant problem.

Key points

- Palliative surgery
- Obstructive jaundice
- ERCP and stent
- Open bypass
- Laparoscopic bypass
- Colon obstruction
- Malignant ascites
- Pain management

Key points

- Minimally invasive surgery
- Port recurrences
- May not be good cancer technique

Preventative surgical oncology

The surgeon may be required occasionally to perform prophylactic surgery in a patient who has not yet developed cancer but who has a high risk of so doing. This arises, for example, in patients with polyposis coli. Patients who have this syndrome will definitely develop cancer of the colon from age 40 years (or sooner). There is a definite role for prophylactic colectomy to be performed around the age of 20 years. A pouch procedure may be used in these patients. Similarly, patients who have a bad family history of breast cancer and who may have the appropriate *BRCA1* and *BRCA2* gene profile, may request a prophylactic mastectomy. This has to be done bilaterally and will diminish greatly (but not totally prevent) the risk of getting breast cancer.

Surgery for metastases

Up to a decade ago patients who developed metastases in lung or liver were offered no further surgery. It is now clear that patients who have secondaries in the liver or lung from certain tumours (if the secondaries are sufficiently small and few in number) may benefit from surgery. Whether or not the patient will benefit will depend on the origin and extent of the primary tumour. Patients who have primary cancer of breast only occasionally benefit from resection of metastases in lung or brain. Patients who develop secondaries from the pancreas and liver rarely benefit from resection of the liver tumour (unless the primary is an endocrine tumour).

However, it is clear that some patients do benefit from resection. These include patients who have tumours that have spread to lung from seminoma of testis. Similarly, for patients who have breast secondaries in lymph nodes, the appropriate treatment is an axillary clearance. Patients with bone secondaries, whilst rarely benefiting from excisional surgery, will benefit from internal fixation, which decreases the risk of pathological fracture; internal fixation also relieves pain. Similarly, in secondary disease in the local lymph glands in a patient with head and neck cancer, it is appropriate to perform a block dissection of the nodes. Liver secondaries from colon cancer are amenable to resection if they are confined to one lobe, or, alternatively, if there are fewer than four, in both lobes. This can give a reasonable 5-year survival of up to 30%. Brain secondaries have not been tackled until recently, but over the past 5 years more centres are resecting brain secondaries from lung and breast. This gives reasonably good palliation, provided there are no widespread secondaries, and the operation can be done with sufficiently low morbidity and mortality. In cancer of the ovary, cytoreduction is very important and the omentum should always be removed to reduce the tumour mass before chemotherapy. Other tumours that benefit from resection of lung secondaries include renal tumours, and bone and soft tissue sarcomas. It is now accepted that with modern techniques and correct patient selection, resection of lung metastases can be performed with a low morbidity and mortality (below 2%). Solitary metastases from a renal cell carcinoma may be amenable to resection and 5-year survival rates up to 35% have been reported.

Vascular access

The surgeon can be involved in establishing long-term vascular access for chemotherapy. This can be done either with a percutaneous technique or an open surgical cut-down. This includes creating a subcutaneous tunnel for a subclavian line, and implantable systems such as the Portacath. Local implanted devices include those for portal vein infusion. Regional vascular access is helpful for patients who require chemotherapy into the hepatic artery for infusion into the liver. One of the useful treatments for melanoma of the lower limb is an infusion of chemotherapy into the femoral artery.

Complications of treatment

The surgeon may be involved in treating his own complications in a cancer patient, such as leaks after an anastomosis. He/she may also be involved in the management of the complications of other treatment modalities. Examples include radiation damage to bowel, which can cause proctitis, colitis, perforation, fistula formation, and stenosis. Radiation damage to the urinary tract can occur, giving rise to cystitis, nephritis, renal hypertension, and ureteric strictures; the surgeon may be involved in the management of these complications. Up to 10% of patients with intestinal tumours of the large bowel develop obstruction and over 40% of patients with ovarian cancer develop bowel obstruction.

Blood transfusion

In cancer patients, blood transfusion during surgery appears to be important as there is a suggestion that it adversely affects the outcome in colorectal cancer. It seems that blood transfusion alters the patient's immunological response but the precise mechanism is unclear. Currently it seems reasonable to avoid a blood transfusion provided this is deemed surgically safe.

General complications of surgery in patients with cancer

Patients with cancer who are undergoing surgery are prone to certain general complications. Patients with jaundice may have deranged coagulation and pre- and intraoperative supplementation with fresh frozen plasma and other blood products may be required. Patients with cancer are prone to deep venous thrombosis and appropriate preventative measures will be required. This applies particularly to pancreatic cancer patients and patients with tumours in the pelvis, where there may be increased venous stasis, owing to pressure on the major veins. Mechanical and pharmacological measures are required to decrease this complication and the serious sequel of pulmonary embolism. Patients with cancer are often malnourished, either from the disease *per se* or inability to absorb nutrients. Such patients will have impaired nutrition and less than optimum healing of wounds and anastomoses.

Nutrition

The surgeon can also be involved in the management of the patient's nutrition. It is preferable to avoid total parenteral nutrition in these patients because of potential complications. It is helpful if the patient is going to require long-term nutrition (and it is appropriate ethically) for the surgeon to insert a feeding jejunostomy. Alternatively, a PEG tube can be inserted to allow gastric feeding. However, before proceeding to long-term nutrition management, it is important to discuss with the patient, the family, and with the other members of the multidisciplinary team whether this is appropriate management, depending on prognosis.

Surgical emergencies in oncology

Cardiac tamponade is due to a malignant pericardial effusion, usually caused by breast or lung carcinoma, or occasionally lymphoma. The acute treatment is that of pericardiocentesis performed under ultrasound control. Long-term management may require surgery, which may include pericardectomy or the formation of a pleuropericardial window.

Acute large airway obstruction can occur with tumours of the oesophagus, bronchus, lung, or thyroid, and laser treatment may be of help if there is insufficient time to administer radiotherapy.

Pulmonary haemorrhage secondary to coagulation problems or infection in pancytopenic patients may be managed with the YAG laser. Occasionally embolization by a radiologist may be required.

Obstructive uropathy in malignant disease usually occurs in the ureters or the bladder neck. The ureters may be obstructed by retroperitoneal lymphatic disease, pelvic tumours, or post-radiation fibrosis. Acute management may involve percutaneous drainage or the insertion of ureteric stents. Long-term management may include permanent urinary diversion via an ileal conduit. Insertion of an urethral or suprapubic catheter is used for bladder outflow obstruction.

Emergencies can be caused by gastrointestinal obstruction, secondary to primary tumour of oesophagus, stomach, or colon; obstruction can be caused by secondary deposits, such as diffuse peritoneal carcinomatosis or by oncological treatment such as radiation. Obstruction due to benign causes such as adhesions can of course arise in the cancer patient. Careful decisions regarding operation are important. Perforation and haemorrhage must be treated on their merit and it should be borne in mind that benign causes can arise in patients with cancer, e.g. peptic ulceration, gastritis, and Mallory–Weiss tears.

Case history

Middle-aged lady with anaemia

Dear Doctor,

Mrs M is 64 years of age and has a haemoglobin of 8.5 g. Please see.

History

Mrs M is age 64 years and has felt tired for the past 3 months. She has lost one stone in weight and has noticed a slight looseness of bowel movement. She has no other symptoms.

Family history

Her mother and grandmother had bowel cancer.

On examination she was pale and looked anaemic. Examination of the abdomen revealed a mass in the right iliac fossa, which was non-tender. Her liver was palpable to two fingerbreadths below the costal margin. Rectal examination was clear.

continued

Case history continued

Investigations
- Haemoglobin 8.5 g
- White cell count normal
- ESR 55 mm/h
- Liver function tests – within normal limits
- Faecal occult bloods positive
- Baseline – CEA normal
- Chest x-ray normal
- Ultrasound of liver showed no secondaries
- Rigid sigmoidoscopy – negative
- Barium enema showed puckering on the medial wall of the caecum, suggestive of tumour.
- Colonoscopy and biopsy confirmed adenocarcinoma of the caecum.

Treatment
The patient was advised of the diagnosis and counselled. She was also advised that her family history was important and that her children, aged 40 and 35 years, may need to be screened and have genetic advice. The patient was happy to proceed to surgery.

The haemoglobin was corrected preoperatively with 3 units of transfused blood.

At operation there was a tumour of the caecum. There were no liver secondaries. Right hemicolectomy was performed and ileum anastomosed to transverse colon. Tumour had penetrated the bowel wall and three nodes were positive.

Post-op
Satisfactory recovery.

Pathology
Dukes' C (stage 3) cancer of the caecum.

Oncology opinion
This patient had a Dukes' C, stage III caecal carcinoma. A CT scan of the abdomen and liver postoperatively confirmed no evidence of secondary deposits in the liver. The patient was offered postoperative adjuvant chemotherapy consisting of 5-fluorouracil (5-FU) and leucovorin. The patient received six cycles of 5-FU–leucovorin therapy, which was tolerated poorly. The complications that occurred included severe mucocytis during the fourth and fifth cycles, associated with profuse diarrhoea. This required hospitalization and improved with conservative management. The patient is now 12 months post-chemotherapy and remains in complete remission.

Case history

Middle-aged woman with a breast lump

Dear Doctor,

This lady has a lump in her breast. Please investigate.

History

Mrs F is age 40 years. She found a lump in her right breast 10 days ago. The lump is painless.

Family history

Her mother had bilateral breast cancer age 45 years and required a bilateral mastectomy.

On examination there was a hard lump in the upper outer aspect of the right breast, measuring 2 cm in diameter, which was not fixed deeply or superficially, but she had two palpable glands in the right axilla. Liver and other glands were not palpable.

Investigations

Bilateral mammograms showed a suspicious lesion in the right breast with a dense spiculate mass with adjacent microcalcification elsewhere in the breast.

Fine needle biopsy

A fine needle biopsy confirmed a diagnosis of breast carcinoma. Chest x-ray was clear. Bone scan and ultrasound scan were not done routinely. The patient was counselled and advised regarding diagnosis by the breast nurse counsellor and the surgeon.

Treatment

Because of the size of the tumour, its proximity to the nipple, and the presence of widespread calcification in keeping with ductal carcinoma in situ (DCIS), the patient was offered and agreed to a simple mastectomy and a level 2 (up to the axillary vein) lymph node clearance.

Pathology

Invasive ductal carcinoma, 3 cm in diameter, with adjacent foci of DCIS. Five nodes out of 12 were positive.

Oncology

The surgical pathological staging on this lady revealed she had a stage IIB breast cancer (T2N1M0). This patient was then offered a choice between four cycles of cyclophosphamide and doxorubicin or six cycles of cyclophosphamide, methotrexate and fluorouracil. The patient chose to have four cycles of cyclophosphamide/ doxorubicin therapy. She tolerated the therapy very well and remains in complete remission 2 years post-therapy. The patient was also treated postoperatively with chest wall irradiation as she was at high risk for local regional failure given that five axillary nodes were deemed positive for cancer.

Further reading

Allen-Mersh, T. G. (1996) *Surgical oncology*. Chapman & Hall Medical, London.

Calman, K. and Hine, D. (1995) *A policy framework for commissioning cancer services*. April 1995.

Davis, C. L. and Wee, B. L. (1997) Recent advances in palliative care. In *Recent advances in surgery 20*, 161–76. Churchill Livingstone, Edinburgh.

Fentiman, I. S. (1995) Management of advanced breast cancer. In *Recent Advances in Surgery 18*, 85–98. Churchill Livingstone, Edinburgh.

McArdle, C. S., Murray, G. D., and Hole, D. (1997) Outcome following surgery for colorectal cancer. In *Recent advances in surgery 20*, pp. 129–44.Churchhill Livingstone, Edinburgh.

McClelland, R. N. (ed.) (1993) General Oncology. In *Selected readings in general surgery*, 1–66. University of Texas, Austin, TX.

Morris, P. J. and Malt, R. A. (91994) *Oxford textbook of surgery*, vol. II, pp. 2577–624. Oxford Medical Publications, Oxford.

Neal, A. J. and Hoskin, P. J. (1997) *Clinical Oncology*, 2nd edn. Arnold, London.

Peckham, M., Pinedo, H. M., and Veronesi, U. (1995) *Oxford Textbook of Oncology*, vols I and II, pp. 865–7, 2193–201. Oxford Medical Publication, Oxford.

Ponsky, J. L. (1997) *Complications of Endoscopic and Laparoscopic Surgery*. Lippincott-Raven, Philadelphia.

Sabiston, D. C. and Lyerly, H. K (1994) *Essentials of surgery*, 2nd edn, pp. 167–72. W. B. Saunders, London.

Taylor, I. (1997) What's new in the journals? In *Recent Advances in Surgery 20*, pp. 259–86. Churchill Livingstone, Edinburgh.

Taylor, I., Cooke, T. G., and Guillou, P. (1996) *Essential General Surgical Oncology*. Churchill Livingstone, Edinburgh.

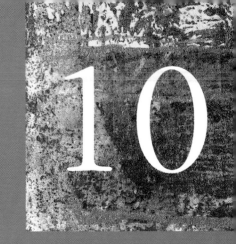

10

The principles of chemotherapy
Patrick G. Johnston

- Adjuvant and neoadjuvant therapy

- General principles of chemotherapy

- Pharmacological aspects of cancer chemotherapy

- New therapeutic approaches to cancer

The principles of chemotherapy

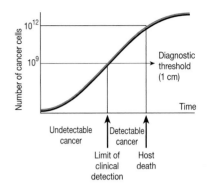

Fig. 10.1 The limit of clinical detection of tumours in patients.

Medical oncology is the cancer speciality that focuses on the systematic management of the cancer patient with chemotherapy and other systemic treatments. The smallest clinically detectable tumour lump is approximately 1 cm in diameter and already contains one billion tumour cells (Fig. 10.1). Therefore, the potential to develop secondary tumours and metastatic disease at distant sites throughout the body is significant, even in the earliest detectable lesion. Patients do not die as a result of local recurrence in the primary organ but due to systemic spread of the disease. Therefore, treatment to eradicate occult cancer cells must include effective systemic treatment. Today, approximately 60–70% of cancer patients will require chemotherapy as part of the treatment of their disease.

Adjuvant and neoadjuvant therapy

Significant improvements in cures have been observed in many types of cancer with the administration of systemic therapy after optimal locoregional therapy (surgery/radiotherapy), even when there is no clinical evidence of metastases. The object of adjuvant therapy is to destroy all occult metastases. In certain circumstances chemotherapy is administered prior to locoregional therapy in an attempt to reduce the tumour cell burden significantly. This approach is termed neoadjuvant therapy.

General principles of chemotherapy

The major biological factors inherent to the treatment of tumours with chemotherapy include an understanding of tumour cell kinetics and the tumour doubling time (Norton and Simon, 1986; Chabner, 1993). A variable proportion of the tumour cells will actively divide at any one time. This may range from 90% in some tumours, for example, lymphomas, to less than 20% in others such as some solid tumours (colon and breast cancer). Chemotherapeutic agents are preferentially toxic towards actively proliferating cells, however, they will also kill non-proliferating cells, but do so less efficiently. Therefore, understanding the growth and cell cycle kinetics of cancer cells is important. The various phases that make up the proliferating phases of the cell cycle are termed G1, S, G2, and M cycle, and the G0 phase, which makes up the resting phase of the cycle (Fig. 10.2).

The G1 phase is the protein synthetic phase. S1 phase is the phase of DNA synthesis, G2/M is the phase of cellular division and G0 is the resting phase of the cell cycle.

Chemotherapeutic agents display differential activity depending on the phase of the cell cycle. These phase-specific agents give rise to biphasic survival curves. The initial phase corresponds to the killing of cells in the most sensitive component of the cycle whilst the second phase is due to killing of cells in the more resistant phase. Agents that do not display any preference for a given phase of the cell cycle are defined as cycle-specific agents (Fig. 10.2). Antimetabolites and

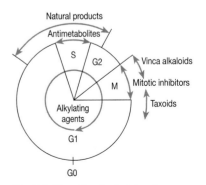

Fig. 10.2 The cell cycle. Activity of chemotherapeutic agents depending on the phase of cell cycle.

anthracyclines are most active in the S phase, whereas vinca alkaloids and taxanes are active in M phase. Alkylating agents are active throughout the cell cycle but are most active at G2 and the G1/S boundary. Other agents, such as nitrosoureas and nitrogen mustards, are active throughout the cell cycle (Fig. 10.2).

The principles of combination chemotherapy include:

- the use of agents with non-overlapping mechanisms of action (non-cross-resistant);
- the simultaneous use of drugs reduces the risk of selecting double-resistant clones;
- the use of agents with non-overlapping toxicities permits the administration of full doses of drugs;
- drug combinations and their sequence of administration are not random but based on additive or greater than additive interactions.

The probability of cure with chemotherapy is inversely proportional to the tumour burden for the following reasons:

- the greater the tumour burden the more cycles of treatment required;
- the greater the tumour burden the higher the likelihood of resistant clones;
- The greater the tumour burden the smaller the growth fraction;
- The greater the tumour burden the higher the probability of metastatic spread.

Chemotherapy dose intensity

The total dose and the overall treatment time are two variables that have a significant impact on the effectiveness of a given drug treatment. For most chemotherapeutic drugs, the relationship between cell kill and dose is very steep. Realization of this has led to the evaluation of dose intensity (total amount of chemotherapy/unit time) of various treatment schedules and generated the concept that high dose intensity should be used. The dose intensity of chemotherapy and the schedule of administration are two important key variables in chemotherapy administration.

Resistance to chemotherapy

The single biggest obstacle to chemotherapy efficacy is the development of drug resistance within tumours (Goldie and Coldman, 1984). The heterogeneous biological characteristics of tumour cells contribute to the development of chemotherapy resistance. Various mechanisms of resistance to chemotherapeutic drugs are now understood (Table 10.1). These mechanisms may overlap and the selection of non-cross-resistant chemotherapy agents is essential for the success of combination chemotherapy. These mechanisms include:

- decreased drug-activating enzymes
- increased drug-inactivating enzymes
- increased DNA repair
- mutations in drug targets
- excretion of drug out of the cells.

Table 10.1 The mechanisms of drug resistance

Mechanism	Drug	Effect
Multidrug resistance	Anthracyclines	Increased drug efflux through active transport
	Vinca alkaloids	
	Etoposide	
	Taxanes	
Impaired transport	Methotrexate	
	Melphalan	Decreased binding sites or carrier activity
Impaired drug activation	Cytarabine	Low cytidine kinase
	Methotrexate	Low polyglutamation
Increased inactivation	Cytarabine	High cytidine deaminase
	Alkylating agents	Increased glutathione and cellular thiols
Improved DNA repair	Platinum compounds	Increased excision
Gene amplification	Methotrexate	Increased dihydrofolate reductase levels
Target alterations	Methotrexate	Increased levels of dihydrofolate reductase, mutations in dihydrofolate reductase
	5-Fluorouracil	Mutations in thymidylate synthase
	Tomudex	Increased levels of thymidylate synthase

The development of drug resistance by tumours has provided some of the rationale for adjuvant chemotherapy of micrometasases. Tumours with a smaller tumour burden would be expected to have fewer drug-resistant variants and possibly be more sensitive to a combination of chemotherapeutic drugs (Fig. 10.3).

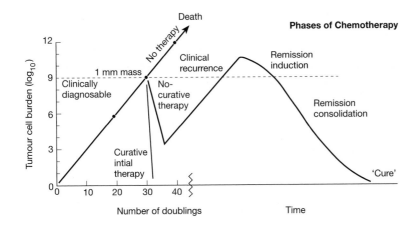

Fig. 10.3 The principles of chemotherapy treatment of tumours.

Intrinsic drug resistance

Intrinsic drug resistance is a frequent problem with the treatment of solid tumours. Cancer cells derived from the gut or renal tract or lung are frequently resistant to chemotherapy. These cells may have intracellular metabolic pathways that are normally used to protect cells against naturally occurring toxic substances. These intracellular pathways may also be used to protect tumour cells from chemotherapeutic drugs.

Acquired drug resistance

A small percentage of resistant tumour cells may survive chemotherapy and subsequently proliferate and constitute the predominant remaining cell type in a tumour. This series of events may explain the relatively frequent observation of initial tumour regression followed by progressive regrowth in spite of the continuous administration of original drug. The probability of this happening is dependent on the tumour cell population size and the mutation frequency as outlined in the Goldie–Coldman hypothesis (Goldie and Coldman, 1984).

Multidrug resistance (MDR)

Julians and Ling (1976) have identified a plasma membrane transport protein (MDR) that is greatly amplified in cancer cells with acquired resistance to certain classes of anticancer drugs. MDR rapidly removes large, complex molecules from the intracellular cytoplasm and increases the drug concentration gradient between the outside of the cell and the cytoplasm. Certain drugs such as calcium channel blockers or drugs such as quinidine, amiodarone, and cyclosporin appear to inhibit the action of the MDR pump.

Intracellular thiols

Many alkylating agents can be inactivated inside the cell by increased levels of glutathione and other non-protein molecules. These sulphur-rich molecules act as radical scavengers, by inactivating active metabolites before the drug can bind to DNA molecules.

Transport resistance

Many active anticancer drugs require facilitated transport to enter cancer cells. Cells in which these transport systems are not abundant and are underrepresented may have a selective advantage over cells in which they are highly expressed. This is one of the major mechanisms of resistance to antimetabolite drugs, which use nucleoside transport systems, and alkylating drugs, which are transported into cells by amino-acid transport systems.

Enhanced DNA repair

Another important mechanism of drug resistance is enhanced and preferential DNA repair. This leads to increased excision of the aberrant nucleotides and repair of DNA strand breaks; moreover, DNA repair may happen at key regulatory sites. This is particularly true in the case of resistance to platinum analogues such as cisplatin where enhanced DNA excision repair is very important in the development of resistance.

Increased target gene expression

Another important mechanism is increased expression and/or mutation of chemotherapeutic drug targets such as thymidylate synthase and dihydrofolate reductase. These are important mechanisms of resistance for the antimetabolite class of drugs.

Patient performance status

The patient performance status is used as an important measure of patient well-being and activity. Performance scales such as the ECOG and WHO scales are commonly used (Table 10.2). Only patients with a performance status of (0–2) should receive chemotherapy.

Classification of antineoplastic chemotherapeutic drugs

Chemotherapeutic drugs are classified into several major families (Table 10.3). These include the following.

Alkylating agents

Alkylating agents form electrophilic carbonium ions that alkylate nucleotide residues of DNA such as guanidine and cause cross-linking of DNA by abnormal base pairing that interferes with DNA replication and function. They also react with sulphydryl phosphate groups in amino acids, resulting in multiple lesions in dividing or non-dividing cells. Examples of alkylating drugs are shown in Table 10.3.

Antimetabolites

Antimetabolites inhibit enzymes such as thymidylate synthase or dihydrofolate reductase involved in purine and pyrimidine nucleotide synthesis and folate metabolism within cells. These drugs are shown in Table 10.3.

Natural products

Other natural products work in a slightly different mode by binding to DNA and causing intercalation of DNA, thus inhibiting DNA and RNA synthesis and causing chromosomal strand breaks. These include agents such as doxorubicin, daunorubicin, bleomycin, dactinomycin, mithromycin, and mitomycin (Table 10.3).

Table 10.2 **ECOG and WHO performance status scale**

Status	Definition
0	Normal activity
1	Symptoms but ambulatory
2	In bed < 50% of time
3	In bed > 50% of time
4	100% bedridden

ECOG, Eastern Co-operative Oncology Group; WHO, World Health Organization.

Table 10.3 Classification of chemotherapeutic drugs

Alkylating agents	Antimetabolites	Mitotic inhibitors	Natural products	Others
Busulfan	Cytarabine	Etoposide	Bleomycin	L-Asparaginase
Carmustine	Floxuridine	Teniposide	Dactinomycin	Hydroxyurea
Chlorambucil	Fluorouracil	Vinblastine	Daunorubicin	Procarbazine
Cisplatin	Mercaptopurine	Vincristine	Doxorubicin	
Cyclophosphamide	Methotrexate	Vindesine	Mitomycin C	
Ifosfamide	Plicamycin	Taxoids	Mitoxantrone	
Melphalan				

Mitotic inhibitors

These drugs tend to interact with microtubulins by interfering with polymerization or depolymerization of cellular tubulins. Examples of these compounds are vincristine, vinblastine, and the taxanes (Table 10.3).

Pharmacological aspects of cancer chemotherapy

The proper administration of cancer chemotherapy drugs to patients **requires** a knowledge of the absorption, distribution, biotransformation, and excretion of these agents.

Absorption, distribution and excretion

Absorption of the drug requires that it is bioavailable and this defines the appropriate route of administration (oral, intravenous, intrathecal, or intramuscular) for a given agent. The rate of absorption affects the concentration achieved and the duration and intensity of exposure. The distribution of the drug depends on its water solubility and will largely determine the half-life of the drug.

Excretion patterns of antineoplastic drugs are also important determinants of toxicity and may require alterations of drug dosage, especially when impaired excretion due to abnormal end-organ function is present, e.g. renal/liver failure. Examples include drugs such as cisplatin and methotrexate.

Biotransformation

Some drugs need to be metabolized in order to become active. 5-Fluorouracil (5-FU) requires activation when it enters a cell in order to become an active anticancer drug. This is the result of conversion of 5-fluorouracil to 5-fluorodeoxyuracil monophosphate by the enzymes thymidine phosphatase and thymidine kinase. Inactivation of drugs must also be considered. 5-FU is inactivated by dihydropyrimidine dehydrogenase.

Chemotherapy-induced toxicities

Cancer clinical trials are designed to detect antitumour activity and to eliminate those drugs or drug combinations that are too toxic to be used in patients. Therefore, the chemotherapy drugs that ultimately enter clinical use usually are well tolerated by patients. Moderate side-effects are usually effectively controlled by proper dosage and the judicious use of other drugs such as anti-emetic agents.

The major toxicities encountered from the use of chemotherapy are as follows.

Bone marrow suppression

Several chemotherapeutic agents such as carboplatin or cytarabine have a tendency to cause severe bone marrow depression. This will occur between 8 and 14 days from the start of the chemotherapeutic cycle. Bone marrow suppression has become less of a major toxicity with the advent of colony-stimulating factors (CSFs). These CSFs mobilize granulocyte and neutrophil precursor cells within the bone marrow and decrease the length of time that the bone marrow is suppressed and the patient is without white cells.

Immunosuppression

Immunosuppression may not be readily apparent during the course of chemotherapy unless specialized tests for immunological reactivity are conducted. While patients are on chemotherapy and are being treated for cancer, one must assume that they are immunosuppressed and therefore susceptible to opportunistic infections.

Nausea and vomiting

Nausea and vomiting are widely associated with cancer chemotherapy and may lead to the patient's refusal to continue therapy. However, nausea and vomiting are now readily controlled using a combination of several emetics and steroids for the most emetogenic chemotherapy agents. The treatment of nausea and vomiting is outlined in Chapter 12.

Alopecia

Loss of hair (alopecia) is especially troublesome with agents such as cyclo-phosphamide, vincristine, doxorubicin, bleomycin, and Taxol. Attempts to reduce hair loss with scalp cooling and tourniquet reconstruction have met with mixed success and are not advisable as they may decrease perfusion of chemotherapy to the scalp, which may harbour metastatic tumour cells.

Renal toxicity

Renal tubular necrosis can result from the use of agents such as cisplatin or methotrexate. Occasionally these side-effects are not reversible and patients will require dialysis.

Cardiotoxicity

This has been associated in particular with anthracyclines such as doxorubicin and daunorubicin. There may be transient electrocardiographic changes owing to the onset of delayed cardiomyopathy with congestive heart failure, particularly when the cumulative dose of doxorubicin approaches 450–550 mg/m^2. This condition is not reversible. Treatment of the chest with radiotherapy may also lead to cardiotoxicity and constrictive pericarditis.

Pulmonary toxicity

Pulmonary toxicity is associated with bleomycin, which causes a decrease in dif-fusion capacity and total lung capacity. This occurs in approximately 10–15%

of patients who receive bleomycin. Such fibrosis is usually only associated with doses of 300–350 units/m^2. However, it may also occur at lower doses and may be irreversible on stopping the drug.

Neurotoxicity

Neurotoxicity is most commonly associated with vincristine and cisplatin. These drugs causes peripheral neuropathy characterized by loss of deep tendon reflexes, paraesthesia, motor weakness, and occasional jaw or other pain. Procarbazine and L-asparagine, used in the treatment of leukaemia and lymphoma, may cause central nervous system symptoms including hallucination and depression. Ifosfamide may lead to the development of encephalopathy, which is usually reversible, but may lead to residual neurological side-effects such as memory loss or drowsiness.

Gonadal damage and sterility

Several drugs, including the alkylating agents or others such as vinblastine, procarbazine and the cytosine analogues, may lead to sterility in both males and females. For young patients receiving these drugs it is wise to consider sperm storage and egg harvesting if they wish to have a family.

New therapeutic approaches to cancer

Immunology

Research into immunology has rapidly expanded our knowledge of the normal function of the immune system. Research in cancer immunology has resulted in components of the immune system being tested as new concepts for anticancer treatment. The primary components of the immune system include T and B lymphocytes, natural killer cells, macrophages as well as small peptide molecules called cytokines.

Biological response modifiers

This is the term that is applied to those agents whose antitumour activity is thought to be exerted through modulation of the host immune function. This term is also applied to a broad range of agents consisting of immune cells or cytokines that have a wide range of effects on the host and the malignant cell. These components of the immune system normally mediate an immune response to foreign peptides or altered cells.

Interferons

Interferons are glycoproteins of cellular origin that have been used as biological response modifiers to mediate antitumour effects. There are several types of interferon (IFN-α, β, γ). They would appear to have significant clinical activity in diseases such as hairy cell leukaemia and some lymphomas and may also be useful in the treatment of malignant melanoma, Kaposi's sarcoma, renal cell carcinoma, and myeloma.

Interleukin-2 and adoptive immunotherapy

Interleukin-2 (IL-2) is a cytokine produced by T-helper lymphocytes after stimulation by mitogens or specific antigenic stimuli. Lymphokine-activated killer

(LAK) cells result from the *in vivo* or *in vitro* exposure of normal lymphocytes to IL-2. To date these studies are at the stage of clinical investigation and have not entered clinical practice.

Colony-stimulating factors

Colony-stimulating factors (CSFs) are growth factors which are responsible for the survival proliferation and maturation of bone marrow stem cells into fully differentiated granulocytes, eosinophils, and monocytes. In addition to their effects on haematopoiesis, CSFs are also important in stimulating chemotaxis, phagocytosis, and antibody-mediated functions. Their clinical use has been primarily restricted to:

* primary bone marrow failure
* immunodeficiency states
* chemotherapy-induced myelosuppression.

Monoclonal antibodies

The technology to allow fusion of specific antibody-producing B lymphocytes and select murine myeloma cells was developed by Kohler and Milstein in 1975. These hybrid cells can produce vast quantities of antibody with defined specificities and can be maintained in culture indefinitely. Monoclonal antibodies can also be developed against tumour-associated antigens and have helped play a major role in tumour diagnosis as well as the development of novel therapeutic strategies. Monoclonal antibodies can bind to tumour-associated antigens and cause direct tumour cytotoxicity by complement or by cell-mediated mechanisms. As antibodies are also foreign proteins, they can elicit an immune response against the tumour. Most clinical trials with antibodies have produced only minor responses (<10%). However, some studies in solid tumours such as colorectal and breast cancer suggest that they may produce a survival benefit when given in the adjuvant disease setting. Monoclonal antibody immunoconjugates such as radiolabelled antibodies have also been undergoing clinical evaluation. These involve antibodies linked to toxins, cytotoxic drugs, or radionucleotides. However, their role has yet to be defined.

Tumour vaccines

Another potential use of biological response modifiers is to activate the immune system of the tumour-bearing host against tumour-associated antigens. Both autologous and allogeneic tumour cells have been utilized as vaccines to stimulate the patient's immune system. The vaccines being used to date include whole tumour cell lysates, virally infected tumour cells, solubilized cell surface antigens, and oncogenic peptides. These vaccines are administered as an injection into the skin along with an adjuvant to increase their immunogenicity. Clinical trials testing these vaccine approaches are ongoing in a variety of tumour types including melanoma and colon and renal cell cancer.

Gene therapy

Gene therapy for cancer is an approach in which a functioning gene is inserted into the tumour cells of a patient to restore the original gene function in these cell. This approach also includes modifying the function of tumour infiltrating lymphocytes to increase their therapeutic efficacy as well as increasing the immunogenicity of the tumour. Tumour cells can be modified to secrete immuno-modulatory cytokines, to secrete chemotactic cytokines to increase the expression of major histocompatibility, HLA class I and II molecules. Two major approaches currently under evaluation are to use the gene-modified cell to increase the concentration of immunomodulatory cytokines in the tumour environment or to use gene-modified cells to stimulate the patient's immune system.

Biological response modifiers have largely been applied to patients with advanced or refractory cancers. However, some of these immunological approaches are now being tested in patients with earlier stage disease (breast and colorectal cancer, melanoma). The use of immunological treatment with other more standard treatments such as surgery, chemotherapy, and/or radiation therapy is also under evaluation. As our understanding of tumour immunology further improves this will lead to a more rational design of immunological approaches to the treatment of cancer.

Case histories

Middle-aged man with cancer of the lung

History
- January 1998 – tumour diagnosis in right apical and paramediastinal region
- Biopsy – non-small cell lung cancer, squamous type
- Treatment – Taxol plus cisplatin.
- February 1998 – readmitted after 2nd cycle with signs of septicaemia and clinical deterioration. Treated successfully with IV antibiotics and received a blood transfusion. CT scan of the chest at that time showed disease progression. Chemotherapy was discontinued.

Family history
The patient lives with his wife who is an ex-nurse. They have three sons, two living locally and one in the USA.

Social history
The patient is a non-smoker. He has a district nurse, home care hospice nurse and a very supportive GP.

- March 1998 – emergency readmission
- Symptoms – related by patient's wife:
  increasing tiredness, weakness and drowsiness
  intermittent confusion
  hallucinations and paranoid ideation
  drenching night sweats
  pain in right shoulder radiating into arm/hand, associated with numbness and tingling in fingers
  muscle jerking

Medications
- MST 40 mg b.d. (this had been decreased by his wife from 60 mg on the day prior to admission because of drowsiness)

continued

Case histories continued

- Diclofenac 75 mg b.d., fluoxetine 20 mg mane, ciprofloxacin 250 mg b.d., co-danthramer 2 b.d.

On examination
- Pale, weak, sweaty, sleepy, pinpoint pupils.
- Multifocal myoclonic jerks.
- Pulse 50, respiratory rate 10/min.
- Positive findings – decreased air entry in the right apex.
- No localizing CNS signs.
- Chest and abdomen NAD.

Investigations
- Full blood count: Hb 9.6; WCC 31.5; ANC 29.
- Liver function tests and urea and electrolytes both within normal limits. Serum calcium checked.
- Sputum C+S, MSU, no growth.
- U/S liver, no metastases.
- CXR: enlargement of right apical lobe and paramediastinal mass.

Treatment Plan

Radiotherapy to right apical lung lesion.

Testicular cancer

Dear Dr

This young man has had a painless lump in his left testis for 4 months. He has no other complaints. Please see urgently and advise.

History
This is a 34-year-old man who found a painless swelling in his left testis 4 months ago. It has slowly increased in size. No other symptoms. No significant past medical history. He is married with one child of 18 months and works as an Air Traffic Controller.

On examination he has a hard craggy mass in his left testis and no groin nodes. The only other abnormal finding is the presence of bilateral gynaecomastia.

Test results
- Full blood count: Hb 15.4; WCC 3.8; platelets 234 000.
- Liver function tests and urea and electrolytes normal.
- Preoperative tumour markers: AFP 123; βHCG 455.
- Ultrasound scan: right testis contains a 3 cm abnormal area of mixed echogenicity consistent with a testicular tumour. The left testis is normal.
- Chest x-ray normal.

He was counselled and had a left radical orchidectomy. Pathological examination revealed a malignant teratoma undifferentiated with trophoblastic elements.

continued

Case histories continued

Postoperative CT scan – chest, abdomen and pelvis
There is a solid mass in the left para-aortic area, just distal to the renal vessels, which is 4 cm in transverse diameter. There are three small peripheral lesions in the right lung and four lesions in the left lung. All lesions are less than 1 cm in diameter.

Conclusion
These findings are consistent with lymph node and lung metastatic spread from a testicular tumour.

Oncology opinion
This young man clearly had a metastatic teratoma and he was offered chemotherapy comprising bleomycin, etoposide, and cisplatin (BEP) for 3–4 cycles depending on response to treatment.

Further reading

Albertini, M. R. and Schiller, J. H. (1992) Biological response modifiers. In Brain, M. C. and Carpone, P. P. (eds), *Current therapy in haematology/oncology*, Vol. 4, pp. 198–203. B. C. Decker, Philadelphia.

American Joint Committee on Cancer (1990) *Manual for staging of cancer*, 3rd edn. J. B. Lippincott, Philadelphia.

Chabner, B. A. (1993) Biologic basis for cancer treatment. *Ann Intern Med* 118, 633–9.

Chabner, B. A. and Longo, D. L. (1996) *Cancer chemotherapy and biotherapy*, 2nd edn. Lippincott-Raven, Philadelphia.

DeVita, V. T., Hellman, S., and Rosenberg, A. (1997) *Cancer: Principles and Practice of Oncology*, 5th edn. Lippincott-Raven, Philadelphia.

Goldie, J. H. and Coldman, A. J. (1984) The genetic origin of drug resistance in neoplasms: implications for systemic therapy. *Cancer Res* 44, 3643–53.

Harnett, P., Cartmill, J., and Glare, P. (1999) *Oncology – a case based manual*. Oxford University Press, Oxford.

Holland, J. F., Bast, R. C., Morton, D. L., Frei, E., Kufe, D. W., and Weichselbaum, R. R. (1997) *Cancer medicine*, 4th edn. Williams & Wilkins, Baltimore.

Julians, R. L. and Ling, V. (1976) A surface glycoprotein modulating drug permeability in Chinese hamster ovary cell mutants. *Biochem Biophy Acta* 455, 1252.

Milstein, C. (1980) Monoclonal antibodies. *Sci Am* 243, 66–74.

Norton, L. and Simon, R. (1986) The Norton-Simon hypothesis revised (Gompertzian kinetics). *Cancer Treat Rep* 70, 163–9.

Peckham, M., Pinedo, H., and Veronesi, U. (1995) *The Oxford Textbook of Oncology*, 1st edn. Oxford University Press, Oxford.

Pinedo, H., Longo, D. L., and Chabner, B. A. (1998) Annual 17. *Cancer chemotherapy and biological response modifiers*. Elsevier, Oxford.

Rubin, P. (1992) *Clinical Oncology – a multidisciplinary approach for physicians and students*, 7th edn. W. B. Saunders, Philadelphia.

Schottenfeld, D. and Fraumeni, J. F. (1997) *Cancer Epidemiology and Prevention*, 2nd edn. Oxford University Press, Oxford.

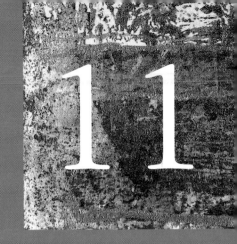

The principles of radiotherapy
Frank Sullivan

- Historical perspective

- Radiobiology

- Medical physics

- Correlation of lung pathology and the chest X-ray appearance

- The Radiation Oncology Department

The principles of radiotherapy

Radiation therapy is a clinical speciality dealing with the use of ionizing radiation on the treatment of patients with malignant neoplasia (and occasionally benign conditions). The aim of radiation therapy is to deliver a precisely measured dose of radiation to a defined tumour volume with as minimal damage as possible to surrounding healthy tissue, resulting in eradication of the tumour, a high quality of life, and prolongation of survival at reasonable cost.

In addition to curative efforts, irradiation plays a major role in cancer management in the effective palliation or prevention of symptoms of disease: Pain can be alleviated, luminal patency restored, skeletal integrity preserved, and organ function re-established, with minimal morbidity in a variety of clinical circumstances. Once a diagnosis of cancer has been established, 50–70% of patients will receive radiation therapy at some time during their illness.

A prominent radiotherapist, Buschke, defined a radiotherapist (radiation oncologist) as a physician who limited his or her practice to radiation therapy. He emphasized the active role of the radiation oncologist:

'While the patient is under our care we take full and exclusive responsibility, exactly as does the surgeon who takes care of a patient with cancer.'

Historical perspective

- Roentgen described x-rays in 1895.
- The Curies reported their discovery of radium in 1898 (almost immediately, the biological effects of ionizing radiations were recognized).
- The first patient to receive radiotherapy, a woman with recurrent breast cancer, was treated by Emil Gubbé in 1896.
- It was not until 1922 at the International Congress of Oncology in Paris that clinical radiation therapy began as a medical discipline.

Radiobiology

This is the study of the effects of ionizing radiation on both normal and malignant cells and goes some way to answering the question 'how does radiotherapy work?' The specific target of radiation damage is DNA.

- Cells are most susceptible to damage during the mitotic, or actively dividing, stage of the cell cycle.
- Damage inflicted on DNA during this stage causes either cell death or loss of the ability to divide.
- The radiation causes either single- or double-strand breaks in the DNA. The latter are more difficult for the cell to repair and thus more likely to result in permanent damage.
- Most radiation used in this way consists of high-energy x-rays which, when they pass through tissue, release a certain amount of energy.

- It is this energy released, the linear energy transfer (LET), which causes electrons to be removed from the outer orbits of nearby molecules.
- These electrons can either damage DNA directly or indirectly by way of free radicals they cause to be formed.
- Although targeted primarily at the cancer, at least some portion of the radiation will cause damage to surrounding normal tissue.
- It is the ability of normal cells, unlike cancer cells, to repair small doses of radiation that enables us to selectively eradicate a cancer population.
- Sufficient time intervals can be left between each radiation treatment to allow normal cells to repair damage but not cancer cells to repopulate.
- Delivering radiation over a longer period of time (fractionation) rather than as a few large doses, facilitates this recovery of normal tissue.

Table 11.1 The '5 Rs' of radiobiology

Radiobiological factor	Mechanism of effect on response	Clinical relevance
Radiosensitivity	Intrinsic radiosensitivity differs between cells of tumours and normal tissue types, and strongly determines final surviving fraction	Can account for variable response of tumours. Curative dose proportional to the log of cell number
Repair	Cells differ in their capacity to repair DNA damage, particularly after small doses of radiation. Repair is usually more effective in non-proliferating cells. The repair process takes at least 6 hours to complete	Repair is maximal in late-responding tissues, given small doses. Treatments need to be well separated in order to avoid compromising the repair
Repopulation	Surviving cells in many tumours normal and in acute-responding tissues proliferate more rapidly once treatment is in progress	Shortened treatment times (accelerated therapy) may be advantageous for some tumours. Acute effects will be increased
Reoxygenation	Hypoxic cells, which occur especially in tumours, are relatively resistant to radiation. Hypoxic surviving cells reoxygenate, becoming radiosensitive, as treatment proceeds	Very short treatment times could lead to resistance due to persistence of hypoxic cells
Redistribution	Cells in certain phases of the proliferative cycle are relatively resistant and survive preferentially. With time between treatments, cells redistribute themselves over all phases of the cycle	Closely spaced treatment fractions could lead to resistance due to persistence of cells in less sensitive phases

There are five main factors controlling tumour response to radiotherapy, the so-called '5 Rs' of radiobiology (Table 11.1). Currently, the most important of these factors is thought to be the intrinsic radiosensitivity of cells and the kinetics of repopulation of surviving cells.

Medical physics

Radiation oncologists use ionizing radiation to eradicate malignancies. Ionizing radiation is composed of electromagnetic and particulate radiation (Fig. 11.1).

- Electrons are the commonest particles used.
- They can either be directed at superficial lesions as they are, or made to strike a target which in turn emits high-energy x-rays.
- This process happens in a linear accelerator (Linac). X-Rays of such great energies have the great advantage of sparing the skin surface while depositing the majority of the dose deep within the body.
- The beams produced by such machines can be shaped with the use of lead blocks to spare surrounding tissue.

The radiotherapy planning process

Pre-planning of treatment

This occurs during the first consultation with the patient. It is at this stage that decisions are made by the oncologist and with the informed consent of the patient. The patient is clinically evaluated (including an assessment of his or her fitness to undergo therapy) and the cancer is properly staged using clinical, radiological, and pathological data. The aim of therapy should be defined at the onset as either curative or palliative. Curative treatment assumes that the patient has a certain probability of surviving after adequate therapy. Palliative treatment, on the other hand, is that which assumes that there is no chance of prolonged survival. Most palliative treatments are therefore aimed at alleviating symptoms.

In curative therapy, a certain incidence of side-effects may be acceptable, as a long-term survival is the goal. However, the same is not true of palliative treatments, in which no major complications should be seen.

Treatment planning

Radiation oncologists seek to maximize the dose absorbed by the tumour and minimize dose delivered to normal tissue. This is the basis of treatment planning. To

---

Radiotherapy planning process

Pre-planning
- TNM staging
- Radical vs palliative intent

Treatment planning
- Description of treatment
- Patient immobilization
- Definition of tumour volumes
- Technique and beam modification
- Calculation of dose distribution

Treatment delivery
- Dose prescription
- Implementation of treatment
- Verification
- Monitoring treatment

Outcome

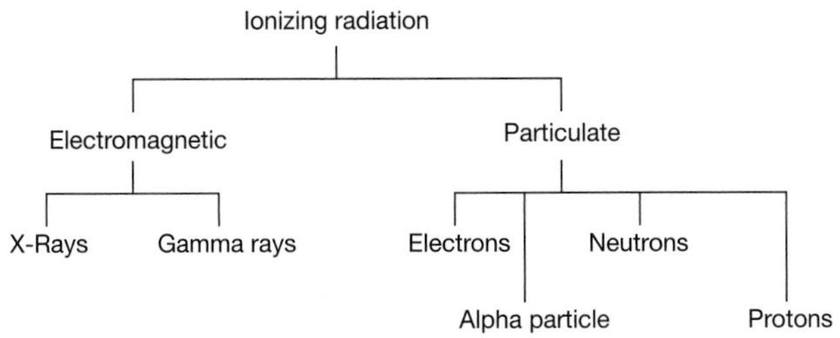

Fig. 11.1 The composition of ionizing radiation.

achieve this, a treatment simulation and planning session is undertaken prior to actual treatment. A simulator is a conventional x-ray unit which simulates the conditions of the therapy beam to be used. It is used to obtain radiographs of the target area and establish basic parameters for treatment planning and set-up. In establishing the target volume, pertinent information regarding the tumour must be available (x-rays, CT scans, surgical reports, pathology reports, etc.). During the planning session, medical physicists and dosimetrists aid the radiation oncologist in establishing the treatment plan. Many variables need to be considered, including the field size, number of treatment beams, beam direction, and use of beam modifiers. Special alloy blocks can be custom-made to block the beam from irradiating normal tissue.

The prescription of radiation is based on the following principles:

- evaluation of the full extent of the tumour (staging) by whatever means available, including radiographic, radioisotope, and other studies;
- knowledge of the pathological characteristics of the disease, including potential areas of spread, that may influence choice of therapy;
- definition of the goals of therapy (cure versus palliation);
- selection of appropriate treatment modalities, which may be radiation alone or combined with surgery or chemotherapy;
- determination of the optimal dose of radiation and the volume to be treated, which is made according to the anatomical location, histology type, stage, and normal structures present in the region;
- periodic evaluation of the patient's general condition, tumour response, and status of the normal tissues treated.

Special treatment planning systems use computer software to determine dose distributions in 3-D. From information available from CT or MRI scans, an accurate definition of the target volume and surrounding normal tissues can be made. Once these volumes are defined, radiation fields can be shaped to 'conform' to the shape of the tumour. Optimization of beam shaping and field arrangement to match the shape of the tumour is known as conformal treatment. Such a treatment plan may allow higher doses to the target volume and/or lower doses to normal tissue, thereby potentially improving the therapeutic ratio (ratio of tumour control to major complications).

The ultimate responsibility for treatment decisions and the technical execution of the therapy, as well as its consequences, always rest with the radiation oncologist. As the patient's physician, he or she has a duty of care to that patient. The need for a large number of other professionals in the planning process does not absolve the oncologist of this responsibility.

Treatment delivery

Following approval by the radiation oncologist, the patient's treatment plan is implemented. This generally entails a number of visits to the radiotherapy department as an out-patient and the actual time spent receiving radiation treatment on each visit is usually quite short. It is essential during the weeks of treatment that there are adequate checks in place to ensure that the target volume remains unchanged and that no modifications to the treatment plan are required. It is an important concept that even though a treatment plan has been approved and started it can still be modified at any time during the treatment and at the discretion of the radiation oncologist.

There are a variety of ways in which radiation may be delivered to a tumour:

- The majority of patients treated with radiation receive their treatment externally, i.e. the radiation is generated in machines and the beams targeted at the patient.
- Radioactive sources may also be placed directly into tumours (interstitial brachytherapy) or into body cavities (intracavity brachytherapy, e.g. vaginal).

Most of the external beam radiation is now generated by linear accelerators (Linacs). As noted in a previous section, these can either generate electrons or high-energy x-ray radiation. Electrons have poor tissue penetration and are therefore used to treat superficial lesions, e.g. skin cancers. High-energy x-rays are used to treat tumours deep within the body. A further source of radiation in most departments is cobalt-60. As this decays, it emits γ-rays and is useful in particular for treating bone metastases.

Outcome

Strategies to improve the therapeutic outcome can be grouped into two main camps. The first uses **biology** to try to improve the results and the second exploits the **physical delivery** of radiation, toward the same end. Both are valid, and complementary. Examples of the biological approaches include the use of drugs as radiation sensitizers, altering the genetic and molecular make-up of the cells to improve killing, improvements in oxygen levels in tumours (see below), and many others. The physical improvements relate to improving the ability to target delivery, such as 3-D conformal therapy, intensity-modulated radiation (IMRT), stereotactic radiosurgery, the use of densely ionizing radiation such as proton beam therapies, etc.

The Radiation Oncology Department

Most patients requiring radiation are ambulatory, and therefore treated as outpatients. Generally, only 5–10% of patients are sick enough to require in-patient radiation care. Therefore, radiation oncology departments are often located outside, but near, cancer hospitals. Due to shielding requirements and the sheer bulk of the equipment, radiation oncology departments are frequently housed at or below ground level.

Proximity to other 'hospital' services, including diagnostic radiology and pathology, can be very useful. The practising radiation oncologist will spend much of the working day consulting with colleagues in these specialties. Additionally, radiation oncologists will be asked to review patients in consultation in the hospital.

There are certain international differences in the way radiation oncology is practised. In Europe and Canada, the radiation oncologist often has admitting privileges, and makes rounds on in-patient services. Furthermore, European radiation oncologists are often cross-trained in medical oncology (then titled clinical oncologists) and many practise both disciplines. In the USA, radiation oncologists do not cross-cover, and are viewed more as 'consultants', leaving in-patient care to the medical and surgical subspecialists.

In either case, a multidisciplinary approach, emphasizing co-operation between the various subspecialists, is considered optimal. One forum for co-operation is the **tumour board**. These periodic meetings, attended by all subspecialists involved in the treatment of the cancer patient, are very useful gatherings. Patient care can be prospectively planned, tissue pathology and radiological studies can be reviewed, and junior staff and students may be taught, in an open environment.

Staffing and patient movement through a radiation oncology department

Most patients reaching a radiation oncology department already carry a diagnosis of cancer, and have generally been though several diagnostic and staging studies. They are therefore somewhat informed as what to expect. However, most are usually quite frightened by the prospect of requiring radiation, and if they have received information from other sources, it is often incomplete and inaccurate. It is vital therefore that they be greeted in a professional, but compassionate way by the receptionists and clerical staff. Accurate demographic information is charted, and the radiation oncologist sees the patient in consultation.

- Often the initial consultation is lengthy (approximately 30–90 minutes), and includes a detailed medical history and physical examination, review of all relevant information including radiology and pathology studies, and operative notes, etc.

- The oncologist will then discuss in detail with the patient whether or not radiation is required, and what the patient might expect from the proposed treatment, including potential toxicities and treatment outcomes.

- The radiation oncologist may wish to confer with other subspecialists prior to making a final recommendation. Family members are often an important part of these consultations, and are encouraged to attend.

If treatment is indicated, a consent form is explained and signed. Nursing staff will also meet with the patient during this initial visit. Prior to beginning therapy, a **simulation** is required. The patient is introduced to the **radiographer**, who will perform this procedure with the oncologist. All the required diagnostic information (CT, MRI, bone scans, plain x-rays, etc.) will be reviewed and used to optimally plan the treatment. A **medical dosimetrist** is often involved in the simulation process, helping the radiation oncologist to select the set-up which optimally covers the target volume (TV), and spares as much normal tissue as possible. The TV is carefully chosen by the physician, with reference to the natural history of the cancer, and the physical and radiographic information as to the cancer's location. The simulation is carefully documented with diagnostic films (sometimes requiring the use of contrast agents), photographs, and chart diagrams. In addition, temporary felt-tip pen marks are often placed on the patient's skin, and permanent freckle-sized tattoo marks, may be placed as a permanent record of the area to be radiated. The entire process may take up to 90 minutes.

- The first day of treatment requires a set-up port film be taken on the treatment table, and compared with the simulation film, to ensure that the daily patient set-up is exactly in accordance with the plan.
- The dose calculation requires the input of a **medical physicist**, who checks the set-up, and dose calculation, verifying the work of the therapist and medical dosimetrist.
- The radiation therapist administers the treatment.
- The treatment course may take from 1 to 7.5 weeks; generally five daily treatments are administered per week.
- The average number of treatments required is approximately 20–25.

During the treatment course, the patient will be seen on a regular basis by the nursing and medical staff. Weekly physician management checks are the norm in most departments. Following completion of therapy, most patients will return for periodic status checks; the first visit is generally approximately 30 days from completion. Written reports of all medical interactions from consultation to follow-up are provided by the radiation oncologist.

Case histories

Case 1

Mr B, a 67-year-old retired schoolteacher, had developed haematuria and lower back pain over a 3-month period.

- X-Rays of his lumbosacral spine demonstrated lytic lesions in L2/3 and his sacrum. A search for the source of his bony metastases revealed an elevated PSA (prostate specific antigen) level and he was diagnosed as having metastatic prostatic carcinoma.
- He was started on monthly injections to prevent androgen release and his PSA level normalized. His back pain also disappeared.
- He remained asymptomatic for 7 months, when his back pain returned, this time associated with numbness in his right leg. Two days later he noticed his right foot dragging and diminished sensation in his right groin. He alerted his GP and was seen that afternoon by an oncologist.
- Probable spinal cord compression was diagnosed. He was admitted to hospital and started on high-dose dexamethasone. PSA had risen.
- Plain x-rays demonstrated a collapsed L3. MRI scans were not readily available, but CT scans confirmed collapse and intrusion of L3 into the spinal canal.
- A 5-day course of emergency radiotherapy covering L1–5 was implemented after careful planning.
- Physiotherapy was started to prevent muscle wastage. Two weeks later most of his power had returned but there was still some reduced sensation. *continued*

Case histories continued

Case 2

Mr S, a 58-year-old engineer, developed nocturia and daytime frequency. He eventually consulted his GP.

- During the course of his examination, the GP checked the patient's PSA level, which was moderately elevated.
- Referral to a urologist was made and a prostatic biopsy was obtained, which confirmed prostatic adenocarcinoma.
- An MRI scan of the pelvis showed no evidence of capsular breach or lymphadenopathy. An isotope bone scan was clear.
- A diagnosis of organ-confined prostate cancer, suitable for radical treatment, was made.
- The patient had a significant history of heart disease and was felt to be an anaesthetic risk. He was referred for radical radiotherapy.
- CT planning localized the target volume and three external beams were employed to give optimum dosage.
- He was treated over 5 weeks. During treatment he developed some cystitis but was otherwise well.
- Over the next 6 months, his PSA level gradually normalized. There was occasional urinary incontinence only.

Further reading

De Vita, V. T., Hellman, S., and Rosenberg, S. A. (1997) *Cancer – principles and practice of oncology*, 5th edn. Lippincott-Raven, Philadelphia.

Hall, E. J. (1978) *Radiobiology for the radiologist*, 3rd edn. Lippincott, Philadelphia.

Khan, F. M. (1984) *The physics of radiation therapy*. Williams & Wilkins, Baltimore.

Mauch, P. M. and Loeffler, J. S. (1994) *Radiation oncology: technology and biology*. W. B. Saunders, Philadelphia and London.

Pass, H. I., Mitchell, J. B., Johnson, D. H., and Turrisi, A. T. (1996) *Lung cancer, principles and practice*, 1st edn. Lippincott-Raven, Philadelphia.

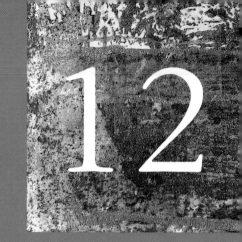

Palliative care in cancer
Sheila Kelly

- Introduction
- Specialist palliative care services
- Common symptoms and their management
- Psychosocial and spiritual care
- Management of the terminal phase of illness

Palliative care in cancer

Introduction

Palliative medicine is defined as the study and management of patients with active, progressive, far-advanced disease for whom the prognosis is limited and the focus of care is quality of life (Doyle *et al.*, 1993).

When care is offered by a multiprofessional team, with core members of doctors, nurses, social workers, chaplains, physiotherapists, and occupational therapists, it is more correct to refer to this as palliative care. Palliative care is the active total care of patients whose disease is not responsive to curative treatment (European Association for Palliative Care, 1989). Palliative care has evolved because of the insights developed within the modern hospice setting, through listening to patients and paying attention to their needs. Since the 1960s, new treatment and new concepts of care are being developed which are relevant to current practice. Palliative care has extended its spectrum of responsibility from care for the dying to caring for patients with irreversible disease at any point in their illness. Although palliative care has focused on the needs of patients with cancer, it is also available to non-cancer patients who have a defined palliative phase such as congestive cardiac failure, motor neurone disease, etc. Palliative care is also defined by the World Health Organization (WHO) as the total care of patients and their families by a multiprofessional team when the patient's illness is no longer responsive to curative treatment (WHO, 1990). Control of pain, of other symptoms, and of psychological, social, and spiritual problems is paramount. The goal of palliative care is achievement of the best possible quality of life for patients and their families. Many aspects of palliative care are also applicable earlier in the course of the illness, in conjunction with anticancer treatment.

WHO (1990) further defines palliative care by its characteristic principles:

- affirms life and regards dying as a normal process;
- neither hastens nor postpones death;
- provides relief from pain and other distressing symptoms;
- integrates the psychological and spiritual aspect of patient care;
- offers the support system to help patients live as actively as possible until death;
- offers a support system to help the family cope during the patient's illness and in their own bereavement.

Specialist palliative care services

Specialist palliative care in-patient units

In-patient units are usually referred to as hospices. They offer specialist palliative care for patients and their families. Patients are referred from general hospitals and from the community when their symptoms require this level of expertise.

The unit is staffed by a multiprofessional team whose members are specialized in palliative care within their own professional role. The core team members usually include a consultant in palliative medicine, specialist nurses, social worker, chaplain, and other therapists. The unit normally offers bereavement and counselling services to patients' families. It may have an out-patient facility and/or a day care facility. It is usually a resource as a centre for audit, research, and education in palliative care.

Specialist palliative care teams within an acute hospital setting

This team is led by a consultant in palliative medicine and includes clinical nurse specialists in palliative care. The service provided by the specialist staff offers advice and support to patients, families, and health professionals. The team complements the skill and resources of the existing hospital ward team. There is an increasing awareness of the patient benefits of joint palliative care clinics with oncology tumour-specific clinics. The members of the specialist palliative care team participate in bedside and in-service training and education programmes.

Palliative day care centre

Patients may be referred to the day care centre from the community or from an in-patient unit. Most centres include core palliative medical and nursing supervision. They also design a carefully thought-out programme of activities focusing on the creative and supportive aspects of care.

Palliative care unit in a hospital

Some hospitals have designated beds for patients needing specialist palliative care. These units are managed by staff with expertise in palliative care.

Home care team

This is a team of specialist palliative care nurses in the community who act as a resource for the primary care team. These nurses professionally liaise with a palliative medical physician. This facilitates patients to be cared for by their families at home for as long as possible and to die at home if that is their choice.

Bereavement service

Bereavement is a normal process and can be greatly facilitated by optimal management of the patient in the terminal phase. However, some can experience what is regarded as 'complicated bereavement'. Bereavement needs play an increasing role in palliative care services towards the terminal phase of the patient's life and after death. Many specialist palliative care services have a 'bereavement risk assessment' tool to pick up potential problems at this time (Parkes and Weiss, 1983). This enables the bereavement counsellors to support and counsel the family members in most need during the anticipatory grief time and after the patient's death. Bereavement care is seen as an important element in the future well-being of the bereaved.

Integral to all the specialist services described is the ongoing commitments to palliative care education, audit, and research.

Common symptoms and their management

Cancer pain

Pain is one of the most feared symptoms in cancer. At diagnosis one-third of patients have pain. This is increased to two-thirds towards the terminal phase of illness. Evidence to date has established that cancer pain can be controlled in the majority of patients. As pain is complex in nature, a multidisciplinary team approach is essential. A combination of pharmacological and non-pharmacological strategies is essential.

The International Association for the Study of Pain defines pain as an unpleasant sensory and emotional experience associated with actual or potential tissue damage, or described in terms of such damage (Saunders, 1989). Pain can be a multidimensional experience. Dr Cecily Saunders, who, in 1969, established St Christopher's in London, one of the first modern palliative care units, introduced the concept of 'total pain', embracing physical, mental, social, and spiritual components. Cancer pain is regarded as a chronic-type pain rather than the acute pain of trauma. The patient may experience it as steadily worsening and totally preoccupying. Severe pain can be associated with anxiety and depression.

Types of pain

Cancer pain can be categorized in many ways. The following is a commonly recognized classification:

- **nocioceptive pain** – this pain may originate in cutaneous or deep tissues. Examples are:
  pain arising from bony metastases;
  visceral pain. This pain is caused by distension, infiltration, or compression of thoracic and abdominal viscera. It may be poorly localized pain. It is frequently associated with nausea and vomiting.

- **neuropathic pain** – this pain results from damage to, or dysfunction of, the nervous system. It is usually caused by tumour compressing or infiltrating peripheral nerves or the spinal cord. It is characterized as a dull ache, a burning or tingling sensation, or shooting pain. Examples of this are brachial or lumbosacral plexopathies.

- **pain unrelated to cancer** – this may arise from other conditions such as arthritis, muscular spasm, intestinal colic.

Not all patients with advanced cancer experience pain. Of those who do:

- one-third have a single pain;
- one-third have two pains;
- one-third have three or more pains (Grond *et al.*, 1996).

Pain management

Aim

The aim of pain management is optimal pain control to maintain maximum quality of life and patient independence.

Principles of pain management

- To recognize and promptly assess patients in pain.
- To diagnose accurately the cause of each pain.
- To reverse each cause of pain if possible.
- To address and alleviate fear.
- To communicate to the patient the likely cause of the pain, and with the patient set realistic goals, i.e. pain relief at night, at rest, and on movement.
- To use regular analgesia in doses titrated to the individual's pain threshold.
- To manage the patient at the lowest effective dose of the most appropriate drug.
- To review regularly, because pain levels change frequently, especially after change in dose or choice of medication.
- To communicate clearly with the patient regarding medication changes, likely side-effects and hoped-for response.
- To choose the most appropriate route of administration. Oral administration is the usual route for patients with chronic pain.
- To remember to attend to the multidimensional aspects of 'total pain'. The 'meaning' of pain varies with each patient, and each culture, and may need to be explored.
- To provide support for family and carers of patients with pain.

Approaches to pain management

Effective pain management may be achieved by any of these components. Frequently a combination may be necessary:
- **retard tumour progression:**
  palliative chemotherapy
  palliative radiotherapy
  palliative surgery
- **analgesics:**
  non-opioids
  opioids
  non-steroidal anti-inflammatory drugs (NSAIDs)
- **adjuvant drugs:**
  anticonvulsants
  corticosteroids
  benzodiazepines
  night sedation
- **TENS (transcutaneous electrical nerve stimulation)**
- **nerve blocks:**
  local nerve block
  epidural
  intrathecal
  sympathetic ganglion block

- **alterations in lifestyle:**
  walking aid
  wheelchair
  restrict pain-precipitating activities.

Pharmacology of cancer pain management

Cancer pain varies in its responsiveness to different classes of analgesia. Analgesics vary in their potency, side-effect profile, and duration of action. These need to be understood before prescribing.

The World Health Organization 3-Step Analgesic Ladder (Fig. 12.1) effectively combines analgesic agents to achieve optimum pain control using a stepwise approach (WHO, 1986). If the first-step analgesia fails to relieve pain, move up the ladder. It is not beneficial to move laterally in the same drug efficacy group.

NSAIDs may be added at any step of the three-step ladder if no contraindication exists and when pain control is not achieved.

- **Step 1 – mild pain**
  Non-opioid
  Paracetamol every 4–6 hours
  Aspirin: not frequently used because of gastric toxicity
  ± Adjuvant drugs
- **Step 2 – moderate pain**
  Weak opioids in combination with non-opioids, e.g. codeine 30–60 mg 4-hourly. There are many preparations of combined non-opioid and weak opioids available. Ensure they are the appropriate dosage and are given
  + Non-opioids regularly.
  ± Adjuvant drugs
- **Step 3 – severe pain**
  Strong opioids. These are required for most patients with cancer pain, but should be commenced only after step 1 and step 2 have failed to achieve optimal pain control.
  + Non-opioids
  ± Adjuvant drugs

The analgesic ladder accurately ensures effective pain control in 80% of patients with chronic cancer pain. Alternative pain management needs to be considered in the remaining 20% (Hanks *et al.* 1996).

Access early referral to specialist palliative care service if pain control is not readily achieved.

Morphine and its use

Morphine remains the opioid most used as a strong analgesic. It is well absorbed by mouth and rapidly distributed throughout the body. Careful dose titration is essential. In appropriate doses it has well tolerated side-effects.

- Morphine is metabolized to morphine-3-glucuronide, and morphine-6-glucuronide. The latter is more potent as an analgesic. Both glucuronides accumulate in renal failure, therefore it should be used with caution in patients with renal impairment and in the elderly.

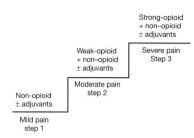

Fig. 12.1 The World Health Organization 3-step analgesic ladder.

- There are a number of opioid receptor subtypes in the CNS. Mu, kappa and delta opioid receptors are involved in analgesia. Morphine is mainly a mu agonist (Hanks and Cherny, 1998). Other strong opioids can differ in their activity and receptor-site affinity. Alternative opioids are therefore available for patients intolerant to morphine.
- For optimal analgesia a non-opioid should be prescribed with a strong opioid.
- A laxative should always be prescribed with morphine.
- Nausea disturbs approximately one-third of patients starting on morphine.
- Morphine dependency has not been documented as a problem in patients taking morphine for cancer pain (Schug *et al.*, 1992).
- Morphine in appropriate analgesic dose does not cause clinically important respiratory depression in cancer patients in pain. It seems that pain is a physiological antagonist to the central depressant effects of morphine (Twycross, 1997).
- Morphine is not always the most effective analgesic for all cancer pain as pain may be:
  (a) opioid responsive;
  (b) opioid semi-responsive, indicating the need to add an adjuvant analgesic;
  (c) opioid resistant, pain not relieved by Morphine.

In the event of pain not being opioid responsive, it is essential to consult the specialist palliative care team for advice. Increasing the opioids results in a patient increasingly distressed by pain, compounded by opioid toxicity. The response of different types of pain to opioids is shown in Table 12.1.

Commencing a patient on morphine The different forms of morphine are shown in Table 12.2.

The immediate-release Oramorph preparation given orally 4-hourly facilitates rapid pain management. It is good practice to commence on a low dose of immediate-release Oramorph, e.g. 2.5–5 mg 4-hourly and titrate up rapidly to achieve pain control. If the patient has been on the maximum dose of weak opioids, e.g. codeine 60 mg q.d.s., start oral Oramorph 10 mg every 4 hours (60 mg/day).

Table 12.1 Response of pain to opioids

Type of pain	Response to opioids
Nocioceptive	
Visceral	+
Soft tissue	+/−
Bone	+/−
Neuropathic	
Nerve compression	+/−

Table 12.2 Forms of morphine

- Oral route
  Immediate release
    Sevredol tablets 4 hourly
    Oramorph solution 4 hourly
  Modified release
    Twice daily dose administration
    MST tablets or suspension (sachets)
    Zomorph capsules
    Single daily dose administration
    MXL capsules

- Rectal route
  24 hours morphine hydrogel suppository

- Parenteral route
  Diamorphine

Dosing frequency Oramorph is usually administered 4-hourly. A double dose can be given at 12 midnight to avoid disturbing the patient at 4 a.m. Less frequent doses may be necessary in the elderly and patients with renal impairment.

Dose increase

- Usually 24 hours should be allowed to reach steady state before increasing the dose.
- If pain persists, the dose should be increased by 30–50%.
- The dose should be titrated upwards until pain is relieved. There is no fixed upper dose limit of morphine preparations.
- When pain control is optimum the patient should be put on 12-hourly or 24-hourly modified-release preparation:
  (a) MST 12-hourly = total 24-hour dose of immediate release divided by two;
  (b) MXL 24-hourly = total 24-hour dose of immediate release.

Breakthrough pain This is defined as pain that occurs before the next regular dose of analgesia is due. When this happens:

- if the patient is on the immediate-release preparation, an extra dose of Oramorph equivalent to the 4-hourly dose should be given;
- if the patient is on modified-release Oramorph, an immediate-release preparation equivalent to one-sixth of the total 24-hour dose should be given.
- The need for frequent breakthrough doses suggests that the total dose of modified-release preparation needs to be increased.
- Achieving rapid control via the parenteral route Diamorphine – this is the preferred drug for parenteral use. It is highly soluble in small volumes and can be given 4-hourly or by syringe driver as a continuous infusion.

The relative potency ratios or the oral administration of morphine are shown in Table 12.3.

Table 12.3 **Relative potency ratios for oral administration of morphine by different routes of administration (Hanks *et al*, 1996)**

Oral morphine to	Ratio
Rectal morphine	1:1
Subcutaneous morphine	1:2
Intravenous morphine	1:3
Subcutaneous Diamorphine	1:3

Side-effects of morphine

- Constipation – a laxative should always be prescribed with opioids.
- Nausea and vomiting – occurs in about 30% of patients first starting on opioids, but is self-limiting. Appropriate antiemetics are haloperidol 1.5–3 mg nocte or metoclopramide 10 mg q.d.s.
- Drowsiness – may occur when starting opioids or increasing the dose. This improves within 3–6 days. Excessive sedation indicates early toxicity.
- Addiction/dependence – is not a problem in clinical practice.

Signs of morphine toxicity

- Persistent drowsiness
- Persistent nausea or vomiting
- Pinpoint pupils
- Myoclonic jerks/seizures
- Respiratory depression

Neuropathic pain

Patients may have great difficulty describing neuropathic pain. The characteristics are:

- burning
- shooting
- stabbing
- numb sensation in area of pain.

Examination may reveal:

- altered sensation in area of nerve damage;
- motor weakness;
- altered reflexes;
- autonomic changes such as pallor or sweating in the affected area.

Treatment Neuropathic pain responds poorly to the analgesic ladder, but it is appropriate to try conventional analgesia, in addition to the adjuvant drugs. It takes

3–5 days before pain relief is noted. Drug titration may be necessary for optimal pain response. Nerve blocks may be necessary. Non-drug measures such as TENS can be helpful. Early diagnosis is essential for optimal management. If pain control proves challenging, an expedited referral to a specialist palliative care team is advised.

Bone pain

Bone pain due to skeletal metastases is nocioceptive type pain. Characteristically, it is described by the patient as a dull aching pain worse on movement and on weight-bearing. On examination, there frequently is bone tenderness at the site of the metastases.

Pain management includes different modalities. Analgesics are the mainstay of treatment. This pain frequently needs step 3 of the analgesic ladder, i.e. opioids ± non-opioid. NSAIDs can greatly enhance bone pain management. Bisphosphonates have been used for their analgesic effects in patients with bone metastases from breast cancer. Hormonal therapy may be effective in bone pain in hormone-responsive tumours, especially of the breast or prostate. If investigations reveal large lytic lesions, an orthopaedic opinion is sought for bone stabilization. Radiotherapy may also play a role.

A summary of cancer pain management is shown in Fig. 12.2.

Respiratory symptoms

The two most common respiratory symptoms encountered in palliative care are dyspnoea and cough.

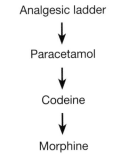

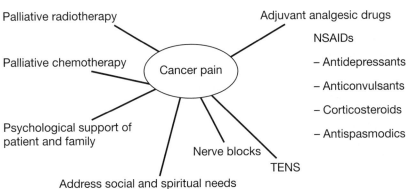

Fig. 12.2 Summary of cancer pain management.

Dyspnoea

Dyspnoea or breathlessness is defined as an unpleasant sensation of difficulty in breathing. It is a subjective experience. It is usually accompanied by tachypnoea.

Dyspnoea is caused by multiple factors. The physical causes may be related to the cancer itself, to the cancer treatment, to the debility associated with cancer, or concurrent illnesses. There is usually a component of fear and anxiety accompanying the physiological causes. This compounds the subjective experience of breathlessness and makes its management more difficult.

As the mechanism of dyspnoea is poorly understood, much of the therapeutic interventions are not evidence based. The evidence is that breathlessness is poorly managed despite standard palliative care interventions (Cowher and Hanks, 1990).

Management of patients with dyspnoea If dyspnoea is of sudden onset, reversible causes such as infection, cardiac failure, effusion, lung collapse, and pulmonary emboli should be ruled out. Causes more directly related to cancer, which may not be reversible, include obstruction of a main bronchus, lymphangitis, or carcinomatosis. As with all symptom management, decisions to investigate and actively treat are made on the general well-being of the patient. Regular review of management is essential.

The common fear in these patients is that they will die by suffocating or choking in one of these episodes of breathlessness. This may be helped by:

- reassuring the patient that staff are constantly and readily available;
- establishing breathing exercises and relaxation therapy;
- increasing local air flow (either by opening the window or turning on a fan);
- anxiolytic medications.

Counselling to allow patients to explore their fears and lessen dyspnoea empowers the patient to cope better and improves quality of life (Corner *et al.*, 1996).

Pharmacological symptom management for dyspnoea

- **Opioids** – Opioids decrease the subjective sensation of dyspnoea. Opioids diminish the sensitivity of the respiratory centre in the medulla to hypercapnia and thus reduce the respiratory drive. Oramorph 2.5–5 mg 4-hourly is given initially. If the patient is already on morphine for pain, the dose can be titrated up to a 50% increase, constantly monitoring response against development of side effects (Cowher and Hanks, 1990).

- **Benzodiazepines** – Diazepam 5–10 mg stat and 5–10 mg nocte can be given. If the patient is unable to take oral medication, diazepam can be given rectally. If already on a syringe driver, midazolam 2.5–5 mg over 24 hours is added. The dose of benzodiazepines in the elderly should be reduced.

- **Oxygen** 4 l/min may be helpful.

- **Nebulized therapies** – If reversible airways obstruction is present, bronchodilators may be helpful. If viscid lung secretions are present, nebulized saline may be helpful. There is no scientific basis to support the use of nebulized opioids.

- **Steroids** – The use of steroids is indicated for lymphangitis carcinomatosa, radiation pneumonitis, endobronchial disease, or superior vena caval obstruction.

Management of daily activities

- The patient should be given adequate help in mobilizing.
- Periods of rest should be increased as required.
- Unnecessary activity such as stairs climbing should be avoided.
- A wheelchair should be used in preference to walking.

Management of dyspnoea in the terminal phase
In acute, irreversible terminal dyspnoea, it is important to ensure that the patient is as comfortable and as unaware as possible. This is achieved by administering midazolam 5–20 mg via the subcutaneous route by syringe driver. If this is not an option, rectal suppositories of diazepam is a useful alternative.

Because of the complexity of dyspnoea, a multiprofessional team approach is essential to address the emotional, physical, psychological, and functional factors involved.

Cough

Cough may be a persistent and distressing symptom for some patients. Fifty per cent of all patients with terminal cancer and 80% of patients with lung cancers experience this symptom.

Types of cough
Productive cough with sputum – This type of cough is related to chest infection, heart failure, and bronchitis. Treatment options for this type of cough include:

- antibiotics
- diuretics/ACE inhibitors
- physiotherapy
- nebulized saline.

Dry cough – Dry cough can be more difficult to manage. The common causes are:

- bronchial tumour mass
- multiple lung metastases
- bronchospasm
- pleural effusion.

Complications of dry cough include:

- exhaustion
- vomiting
- insomnia.

As most of the causative factors for dry cough are irreversible, good symptom management is essential. The management approach includes:

- **cough suppressant**
  simple linctus 10 ml every 2–4 hours
  codeine linctus 30–60 mg every 4 hours

methadone linctus if codeine linctus is not effective.

- **nebulized saline** may help if the patient is struggling to expectorate tenacious secretions.

- any bronchospasm present can be treated with **nebulized bronchodilators**.

- depending on the general well-being of the patient, the possibilities of **disease modification** should be reviewed:
  radiotherapy
  chemotherapy
  corticosteroids.

- **related symptoms**
  if the patient is anxious, an anxiolytic can be prescribed;
  if insomnia is present, night sedation can be prescribed;
  if nausea or vomiting are present, an anti-emetic can be prescribed.

Gastrointestinal symptoms

Patients with cancer encounter the following gastrointestinal symptoms:

- anorexia, malaise, weakness

- nausea and vomiting

- intestinal obstruction

- constipation.

Despite the growing research interest into the pathophysiology and management of gastrointestinal symptoms, we still have many gaps in our knowledge. Nevertheless, there is a body of growing international consensus with general accepted management guidelines increasingly available.

Anorexia, malaise, and weakness

Anorexia is a common symptom in patients with cancer. It frequently diminishes a sense of well-being and reduces quality of life. The patient's inability or unwillingness to eat can be a cause of great distress for the family/carer.

Anorexia is usually associated with malaise/weakness. There frequently is an associated anxiety or depression.

There is a recognized syndrome of cancer cachexia, consisting of anorexia, weakness, and weight loss. Some 50% of patients may already have a degree of cachexia at diagnosis.

Factors contributing to cancer cachexia

- Poor nutrition – this may be related to nausea, vomiting, and malabsorption.

- Metabolic abnormalities – studies confirm abnormalities in protein, carbohydrate, and lipid metabolism (Keller, 1993). Abnormalities include triglyceride and cholesterol with reduced protein levels. There is evidence of hypermetabolism. Loss of body fat occurs because of increased lipolysis and reduced lipid synthesis.

- Humoral factors – these factors, which are capable of producing cachexia, may be produced by the tumour or by the host in response to the tumour. Tumour necrosis factor and interleukin-1 are humoral factors called cytokines produced by the host in response to the presence of cancer cells. They are mediators of the anorexia/cachexia syndrome (Hocknell, 1997).

Management of anorexia, malaise, and cachexia There is at present no specific treatment. Management aims at addressing the associated symptoms. The management approach includes the following.

- **Careful assessment of symptoms** – That there are no reversible causes, such as mouth infection or gastrointestinal pathology, should be determined. If oral candida is present, it is treated with nystatin or oral fluconazole. If nausea or vomiting is present, administration of a prokinetic anti-emetic, e.g. metoclopramide, is appropriate.

- **Careful attention is given to presentation of food and environment.** Advice from a dietitian should be sought. There is anecdotal evidence that alcohol stimulates the appetite. It may be helpful to link meals with normal social activities, rather than eating for the nutritional benefits during illness.

- **Drug therapy** – Research has demonstrated that corticosteroids are appetite-enhancing. This is associated with an increased sense of well-being. Unfortunately, the appetite improvement lasts only a few weeks (Bruera, 1992). This brief increase of appetite is not associated with weight gain. Megestrol acetate has been shown to increase appetite and weight in women with breast cancer.

- **Physiotherapy and occupational therapy** – These play a role in maintaining independence for as long as possible.

- **Art and diversion therapy** – These can enhance creative capacity, quality of life, and decrease the sense of isolation associated with anorexia/cachexia.

Nausea and vomiting

Nausea and vomiting affect between 40 and 70% of patients with advanced cancer (Dunlop, 1989). Approximately one-third of hospice admissions are for patients with intractable nausea and vomiting.

Management of nausea and vomiting The aim of symptom management is rapid control of nausea and vomiting. Most patients find nausea more intolerable than vomiting. Therefore the initial aim is to completely reverse nausea. In certain conditions, vomiting cannot be completely reversed but patients can tolerate infrequent vomiting once nausea has been successfully managed. A good understanding of the causative factors of nausea and vomiting, the pathogenesis, and the antiemetic classifications are necessary to achieve this aim.

Assessment of causes of nausea and vomiting

- Accurate history taking and physical examination are essential. A clear knowledge of the pattern, frequency, volume and content of vomitus, exacerbating and relieving factors are helpful clues to the actual cause of nausea and vomiting.

- The patient's drug regimen should be reviewed to ensure symptoms are not drug related.

- Fundi should be checked for papilloedema.

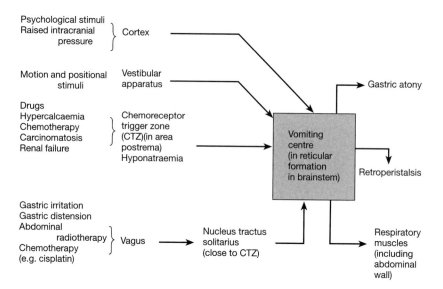

Fig. 12.3 Pathogenesis of nausea and vomiting (reproduced with permission from Twycross, 1995).

- Plasma concentrations of urea, creatinine, calcium, albumin, and digoxin should be checked if the patient's well-being allows for interventional investigation.

- Radiological investigations may be helpful if appropriate to undertake.

Pathogenesis of nausea and vomiting The vomiting centre in the reticular formation in the brain stem co-ordinates this process. It receives and integrates input from several peripheral sources. Vomiting is a reflex process involving co-ordinated activities of the gastrointestinal tract, diaphragm, and abdominal muscles. Nausea is mediated through the autonomic nervous system. Vomiting is mediated via the somatic nerves. Fig. 12.3 represents this pathogenesis. It connects the causative factors with the stimulation of the vomiting centre, resulting in the act of vomiting.

Treatment of nausea and vomiting The general approach for the treatment of nausea and vomiting encompasses the following points:

- If a reversible cause is identified, it should be actively treated.

- If indicated, non-drug measures should be considered to address the level of anxiety.

- Factors that precipitate nausea, e.g. smell or sight of food, should be avoided.

- Small and frequent meals should be arranged.

- The use of acupuncture techniques may be helpful.

- An appropriate anti-emetic drug should be chosen. Anti-emetic drugs are classified according to their affinities for neurotransmitter receptor site.

The specific approach for the treatment of nausea and vomiting is with anti-emetics, as illustrated in Table 12.4.

Symptom management should be as follows:

- Anti-emetics acting principally in the vomiting centre – In mechanical bowel obstruction or raised intracranial pressure, cyclizine 50 mg t.d.s. orally or

Table 12.4 The treatment of nausea and vomiting using anti-emetics

Site of action	Anti-emetic classification	Example
Gastrointestinal tract		
Prokinetic	Dopamine (D_2) antagonist	Metoclopramide, domperidone
	$5HT_4$ agonist	Metoclopramide
Vagal blockade	$5HT_3$ antagonist	Granisetron, ondansetron.
Central nervous system		
Vomiting centre	Antihistaminic	Cyclizine
	Anticholinergic	Hyoscine hydrobromide
	$5HT_2$ antagonist	Methotrimeprazine
Chemoreceptor trigger zone	Dopamine (D_2) antagonist	Haloperidol, metoclopramide
Cerebral cortex	Benzodiazepine	Lorazepam
	Corticosteroid	Dexamethasone

100 mg t.d.s. rectally or 150 mg per 24 hours by subcutaneous infusion is used (Twycross and Back, 1998).

- Anti-emetics acting principally in area postrema CTZ for chemical causes of vomiting, e.g. hypercalcaemia, renal failure, drugs – haloperidol 1–5 mg nocte orally or 5 mg per 24 hours by continuous subcutaneous infusion is used.

- Anti-emetics acting principally on the gastrointestinal tract, e.g. prokinetic agents for gastric stasis, functional bowel obstruction – metoclopramide 10 mg q.d.s. orally or subcutaneously 40–100 mg per 24 hours by continuous subcutaneous infusion is used.

- If the first-line anti-emetic drug dose is optimized and symptoms persist after 24–48 hours, it is necessary to review the drug regimen. Where the aetiology of nausea and vomiting is multifactorial, an anti-emetic combination could prove more appropriate. Approximately one-third of patients need more than one anti-emetic for optimal symptom management. Because of the neurotransmitter receptor-site activities, a combination of haloperidol with cyclizine gives a good broad-spectrum anti-emetic activity without unduly increasing the side-effect profile.

- Response to change in medication should be continually assessed. Should symptoms persist for a further 24–48 hours after anti-emetic changes, an alternative second-line substitute may be appropriate. Current practice suggests that dual-agent therapy with haloperidol and cyclizine may be replaced by methotrimeprazine (levomepromazine). This is a broad-spectrum anti-emetic; 6.25–12.5 mg subcutaneously over 24 hours is a usual starting dose. Postural hypotension and drowsiness are increasingly likely at higher doses (Twycross *et al.*, 1997).

- During the initial period of gaining control over nausea and vomiting, it is good clinical practice to prescribe an anti-emetic on an as-needed (*pro re nata*, prn) basis. It is preferable that this prn anti-emetic has different receptor-site affinity activity from the anti-emetic in regular use.

- Depending on the symptom response, and the general condition of the patient, if the anti-emetic has been commenced in the syringe driver by subcutaneous route, close assessment of the patient's response and disease status will help decide if/when the patient is ready to resume the anti-emetic regimen via the oral route.

If satisfactory symptom management is not achieved following the above suggestions, it may be helpful to call in the specialist palliative care team.

Intestinal obstruction

This is caused by an occlusion of the lumen of the gut, or a lack of normal pro-kinetic movement, delaying or preventing intestinal contents from passing along the gastrointestinal tract.

The most common primary tumours associated with intestinal obstruction are ovarian or large bowel (Parker and Baines, 1996). In studies of patients with advanced ovarian cancer, 25–42% developed obstruction (Beattie *et al.*, 1989).

Management of patients with intestinal obstruction Depending on the causative factors and the level of obstruction, the symptoms and clinical findings will vary. It is important to differentiate between bowel dysfunction, associated constipation, and a true obstruction. To do this, investigation may be indicated but should only be carried out if the results will influence the treatment planned.

Treatment options A small number of patients may benefit from surgical intervention. It is important to consider this modality of treatment, but disease status and poor prognostic factors are usually contraindications for surgery.

The alternative to surgery is medical management and the principles are:

- the relief of intestinal colic using an antispasmodic, such as hyoscine butyl-bromide 40–100 mg by syringe driver over 24 hours;

- treating continuous pain with adequate analgesia such as diamorphine;

- treating nausea and vomiting with centrally active anti-emetics such as cyclizine 150 mg daily and/or haloperidol 5–10 mg daily. These anti-emetics can be administered singly or in combination by continuous route in a syringe driver. A second-line anti-emetic, e.g. methotrimeprazine commencing at –6.25 mg by syringe driver over 24 hours, is an alternative choice.

- octreotide, which is a synthetic stable analogue of somatostatin, can enhance symptom management. It reduces the volume of gastrointestinal secretions by increasing the absorption of water and electrolytes and inhibiting their secretion. Its use therefore is indicated in upper gastrointestinal obstruction with irreversible large volume vomitus. Initial recommended dose is 300 μg increasing to 600 μg over 24 hours. This can be given in single subcutaneous doses three times a day or as a continuous subcutaneous infusion in the syringe driver. Octreotide has been mixed with morphine, haloperidol, midazolam, and hyoscine in the syringe driver with no apparent effect on its efficacy (Riley and Fallon, 1994).

A small subgroup of patients with intestinal obstruction who do not respond to pharmacological management and continue to complain of nausea and vomiting may benefit from a decompression or venting procedure (venting gastrostomy). These patients usually have a high small-gut obstruction and continue to present with episodes of nausea relieved by projectile large-volume vomitus. A venting gastrostomy not only alleviates these symptoms, but also allows the patient to take a light diet and liquids while the gastrostomy tube is clamped (Ashby *et al.*, 1991).

Nutrition and hydration are rarely problems for the patient. When the nausea and vomiting are adequately controlled, patients are able to take fluids and a light diet. These are mostly absorbed in the proximal part of the gastrointestinal tract and maintain the patient's nutrition and hydration satisfactorily. A recurring dry mouth can be treated with local measures. In a small group, fluid loss may become a problem. This may be overcome with intermittent fluid replacement either intravenously or subcutaneously. When subcutaneous fluid replacement is carried out overnight, the patient retains normal mobility throughout the day (Fainsinger *et al.*, 1994).

As patients with irreversible intestinal obstruction deteriorate, they need to be reviewed regularly for adjustments to their medication. With the above recommended regimen they can have good symptom management and optimal quality of life in this pre-terminal phase of their illness.

Psychosocial and spiritual care

At the core of palliative medicine is holistic care of the patient and family. Whilst optimal management of pain and other symptoms is central, palliative care also extends beyond the physical symptoms to address psychological, social, and spiritual needs. These needs are expressed in and through:

- the patient's grief resulting from the anticipatory loss of family, friends, and all that is familiar;
- the social changes in a family relationship as it adjusts to the imminent loss;
- the ontological questions that arise irrespective of the patient's or relative's religious or belief systems, e.g. 'why me?', 'what have I done to deserve this?'

The underlying ambition of palliative medicine is to alleviate as far as possible physical symptoms and distress so that the patient and family are empowered to deal with their more personal and vulnerable psychosocial losses and spiritual questions.

Addressing these areas of need with the patient and family is a challenging experience for clinicians. These skills are best taught and learned in reflective clinical practice.

Patients with non-responsive cancer and their families are particularly vulnerable. Optimal management of their care in these circumstances demands sensitive and skilful interacting. Basic to this clinical exchange is good communication skills. This involves:

- allowing time for patients to talk;
- checking out their understanding of their illness if that is their area of concern;
- being aware of the challenge in 'breaking bad news'; despite it being done in the most appropriate and sensitive manner, patients still experience it as 'bad news';

- being aware of, and receptive to, the range of deep emotions patients touch during these vulnerable weeks/days;
- using language that the patient can easily understand.

Within the multi-professional team, doctors in particular find this level of presence to, and communication with, patient and families difficult. This may be as a result of inadequate skill at handling sensitive communication with vulnerable patients. It may also relate to the fact that the doctor feels he or she has to produce a solution or an answer to the questions raised. Very often the patient and family are more helped by sympathetic listening than suggesting solutions or giving answers.

> Palliative medicine is about curing symptoms while simultaneously preparing the conditions where healing may happen, and the healing on offer may be there not just for the patient and his family, but also for us as people who are physicians. (Kearney, 1992)

By effectively supporting patients at this level of their need it is hoped that they are enabled to move towards the phase which Kubler-Ross (1977) calls 'acceptance'.

In palliative medicine more so than any other speciality, issues of cultural beliefs and taboos are encountered. This has a direct bearing on how we manage the psychosocial spiritual care of patients and families. This will demand from us a knowledge and understanding of cultural differences, a sensitivity towards them and deep respect for our patients.

Management of the terminal phase of illness
Definition

The terminal phase of illness refers to the last few days of the patient's life. If a person has been deteriorating slowly, recognizing the 'terminal phase' may not always be easy.

Signs that may be helpful in recognizing this phase are:
- loss of interest
- increasing drowsiness
- intermittent confusion
- losing interest in food and drink
- weakness associated with difficulty in swallowing medications.

If all or any combination of the above signs and symptoms have an acute onset it is necessary to rule out reversible causes such as:
- hypercalcaemia
- drug toxicity
- septicaemia
- dehydration
- uraemia.

These conditions may be potentially reversible and may enable the person to have further quality time. However, depending on the stage of advancement in the person's illness, the patient's choice regarding resuscitative measures, and in light of the team's clinical and ethical judgements, the best decision is reached.

If there are no reversible causes contributing to the physical deterioration and the terminal phase is established, active management of the patient and family is essential. This management is the same whatever the cause of the terminal phase of illness.

Palliative care of the terminal phase ensures good symptom management and comfort for the patient. It also addresses the concerns and grief of the carers and relatives. The manner of dying can have major effects on subsequent family bereavement (Fakhoury *et al.*, 1997).

Aims of care in the terminal phase

The aims of care in the terminal phase are:

- to facilitate the patient's awareness of the final phase of illness;
- to optimize the patient's comfort;
- to maintain the patient's dignity;
- to prepare the patient's family/carers for this final phase of illness;
- neither to shorten nor to prolong the dying process.

Symptoms in the terminal phase

Table 12.5 presents the frequency of symptoms in the last 48 hours of life, from a survey of 200 consecutive hospice patients (Lichter and Hunt, 1990).

Approach to symptom management

- Rationalizing regular medication – As many dying patients can find swallowing burdensome, unnecessary medications should be discontinued, e.g. thyroxine, iron, hormones, hypoglycaemics. Drugs that are contributing to the patient's comfort should be continued.

Table 12.5 Frequency of symptoms in the final 48 hours of life

Symptom	Frequency (%)
Noisy and moist breathing	56
Pain	51
Restlessness and agitation	42
Incontinence of urine	32
Dyspnoea	22
Retention of urine	21
Sweating	14
Nausea and vomiting	14
Jerking, twitching, plucking	12
Confusion	9

- Reviewing the route of administration of medications – If oral medication is burdensome for the patient, alternative routes should be considered. Subcutaneous administration via the syringe driver is an appropriate route. Rectal or intravenous routes are alternative choices. Prior to converting to the subcutaneous route, it is wise to ensure that the patient and family understand this change together with its indications and benefits; otherwise it can be misinterpreted as contributing to the patient's rapid deterioration.

- Reviewing potentially reversible causes of distress, e.g. checking for retention of urine, impacted rectum, metabolic disorders, infection, and fear.

Management of the terminal phase is influenced by the patient's condition and the patient's needs. It may be necessary to:

- explore the fear of dying if appropriate;

- explore the patient's views on resuscitation if indicated (ideally this is best done long before the terminal phase);

- discuss any unfinished business. This may lie in the legal, financial, interpersonal or spiritual areas. It may be necessary to seek help from the wider multiprofessional team or from outside professionals to address these areas.

- discuss, if appropriate, the place of care – hospital, hospice, home – taking into account the needs or wishes of the patient and the family. The earlier this is discussed the better so as to avoid transferring the patient at the later stage of the terminal phase.

- address the needs of the family/carers. These needs may vary from very little to very complex needs. Sensitive and open communication is essential. Missed opportunities for reconciliation and for farewells can be the cause of complicated bereavement. It is therefore necessary to take the time to explain any changes in the patient's condition, or management, during this phase and to answer any questions families may have. Because of the uncertainty of prognostication it is wise to leave relatively wide limits when informing patients about the exact length of time left.

- frequently review symptoms and alter management when necessary as this phase is a dynamic not a static one. It is important to remember that professional carers also need to acknowledge and share the feelings emerging regarding their experience of this stage of the patient's illness. Mutual support and teamwork are essential for good palliative care (Twycross and Lichter, 1998).

Management of common symptoms
Anxiety, restlessness, and agitation

These symptoms can prove challenging for the doctor (Store *et al.*, 1997). If restlessness and agitation are interpreted by the family or clinical team as increase in pain, an escalation of opioids is indicated. If this is a misinterpretation, opioid toxicity ensues. This may result in further agitation, confusion, and myoclonic jerks. Therefore, accurate clinical assessment of the indication to increase opioids is essential.

If any causative agents for anxiety and restlessness cannot be identified and reversed, they are best managed by benzodiazepines. Midazolam is anxiolytic, sedative, anticonvulsant, and muscle relaxant. It is short acting. The normal starting dose is 2.5–5 mg given either as a bolus or subcutaneously, or via the subcutaneous syringe driver over 24 hours. This dose can be increased and titrated against response. If adequate control of the agitation and restlessness is not achieved by 80 mg in 24 hours, it may be necessary to use an alternative drug. Haloperidol or methotrimeprazine are both sedative and antipsychotic, and may be indicated if adequate clinical response has not resulted from increased midazolam. Haloperidol 1.5–10 mg in 24 hours is given by subcutaneous syringe driver. Methotrimeprazine 12.5–100 mg in 24 hours is given by subcutaneous syringe driver. To achieve a rapid response it is advisable to give an initial bolus dose of either haloperidol or methotrimeprazine.

Death rattle

This is caused by bronchial or pharyngeal secretions in a patient who is no longer able to cough or swallow. It frequently causes distress to family/carers. There is no evidence that it distresses the patient. Hyoscine hydrobromide 0.4 mg subcutaneously to a maximum of 2.4 mg in 24 hours as an antisecretory drug may be helpful in preventing this noisy breathing. Hyoscine can be given as bolus subcutaneous injections or can be added to a syringe driver and given subcutaneously over 24 hours. Hyoscine hydrobromide has both sedative and anti-emetic action. Paradoxical agitation has been reported in some patients.

Other common symptoms

Other common symptoms, such as nausea, vomiting and pain, are managed as already described in the relevant sections.

The role of hydration in the terminal phase

Artificial hydration (IV fluids) may not contribute to a patient's comfort. Dry mouth and thirst relate to adequacy of mouth care rather than electrolyte imbalance. Possible benefits of withdrawing artificial hydration/nutrition are:

- less bronchial rattle
- less vomiting
- less incontinence
- helps family to recognize that death is imminent
- reduces barriers between patient and family.

In reviewing the use of intravenous fluids at this stage of illness, it is important to remember that there are no definite studies to demonstrate that intravenous fluids influence the prognosis of dying patients. One also needs to question whether the administration of intravenous hydration is prolonging life or prolonging the dying process (Dunlop *et al.*, 1995).

It is important to keep open discussions with relatives concerning the administration of hydration if this is an issue for them.

Cultural issues and religious practices

These may be very important to some patients and their families around the time of death. It is essential to be open, respectful, and responsive to these needs.

Good terminal care involves frequent and open communication between patients, families, and professionals. Attention to detail is a central value. If any aspect of management of the terminal phase proves challenging it is important to seek advice from specialist palliative care service or team.

After the patient's death, it is good practice to:

- complete the death certificate promptly and be available to talk to relatives. They frequently have unanswered questions;
- sympathize with relatives and offer bereavement support if appropriate;
- phone the patient's GP as soon as possible to inform him/her of the patient's death.
- discuss aspects of management of the terminal phase, if this has been problematic, with the multidisciplinary team as a means of personal support.

Case histories

Case 1

Agnes, a 62-year-old woman with a 5-month history of an inoperable gastric carcinoma was admitted for pain management and terminal care. She was mobile, cachectic and pale on admission. She had a large palpable mass in her epigastrium. She was fully aware of her condition and her only wish was to be pain free, and as alert as possible to spend the remaining quality time with her family.

She was on MST 200 mg b.d., which gave her moderate pain relief at rest. Her pain greatly increased on moving. She took Sevredol 50 mg for breakthrough pain. Further pain relief was not achieved nor did she develop signs of toxicity on increasing the opioid dose. On changing to the subcutaneous route using morphine to diamorphine 1:3 ratio, she had excellent pain relief at rest. This change of administration route was made on the assumption that because of her gastric tumour and cachexia, she may not have been adequately absorbing the oral opioid.

She continued to have severe pain on movement. Her dose of opioid was increased, to the level of optimal pain relief but with unacceptable drowsiness.

In discussion with her, the opioid was reduced, and a non-opioid added (soluble paracetamol). She was more alert and had acceptable (to her) pain relief for 2 days. As the pain further increased and the terminal phase was imminent, we took the risk of adding a NSAID suppository as an adjuvant drug (Piroxicam 20 mg daily). She remained pain free and fully aware, without the necessity of further increasing the diamorphine in the syringe driver.

This was the last change in her medication as she died peacefully 2 days later.

Case 2

In mid-December, William, a 70-year-old gentleman who had intra-abdominal recurrence of adenocarcinoma in his transverse colon was admitted to a specialist palliative care unit for symptom management and terminal care. He had a 3-week history of nausea, vomiting, and increasing weakness. He had been constipated for 3 days. Physical examination revealed a drowsy, moderately dehydrated, withdrawn, cachectic man. It was difficult to hear his voice as his weakness was all pervading. He did state he felt so weak 'he was better off dead'. A large central modular abdominal mass was palpable with hyperactive bowel sounds.

He had had cyclizine and haloperidol prior to admission, with poor response. A functional small bowel obstruction was the likely diagnosis.

Case histories continued

After some team discussion, a decision was made to commence 24 hours intravenous hydration and a syringe driver with metoclopramide was set up. He was too nauseated initially to tolerate a faecal softener laxative.

His nausea had subsided within 24 hours and he was able to recommence oral intake. He continued to have one large vomitus daily. His bowels began to function again.

The nausea recurred and on the third day his anti-emetic was changed from metoclopramide to methotrimeprazine 12.5 mg in 24 hours in the syringe driver. His nausea was fully reversed but the vomiting continued, though less frequent.

Octreotide 300 μg in 24 hours was added. There was no further recurrence of the vomiting and his mood was noticeably brighter. During his subsequent 4 days stay in the hospital he remained free of gastrointestinal symptoms, his bowels moved intermittently. As he became free of symptoms, his mood lifted and he asked to be allowed home for Christmas day, although still very weak. He had gradually resumed light diet, and despite his ongoing partial bowel obstruction, he felt able to participate with his family in a Christmas dinner.

Further reading

Ashby, M. A. Game, P. A., Devitt, P. *et al.* (1991) Percutaneous gastrostomy as a venting procedure in palliative care. *Palliat Med* 5, 147–50.

Beattie, G. J., Leonard, R. C. F., and Smyth, J. F. (1989) Bowel obstruction in ovarian cancer: a retrospective study and review of the literature. *Palliat Med* 3, 275–80.

British Medical Association (1993) *Medical ethics today: its practice and philosophy*. BMJ Publishing Group, London.

Bruera, E. (1992) Current pharmacological management of anorexia in cancer patients. *Oncology* 6, 125–30.

Buckman, R. (1992) *How to break bad news: a guide for health-care professionals*. Pan Books in association with Macmillan, London.

Corner, J., Plant, H., A'Hern, R., and Bailey, C. (1996) Non-pharmacological interventions for breathlessness in lung cancer. *Palliat Med* 10, 299–305.

Cowher, K. and Hanks, G. W. (1990) Longterm management of respiratory symptoms in advanced cancer. *J Pain Symptom Management* 5, 320–30.

Doyle, D., Hanks, G., and Macdonald, N. (eds) (1998) 2nd ed. *Oxford textbook of palliative medicine*. Oxford University Press, Oxford.

Dunlop, G. M. (1989) A study of the relative frequency and importance of gastro-intestinal symptoms, and weakness in patients with far-advanced cancer. *Palliat Med* 4, 37–43.

Dunlop, R. J., Ellershaw, J., Baines, M. J., Sykes, N., and Saunders, C. M. (1995) On with-holding nutrition and hydration in the terminally ill: has palliative medicine gone too far? *J Med Ethics* 21, 141–3.

European Association for Palliative Care (1989) *Newsletter* No 1.

Fainsinger, R. L., MacEachern, T. and Miller, M. J. *et al.* (1994) The use of hypodermoclysis for rehydration in terminally ill cancer patients. *Journal Pain and Symptom Management* **9** (5), 298–302.

Fakhoury, W., McCarthy, M., and Addington-Hall, J. (1997) The effects of the clinical characteristics of dying cancer patients on informal care givers' satisfaction with palliative care. *Palliat Med* **11**, 107–15.

Ford, G. and Lewin, I. (eds) (1996) *Managing terminal illness*. Royal College of Physicians, London.

Grond, S., Zech, D., Diefenbach, C., Radbruch, L., and Lehmann, K. A. (1996) Assessment of cancer pain: a prospective evaluation in 2266 cancer patients referred to a pain service. *Pain* **64**, 107–14.

Hanks, G. (1998) Opioid analgesic therapy. In Doyle, D., Hanks, G., and Macdonald, N. (eds), *Oxford textbook of palliative medicine 2nd ed.*, p. 332. Oxford University Press, Oxford.

Hanks, G. W., de Gorro, F., Ripamanti, C. *et al.* (1996) Morphine in cancer pain: modes of administration. Expert Working Group of the European Association for Palliative Care. *BMJ* **312**, 823–6.

Higginson, I. (ed.) (1993) *Clinical audit in palliative care*. Radcliffe Medical Press, Oxford and New York.

Hocknell, J. (1997) Anorexia and weakness. In Kaye, P. (ed.), *Tutorials in palliative medicine*, pp. 171–88. EPL Publications, Northampton.

Hull, R., Ellis, M., and Sargent, V. (1989) *Teamwork in palliative care*. Radcliffe Medical Press, Oxford.

Kaye, P. (1992) *A to Z of hospice and palliative medicine*. EPL Publications, Northampton.

Kearney, M. (1992) Palliative medicine just another speciality? *Palliat Med* **6**, 39–46.

Kearney, M. (1996) *Mortally wounded*. Marino Books, Dublin.

Keller, U. (1993) Pathophysiology of cancer cachexia. *Support Care Cancer* **1**, 290–4.

Kubler-Ross, E. (1969) *On death and dying*. Macmillan, New York.

Kubler-Ross, E. (1977) Fifth stage: acceptance. In *On death and dying*, pp. 112–13. Macmillan, New York.

Lichter, I., and Hunt, E. (1990). The last 48 hours of life. *Journal of Palliative Care* **6** (4), 7–15.

Parker, M. C. and Baines, M. J. (1996) Intestinal obstruction in patients with advanced malignant disease. *Br J Surg* **83**, 1–2.

Parkes, C. M. and Weiss, R. S. (1983) Appendix 5. *Recovery from bereavement*. Basic Books, New York.

Randal, F. and Downie, R. S. (1996) *Palliative care ethics: a good companion*. Oxford University Press, London.

Regnard, C. and Tempest, S. (1998) *A guide to symptom relief in advanced disease*, 4th edn. Hochland and Hoschland Ltd, Hale.

Riley, J. and Fallon, M. T. (1994) Octreotide in terminal malignant obstruction of the gastrointestinal tract. *European Journal of Palliative Care* **1**, 23–5.

Ripamanti, C., Bruera, E. (1997) Dyspnoea: Pathophysiology and assessment. *Journal Pain Symptom Management* **13**, 220–32.

Saunders, C. (1989) The philosophy of terminal care. In Saunders, C. (ed.), *The management of terminal malignant disease*, 2nd edn, p. 232. Edward Arnold, London.

Saunders, C. and Sykes, N. (eds) (1993) *The management of terminal malignant disease*, 3rd edn. Hodder and Stoughton, London.

Schug, S. A., Zech, D., Grond, S., Jung, H., and Stobbe, B. (1992) A long term survey of cancer pain patients. *J Pain Symptom Management* 7(5), 259–66.

Stedeford, A. (1984) *Facing death: patients, families and professionals.* Heinemann Medical Books, Oxford.

Store, P., Philip, C., Spruyt, O., and Waight, C. (1997) A comparison of the use of sedatives in a hospital support team and in a hospice. *Palliat Med* 11, 140–4.

Twycross, R. (1997) *Symptom management in advanced cancer.* 2nd ed. Radcliffe Medical Press, Oxford.

Twycross, R. (1997) Symptom management 1. *Introducing palliative care*, 2nd edn, p. 64. Radcliffe Medical Press Ltd, Oxford.

Twycross, R. and Back, I. (1998) Nausea and vomiting in advanced cancer. *Eur J Palliat Care* 5(2), 39–45.

Twycross, R. G., Barkby, G. D., Hallwood, P. M. (1997) The use of low dose levomepromazine (methotrimeprazine) in the management of nausea and vomiting. *Progress in Palliative Care* 5 (2), 49–53.

Twycross, R. G. and Lichter, I. The terminal phase. (1998) In Doyle, D., Hanks, G. W. C., and Macdonald, N. (eds), *Oxford textbook of palliative medicine*, 2nd ed. p. 977–979. Oxford University Press, Oxford.

Waller, A. and Caroline, N. (1996) *Handbook of palliative care in cancer.* Butterworth-Heinemann, Boston.

WHO (1986) Cancer pain relief and palliative care. *WHO Tech Rep Ser* No. 804. WHO, Geneva.

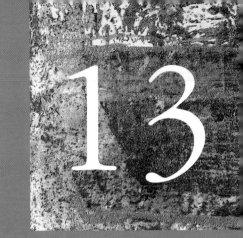

Skin cancer

Ronnie J. Atkinson

- Introduction

- Aetiology of skin tumours

- Diagnosis

- Treatment

- Melanoma

Skin cancer

Introduction

The skin is unique in three ways. First, it is a living covering for the body to protect it from loss of water and injury from light, heat, chemicals, and infectious organisms. Second, it is the main organ for regulating body temperature. Last, apart from the eye, it is the only organ easily visible, making it an excellent model for early diagnosis treatment and prevention.

An understanding of the structure of the skin is important. It has two layers, the epidermis and the dermis, with a basement membrane separating them. The dermis also has two layers – the papillary dermis, adjacent to the basement membrane, and the reticular dermis, next to the subcutaenous fat. This second layer of the dermis consists of connective tissue, blood vessels, lymphatics, nerves, and muscle fibres. The cell types represented in the skin are shown in Table 13.1. Whilst cancers may arise from most of these, only those commonly seen from the epidermis are discussed in detail in this chapter.

Overall, external physical and chemical agents are the most important causes of cancer and the skin is no exception. Again, like most other human cancers, the numbers of skin tumours increases steadily with age. As the age profile of the population becomes more elderly, so skin cancer incidence is increasing. In addition, the erosion of the ozone layer has allowed a significant increase in the amount of UV light to pierce the atmosphere and reach exposed skin. These, plus other social factors, have produced a 3% per year increase in the most dangerous form of skin cancer – melanoma – which seems set to continue for the foreseeable future. This is in stark contrast with a decrease in cancer of another site, the uterine cervix, by 7% per year.

Skin cancer is the most common cancer diagnosed in the UK as well as many other countries. Ironically, many of the common cancers of the skin, apart from

Table 13.1 Cell types in the skin

Epidermis

Squamous

Basal

Melanocytes

Langerhans – immunological, no tumours

Merkel – mechanoreceptors, APUD system

Dermis

Connective tissue – blood vessels, lymphatics, nerve supply

Appendages – hair follicles, sebaceous and exocrine glands

Table 13.2 Tumour aetiology

- Ultraviolet (UV) light
- Genetics
- Atrophic skin lesions
- Chemical carcinogenesis
- Radiation exposure
- Immunosuppression

melanoma, are easily treated and the death rate is low compared to that for other solid tumours. For this reason, skin cancers are often disregarded in solid cancer 'league' tables so, for instance, lung cancer is shown as the leading cancer in males and, more recently, in females. There are more than 40 000 new cases of skin cancer annually in the UK. Most, around 90%, are non-melanomatous cancers.

This chapter looks briefly at some of the common non-melanomatous skin cancers, but will highlight melanoma because it represents such a serious public health problem.

Aetiology of skin tumours

The causes of tumours of the skin are listed in Table 13.2 and are dealt with individually here.

Ultraviolet (UV) light

The UVB spectrum (290–320 nm) is the major carcinogenic wavelength. Basal cell carcinomas (BCC), in particular, but also squamous cell carcinomas (SCC) are more prevalent on light-exposed areas of the body, especially the dorsum of the hands and the face. Many of these are linked to occupation, e.g. farmers and outdoor workers. Areas of vitiligo (depigmentation) lead to increased susceptability. Normally the ozone layer in the stratosphere absorbs UVB from sunlight. Fluorinated hydrocarbons have unfortunately reduced the thickness of the ozone layer, allowing more UVB to pierce the lower layers of the atmosphere and reach ground level (Blumthaler, 1990). Skin is therefore more exposed than ever before to UVB and this is thought to be responsible for some of the increase in skin cancer.

A condition called xeroderma pigmentosa, where there is difficulty in repair of DNA damaged by UV light, is of special interest since skin cancer is increased in these individuals.

Genetics

This is discussed in the section on risk factors for melanoma.

Atrophic skin lesions

As in any other epithelium of the body, cancer can result from skin damage which leads to atrophic lesions. It may also arise in chronic ulceration – breakdown of the epithelium in a recurring cycle of repair and ulceration.

Chemical carcinogenesis

In 1775, Sir Percival Pott described the first occupational skin cancer, that of the scrotal skin in boy chimney sweeps. The cancer was later shown to be due to coal tar irritation of the scrotal folds.

Radiation exposure

In the past, radiotherapy was used to treat the benign conditions of acne and tinea capitis. Later it was found that there was an increased incidence of skin cancer in the treated areas. Because of the inherent dangers, this use of radiation has now been abandoned.

Immunosuppression

Immunosuppressive drugs used to prevent rejection of transplants can cause lymphomatous conditions of the skin such as mycosis fungoides. Recently, the increasing incidence of HIV infection has produced a rise in Kaposi's sarcoma. The appearance of these lesions on the face and neck are a constant reminder to the patient of their disease, as well as leading to the unmasking of the diagnosis socially.

Diagnosis

As with all other medical conditions, good history-taking and clinical examination are paramount. A full general examination of the skin in good light should be carried out, with a meticulous examination of each particular lesion together with the associated regional lymph node drainage areas.

Benign lesions

There are a number of these which do not usually require biopsy.

Seborrhoeic keratosis

These are common and increase in incidence with age. They are brownish lesions, round to oval in shape with a slightly irregular non-shiny surface and a 'waxy or greasy' quality. They often appear to be stuck, like a limpet, on to the skin of the face and trunk. They can usually be treated with liquid nitrogen. Alternatively, curettage may be used with light cautery to achieve haemostasis.

Warts

These are common, viral-induced lesions that often resolve spontaneously. Occasionally biopsy may be required for definitive diagnosis. If persistent, they are treated with liquid nitrogen, though a number of applications may be necessary to achieve success.

Adenoacanthoma

This is a hyperkeratotic tumour, which clinically resembles a squamous cell carcinoma. It usually arises on sun-exposed skin in the central face but also may be seen on the dorsum of the hands and forearms. It is characteristically dome shaped with a central plug of keratin. It usually has a short history of 2–4 weeks and tends to involute spontaneously over the next 4–5 months, often leaving a scar. These features distinguish it from squamous carcinoma, which has a longer history. If there is doubt a wedge biopsy may be necessary.

Pre-malignant lesions

Solar (actinic or senile) keratosis

UVB damages the keratinocytes leading to multiple, red, and rough papules of 1–3 mm in diameter. They tend to arise on sun-exposed areas, especially on the dorsum of the hand, face, neck, and nose. Over a long time they may progress to squamous cell carcinoma. Heaped up lesions require a biopsy but otherwise a watch policy is reasonable.

Malignant lesions

The two most common lesions are the basal cell carcinoma and the squamous cell carcinoma. Of these, the basal cell is the commonest.

Basal cell carcinoma

This starts as a painless translucent pearly nodule with telangiectasia on a sun-exposed area. It grows slowly with local invasion over many years. As it enlarges, it ulcerates, bleeds, and develops a rolled, shiny border. For these reasons, it is often termed a rodent ulcer. Fortunately, metastases are rare. The face is the commonest site.

Squamous cell carcinoma

These are red, irregular, hyperkeratotic tumours that ulcerate late and develop a crust. They generally occur on sun-exposed areas of the head and neck and dorsal extremities. Metastases to local lymph nodes are rare – amounting to 1–2% of cases.

Paget's disease

This important lesion appears as an erythematous, slightly scaly patch that may be pigmented, particularly on the nipple or the genital area, and is easily confused with dermatitis. Biopsy is essential for diagnosis. At the nipple the lesion is usually due to malignant cells having migrated along the ducts from a breast carcinoma to lie in the skin.

Skin metastases

These are subcutaneous tumours that have seeded to the skin from another primary site. The diagnosis is usually made on a biopsy and by a process of exclusion. A thorough search must be made for the primary site since it may be treatable, e.g. a lymphoma.

Treatment

Treatment is usually tailored to suit the situation, with the aim of eradicating the local disease and obtaining the best functional and cosmetic result. Cure rates for non-melanomatous lesions are in the 90–99% range.

The main modes of treatment are surgery and/or radiotherapy to achieve local control. Decisions are usually based on size, location, and aggressiveness of the tumour, as well as patient suitability for the procedure. All tumours should have histological confirmation.

Surgery

Surgery offers a single procedure with a high cure rate. The aim is to remove the lesion completely. Frozen section examination can give immediate indication of marginal involvement. If the margins are not clear, then further excision must be carried out as soon as possible. Healing may be by primary closure or secondary intention.

Radiotherapy

Radiotherapy, using an electron beam which has limited depth of penetration (the exact depth is dependent on energy selected), can produce excellent results but needs to encompass the lesion and provide a margin of 10–15 mm surrounding it. Usually multiple visits to the radiotherapy centre are needed for fractions of treatment. A total dose of 45 Gray over 3 weeks in 3 Gray daily fractions would be a typical example. Where biologically equivalent doses are given in shorter periods of time, the cosmetic result tends to be less satisfactory but such a compromise may be necessary in elderly patients or where long distance of travel is a problem.

Radiotherapy is a good choice for a patient who would not be keen or fit for surgery. It is less suitable where bone, cartilage, or tendons are involved because of the danger of radionecrosis. Radiation is used in locations such as the eyelids and tip of the nose where surgical excision involves extensive reconstruction. It is also useful where, following surgery, the histology shows tumour involvement of the surgical margins. Individual lead shields are made for each patient to protect the adjacent skin.

Melanoma

Melanoma is a neoplasm of the epidermal melanocyte whose primary function in the skin is to protect the body from excessive UV light. Embryologically, melanocyte stem cells migrate from the neural crest in the fetus to the dermo-epidermal junction. They are also found at non-cutaneous sites, e.g. mucous membranes, the eye, in the CNS, and in lymph node capsules. Therefore, although growth abnormalities most commonly occur in the skin, they can sometimes become manifest in any of these other sites. The melanocyte produces the brown-black pigment melanin from tyrosine via dehydroxyphenylalanine (DOPA). It has a protective effect, absorbing UV photons and reactive oxygen radicals produced by sunlight. The melanin is secreted into melanosomes and transported to the surrounding keratinocytes by dendritic projections. In cells the melanin forms supranuclear 'caps', which protect the nuclei from UV damage. The pathway is usually activated by UV radiation – a single exposure gives an increase in activity and size of existing melanocytes. Repeated exposure gives a further increase and eventually causes melanocyte numbers to increase. Negro melanocytes constantly produce large amounts of melanin.

Skin melanomas were comparatively rare but have recently assumed greater importance because of the year-on-year increase in incidence of some 2–5% in white people. This is a greater rate of increase than that of all other malignancies except lung cancer in females. In the UK, melanomas increased from 2239 cases annually to 4114 cases between 1980 and 1989 – a rise of 84% (Cancer Research Campaign, 1995). There has been a steady, though lower, increase in death rates. The increase is worldwide and has affected men more than women. Figures from the American Cancer Society for 1995 show 34 100 new cases of melanoma and approximately 7200 deaths (Wingo *et al.*, 1995).

The lesions tend to behave more aggressively than either BCC or SCC. In contrast to BCC and SCC, young adults are affected as well as older age groups; 45% occur in the under 60s compared with 20% of other skin cancers. The incidence varies around the world and correlates with latitude. Australia currently has the highest incidence of 17 cases per 100 000 per year. Studies, especially from Australia, have shown that prevention as well as early removal of thin skin lesions could significantly improve morbidity and mortality. Sadly, apart from these two measures, there has been little progress in treatment.

Risk factors

Skin types

Of those shown in Table 13.3, people with fair skin, which tends to burn easily and tan poorly, are at greatest risk. The closer to the equator, the higher the incidence of melanoma for similar skin colour. Severe sunburns, similar to radiation damage, appear to be cumulative, particularly in childhood. The skin may be permanently damaged in that area so that it loses its elasticity, becomes thinner, and is more likely to develop pigmented moles or naevi. It is hypothesized that melanoma is induced by acute sun exposure after a long period of non-exposure – the typical annual sunshine holiday that has become so popular over the last several decades. By contrast, BCC and SCC are caused by the prolonged sun exposure seen in outdoor workers (Gilchrest *et al.*, 1999).

Moles may arise in normal skin, in benign pigmented naevi, dysplastic naevi or congenital melanocytic naevi. The last two are thought to be melanoma precursors. Moles (naevi) are thin lesions – no more than 1 mm in depth but with a diameter usually greater than 5 mm. They are rare in children. In female adults they

Table 13.3 Six skin types

Type 1	Always burns, never tans – white skin
Type 2	Initially burns, difficult tanning – white skin
Type 3	Rarely burns, easily tanned – white skin
Type 4	Never burns, always tans – white skin
Type 5	Brown skin
Type 6	Black skin

occur mainly on the lower extremities and in males mainly on the trunk. Wherever they arise, although initially benign, they may undergo change to become established melanomas. This is often imperceptible. Most melanomas are thought to arise in a single transformed melanocyte. The growth is initially in the horizontal axis at the basal lamina, known as the radial growth phase, and is non-metastatic. The duration of this phase varies with aggressiveness. Eventually, dermal invasion ensues as the vertical growth phase takes over, leading to metastatic potential.

Genetics

Individuals with a family history of melanoma are at greater risk of developing the disease. In addition, they have an earlier age of onset and a higher incidence of developing multiple primary melanomas. Around 10% of patients with melanoma have a family history and an autosomal dominant gene with incomplete penetrance is likely. Xeroderma pigmentosa (mentioned above) is an autosomal recessive condition.

Chromosomal alterations of the short arm of chromosome 1 as well as both arms of 6 and 7 and a 9p21 deletion have been found in melanoma tumours and cell lines (Goldstein *et al.*, 1994). Interestingly, some of the mutations in *MTS1*, a tumour suppressor gene identified by Kamb *et al.* (1994) and mapping to 9p21, are specific for ultraviolet-induced DNA damage.

Melanoma types

There are four types classified on growth patterns – superficial spreading, nodular, lentigo maligna and acral lentiginous. Each has a unique natural history and features.

Superficial spreading or flat melanoma (SSM)

This is the commonest type at about 70% (Fig. 13.1). It usually arises in a pre-existing naevus or dysplastic naevus and develops over 3–5 years. The shape changes, the edge becoming irregular. The surface shows dark areas with colour variation and it becomes rough or even ulcerated. The lesion develops over a number of years.

Nodular

Whilst relatively rare at 10–20%, this is the second most common type and the most aggressive (Fig. 13.2). It usually appears on normal skin and grows quickly; the volume may double in a few months. It is typically blue/black, raised, or dome shaped, and may look as if it is stuck on to the skin. This is because it lacks the radial growth phase. There are no melanocyte abnormalities in the adjacent epidermis, so the margins are clearly demarcated. The exception to this is where a nodule develops in a superficial spreading melanoma though the nodule growth rate is again aggressive.

Lentigo maligna melanoma (LMM)

LMM (4–10% of melanomas) is usually seen on sun-exposed skin, especially on the face in the elderly and often in females. It arises in a lentigo maligna (melan-

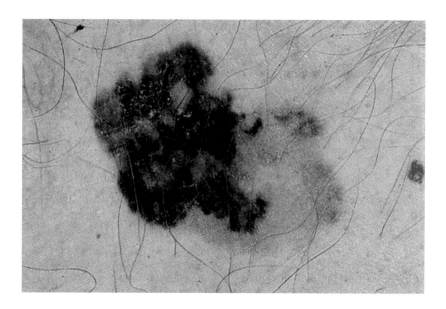

Fig. 13.1 Superficial spreading melanoma.

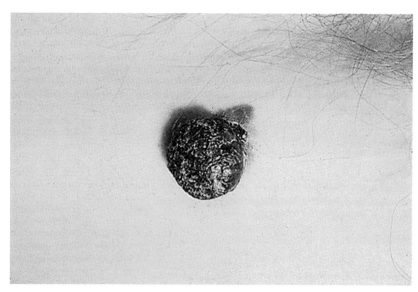

Fig. 13.2 Nodular melanoma.

otic freckle) that has been present for a long time. Since there is a prolonged radial phase, the lesions are generally flat, irregular in shape and large – up to 3 cm. The colour tends to be light to dark brown. The lesions develop over decades.

Acral lentiginous melanoma (ALM)

ALM (2–8% in whites but 35–60% in blacks) occur on the palms, soles, and sub-ungal areas, and are usually large (> 3 cm diameter) and aggressive. The subungal lesions have a particularly evil reputation. Early lesions may appear similar to LMM, but late lesions have a rapid vertical growth phase, giving ulceration and fungation. Metastatic spread of such a lesion, following amputation, is shown in Fig. 13.3.

Melanomas may arise at 'hidden sites' such as the vulva as well as at extra-dermatological sites, e.g. mucosal surfaces and in the orbit. These will not be discussed further here.

Clinical presentation

Clinically the lesions become larger, darker, and gradually develop an irregular outline. They also become thicker and gradually rise above the skin surface to become palpable. Like an iceberg, a lesion palpable above the surface is likely to have a much larger component below. This invades into the dermis to gain early access to lymph vessels and the bloodstream, enabling systemic spread to other organs such as liver, lungs, brain, and bone. On close inspection, in a good light, the surface of a melanoma often has a mottled appearance. The dark areas represent actively growing disease and are overproducing pigment, whereas the adjacent light-coloured areas have undergone regression with some resolution of pigment. Eventually bleeding from the surface may occur. This is usually a late and sinister sign since it indicates dermal spread and vascular involvement.

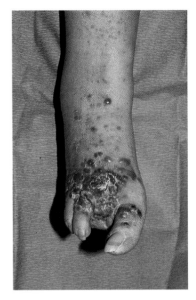

Fig. 13.3 Metastatic spread.

Clinical Diagnosis

Clinical diagnosis is based on appearance. No symptoms are expected with early lesions.

There are four criteria (ABCD) for diagnosis of melanoma in a mole (Cascinelli *et al.*, 1987):

- A – asymmetry of shape;
- B – border notching (sharp and irregularly serrated);
- C – colour darkening (brown, black, or dark blue with uneven distribution);
- D – diameter enlargement (usually in excess of 7–9 mm).

Clinical examination should include examination for satellite lesions in the skin between the lesion and the regional lymph nodes, nodal enlargement, distant skin metastases, or hepatosplenomegaly.

Staging

This has advanced from the older anatomical staging of localized, regional, and disseminated to TNM staging and on to more refined systems of measurement that accurately describe the histological extent within the excised skin. The depth of invasion, thickness in millimetres, any ulceration, and growth patterns are all important features. Where there is no lymph node involvement, thickness in millimetres is of over-riding importance, correlating well with prognosis.

Clark *et al.* (1969) developed the first system of depth measurement known as Clark levels. There are five levels of invasion. Level 1 (melanoma in situ) lies totally within the dermis and shows no invasion. Invasion into the papillary dermis is level 2, to the papillary-reticular dermis function is level 3, to the reticular dermis is level 4 and finally to the subcutaneous fat is level 5. These are shown in Fig. 13.4.

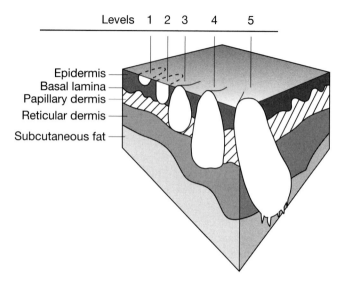

Fig. 13.4 Clark levels.

Breslow (1970) made the depth measurement more accurate and reproducible by using an ocular micrometer to document it in millimetres. The vertical thickness (Breslow thickness) is measured from the epidermal granular layer (or the base of the lesion if there is ulceration) to the deepest melanoma cell identified.

Anatomical stage, TNM stage, Breslow measurement and Clark level have all been combined by the American Joint Committee on Cancer (AJCC) as shown in Table 13.4.

Table 13.4 New staging system for melanoma adopted by the American Joint Committee on Cancer

Stage	Description
1A	Localized melanoma 0.75 mm or level II* (T1N0M0)
1B	Localized melanoma 0.76–1.5 mm or level III* (T2N0M0)
IIA	Localized melanoma 1.5–4 mm or level IV* (T3N0M0)
IIB	Localized melanoma > 4 mm or level V* (T4N0M0)
III	Limited nodal metastases involving only one regional lymph node basin, or fewer than 5 in-transit metastases without nodal metastases (any T.N1M0)
IV	Advanced regional metastases (any T.N2M0) or any patient with distant metastases (any T, any N, M1 or M2)

*When the thickness and level of invasion criteria do not coincide within a T classification, thickness should take precedence.

Used with the permission of the American Joint Committee on Cancer (AJCC), Chicago, Illinois. The original source for this material is the AJCC Cancer Staging Manual, 5th edition (1997) published by Lippincott-Raven Publishers, Philadelphia, Pennsylvania.

Table 13.5 Prognostic factors in melanoma

Depth
Sex
Age
Site
Type
Ulceration
Regression
Clinical stage

Prognosis

Balch *et al.* (1992) carried out a prognostic analysis on 8500 patients with cutaneous malignant melanoma. The main factors are summarized in Table 13.5 and elaborated below.

Depth (thickness)

This is the most important factor affecting prognosis. The survival of patients with melanomas up to 0.75 mm is excellent. Fig. 13.5 shows that survival with thin lesions (< 1.5 mm) where the chance of metastasis is low, is good with 5-year survival in excess of 90%. For a number of reasons, diagnosis tends to be delayed and most lesions when excised are thicker than this. The deeper the lesion, the worse the outlook. Overall, the 5-year relative survival is therefore much lower at 52% for men and 75% for women.

Sex

The incidence tends to be equal for both sexes where sun exposure is the predominant factor in aetiology, e.g. USA and Australia. However, there is an excess of females in many countries where the climate has less sunshine. Females have a better prognosis than males, independent of other variables.

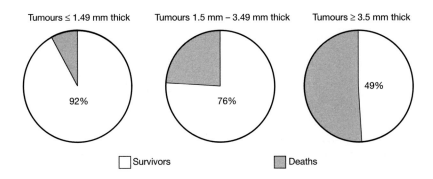

Fig. 13.5 Survival related to depth of invasion (reproduced with permission from Cancer Research Campaign (1995).

Age

Melanoma is extremely rare in childhood but it does affect young adults. Twenty per cent of cases occur in the age group 15–39 years. Males over 50 years have the worse prognosis.

Site

In contrast to non-melanomatous skin cancers, which mainly occur on the head and neck, a high percentage of melanomas occur on unexposed sites. The most common site for males is the trunk and for females the lower limb. Extremity sites (limbs) have a better prognosis than axial sites, e.g. head, neck, and trunk.

Type

A nodular melanoma (see Fig. 13.2) or a nodular component within the lesion is usually the fastest growing element and should be treated with respect, remembering that projection above the surface is a sign of greater growth below it.

Ulceration

This is late in the history of the lesion and is a bad prognostic sign, especially if accompanied by bleeding, since it almost certainly means that there has been invasion into the deep layers of the dermis.

Stage

Thin lesions have a better prognosis than thick ones as shown in Fig. 13.5.

Management

Surgery is the treatment of choice, first, to make a definitive diagnosis, and second, to remove the lesion. Pigmented naevi are best excised *in toto*. Local anaesthetic is used and a diagnostic excision is performed. An ellipse of skin is incised 1–2 mm clear of the margins in a downward 'V' shape extending below the lesion to the subcutaneous fat. Once removed, direct closure of the 'V' deficit can be achieved.

If histology confirms a diagnosis of melanoma of less than 2 mm depth and clear margins then the patient can be followed up. If the margins are clear and it is thicker than 2 mm or where the lesion is clinically an obvious melanoma then a wider excision is carried out and the patient followed up. Where the lesion is on the distal region of a digit, then amputation of the finger or toe is the best way to achieve adequate clearance.

Where cervical, axillary, or inguinal/iliac lymph nodes are enlarged, fine needle aspiration of the nodes can be performed as well as investigation for evidence of widespread disease. If the nodes prove positive with no evidence of other disease, then radical dissection of the appropriate group is performed. Unfortunately, these are mutilating operations with considerable extra patient morbidity.

Recently, an innovative procedure has been introduced to provide a more precise approach to lymphadenectomy. Lymphoscintigraphy (Morton *et al.*, 1992) is used to identify the first drainage or 'sentinel node(s)' within a group of nodes. Sentinel node biopsy gives material for histology, immunohistochemical or other detection such as molecular examination. If positive, the nodal metastases can then be treated by regional lymphadenectomy.

Local recurrences

These can be surgically excised. Depending on the size of the deficit, skin graft may be required. A thorough search must be made for distant metastases.

Distant metastases

In spite of the apparent immunological phenomena associated with the disease, melanoma has been notoriously resistant to treatment with any other modality. With radiotherapy, for instance, a 'shoulder' of resistance has to be overcome by increasing the fractional dose before response is seen. Individual lesions can be made to shrink using this technique. It is an important treatment to avoid skin ulceration, stop bleeding, or relieve pain, and so is mainly used for palliation.

Treatment

This involves health care workers as well as every member of the general public having a high index of suspicion and reporting any change in moles. If a lesion is suspect then it must be excised *in toto* with a margin of 1 cm for lesions up to 1 mm and 3 cm for thicker lesions with submission for histology. It is too dangerous to cut it off without histology or to take a piece of the lesion as a biopsy.

Adjuvant therapy

Patients with thick lesions or nodal involvement are at greater than 50% risk of recurrence, systemic disease, and death within 5 years, so adjuvant therapy should be considered as part of a good clinical trial where full assessment is being carried out.

This is the one cancer where historically there is more documented evidence of spontaneous regression than any other (Everson and Cole, 1966). The regressions are thought to be due to the expression of antigens recognized as foreign on the melanoma cells by the immune system, which then mounts an attack against them. The mottled appearance of the lesions clinically, with evidence of regression under the microscope, bears further testimony to the phenomenon.

Many attempts have been made to try to enhance the host recognition and/or immunological response to melanoma cells. Historically the literature abounds with reports that non-specific immunostimulants such as Bacillus Calmette–Guérin (BCG) and *Corynebacterium parvum* (*C. parvum*) can cause regression. Unfortunately, in most instances the individual lesions which were injected regressed, but the systemic disease was unaffected to eventually become manifest elsewhere. No survival advantage has been shown so far with or without chemotherapy. Similarly, immunomodulators such as levamisole as single agents or in combination with chemotherapy have not proved effective.

In the early 1980s it was hypothesized that high-dose adjuvant recombinant interferon (rIFN-α) might reduce the recurrence rate in stage III patients who were at high risk following curative surgery. Large multicentre trials were initiated in Europe and the USA between 1983 and 1990 to answer as many of the questions posed as possible. The Eastern Cooperative Oncology Group (ECOG) study, E1684, was the only study to show significant benefit. This compared 20 MIUs/m^2 rINF-α2b given IV 5 days per week for 4 weeks, followed by maintenance of 10 MIUs/m^2 SC three times weekly for the remainder of one year to an observation group (Hillner *et al.*, 1997). However, interim results of a more recent study are less encouraging and the final results are eagerly awaited.

Treatment of metastatic melanoma

Resistance to chemotherapy has been almost universal with all the available agents. Response rates of 15–20% to dacarbazine, considered the most effective drug, have been achieved. Multidrug therapy or high-dose therapy with stem-cell harvest generally has not shown better responses and is usually associated with greater toxicity.

Because of this, effort has concentrated on imaginative manipulation of the immune system. This has usually consisted of attempts at mimicking the physiology of the immune response to raise it beyond the normal and so make it more effective. Lymphocyte-activated killer (LAK cells) have been extracted from peripheral blood or tumour-infiltrating lymphocytes (TILs) have been extracted *in vitro* from tumour masses, incubated with interleukin-2 (IL-2) and re-infused. Unfortunately IL-2 causes capillary leak syndrome and in addition the LAK cells may not be specific enough. While some spectacular regressions have been achieved, many severe life-threatening side-effects have ensued. The results are not reproducible and the procedures remain complex, expensive, and controversial. IL-2 and LAK cells have been almost totally abandoned. There is, however, still interest in TIL cells since they appear to be more specific. Rosenberg *et al.* (1988) achieved a clinical response rate of 60% in 15 patients and 40% in 55 evaluable patients. However, the disease tends to recur in almost all patients within months.

In a less aggressive approach, interferon has been used for advanced disease and has produced regressions. A dose of 3–10 million International Units (MIU) subcutaneously (SC) three times per week has been found to be well tolerated and gives responses in about one-third of patients. The patient or district nurse can give the treatment at home, so avoiding hospital admission.

In another approach, vaccines made from partially purified melanoma antigens extracted from melanoma cell lines have been combined with adjuvants to try to boost their effectiveness when given to patients with advanced disease. At the time of writing they still remain investigational and they are not in routine clinical use. Entry of patients to properly organized clinical trials is essential to progress in our understanding of the effectiveness or otherwise of these innovations.

Prevention

Because treatment of the established disease is so limited, primary prevention has assumed great importance. Australia, with the highest incidence, has targeted children and adolescents with primary prevention programmes to protect them from excessive sun exposure. This has included sunscreen sprays on the beach, although sunscreens, whilst useful, should not be used as the sole protection. Natural protection, by avoidance of the sun during the two hours around mid-day, use of wide brimmed hats and clothing, as well as natural shade, are all useful measures. Local planning authorities need to be constantly reminded of the need to provide adequate shade.

In most instances, the condition is preventable by early detection and excision so this offers a second approach. Public awareness campaigns have been mounted in the UK (Mackie and Hole, 1992) with some success in terms of the removal of increased numbers of thin lesions, a fall in the number of thick lesions and a reduction in melanoma-related mortality amongst women. Such campaigns cause a significant rise in clinic workload (Melia *et al.*, 1995). In the USA, similar programmes have been attempted and Wender (1995) has summarized some of the obstacles encountered.

Case history

This patient has a pigmented skin lesion on the posterior aspect of his left knee. Please see and advise.

History

The patient was a male age 35 years who played rugby. He had noticed a pigmented lesion behind his left knee but it had been present 'for as long as he could remember'. Other members of the team had noticed the lesion becoming more prominent. Indeed, a colleague had jokingly mentioned to him that he could be recognized in the scrum by the mole. Recently it had become larger, darker, as well as itchy, and had bled on one occasion.

Examination

There were two abnormalities on clinical examination:

- a black pigmented lesion 1.5 cm in diameter on the skin of the posterior aspect of the left knee, elevated above the skin surface with a rough crust and an irregular margin.
- a single mobile, non-tender enlarged lymph node in the left groin which the patient claimed he had not noticed.

Management

A presumptive diagnosis of melanoma was made. An urgent chest x-ray and CT scan were requested. Routine blood tests were checked including liver function tests. No abnormalities were noted in any of these.

Arrangements were made, in parallel to these tests, for excision biopsy of the lesion with a 3 cm margin. Fine needle aspiration of the groin nodes was carried out. Histology showed the skin lesion to be Clark level 3 and cytology on the aspirate was positive for melanoma cells.

Case history continued

A radical dissection of the lymph nodes from the left groin followed. Three out of seven nodes were infiltrated with melanoma.

Since the best treatment following surgery for advanced disease is unknown, the situation was discussed fully with the patient and his wife by the surgeon and oncologist together. The patient sought information from other sources including 'alternative medicine' and the internet. He eventually decided to enter a clinical trial of interferon, which was one of the options offered by the oncologist. He remained well for 18 months and had a good quality of life (ECOG1) on the interferon. However, he gradually developed loss of power in the right hand. CT scan of brain demonstrated two metastases in the left cerebral hemisphere. He obtained good symptom relief from dexamethasone 4 mg q.i.d. followed by cranial irradiation and lived a further 6 months.

Notes

Because of the unusual site of the lesion, this patient was not as aware of the changes occurring as he might have been. If his rugby colleagues had mentioned it earlier and especially the fact that it was becoming more obvious, the whole scenario could have been prevented by early surgical excision. Prevention is always better than cure.

Further reading

Balch, C. M., Soong, S. -J., Shaw, H. M., Urist, M. M., and McCarthy, W. H. (1992) An analysis of prognostic factors in 8500 patients with malignant melanoma. In Balch, C. M., Houghton, A. N., Milton, G. W., Sober, A. J., and Soong, S.-J. (eds), *Cutaneous melanoma*, 2nd edn. pp. 165–87. J. B. Lippincott, Philadelphia.

Blumthaler, M. and Ambach, W. (1990) Indication of increasing solar ultraviolet B radiation flux in alpine regions. *Science* 248, 206–8.

Breslow, A. (1970) Thickness, cross sectional areas and depth of invasion in the prognosis of cutaneous melanoma. *Ann Surg* 172, 902–8.

Cancer Research Campaign. (1995) Factsheet 4.1/4.2. obtainable from 10 Cambridge Terrace, London NW1 4JL.

Cascinelli, N., Clementie, C., and Belli, F. (1995) Cutaneous melanoma. In Peckham, M., Pinedo, H., and Veronesi, U. (eds), *Oxford textbook of oncology*, Vol. 1, pp. 902–29. Oxford University Press, London.

Clark, W. W., Bernardino, E. A., and Mihm, M. C. (1969) The histogenesis and biological behavior of primary human malignant melanoma of the skin. *Cancer Res* 29, 705–27.

Everson, T. C. and Cole, W. H. (1966) *Spontaneous regression of cancer*. Saunders, Philadelphia.

Gilchrest, B. A., Eller, M. S., Geller, A. C., and Yaar, M. (1999) Mechanisms of disease: the pathogenesis of melanoma induced by ultraviolet radiation. *N Engl J Med* 340, 1341–8.

Goldstein, A. M., Dracopoli, N. C., Engelstein, M., Fraser, M. C., Clark, W. H. Jr, and Tucker, M. A. (1994) Linkage of cutaneous malignant melanoma/dysplastic nevi to chromosome 9p, and evidence for genetic heterogeneity. *Am J Hum Genet* 54, 489–96.

Hillner, B. E., Kirkwood, J. M., Atkins, B. M., Johnson, E. R., and Smith, T. J. (1997) Economic analysis of adjuvant interferon alfa-2b in high-risk melanoma on projections from Eastern Cooperative Oncology Group 1684. *J Clin Oncol* **15**, 2351–8.

Kamb, A., Gruis, N. A., Weaver-Feldhaus, J., *et al.* (1994) A cell cycle regulator potentially involved in genesis of many tumor types. *Science* **264**, 436–40.

MacKie, R. M. and Hole, D. (1992) Audit of public education campaign to encourage earlier detection of malignant melanoma. *Br Med J* **304**, 1012–15.

Melia, J., Cooper, E. J., Frost, T., *et al.* (1995) Cancer Research Campaign health education programme to promote the early detection of cutaneous malignant melanoma. I: Work-load and referral patterns. *Br J Dermatol* **132**, 405–13.

Morton, D. L., Essner, R., Kirkwood, J. M., and Parker, R. G. (1996) Malignant melanoma. In Holland, J. F. (ed.), *Cancer medicine*, pp. 2467–97. Williams & Wilkins, Baltimore.

Rosenberg, S. A., Packard, B., Aerbersold, P. M., *et al.* (1988) Use of tumor-infiltrating lymphocytes and interleukin-2 in the immunotherapy of patients with metastatic melanoma. A preliminary report. *N Engl J Med* **319**, 1676–80.

Wender, R. C. (1995) Barriers to effective skin cancer detection. *Cancer* **75**, 691–8.

Wingo, P. A., Tong, T., and Bolden, S. (1995) Cancer statistics *CA* **45**, 8.

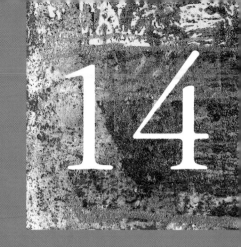

14

Head and neck cancer
Ruth Eakin

- Introduction

- Epidemiology

- Aetiology

- Prevention

- Anatomy

- Pathology

- Presentation

- Examination

- Diagnosis

- Staging

- Treatment

- Side-effects of treatment

- Prognosis

Head and neck cancer

Introduction

Cancers of the head and neck account for 4% of all malignancies. They are a heterogeneous group of tumours, and can be divided into the following sites:

- skin and lip
- oral cavity
- oropharynx
- larynx
- hypopharynx
- nasopharynx
- salivary glands
- nasal cavity and paranasal sinuses
- external auditory meatus and middle ear.

The impact of these cancers on psychological, physical, and social functioning cannot be understated. The disfigurement from the disease or treatment can be enormous, although continuing improvements in surgical techniques and prostheses are resulting in better cosmetic results. It is hoped that improvements in radiotherapy, such as altered fractionation and 3-D conformal therapy, will also help to reduce treatment related morbidity.

Epidemiology

There are more than 5000 new cases of head and neck cancer per year, throughout the UK, with around 2000 registered deaths per annum. It is up to three to four times more common in males than in females, and most cases tend to occur from the fifth decade of life onwards. Some of the rarer tumours, such as nasopharyngeal carcinomas and salivary gland tumours, occur in the younger age groups. The overall incidence is currently rising in females and declining in males. Oral cancer is commonest worldwide in the Indian subcontinent, and this is thought to be related to the high incidence of betel nut chewing. More than 20% of patients develop a second or third primary tumour, most often within the oral cavity, because of the susceptibility of the mucosa to carcinomatous change.

Aetiology

Tobacco

This is the main factor associated with the development of head and neck cancers, with 90% of patients giving a history of smoking. Over 30 carcinogenic agents have been identified in tobacco smoke, and the larynx is the most vulnerable site in the head and neck. The floor of mouth is also a high-risk site, from cigarette smoke. Pipe smoking is particularly associated with carcinoma of the lip, tongue, and floor of mouth. Snuff and chewing tobacco, are also implicated.

Alcohol

The fact that smokers often drink significant amounts of alcohol makes it difficult to assess how much risk is contributed from either factor alone. In any case, they are thought to act synergistically. Alcohol intake predisposes to oral cavity and hypopharyngeal tumours, whilst the combination of alcohol and tobacco increases the risk of all forms by as much as 15 times.

Environment

Given the close physical association of our environment to structures of the head and neck, it is not surprising that environmental factors are important. Air that is breathed, food and drink that are consumed, smoking and chewing, all interact directly, but the combination of tobacco and alcohol appears to be the most prominent. There is also a well-recognized association between the furniture industry and malignancies of the paranasal sinuses. Exposure to polycyclic hydrocarbons, as in the textile industry, has been linked to tumours of the oral cavity.

Diet

There is much less certainty around dietary factors, although there is some suggestion that poor nutrition plays its role. This may well be linked to insufficient intake of vitamin A or C, or β-carotene. Aetiological studies are difficult to carry out in this area because of changing eating habits and inherent difficulty in gathering precise data. Nonetheless, iron-deficiency anaemia has been shown to be a predisposing factor for post-cricoid carcinomas.

Viruses

Human papilloma virus (HPV) has been detected in squamous cell carcinomas of the head and neck, and Epstein–Barr virus (EBV) is well recognized in association with nasopharyngeal carcinoma (see below).

Genetics

Genetic susceptibility to head and neck cancer has been studied, and needs to be considered as a possible factor, either alone or in conjunction with tobacco smoking. It can be manifest in the inheritance of clearly defined cancer-susceptibility syndromes, DNA repair defects, alterations of carcinogen-metabolizing capabilities, or changes in host immunological responses. The activity of glutathione-S-transferase μ (GST-μ), a detoxifying enzyme, when reduced in smokers, has been found to correlate with an increased risk of developing laryngeal cancer.

Nasopharyngeal carcinomas (NPC) are aetiologically distinct. Association with the presence of EBV is unique. High antibody titres against the EBV-viral capsid antigen (VCA) and the EBV-induced diffuse component of the early antigen complex occur commonly in undifferentiated NPC. These titres have proved useful not only in diagnosis, but also in monitoring disease progress, and in follow-up. Predicting relapse after initial therapy and the possible use of titres in screening have also been investigated. Unlike other tumours of the head and neck, NPC are not associated with significant tobacco and alcohol consumption, and there is no increased risk of second primary tumours in those patients who have been treated for NPC. Diets rich in salted fish have been implicated, hence the increased incidence in the Far East. Environmental factors are thought to play more of a role than genetic factors such as histocompatibility antigens.

Prevention

- Reduction of cigarette smoking, especially combined with alcohol intake, would do more in the way of prevention than any other approach.
- Improving the nutritional status, particularly of the lower socioeconomic groups, could well help to reduce the incidence in this high-risk group.
- Retinoids have been used in an attempt to suppress the carcinogenic pathways. Although there have been some encouraging reports of reduced risk of secondary carcinomas in those patients who have been treated with surgery or radiotherapy for squamous cell carcinomas of the oral cavity, oropharynx, larynx, and hypopharynx, the place of this type of treatment is still not yet adequately defined.

Anatomy

The anatomy of the head and neck region is complex, yet a clear, three-dimensional concept is very important for the understanding of the location of tumours, potential areas of local spread, and lymphatic drainage (Fig. 14.1). A full description of the anatomy is outside the scope of this text, although a few key points are worth making.

- The posterior one-third, or base of tongue, is not mobile, and tumours involving this part are much more likely to spread to local lymph node stations at an earlier stage of the natural history. They also have more of a tendency to spread bilaterally, because of extensive lymphatic pathways which cross the midline.
- The maxillary sinus is bounded by the following:
superiorly – floor of orbit and infra-orbital nerve
inferiorly – hard palate and alveolar process of the maxilla
medially – lateral wall of nasal cavity
anterolaterally – skin and fascia of cheek
- The nasopharynx is formed into the shape of a truncated pyramid, being related superiorly to the sphenoid sinus and basal part of the occipital bone. The third and sixth cranial nerves run in the cavernous sinus in this region, thus extension of a nasopharyngeal tumour superiorly may cause cranial nerve palsies. The inferior boundary is the hard and soft palate, and posteriorly lies the retropharyngeal space containing nodes of Rouviere, which are directly anterior to the lateral processes of atlas. In this region, the ninth and twelfth nerves run through the carotid sheath. The lateral walls are where the Eustachian tubes emerge, in the fossa of Rosenmuller, through which spread can occur into the parapharyngeal space and pterygoid muscles.
- The major lymphatic chains in the neck run parallel to the jugular veins, accessory nerve, and facial artery, through to the submandibular triangle (Fig. 14.2). Regions of the neck are subdivided into levels as follows:

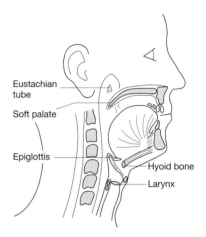

Fig. 14.1 Anatomical relationships of the head and neck structures.

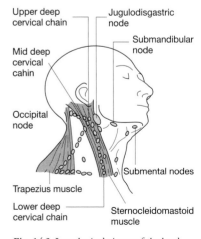

Fig. 14.2 Lymphatic drainage of the head and neck.

level I – submental and submandibular triangles, bordered by the midline, anterior and posterior belly of the digastric muscle, mandible and hyoid bone;

level II – subdigastric area down to the carotid bifurcation, and from the jugular foramen to the posterior border of sternocleidomastoid muscle. It also includes the upper posterior cervical triangle;

level III – from the posterior border of sternocleidomastoid to omohyoid muscle, stretching along the jugular vein between the carotid artery and its bifurcation;

level IV – below omohyoid muscle down to the level of the clavicle, anterior to omohyoid and posterior to the carotid vessels;

level V – from posterior edge of sternocleidomastoid muscle to trapezius muscle, and between the posterior belly of omohyoid to entrance of the spinal accessory nerve. This is the posterior cervical triangle.

Pathology

Approximately 90% of all malignant tumours of the head and neck are squamous cell carcinomas of variable differentiation. Well-differentiated tumours show a large degree of keratinization, whereas poorly differentiated tumours are sparsely keratinized. There are variants as well, such as verrucous carcinoma, which occurs most commonly on the larynx. Other important factors are presence of vascular or lymphatic channel invasion, degree of inflammatory infiltrate, and appearance of the tumour edges.

Pre-malignancy

Leukoplakia is the commonest form of premalignant lesion, and appears as a white plaque. It consists of hyperkeratosis associated with different degrees of underlying epithelial hyperplasia, and progresses to carcinoma in situ or invasive malignancy in up to 40% of cases. If there are no associated dysplastic changes, the chance of transformation is markedly reduced.

Salivary gland tumours
Pleomorphic adenoma

This benign tumour accounts for 75% of all parotid tumours, and is commonly located in the superficial lobe of the parotid gland. The histological features are typically varied, but there are usually mixed features of epithelial and mesenchymal elements. Careful histological examination is required in order to rule out any malignant foci.

Papillary cystadenoma lymphomatosum (Warthin's tumour)

This is a cystic, slow-growing tumour which arises in the lower pole of the parotid gland.

Monomorphic adenoma (oncocytoma)

This has a more lobulated appearance macroscopically, and tends to be well encapsulated. It occurs mostly in the parotid glands, but is also seen in some of the minor salivary glands around the upper lip.

Acinic cell carcinoma

This is a low-grade tumour, probably arising from acinar cells. The longer the tumour has been present, the more malignant it is likely to be.

Adenoid cystic carcinoma

This is a low-grade tumour most commonly arising in the submandibular glands. It characteristically invades along perineural spaces.

Mucoepidermoid carcinoma

This tumour tends to arise from major salivary gland ducts, and is composed of mucin-secreting acinar cells. One-third of these tumours are high grade.

Undifferentiated carcinoma

This is an uncommon tumour, and as suggested by its name, has no clear histologically identifiable features. It often presents with facial nerve palsy.

Malignant mixed carcinoma

This is a pleomorphic adenoma in which malignant cells are found.

Sarcomas

See Chapter 20.

Esthesioneuroblastomas

These are neuroblastomas of the olfactory nerve. They are composed of small round cells, and are prone to local invasion into the ethmoid sinus. Homer Wright rosettes are a characteristic feature.

Extramedullary plasmacytomas

These are most often found in the mandible, maxilla, and maxillary sinus. A full screen for multiple myeloma must be performed, so that myeloma can be excluded before this diagnosis can be made.

Melanomas

These mostly occur on the external skin of the head and neck region, but up to 4% may arise on the mucosal surfaces of the nose and paranasal sinuses.

Chemodectomas

These are glomus jugulare tumours located within the temporal bone, and are histologically highly vascular. They do not metastasize, but are locally very invasive.

Nasopharyngeal carcinomas (NPC) are also pathologically distinct. The most common type is lymphoepithelioma, which can appear morphologically similar to lymphoma, but is most often poorly differentiated squamous cell carcinoma with a prominent lymphocytic infiltrate. They are rarely adenocarcinomas, similar to salivary gland tumours.

Presentation

Cancers of the head and neck can present with a variety of symptomatology, depending on the tumour site. They can also be found incidentally and patients are not uncommonly referred by their dentist, or orthodontist. Laryngeal carcinomas often present early, because it may only take little in the way of irritation to cause the most common symptom of hoarseness. By contrast, nasopharyngeal tumours, and carcinomas of the hypopharynx, tend to present late in the course of their natural history, either with palpable cervical lymphadenopathy, or in the case of hypopharyngeal carcinoma, with dysphagia. Other difficult sites, where presentation tends to be 'silent', are base of tongue, supraglottic larynx, pyriform sinus, and paranasal sinuses. Symptoms such as persistent sore throat, earache or an ill-defined swelling should be followed up carefully. The most common presentations are as follows:

- palpable swelling or non-healing ulcer (oral cavity)
- cervical lymphadenopathy – jugulodigastric is the most common
- dysphagia or odynophagia (oropharynx)
- otalgia (may be direct or referred pain)
- stridor (larynx or hypopharynx)
- persistent hoarseness (larynx)
- epistaxis, nasal obstruction, conductive deafness (nasopharynx)
- cranial nerve palsy, e.g. diplopia
- facial pain or swelling (paranasal sinuses).

Examination

A full ENT examination is mandatory. Careful inspection of the oral cavity, buccal mucosa, and under the tongue, followed by palpation and indirect laryngoscopy (Fig. 14.3) can be performed in the out-patient department on the initial visit. Inspection of the nasopharynx and external auditory meatus, and palpation for cervical or supraclavicular lymphadenopathy are also carried out. If indicated, direct laryngoscopy with inspection of the nasal cavity can be done as well, using local anaesthetic spray on the posterior pharyngeal wall. If a lesion is directly visualized, a detailed description of site, size, boundaries, and appearance, needs to be documented. Tumours of the head and neck tend to grow as ulceration of the mucosal surface, with raised indurated edges. Palpation may be the best way of identifying the more subtle endophytic lesions, which tend to be more aggressive than the easily visible exophytic lesions. The cranial nerves should be systematically tested, including the infraorbital nerve if a tumour of the maxillary sinus is suspected. The presence or absence of lymphadenopathy must be noted, and any palpable nodes should be categorized and measured. A simple sketch of the findings can be very helpful. It is important to take into account dental appearance and nutritional status of the patient.

Diagnosis

To make the final diagnosis, a biopsy of the lesion is required, and often this will be done during an ENT examination under anaesthetic. If the patient presents with cervical lymphadenopathy and a primary site cannot be identified, fine needle aspiration (FNA) of a lymph node may need to be carried out, after a thor-

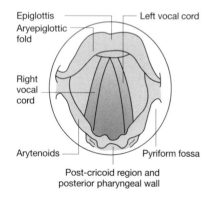

Epiglottis — Left vocal cord

Aryepiglottic fold

Right vocal cord

Arytenoids — Pyriform fossa

Post-cricoid region and posterior pharyngeal wall

Fig. 14.3 Mirror view on indirect laryngoscopy.

ough ENT examination with blind biopsies of the nasopharynx. CT scan, or, more commonly, MRI scan, can be particularly helpful for outlining the full extent of the primary tumour (Fig. 14.4) and also for identifying impalpable, but none-theless enlarged, neck nodes (Fig. 14.5). Positron emission tomography (PET) scanning is the latest tool to be employed in helping to assess the involvement of nodes. Its place is not yet clearly defined in current clinical practice.

Staging

Staging is defined by a site-specific TNM (tumour, node, metastasis) system, as devised by the American Joint Committee on Cancer (AJCC), and has different specifications for each primary site. It relies on clinical and radiological evaluation, and increasing T stage generally indicates increasing size of primary tumour (Table 14.1). Lymph node staging is uniformly applicable across tumour sites (Table 14.2). Limitations are recognized because of individual interpretation, as with more advanced lesions, it may be difficult to tell where the exact site of origin is, and whether more than one subsite is anatomically involved. All patients should be clinically staged (Table 14.3).

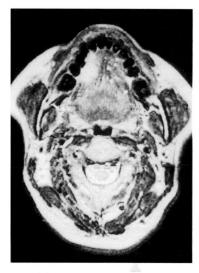

Fig. 14.4 Axial image showing lateral tongue tumour (courtesy of Professor M.I. Saunders, Marie Curie Research Wing, Mount Vernon Hospital, Middlesex).

Table 14.1 T Staging for head and neck cancer

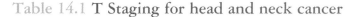

Site	T1	T2	T3	T4
Lip, oral cavity	≤ 2 cm	2–4 cm	> 4 cm	Invades adjacent structures
Oropharynx	≤ 2 cm	2–4 cm	> 4 cm	Invades bone, muscle, etc.
Larynx	Limited but mobile (a) One cord (b) Both cords	Extends to supra- or subglottis/ impaired mobility	Cord fixation	Extends beyond larynx
Supra- and subglottis	Limited/ mobile	Extends to glottis/mobile	Cord fixation	Extends beyond larynx
Hypopharynx	One subsite	> One subsite or adjacent site, without larynx fixation	With larynx fixation	Invades cartilage/ neck, etc.
Nasopharynx	One subsite	> One subsite	Invades nose/ oropharynx	Invades skull/cranial nerve
Maxillary sinus	Antral mucosa	Infrastructure, hard palate, nose	Cheek, floor of orbit, ethmoid, posterior wall of sinus	Orbital contents and other adjacent structures
Salivary glands	≤ 2 cm (a) No extension (b) Extension	2–4 cm	> 4 cm	> 6 cm

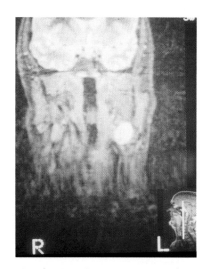

Fig. 14.5 Coronal MRI scan showing left cervical node (courtesy of Professor M.I. Saunders, Marie Curie Research Wing, Mount Vernon Hospital, Middlesex).

Table 14.2 **N Staging for head and neck cancer**

	N1	N2	N3
All sites	Ipsilateral single ≤ 3 cm	(a) Ipsilateral single > 3–6 cm	> 6 cm
		(b) Ipsilateral multiple ≤ 6 cm	
		(c) Bilateral, contralateral ≤ 6 cm	

Table 14.3 **Clinical stage grouping for head and neck cancer**

Clinical stage	TNM
0	Tis (carcinoma in situ) N0 M0
I	T1 N0 M0
II	T2 N0 M0
III	T3 N0 M0, T1–3 N1 M0
IV	T4 N0–1 M0, any T, N2–3 M0, any T any N M1

Table 14.4 **Clinically positive lymph nodes (N1–N3) on presentation, for each primary site**

Oral tongue	35%
Floor of mouth	30.5%
Retromolar trigone/anterior faucial pillar	45%
Soft palate	44%
Tonsillar fossa	76%
Base of tongue	78%
Oropharyngeal walls	59%
Supraglottic larynx	55%
Hypopharynx	75%
Nasopharynx	87%

Treatment

Treatment options are surgery, radiotherapy, chemotherapy, or a combination of these. Factors relating to disease site, stage, and anatomical accessibility of the tumour, must be considered, along with those relating to the nutritional status and overall well-being of the patient. Current surgical techniques employ primary closure where possible, but can allow for extensive resections by performing immediate reconstructions using free flaps from skin, fascia, muscle, or bone. Local or distant flaps can be used, as well as skin or bone grafting. Tissue viability can be a problem, but a satisfactory vascular supply can be achieved in the majority of patients. If neck dissection is required, the degree of dissection will be determined by the risks of nodal involvement (Table 14.4).

Radiation therapy can be used as the primary treatment, or in the adjuvant postoperative setting. Indications and technique will depend on anatomical location of the tumour, and the need to include sites of lymphatic drainage.

Standard dose and fractionation for radical treatment in the UK is 66 Gy in 2 Gy fractions over 6–7 weeks, and there is significant interest in altered fractionation regimes, treating 2 or 3 times per day. In CHART (Continuous Hyperfractionated Accelerated Radiotherapy), radiotherapy is delivered using 1.5 Gy fractions three times per day at 8-hourly intervals, over 12 consecutive days, with no breaks for weekends. This has produced encouraging results in terms of improved local control, particularly in the more advanced T3/T4 squamous cell carcinomas, but as yet is not offered routinely in UK oncology centres. CHARTWEL (Weekend-Less) is also being studied – this allows slightly higher doses to be given overall in a much shorter time-frame, but is not so disruptive to hard-pressed radiotherapy departments. While several on-going trials continue to explore optimum dose-fractionation schedules, conformal radiotherapy or accurate computer-assisted beam shaping is being increasingly used in the UK so that improvements in technical radiotherapy can achieve better outcomes, giving higher doses without additional toxicity.

The use of chemotherapy is much less clear cut, and the subject of many clinical trials, looking at neoadjuvant chemotherapy, concurrent chemoradiotherapy, and palliative chemotherapy. Response rates are generally high, but are not sustained and have not so far been shown to influence survival. Dental assessment prior to any treatment is important, but particularly because of the potential for delayed healing and abscess formation following radiation. The overall aim must be to offer the best possible way to eradicate tumour, whilst maintaining the best

Table 14.5 Types of neck dissection

Radical neck dissection	Procedure against which all other dissections are compared. Ipsilateral nodes are removed *en bloc*, along with internal jugular vein with sternocleido-mastoid muscle and accessory nerve
Modified neck dissection	One or more non-lymphatic structures are preserved. May be required on the contralateral side, as one internal jugular vein needs to be preserved.
Selective neck dissection	One or more groups of lymph nodes are preserved
Supra-omohyoid	Levels I–III removed
Posterolateral neck	Suboccipital, retroauricular plus levels II–V
Lateral neck	Levels II–IV
Anterior compartment	Pretracheal, paratracheal, perithyroid, and pre-cricoid removed
Extended radical neck dissection	One or more additional structures, lymphatic or non-lymphatic

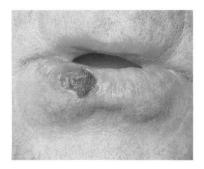

Fig. 14.6 Basal cell carcinoma of the lower lip, suitable for radical radiotherapy.

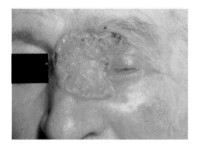

Fig. 14.7 Large basal cell carcinoma around inner canthus.

function and cosmesis, taking into account tumour-related factors, such as stage, and patient-related factors, such as co-morbidity. Management decisions are best made in the multidisciplinary setting, where the relative advantages and disadvantages of the options can be discussed with each individual patient, and this is increasingly done in a combined clinic.

In general, small primary lesions are best treated with surgery or radiation therapy alone. If surgery is used, the neck can be treated by the appropriate level of neck dissection (Table 14.5). If radiotherapy is used, the neck can be treated with radiation in continuity with the primary. More advanced lesions (T3/T4) are more likely to need both modalities, the sequencing of which will be determined by the individual situation. Nasopharyngeal tumours are the exception (see below).

Patients who develop new primaries, or relapse of disease, need to be considered on their merits. Further surgery is sometimes possible, but not always desirable. Radiotherapy is often reserved for relapse after primary surgery, and vice versa. Occasionally it is possible to give additional radiotherapy, but tolerance of surrounding normal tissue is generally prohibitive.

Skin and lip

Squamous cell carcinomas are most common, but basal cell carcinomas and rarer tumours occur as well. They are often curable with surgical excision or radical radiation (Fig. 14.6) and so cosmetic and functional result are also important. If presentation is late, potentially curative surgery or radiation therapy becomes difficult (Fig. 14.7).

Surgical excision is preferable in the following circumstances:

- large lesions (> 5 cm) with or without significant tissue destruction;
- tumours invading bone or cartilage;
- lesions of the upper eyelid, or inner canthus (overlying the nasolacrimal duct);
- relapse after irradiation;

Radiotherapy is preferable in the following circumstances:

- sites where primary closure is difficult, e.g. temple, forehead, nose;
- lesions of the lower eyelid or outer canthus;
- elderly patients, or whenever the risk of general anaesthetic is high;
- if excision has been incomplete, or there is recurrence after surgery.

Oral cavity

Primary sites within the oral cavity include the anterior two-thirds of tongue, posterior one-third or base of tongue, buccal mucosa, upper and lower alveolus, hard palate, retromolar trigone, floor of mouth, and oropharynx. Both surgery and primary radiation therapy can be curative in early-stage disease, and the decision for each patient should be made on the basis of local extent of disease and the general condition of the patient. Sometimes there may be no clinical reason to offer one modality rather than the other, in which case patient preference may be the deciding factor. In advanced disease, cure is less likely, and often surgery with neck dissection and immediate or stepped reconstruction will be recommended. Speech therapy is a major part of the rehabilitation process. In some circumstances, postoperative radiotherapy is given. Although this may improve local control, it may increase morbidity significantly. Where radical radiotherapy is the treatment of choice, surgery can be reserved for relapse, and vice versa. Patients should be advised to stop smoking prior to definitive treatment, as continuation will increase the risks from anaesthesia, and morbidity with radiotherapy.

Surgery

This is often the treatment of choice in more advanced lesions, i.e. T3/T4 tumours, or those invading bone or cartilage. Radiotherapy can cause osteoradionecrosis, and is therefore not recommended when bone invasion is present. Surgical resection aims to remove the whole tumour, with a margin adequate to allow for removal of surrounding microscopic invasion. In many circumstances, a neck dissection will also be appropriate, depending on the site, stage, and location of the tumour. Postoperative radiotherapy will be offered if there are ≥ 3 positive nodes removed, or there is extracapsular spread.

Radiotherapy

The major potential advantage of radiotherapy is functional preservation, particularly of speech and swallowing. It can be given as external beam therapy, interstitial brachytherapy using iridium hairpins, or as a combination of these. Brachytherapy is given over a shorter time period (48 hours vs 5–7 weeks for external beam radiotherapy), requires a general anaesthetic, and avoids treating much of the oral mucosa, but is less readily available throughout the UK at present (Figs 14.8 and 14.9). It can only be used for small lesions with a low risk of nodal metastases, as external beam therapy is required to treat the locoregional lymphatics in continuity with the primary site.

Radiotherapy is inappropriate for locally advanced or bulky disease, but can be used in the palliative setting where bleeding or ulceration are problematic symptoms. For external beam treatment, an immobilization shell is required in order to achieve reproducibility of set-up for daily treatments (Fig. 14.10).

Chemotherapy

Agents such as 5-fluorouracil, cisplatin and methotrexate can produce high response rates; however, responses tend to be short-lived, regrowth is often rapid, and there is no evidence to show any survival benefit. Chemotherapy in the neoadjuvant setting, and concurrent with radiotherapy, along with newer agents, are the subject of current clinical trials.

Oropharynx

The oropharynx extends from the junction of the hard and soft palate, down to the hyoid bone. It includes the tonsillar fossae, soft palate, posterior pharyngeal wall, posterior one-third of the tongue, the valleculae, and the mobile epiglottis. Almost two-thirds of oropharyngeal tumours arise in the tonsils, a quarter in the base of tongue, 10% in the soft palate, and less than 5% from the other sites. Most of these structures have a rich bilateral lymphatic drainage, increasing significantly the risk of ipsilateral and contralateral nodal spread. Tumours of the tonsillar fossae and soft palate have less tendency to spread to the contralateral nodes.

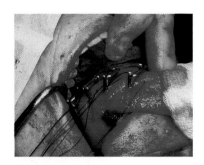

Fig. 14.8 Hairpin needles for brachytherapy (courtesy of Professor M. I. Saunders, Marie Curie Research Wing, Mount Vernon Hospital, Middlesex).

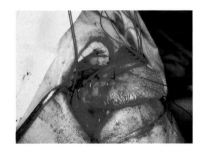

Fig. 14.9 Live iridium sources in place (courtesy of Professor M. I. Saunders, Marie Curie Research Wing, Mount Vernon Hospital, Middlesex).

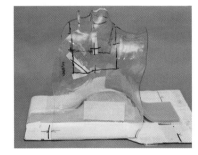

Fig. 14.10 Immobilization shell for radiation therapy.

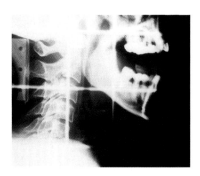

Fig. 14.11 Lateral external beam fields for phase I treatment of carcinoma of the oropharynx.

Surgery

For T1 and T2 tumours, extensive resection with or without mandibular osteotomy, plus or minus neck dissection, is commonly required. Surgery is extremely difficult and hazardous for larger tumours.

Radiotherapy

For bulky or locally advanced tumours, radiotherapy is the treatment of choice. Portals are arranged to include the primary site plus all draining lymph node stations bilaterally, and in continuity (Fig. 14.11). In some circumstances where the risk of contralateral nodal spread is low, such as a tonsillar tumour, the target area can be reduced. In such cases, avoidance of radiation to the contralateral neck will significantly lessen both early- and late-term morbidity.

Larynx

Unlike many other head and neck cancers, most laryngeal tumours present relatively early. Lymphatic drainage is also comparatively poor, and so many are T1 or T2 and N0 at presentation. Radiotherapy can be confined to the larynx, plus a margin, and is the treatment of choice. It can also be used for T3 tumours, with careful follow-up, so that relapse can be detected early and salvage surgery offered. T4 tumours require total laryngectomy, very often with postoperative radiotherapy. Radiotherapy or supraglottic laryngectomy can be used for small tumours of the supraglottis, as the functional result of this operation is generally acceptable.

Hypopharynx

This region is divided into three sites, with the whole structure extending from the aryepiglottic fold down to the lower level of the cricoid cartilage. It includes:

- pyriform fossa
- post-cricoid region
- posterior pharyngeal wall.

The majority of patients present with advanced nodal disease and will require radical surgery with postoperative radiotherapy. Laryngopharyngectomy is the most common procedure, particularly for post-cricoid tumours which have either no lymphadenopathy, or a small, mobile, unilateral lymph node. If the patient has a posterior pharyngeal wall tumour, or is unfit for surgery, radical radiotherapy can be given as primary treatment, reserving surgery for relapse. If the thyroid cartilage is involved, surgery is the preferred option. Twenty per cent of patients with locally advanced disease have distant metastases at presentation.

Nasopharynx

The vast majority of patients have nodal disease at presentation. Unlike other head and neck cancers, the treatment of choice for nasopharyngeal carcinoma is primary radiation therapy, often in combination with chemotherapy. Radiotherapy portals encompass the whole neck, and extend from base of skull down to include the supraclavicular fossa. A smaller boost volume is required in order to keep the spinal cord dose within tolerance.

Salivary glands

Although these tumours have widely varying size, histopathology, and site, they are generally best treated by excision where possible. The exceptions tend to centre around the parotid tumours, where proximity to the facial nerve may make the risks of surgery too high. In these sorts of circumstances, radiotherapy is indicated. Each tumour requires individual planning.

Nasal cavity and paranasal sinuses

For the small proportion of these tumours which present early, surgical resection should be offered. Most, however, present at a locally advanced stage, where extensive surgery may still be possible but primary radiation therapy is often the preferred option.

External auditory meatus and middle ear

Surgery or radiotherapy can be used as a primary curative procedure. If surgically resected tumours have positive margins, then postoperative radiotherapy can also be used.

Side-effects of treatment

Surgery

The site and extent of surgery will define the likely morbidity. Operations on the tongue and oral cavity may impair speech and swallowing, and rehabilitation is important in the postoperative phase.

Radiotherapy

External beam radiotherapy will inevitably affect the sensitive normal tissues of the oral cavity and pharynx. Acute skin reactions are common and often require simple measures such as the application of hydrocortisone 1% cream (Fig. 14.12). Mucositis tends to be maximum from the third week of treatment onwards, and may last for 1 or 2 weeks after radiotherapy is completed (Fig. 14.13). Symptomatic measures, needed for most patients, include mouthwashes, analgesics, and antifungal therapy. Maintaining adequate nutrition throughout is essential in order to maximize normal tissue repair.

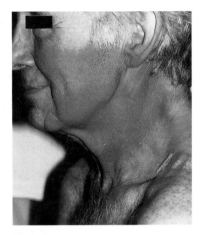

Fig. 14.12 Acute skin reaction.

Chemotherapy

Myelosuppression and mucositis are the most common dose-limiting toxicities, and combining modalities almost inevitably enhances the normal tissue reactions.

Prognosis

Prognosis varies with disease site, histology, and stage. In general, there is a good prospect of long-term remission in early T1–T2, N0–N1 tumours, with between 60% and 90% 5-year survival rates. By contrast, patients with T4 disease can expect no higher than 30% 5-year survival.

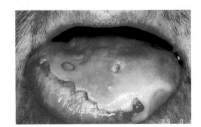

Fig. 14.13 Confluent mucositis (courtesy of Professor M. I. Saunders, Marie Curie Research Wing, Mount Vernon Hospital, Middlesex).

Skin and lip

Cure rates for basal cell carcinomas are generally high, with only a 5–10% recurrence rate. Squamous cell carcinomas have a slightly higher relapse rate, and must be followed up carefully after primary treatment, as salvage surgery or radiotherapy may be required.

Oral cavity

A high proportion of T1/T2 tumours are successfully treated by primary radiation therapy. Salvage surgery is possible in about half of those who relapse. For T3 tumours, the control rate drops to approximately 50%, and relapse is more difficult to treat.

Oropharynx
Tonsil and soft palate

Control rates for T1/T2 tumours are good, as bilateral drainage is less likely. Five-year survival is 75% in node-negative tumours, and about 40% if there is nodal disease at presentation.

Base of tongue

Overall 2-year control rates are poor, around 30%, attributed to late presentation and propensity for bilateral nodal drainage.

Larynx
Glottis

As laryngeal carcinomas often present early, radical radiotherapy can produce up to 95% 5-year survival for T1 tumours, and 80% for T2. Laryngectomy may be required for the small number of patients who relapse. For T3 tumours, surgery or radiotherapy give similar results, with 50% ultimately relapsing.

Supraglottis

Cure rates are not quite as high as for glottis, with 5-year survival reaching 80% for T1N0 disease, and 70% for T2N0 disease. If the primary tumour is more advanced, or there is nodal involvement, then these rates drop to 55%.

Subglottis

Subglottic disease is the most difficult to treat effectively, reflected by overall survival rates of no more than 40%.

Hypopharynx

As the majority of patients present with locally advanced disease, prognosis overall for hypopharyngeal tumours is relatively poor. Radical radiotherapy results in a 15–20% 5-year survival rate, but in those patients who are suitable for surgery, this can be increased to 35%.

Nasopharynx

In the minority of patients who present with N0, localized, well-differentiated tumours, radical radiotherapy can achieve up to 80% 5-year survival. However, most presentations are with cervical lymphadenopathy and locoregionally advanced disease. For these patients, an overall 5-year survival of 60% is possible; however, local control is a major problem with about half of these patients relapsing in the nasopharynx.

Salivary glands

Prognosis is variable and depends on stage or extent of disease, and histological type of the tumour. Five-year survival varies from 20% in high-grade mucoepidermoid and undifferentiated carcinomas, up to 80% for low-grade mucoepidermoid and acinic cell tumours.

Nasal cavity and paranasal sinuses

Radical radiotherapy can achieve 70% 5-year local control rates for nasal cavity tumours. By contrast, results for cancer of the ethmoid sinus are or the order of 30% 5-year survival. Prognosis for tumours of the maxillary sinus ranges from 30 to 65%, depending on stage of disease.

External auditory meatus and middle ear

Prognosis for these tumours is generally poor, especially if there is local bone invasion. Primary radiotherapy can achieve 15–20% 5-year survival, and postoperative radiotherapy can confer up to 40% 5-year survival.

Given the poor prognosis of many of these patients, and the potential suffering that may be endured in the incurable setting, the increasing involvement of Palliative Medicine in the multi-displinary management team, is important to encourage and facilitate. Prevention, improving cure and survival rates, reducing toxicity of single or combined modality therapy, and helping patients to deal with all aspects of their disease at all times in this often difficult cancer journey, must be our aim.

Key points

- A detailed history and careful clinical examination are of paramount importance in the diagnostic and staging procedures.
- Treatment decisions are often complex, and may result in primary surgery or primary radical radiotherapy. Reserving surgery for relapse after primary radiotherapy is a reasonable option for locally advanced tumours.
- Chemotherapy has high initial response rates, but has no impact on overall survival. Nonetheless, combined modality therapy has produced some encouraging results.
- Managing side-effects of treatment, including second malignancies, is an important part of individual patient care.
- Multidisciplinary management is essential, and best done in the setting of a combined clinic with an ENT surgeon and oncologist. Dietitian, dental practitioner, speech therapist, physiotherapist, specialist nurse, and other members of the team should also be available.

Case history

My patient has been complaining of hoarseness for 4 weeks. Please advise.

History

This 51-year-old politician, who has smoked 20 cigarettes per day since he was 15 years old, and who drinks 7 or 8 pints of beer per night on weekends, developed persistent hoarseness. He lives with his wife and has two married sons.

Examination

He appears well nourished, and is of good performance status. There is no cervical lymphadenopathy. On indirect laryngoscopy, there is a small lesion on the right vocal cord, extending to the anterior commissure but not onto the left vocal cord, nor into the supra- or subglottis. There is partial immobility of the left cord, but no fixation.

Investigations

Chest x-ray is normal. Biopsy confirmed well-differentiated invasive squamous cell carcinoma.

Management

This man has a T2N0 squamous cell carcinoma of the larynx and he should be offered radical radiotherapy.

Notes

Equivalent cure rates of 70% can be achieved with laryngectomy, or radical radiation therapy. For this man, the significant advantage of radiotherapy is voice preservation. Chest x-ray is important to exclude a primary simultaneous lung carcinoma in these patients, who are at high risk.

Further reading

Price, P. and Sikora, K. (1995) *Treatment of cancer*, 3rd edn. Chapman & Hall, London.

Peckham, M., Pinedo, H., and Veronesi, U. (eds) (1995) Section 6 – Skin cancer and tumours of the head and neck. *Oxford textbook of oncology*, pp. 891–1083. Oxford University Press, London.

DeVita, V. T., Hellman, S., and Rosenberg, S. A. (eds) (1997) Head and neck cancer. In *Cancer – principles and practice of oncology*, 5th edn. Lippincott-Raven, Philadelphia.

Million, R. R. and Cassisi, N. J. (1984) *Management of head and neck cancer: a multidisciplinary approach*, 2nd edn. Lippincott, Philadelphia.

Munro, A. J. (1995) An overview of randomised controlled trials of adjuvant chemotherapy in head and neck cancer. *Br J Cancer* 71, 83–91.

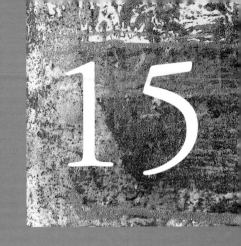

Gynaecological malignancy
John H. Price

- Introduction
- Carcinoma of the vulva
- Endometrial cancer
- Cancer of the uterine cervix
- Carcinoma of the vagina
- Cancer of the ovary

Gynaecological malignancy

Introduction

Gynaecological cancers account for one in seven cancers in women. Approximately one in 20 women will develop a gynaecological malignancy and one in 40 will die of the disease. In the UK, ovarian cancer is now the commonest gynaecological cancer, although worldwide, cervical cancer remains the most important.

Carcinoma of the vulva

Epidemiology

Vulval cancer is a rare tumour, accounting for less than 5% of gynaecological cancers with approximately 750 new cases being diagnosed in the UK per annum. The disease usually presents in the elderly with the commonest age being the seventh decade.

Aetiology

Although there is no clear aetiological cause for this cancer, there is an association with chronic pruritus and it is frequently found in patients with a past history of vulval dystrophy. However, in studies of patients with vulval dystrophy, only 5–10% have been shown to develop vulval cancer on follow-up. There is also an association with vulval intraepithelial neoplasia (VIN) and the development of tumours in younger women where tumours are of a multifocal nature; human papilloma virus has been suggested as a possible causal factor.

Pathology

The vast majority (90%) are squamous cell in origin with 5% being melanomas and the remainder being very rare tumours such as Bartholin's gland sarcomas.

Squamous tumours include basal cell carcinomas and verrucous tumours, which can become very large but usually remain locally invasive only, and are therefore easily managed despite their large size. Prognosis in vulval cancer is closely related to tumour size, differentiation, and spread to the regional lymph nodes. Squamous tumours of the vulva in general are fairly slow growing and spread by lymph channel embolization to the superficial and deep inguinal lymph nodes of the groin. Evidence of spread to the regional lymph glands is present in 43% of patients at diagnosis.

Presentation

Most patients present with a history of irritation and pruritus vulvae, usually of at least 3 months duration or longer, before they seek help. Because of a general reluctance to be examined, the elderly patients who develop carcinoma of the vulva often delay seeking help, leading to a delay in diagnosis. Other reported symptoms include pain, a lump, bleeding, and discharge.

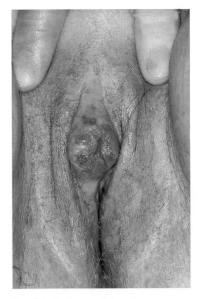

Fig. 15.1 Carcinoma of the vulva.

Examination

Patients presenting with vulval carcinoma are frequently elderly and frail; therefore, a full clinical assessment to ensure fitness for an anaesthetic and surgery is essential.

Patients are frequently reluctant to be examined; nevertheless, careful documentation of the site, size, and fixity of lesion, also whether it is multifocal, is important in deciding management. A diagram is helpful to record findings, as is a description as to whether the tumour involves the clitoris, urethra, vagina, or reaches the anal margin as all these influence staging and management. A careful palpation of peripheral lymph nodes, especially the groin nodes, must be carried out, although the clinical accuracy of such an examination is only 50%.

Diagnosis

Whilst most tumours will be clinically obvious, a clinical examination, a biopsy, and histological examination of the lesion are mandatory to confirm the diagnosis of malignancy, cell type, degree of differentiation, and the presence of lymphovascular channel involvement in order to plan treatment.

Ideally, the biopsy should include a margin of the tumour as this will aid pathological assessment.

Staging

In keeping with other gynaecological cancers, FIGO has developed a tumour staging classification. For vulval tumours this is based upon the TNM system (Table 15.1).

Table 15.1 International Federation of Gynaecology and Obstetrics (FIGO) classification for the stages of carcinoma of the vulva

Stage 0	Carcinoma in situ, intraepithelial carcinoma
Stage I	Lesions 2 cm or less in size confined to vulva or perineum. No nodal metastasis
Stage Ia	Lesions 2 cm or less in size confined to the vulva or perineum and with stromal invasion no greater than 1.0 mm.* No nodal metastasis
Stage Ib	Lesions 2 cm or less in size confined to the vulva or perineum and with stromal invasion greater than 1.0 mm.* No nodal metastasis
Stage II	Tumour confined to the vulva and/or perineum; more than 2 cm in greatest dimension; no nodal metastasis
Stage III	Tumour of any size with adjacent spread of the lower urethra and/or the vagina, or the anus, and/or unilateral regional lymph node metastasis
Stage IVa	Tumour invades any of the following: upper urethra, bladder mucosa, rectal mucosa, pelvic bone, and/or bilateral regional nodal metastasis
Stage IVb	Any distant metastasis, including pelvic lymph nodes

* The depth of invasion is defined as the measurement of the tumour from the epithelial-stromal junction of the adjacent most superficial dermal papilla to the deepest point of invasion.

Whilst this is helpful in determining prognosis, it is hampered by being a clinical staging process and does not consider the effect tumour site has on prognosis or the inaccuracy of clinical assessment of lymph node status.

Treatment

Before 1906, vulval cancer was universally fatal until a French medical student called Basset suggested that, although the original tumour could be removed, patients died with terrible tumours in the groins and suggested removal of those also. This was adopted by Bonney in the UK and Taussig in Chicago with dramatic effect. Despite high morbidity and mortality from the drastic surgery of radical vulvectomy and extensive *en bloc* lymph node dissection, the survival rate became 60%.

The principles of treatment remained unchanged for 60 years and only in the past 25 years have attempts been made to reduce morbidity by achieving primary wound closure, and more recently by performing groin node dissections through separate incisions. Now, small laterally sited tumours away from the clitoris may be managed by wide local excision and ipsilateral separate groin node dissection without compromising outcome.

Surgery remains the mainstay of treatment with the principle of surgery being to perform a wide excision of the tumour and achieve a disease-free margin of 1 cm in all directions. If necessary, excision may extend deeply into the underlying muscle, reach the underlying bone, or involve removing the distal third of the urethra. This latter procedure may be performed without compromising urinary continence.

Groin node dissection should be subfascial and remove all superficial and deep inguinal and femoral triangle nodes. The femoral canal should be explored and the nodes frequently found there removed (the node of Cloquet or Rosemuller).

Postoperatively, the patient needs careful management to prevent wound infection and thromboembolic disease. Long-term problems include chronic leg oedema and loss of sensation or paraesthesia in the distribution of the femoral nerve.

Adjuvant therapy

Radical surgery remains the most effective treatment for carcinoma of the vulva, even when patients are elderly and infirm. Radiotherapy gives disappointing results when directed to treatment of the primary lesion (10% survival rates have been quoted). It is best reserved therefore for the treatment of deep pelvic nodes given by external beam in the those patients in whom Cloquet's node is found to be positive for tumour or for the control of groin and pelvic node metastases, especially if the patient is unfit for extensive surgery.

Chemotherapy has been found to be ineffective in the treatment of vulval tumours and its use is currently best confined to clinical trials.

Prognosis

The prognosis of carcinoma of the vulva has been extensively studied and there is a clear connection between tumour size and the risk of regional lymph node metastases. This is reflected in reported 5-year survival rates. Small tumours (< 2 cm) with negative nodes after radical surgery can expect a 5-year survival of over 90%.

This falls to 50–55% even for small tumours if lymph node spread is identified in the groin nodes and even further to 20% if deep pelvic nodes are involved. Thus excision of not only the complete tumour but also the regional lymph nodes plays an important part in survival.

It has been reported that tumours involving the clitoris have a poorer survival because of the rich lymphovascular network leading to earlier spread. From a histological viewpoint, well-differentiated tumours and those where a strong immunological host response is identified have an improved survival rate independent of other factors.

Overall, provided patients are treated adequately, carcinoma of the vulva is a slow-growing tumour that can be cured by surgery alone. All patients should therefore be referred to a cancer centre for investigation and treatment.

Endometrial cancer

Epidemiology

The incidence of endometrial cancer is gradually increasing and has now overtaken cervical cancer in incidence in the UK and USA where it affects 3% of women. In South Africa, the ratio of endometrial cancer to cervical cancer is 2.5:1 in whites whilst in blacks it is 1:8. This variation is thought to be due to better socioeconomic status, better availability of health care, more women reaching advanced age, and better prevention and or detection of cervical cancer in the white population.

Endometrial cancer is almost always a disease of postmenopausal woman (age range 55–70 years) and is very rare under the age of 40.

Aetiology

Endometrial cancer is closely associated with obesity, low parity, and late menopause; it is also associated with hypertension and diabetes.

In the 1970s in the USA there was a documented rise in the incidence of endometrial cancer, which was found to be linked with the administration of unopposed oestrogens to postmenopausal women to control climacteric symptoms. There is also clinical evidence of the association between endometrial carcinoma and high circulating oestrogen levels, e.g. polycystic ovarian syndrome (PCOS) and oestrogen producing tumours, where chronic anovulation with raised oestrogen production causes endometrial abnormalities.

More recently, concern has been expressed about the long-term administration of tamoxifen to breast cancer suffers. Although this drug is described as an anti-oestrogen because it blocks oestrogen receptors in breast tissue, there is evidence that it has oestrogen-like activity at endometrial level and long-term administration has been associated with endometrial abnormalities, including benign polyps, hyperplasia, and malignant tumours, including carcinosarcomata.

Pathology

Approximately 60–70 % of endometrial malignancies are adenocarcinomas. Other tumours described are adenocanthoma, adenosquamous, clear cell and mixed mullerian (carcinosarcomas). Rarely, papillary adenocarcinomas and squamous cell carcinomas occur.

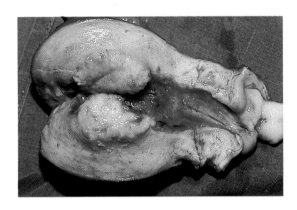

Fig. 15.2 Carcinoma of the endometrium with tumour confined to the inner half of the myometrium.

The microscopic appearances of adenocarcinoma range from very well differentiated tumours (50%) indistinguishable from atypical hyperplasia through moderate differentiation (30%) to very poorly differentiated or anaplastic lesions, which have lost virtually all glandular patterns (20%). Because of the influence of differentiation on management strategies, lesions should be labelled according to the worst grade of differentiation found.

Presentation

Classically, endometrial tumours present with postmenopausal bleeding and all women experiencing abnormal bleeding in the perimenopausal years or afterwards must have investigations to exclude malignancy.

Diagnosis

Patients with postmenopausal bleeding should have a vaginal ultrasound to identify endometrial thickness (normally < 4 mm after the menopause) and an endometrial sample taken for histological examination. This latter investigation is the subject of some controversy as some investigators question its accuracy.

Table 15.2 FIGO classification for the stages of carcinoma of the endometrium

Stage Ia G123	Tumour limited to endometrium
Stage Ib G123	Invasion to less than half the myometrium
Stage Ic G123	Invasion to more than half the myometrium
Stage IIa G123	Endocervical glandular involvement only
Stage IIb G123	Cervical stromal invasion
Stage IIIa G123	Tumour invades serosa and/or adnexae and/or positive cytological findings
Stage IIIb G123	Vaginal metastases
Stage IIIc G123	Metastases to pelvic and/or para-aortic lymph nodes
Stage IVa G123	Tumour invasion of bladder and/or bowel mucosa
Stage IVb	Distant metastases, including intra-abdominal and/or inguinal lymph nodes

The main diagnostic investigation is hysteroscopy and biopsy, which may be performed under local or general anaesthetic. This has the advantage of identifying the site of the lesion and obtaining a directed biopsy.

Staging

FIGO staging of endometrial cancer (Table 15.2) takes into consideration tumour site, differentiation (grade), and evidence of spread. This is reasonably accurate in predicting outcome and therefore as much information as possible should be gathered whilst planning treatment.

Investigation

Hysteroscopy should be performed in all cases of suspected endometrial cancer. This will determine the site of the lesion, i.e. fundal or involving the cervical os. It will also enable a directed representative biopsy to be performed, an estimation of uterine cavity size, and the presence or absence of other uterine pathology.

A bi-manual examination should also be carried out to assess for adnexal pathology (there is a 5% incidence of concomitant tumours of the ovary).

Once the diagnosis is confirmed, an MRI or spiral CT scan should be carried out. The former is useful in determining the depth of tumour invasion preoperatively and also assessing lymphadenopathy in the pelvis, whilst the latter is more useful in visualizing abdominal lymph nodes and chest metastases (a chest x-ray would probably suffice, however, in the majority of cases).

It should be remembered that many of these patients are obese and some have hypertension and/or type II diabetes. Therefore, preoperative investigations to ensure fitness for surgery should be performed.

Treatment

The standard treatment for the past 25 years for endometrial cancer has been total hysterectomy and bilateral salpingo-oophorectomy (TAH & BSO) followed by radiotherapy if adverse prognostic factors are identified at histology, i.e. cervical extension, poor differentiation, and deep myometrial involvement. With improved preoperative assessment, most of this information should now be known and patients more carefully selected for treatment.

Patients with early stage I disease without deep myometrial involvement and well-differentiated tumours may be treated by total hysterectomy and bilateral salpingo-oophorectomy alone. More advanced stage I disease and stage II tumours need adjuvant radiotherapy or else the patient should have a radical hysterectomy and lymph node sampling and only have postoperative radiotherapy depending on the presence or absence of microscopic spread. Currently Medical Research Council trials are addressing this issue to determine a more coherent strategy of treatment.

More advanced disease should be treated by radiotherapy, both intracavity and external beam, followed by surgery if residual central disease persists.

Conventional chemotherapy gives very poor cure rates in this disease and is rarely used outside clinical trials except in occasional palliative circumstances. Ever since it was reported that progestogens obtained a 37% objective response rate in metastatic disease, it became in vogue to give these preparations postoperatively to all patients to prevent recurrence. It has since been reported that these drugs act best on well-differentiated tumours, which are the lesions least likely to recur. It should also be remembered that the progestogens recommended are associated with weight gain and raised cholesterol levels and this has led to a decrease in their use, which is now largely limited to the chemotherapy of advanced and recurrent disease.

Prognosis

Because endometrial carcinoma tends to present at an early stage with postmenopausal bleeding and is commonly a stage I, well-differentiated lesion, the overall prognosis is 70% 5-year disease-free survival. This has led to a degree of complacency among gynaecologists who believe that a TAH & BSO will cure almost all patients. This is not the case and stage for stage this disease is just as fatal as other gynaecological cancers.

Poor differentiation, deep myometrial invasion, and lymph node metastases all confer an adverse prognosis and it is this group that should be identified pre-operatively if possible and selected for a more aggressive treatment strategy.

One other group in which a poor outcome may be expected are those patients with carcinosarcomas. These tumours behave in a very aggressive manner and there may be micrometastases in the lung or brain by the time of diagnosis, making effective therapy almost impossible.

Cancer of the uterine cervix

Epidemiology

Cervical cancer is a disease which predominately affects women over 45 and is the second commonest cancer in women worldwide. Whilst the incidence is decreasing in the countries with a well developed cervical screening programme, the incidence and mortality worldwide remain a major problem.

The age-standardized incidence in Sao Paulo, Brazil is 50/100 000 compared to 10/100 000 in Scotland.

Aetiology

Epidemiological studies indicate that sexual contact is important in the development of cervical cancer. Early intercourse, multiple partners, and male promiscuity all indicate the likelihood of a sexually transmitted oncogenic factor. Prevalence studies reveal that infection with human papilloma virus (HPV), particularly type 16, is strongly associated with cervical intraepithelial neoplasia (CIN) and invasive cancer. Other important associations are low socioeconomic class, smoking, and high parity.

So far research has failed to pinpoint one single cause and it seems likely that more than one aetiological factor is responsible. It has been established, however, that cervical cancer is a preventable disease by population screening as evidenced by screening programmes in Canada and Finland. In the UK in 1988 a national screening programme was initiated with the aim of screening over 80% of the eligible female population aged between 25 and 65 years of age within 5 years and reducing the mortality rate from disease by the year 2000.

Key points

- Commonest presentation is postmenopausal bleeding.
- All patients with post-menopausal bleeding must be investigated.
- Association with unopposed oestrogen therapy.
- Association with obesity, low parity, diabetes, hypertension.
- Hysteroscopy and biopsy are diagnostic investigations of choice.
- Careful preoperative investigation will lead to better treatment strategy.
- Prognosis depends on stage, differentiation, tumour size, and treatment given.

The first part of the programme has been achieved and the year 2000 results are not available. One disturbing aspect of this screening programme has been highlighted by an audit in the United Kingdom where 50% of cervical cancers in 1995/96 arose in women who have either never had a smear or none within 5 years. Many of these women fall within the high-risk group aetiologically and have not responded to cervical screening invitations. Therefore, much work needs to be done in identifying and persuading these women to attend for screening if cervical cancer is to be conquered.

Pathology

Approximately 75% of cervical cancers are squamous in origin – 15% are adenocarcinomas and the remainder are made up of adenosquamous, clear cell and undifferentiated tumours.

Squamous tumours arise from the cervical squamo-columnar junction due to malignant transformation of metaplastic cells and frequently cervical intra-epithelial neoplasia is found at the margins of the tumour. Tumour spread is by direct invasion into surrounding stroma, into the vaginal epithelium, and directly into the paracervical tissues towards the pelvic side wall. Penetration of tumour into lymphovascular spaces allows tumour embolism to occur along the para-cervical lymph channels to the deep pelvic lymph node groups of the internal and external iliac and obstructor nodes. Spread thereafter is upward along the common iliac and para-aortic chain. Bloodborne spread is less common but may occur in some more aggressive lesions.

Presentation

Pre-malignant disease of the cervix is by its nature asymptomatic and may only be detected by cytology, colposcopy, and histological examination.

When invasive disease is present and a clinically obvious tumour develops, the cardinal symptom is abnormal vaginal bleeding. Usually this takes the form of

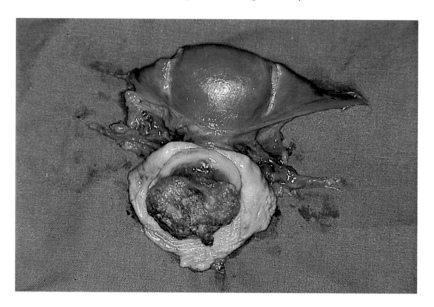

Fig. 15.3 Four centimetre cervical cancer arising from the posterior lip of the cervix removed by radical hysterectomy.

post-coital or intermenstrual bleeding. As the latter is a relatively common event, especially for patients on oral contraception or in the perimenopausal years, this can lead to a delay in diagnosis, either due to ignorance or complacency on behalf of the patient or her medical practitioner. All women who report abnormal bleeding must therefore have a pelvic examination and visualization of the whole of the cervix even if her last cervical smear was normal.

Other symptoms reported are excessive vaginal discharge, which may be mucoid or offensive, dyspareunia, and pelvic discomfort. Sinister late symptoms are unilateral leg oedema, deep pelvic pain, and sciatica, suggesting blockage of lymphatics and nerve root entrapment, respectively.

Examination

A speculum examination will reveal a polypoid mass or an infected ulcerated lesion in advanced disease. On bimanual examination the cervix will feel hard and craggy; mobility will be reduced in advanced disease. A combined vaginal and rectal or rectal examination will help gauge the extent of spread into the parametrial tissues.

Table 15.3 FIGO classification for the stages of carcinoma of the cervix

Stage 0	Carcinoma in situ, cervical intraepithelia neoplasia grade III
Stage I	The carcinoma is strictly confined to the cervix (extension to the corpus would be disregarded)
Stage Ia1	Measured stromal invasion of not more than 3.0 mm in depth and extension of not more than 7.0 mm
Stage Ia2	Measured stromal invasion of more than 3.0 mm and not more than 5.0 mm with an extension of not more than 7.0 mm
Stage Ib	Clinically visible lesions limited to the cervix, uteri, or subclinical cancers greater than stage Ia
Stage II	The carcinoma extends beyond the cervix but has not extended to the pelvic wall. The carcinoma involves the vagina but not as far as the lower third.
Stage IIa	No obvious parametrial involvement
Stage IIb	Obvious parametrial involvement
Stage III	The carcinoma has extended to the pelvic wall. On rectal examination, there is no cancer-free space between the tumour and the pelvic wall. The tumour involves the lower third of the vagina. All cases with hydronephrosis or non-functioning kidney are included, unless they are known to be due to other causes
Stage IIIa	No extension to the pelvic wall
Stage IIIb	Extension to the pelvic wall and/or hydronephrosis or non-functioning kidney
Stage IV	The carcinoma has extended beyond the true pelvis or has clinically involved the mucosa of the bladder or rectum. A bullous oedema as such does not permit a case to be allotted to stage IV
Stage IVa	Spread of the growth to adjacent organs
Stage IVb	Spread to distant organs

An overall general examination must be performed to determine the health of the patient, looking especially for anaemia, lymphadenopathy, oedema, or signs of any intercurrent illness which may affect an anaesthetic or subsequent treatment.

Diagnosis and staging

FIGO have modified staging criteria over the years but have retained a clinical basis in order to allow worldwide participation. Early-stage disease is subdivided as stage 1a1 and 1a2 to differentiate between those patients with very early stromal penetration through the basement membrane of the epithelium to a depth of less than 3 mm, which may be amenable to conservation treatment, and patients with microcarcinomas where there is a very small risk of lymph node metastasis (Table 15.3).

In general the greater the depth of stromal invasion the greater the likelihood of nodal spread.

The staging process involves examination under anaesthetic to determine whether there is spread into the paracervical tissues, cystoscopy looking for tumour invasion and imaging techniques. IVU may be performed and if a hydroureter is found this automatically stages the patient as IIIb.

In the UK, MRI and or CT scans have largely replaced IVU as these techniques can also allow identification of enlarged lymph nodes and evidence of spread within and outwith the pelvis, which may be missed clinically.

Treatment

The mainstay of treatment throughout the world is radiotherapy. In countries where good surgical facilities exist, patients with early-stage disease (stage I–IIa) are offered the choice of radiotherapy or radical surgery. Both offer comparable cure rates of 75% 5-year disease-free survival and both have associated morbidity of 5%. In general, the majority of patients opt for surgery as it can allow preservation of ovarian function, most morbidity is short term, and the patient psychologically feels she has been cured as the tumour has been removed.

Radical hysterectomy and node dissection involves dissection of the ureters from the pelvic brim to the bladder base, removal of the uterus, cervix, upper third of the vagina, parametrial tissues, and dissection of the external iliac, internal iliac, and obturator lymph node groups and biopsy of the lower para-aortic chain of nodes.

Postoperatively there may be decreased bladder sensation leading to voiding difficulties which usually settles spontaneously within a few months. Leg oedema, constipation, and shortened vagina have also been reported.

Radiotherapy was first used to treat cervical cancer in 1901, first with intravaginal cones, and has now evolved into a combination of external beam irradiation delivered by a linear acceleration and intracavity caesium. The total dose of radiation is calculated (usually 45–50 Gy) and delivered in small fractions of over 4–5 weeks. This is followed by examination under anesthetic and hollow plastic tubes are inserted into the uterine cavity and vaginal fornices. An afterloading device then inserts the caesium sources once the patient has returned to her room and these are left *in situ* for a calculated length of time (24–48 hours).

The cure rates for the late stages of cervical cancer are poor. Attempts have been made to improve these by using chemotherapy in recent years. Combination treat-

Key points

- Commonest gynaecological cancer worldwide.
- Incidence declining in the developed world.
- HPV 16, smoking, multiple sexual partners are important aetiological factors.
- Screening reduces incidence.
- Clinical staging is important in determining management.
- Early disease is treated by radical hysterectomy and pelvic node dissection.
- Late disease is treated by radiotherapy.
- The prognosis is good if pelvic lymph nodes are not involved.

ments involving Ifosfamide and cisplatin have been the most promising in achieving tumour responses, but unfortunately gave disappointing long-term cure rates.

Recently, further trials have taken place in an attempt to shrink tumours using chemotherapy in combination with radiotherapy and follow this up with surgery. Promising results using platinum-based drugs have been reported. In the USA and UK some centres are now using chemo-radiation as their standard treatment.

Prognosis

Patients who present with small tumours with no evidence of lymph node spread have an excellent chance of survival and now attempts are being made to treat these patients surgically and preserve function by removing the cervix and lower parametrial tissue and preserving the uterine body in the hope that the patient can achieve a pregnancy at a later date. This is called radical trachelectomy and shows promise in a highly selected group. In the main, however, standard treatment of radical hysterectomy and node dissection or radiotherapy can offer reasonable cure rates. The long-term hope remains that prevention of disease and early detection will mean that this most distressing disease will become a less important cause of morbidity and death in the future.

Carcinoma of the vagina

Epidemiology

Primary vaginal carcinoma is a rare disease, most vaginal tumours being secondary to either cervical, vulval, bowel, or endometrial cancer.

The age range at presentation is very wide, although the majority occur in women in their 60s. Over 90% are squamous in origin apart from a few adenocarcinomas and clear cell adenocarcinomas. The latter group occur in young women with a history of maternal ingestion of stilboestrol in pregnancy and have occurred mostly in the USA.

Aetiology

No single agent has been identified in the development of this disease, although there does seem to be an association with a previous history of having had an abdominal hysterectomy for CIN in the past. This raises two possible aetiological possibilities: first, incomplete excision of the original CIN lesion, which has persisted and progressed to invasive disease; and second, the possibility of multicentric disease involving the cervix, vagina, and possibly the vulva. Indeed, the association between separate vaginal and vulval tumours is well documented and investigation of these with regard to implicating HPV virus as a cause has been considered.

Pathology

Over 90% of vaginal cancers are squamous cell in origin and spread is via local lymphatics and vascular capillaries. The lymph channels drain to the pelvic lymph nodes in a similar pattern to cervical tumours unless the tumour is very low, and spread may be downwards towards the vulva and inguinal glands. Because of the rich blood supply to the vagina, bloodborne metastases occur relatively early in this disease.

Direct tumour extension into adjacent organs such as the bladder, urethra, or rectum is common and frequently leads to therapeutic difficulties.

Examination, diagnosis, and staging

A speculum examination will reveal a bleeding lesion, which will make the diagnosis fairly obvious. Occasionally asymptomatic patients may present with abnormal cytology and vaginoscopy and biopsy will be required to differentiate between vaginal intraepithelial neoplasia (VAIN) or invasive disease.

To confirm the diagnosis, patients should be examined under anaesthetic and the site, size, and spread of the tumour to involve adjacent organs established. This should include cystoscopy and sigmoidoscopy. The lesion should be biopsied to include the margin or, if superficial, an excision biopsy with 1 cm margin obtained.

Treatment

Radiotherapy is the main method of treatment as this can achieve primary disease control with maintenance of vaginal function. The technique used is similar to treatment of cervical tumours.

Surgery has been used to treat this disease in its earliest stages in the form of partial or total vaginectomy and lymphadenectomy or in advanced or recurrent disease by way of exenteration.

Prognosis

Survival rates for stage I disease are good; 65–85% are cured at 5 years. However, the majority of patients are later than this at presentation and the overall cure rate is under 50%.

Cancer of the ovary

Ovarian cancer is really a collection of many different histological tumour types. Epidemiologically they all have a similar distribution, affecting women in industrialized societies of higher socioeconomic class. The disease in general affects women after the menopause with a peak incidence of around 60 being rare, below the age of 40. Germ cell and malignant teratomas are the exception to this in that they tend to affect younger women.

Ovarian cancer is now the commonest gynaecological cancer in the UK with a rising rate of incidence affecting over 4000 women annually with a 5-year survival of only 25%, making it the worst gynaecological cancer in terms of outcome.

Aetiology

There has been considerable interest in trying to determine the cause of epithelial ovarian cancer in recent years and, in particular, trying to identify a familial link. Only 5% of sufferers have a family history of two or more relatives who have had the disease, although a similar number have a history of one relative with ovarian cancer and other family members who have a history of either breast, endometrial, or bowel cancer.

Genetic investigations have identified so far two genes, *BRCA1* and *BRCA2*, which are identified as putting carriers at risk of developing one of these cancers and families can now be offered investigation to determine risk.

The vast majority of ovarian cancers, however, are not genetically linked and whilst many causal factors such as asbestos, talc, coffee, and high-fat diet have been suggested, none has been proved. The association with low parity has, however, been clearly identified as also has been its negative association with combined oral contraceptive pill (COCP) use. These observations have led to the theory that incessant ovulation is an important cause of epithelial ovarian cancers, introducing the concept of repeated damage and repair leading to malignant change. Concern has also been expressed as to whether ovarian stimulation in infertility treatment may be a risk factor; however, so far this has yet to be proved.

Given this evidence, it would seem logical that targeted screening could perhaps prevent ovarian cancer and several trials are currently being undertaken. Several obstacles, however, remain before a screening programme is likely to work. Included in these are the fact that a pre-malignant phase in ovarian cancer development is very difficult to identify and ovarian cancer usually presents at a late stage.

There are two screening methods in current use. Ultrasound has high sensitivity (98%) and when coupled with colour flow Doppler also has high specificity (97%); however, it is expensive.

Serum CA-125 has a sensitivity of 70–80% and specificity of 98%. Each investigation alone has not yet proved to be suitable for mass population screening and at present a combination of the two are being used for limited screening of women perceived as being at high risk.

Pathology

Over 90% of primary ovarian malignancies are epithelial adenocarcinomas arising from the surface epithelium. Within this group several specific histological types can be identified. The commonest of these is serous adenocarcinoma (40–50%) followed by endometroid (15–30%). Mucinoid and clear cell represent approximately 10–15% each whilst Brenner tumours account for a very small number

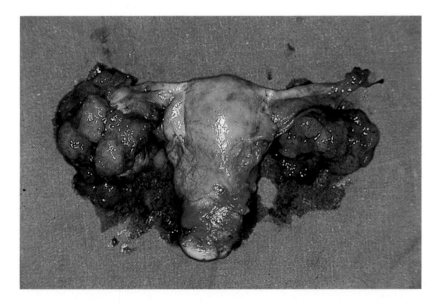

Fig. 15.4 Bilateral ovarian cancers which have breached the capsule of the ovary.

(the majority of this variety are benign). Most of the epithelial tumours are multicystic in appearance with solid elements. The surface may be smooth or have papillary fleshy growths and in the more advanced stages adhere to and grow directly onto the peritoneum of adjacent structures.

Histologically, there is a wide variety in tumour differentiation and papillary patterns of growth are common. Endometroid tumours often mimic endometrial tumours. Psammoma bodies (small dark appearing calcospherites) are characteristic but not diagnostic of primary ovarian tumours and their appearance is often sought when the primary origin of an adenocarcinoma within the abdominal cavity is uncertain, to help distinguish it from bowel, stomach, or pancreatic primary tumours.

Spread of ovarian cancers is primarily to other organs within the peritoneal cavity, and deposits in the omentum, uterus, colon, appendix, and small bowel are common. There may also be malignant ascites and tumour on the parietal peritoneum and the surface of the liver and spleen. Later spread may be to the chest, giving rise to a pleural effusion and the parenchyma of the liver.

Presentation

One of the most frustrating problems in the management of ovarian cancer is the lateness of presentation. The ovary is the only organ in the abdominal cavity not to have a peritoneal covering, which allows it to hang freely. It is also poorly supplied with nerve fibres. This combination of properties allows the ovary to grow quite large without the patient being aware. Many women with huge ovarian cysts the size of a full-term pregnancy go for many months unaware of their condition. It may not be until the tumour is pressing onto or growing into other organs that symptoms occur. Often patients present with vague symptoms such as dyspepsia, abdominal discomfort, increasing abdominal girth, weight loss, dyspnoea, poor appetite, or change in bowel habit. For this reason more than 50% of patients are not referred directly to a gynaecologist, leading to a delay in diagnosis.

Examination and diagnosis

When a woman is suspected of having an ovarian tumour she should have a full clinical history taken and careful examination. Evidence of abdominal distension should make one suspicious and attempts made to clinically distinguish between fat, flatus, fluid, and tumour on abdominal palpation. This should be aided by a vaginal and rectal examination. Clinical suspicions should then be confirmed by an ultrasound examination and serum CA-125.

The presence of a multiloculated cystic and solid pelvic mass with CA-125 over 100 U/ml is most likely to indicate an ovarian cancer. In a young woman (under 35 years) serum α-fetoprotein (AFP) and β-subunit human chorionic gonadotrophin (β-HCG) should also be measured as these can be raised in malignant teratomas and germ cell tumours.

Once the diagnosis is suspected, the patient must be counselled regarding the need for surgery and further investigations ordered, including chest x-ray, CT scan of abdomen, full blood count (FBC), urea and electrolytes (U&E), and liver function tests. On occasions it may be necessary to perform an abdominal tap or pleural tap to relieve symptoms or confirm the diagnosis of malignancy cytologically.

Table 15.4 **FIGO classification for the stages of carcinoma of the ovary**

Stage I	Growth limited to the ovaries
Stage Ia	Growth limited to one ovary; no ascites present containing malignant cells. No tumour on the external surface; capsule intact
Stage Ib	Growth limited to both ovaries; no ascites present containing malignant cells; no tumour on the external surfaces; capsules intact
Stage Ic	Tumour stage Ia or Ib but with tumour on surface of one or both ovaries; or with capsule ruptured; or with ascites present containing malignant cells or with positive peritoneal washings
Stage II	Growth involving one or both ovaries with pelvic extension
Stage IIa	Extension and/or metastases to the uterus and/or tubes
Stage IIb	Extension to other pelvic tissues
Stage IIc	Tumour stage IIa or IIb but with tumour on surface of one or both ovaries; or with capsule(s) ruptured; or with ascites present containing malignant cells or with positive peritoneal washings
Stage III	Tumour involving one or both ovaries with peritoneal implants outside the pelvis and/or positive retroperitoneal or inguinal nodes; superficial liver metastases equals stage III. Tumour is limited to the true pelvis but with histologically proven malignant extension to small bowel or omentum
Stage IIIa	Tumour grossly limited to the true pelvis with negative nodes but with histologically confirmed microscopic seeding of abdominal peritoneal surfaces
Stage IIIb	Tumour of one or both ovaries with histologically confirmed implants of abdominal peritoneal surfaces, none exceeding 2 cm in diameter; nodes are negative
Stage IIIc	Abdominal implants greater than 2 cm in diameter and/or positive retroperitoneal or inguinal nodes
Stage IV	Growth involving one or both ovaries with distant metastases. If pleural effusion is present there must be positive cytology to allot a case to stage IV. Parenchymal liver metastasis equals stage IV.

Staging

FIGO staging for ovarian cancer is based on surgical findings and is a useful prognostic indicator. (Table 15.4). Stage for stage, patients with ovarian cancer do not fare much worse than other cancers. Unfortunately, the disease predominately presents at stage III, by which time the tumour has spread throughout the abdominal cavity, giving a poor outlook. The method of tumour spread does not depend so much on lymphatic and vascular spread as other tumours; therefore, staging is related to tumour spread through the capsule of the ovary, whether one or both ovaries is involved, and on the presence or absence of ascites (stage 1a–IIc). Spread throughout the abdominal cavity except the liver parenchyma remains stage III with secondary deposits in the liver and outside the abdominal cavity being stage IV.

Treatment

The main principle of treatment of ovarian cancers is to remove as much tumour as possible surgically and then follow this up with chemotherapy. It has been shown by many surgical studies over the past 20 years that not only does the bulk of tumour preoperatively have a bearing on ultimate survival but so also does the amount left postoperatively. If no visible disease is present after surgery, the outcome is better than if disease remains no matter what further treatment is given.

The primary aim, therefore, of surgery is to remove all visible tumour if possible. This usually involves performing a hysterectomy, BSO, and omentectomy. Other tumour deposits present should be removed, if possible; as this could involve bowel resection, patients ought to be informed of this and the possibility of having a colostomy explained and permission sought preoperatively. If it is not safe or technically possible to remove all visible tumour, then the secondary aim is to leave no single deposit greater than 1 cm diameter.

The surgical findings and procedure performed must be carefully documented to help further treatment planning.

The exceptions to this strategy are the rare germ cell tumours and malignant teratomas. These respond well to chemotherapy to the extent that these young patients may be cured and go on to have children. If, therefore, one of these tumours is suspected preoperatively, a more consecutive approach is justified, to try and preserve reproductive function without compromising outcome.

Once the patient has recovered from surgery, the diagnosis must be discussed and arrangements made to start chemotherapy. For many years cyclophosphamide was the standard chemotherapy; this was superseded by platinum-based drugs, either single agent or in combination with others such as cyclophosphamide or doxorubicin.

All these drugs have toxic side-effects, which limits the dose, and should be given in a Cancer Centre by a medical oncologist. Almost 50% of patients respond to these regimens for stage III disease and whilst the 5-year survival rate is approximately 30%, the average time to relapse is 2 years. Unfortunately 5-year survival rates are poor at < 30%.

Recently, a new group of drugs, the taxanes, derived from the Pacific yew tree, have shown a promising response rate and are now used as front-line drugs in combination with either cisplatin or carboplatin. Mean response rates of 3 years have been obtained in trials and this must now be seen as the most effective treatment available.

Currently, radiotherapy has virtually no part to play in first-line treatment of ovarian cancer, although it may be used to direct treatment at a solitary pelvic recurrence or to treat bone secondaries.

Prognosis

As stated above, the reported outcome for ovarian cancer generally is very poor compared with other cancers, due to the late stage at diagnosis. This has led to a negative attitude to the disease by the medical profession and as a result many women have in the past had less than adequate treatment. In the UK, with the development of gynaecological cancer centres and the adoption of a multidisciplinary team approach,

---

Key points

- Commonest gynaecological cancer in UK and has the worst prognosis.
- 5% are familial.
- Associated with low parity and incessant ovulation.
- Most present at stage III.
- 90% are epithelial in origin.
- Primary aim of surgery is to remove as much tumour as possible.
- Cisplatin and Taxotere in combination give 50% response rate.
- Rare germ cell tumours and malignant teratomas tend to occur in young women and respond well to chemotherapy.
- Screening for ovarian cancer by ultrasound and serum CA-125 has yet to prove its usefulness.

patients should now have better evaluation of their disease, surgery performed by specially trained surgeons, state of the art chemotherapy administered by medical oncologists, and patients, if possible, entered in clinical trials.

Unfortunately, at present this approach, whilst optimizing each individual's treatment, will still not cure the majority of patients. To achieve overall better outcomes, progress must be made in the future to develop adequate screening and thus prevent, or at least diagnose at an earlier stage, this most distressing disease.

Case histories

Case 1

'I've had this itch for 2 years and nothing seems to help.'

Miss EH is a 72-year-old retired shopkeeper who lives alone. She has noted an itch in the vulval region for more than 2 years. Being a very private woman, she was reluctant to seek help and applied various creams to the area. She only sought help from her GP when the itch became so unbearable that she broke the skin whilst scratching, causing her to bleed. Her GP prescribed oestradiol cream b.d. for 3 weeks. Six weeks later she returned because there was no improvement.

Examination
The vulval region was markedly atrophic with white patches of skin covering the labia minora, clitoris and fourchette. There was a 3 cm raised lesion on the left side of the labium minus and majus with a central area of ulceration.

There was no palpable lymphadenopathy.

Management
On referral to hospital, Miss H was admitted for biopsy of the lesion under general anaesthetic. This confirmed the presence of a moderately differentiated squamous cell carcinoma of the vulva.

After appropriate counselling, a radical vulvectomy and groin node dissection was performed, employing separate incisions.

Histopathology confirmed the diagnosis and that the tumour had been completely excised with adequate margins. The surrounding skin showed lichen sclerosis et atrophicus. All lymph nodes were free of disease. After recovery from surgery, the patient was followed up on a 3-monthly basis for 2 years and at gradually increasing intervals thereafter. *continued*

Case histories continued

Case 2

'My periods have returned after 10 years – I did not think this was possible.'

History

Mrs SN is a 65-year-old married woman who has had two children. She weighs 97 kg, is taking a β-blocker for moderate hypertension and is a non-insulin-dependant diabetic controlled by diet alone. She had a delayed menopause but never took hormone replacement therapy. She noticed blood on her pants after attending the funeral of her sister who had died after a long battle with breast cancer and thought that it was due to shock. The bleeding persisted and became like a period lasting 6 days.

Examination

Mrs N is markedly obese and abdominal palpation is unrewarding.

Speculum examination shows a cystocele and normal cervix. There is blood coming through the cervical os.

Management

Mrs N is referred to her local gynaecologist who performs a vaginal ultrasound, finding an enlarged uterus and thickened endometrium.

An out-patient endometrial sample reveals cheesy endometrium which on histological examination shows adenocarcinoma cells.

A hysteroscopy under anaesthetic shows an enlarged uterine cavity (9 cm) and a polypoid pale lesion arising from the uterine fundus. A biopsy was performed which confirmed the diagnosis and showed a poorly differentiated adenocarcinoma.

A chest x-ray and MRI scan were organized. The latter showed that the tumour did not invade more than a third of the way into the myometrium; no lymphadenopathy was detected.

Because of poor tumour differentiation and high anaesthetic risk, the patient was referred to the gynaecological cancer centre for surgery and an extended hysterectomy, bilateral salpingo-oophorectomy and pelvic and para-aortic node dissection was performed.

Histology revealed that the tumour had poorly differentiated elements, invasion was confined to the inner third of the myometrium and all the lymph nodes were normal. After discussion it was decided not to give adjuvant treatment as the tumour did not show evidence of spread and 5 years later Mrs N remains well and disease free.

Case 3

'I bleed sometimes after we have intercourse.'

Mrs PB is a married woman aged 32 and runs her own business. She has a 4-year-old child and, whilst she takes the combined oral contraceptive pill, plans to have another baby in the near future. For the past 4 months she has been having some light bleeding between her periods and puts this down to occasionally forgetting to take her 'pill'. On several occasions in the past 2 months she has experienced painless bleeding after sex and this has prompted her to attend her general practitioner. She is not unduly alarmed as she had a 'normal cervical smear' 3 years ago. *continued*

Case histories continued

Her GP performs a speculum examination and sees a 2 cm warty lesion on the anterior lip of the cervix which is bleeding. She makes an immediate referral to the colposcopy clinic at the regional gynaecological cancer centre where she is seen and a colposcopic assessment is made. This includes a cervical biopsy. When the result is available, an appointment is arranged for Mrs B. and her husband to meet the consultant gynaecological oncologist who explains the diagnosis is cervical cancer and what investigations are required to determine the appropriate treatment.

Initially an examination under anaesthetic, cystoscopy, and cold knife biopsy of the cervix are performed (staging procedure). This is followed up by an MRI scan of the pelvis. The FIGO clinical stage of the tumour is 1b and at further consultation Mrs B is offered a radical hysterectomy and pelvic node dissection, which she accepts. The operation is performed 2 weeks later without complication. The histology report indicates a completely excised squamous carcinoma with lymph channel involvement and microscopic tumour deposits in two small lymph nodes.

This finding is discussed at the multidisciplinary oncology meeting and it is decided to offer Mrs B adjuvant radiotherapy, which she accepts. After the radiotherapy is complete, Mrs B is reviewed at the gynaecological oncology clinic and it is apparent that she is unhappy. After a lengthy consultation, it emerges that Mrs B has several unanswered questions, which up to now she has not asked. These include: Why did my last smear not diagnose the cancer? What caused the cancer? Will it come back? She also has fears related to running her business, sex, hormone replacement therapy, bladder and bowel functions, and expresses anger and frustration at being unable to have further children. As many of these questions as possible are answered and with the patient's permission she is referred to the oncology counselling team.

Case 4

'I seem to be losing weight yet my skirt size is getting bigger.'

Presentation

Mrs JM is 57 and lives with her husband; they have one grown up daughter. She has lost her appetite and experienced dyspepsia for the past 5 months. She has also noticed increasing constipation and occasional tenesmus. Her GP has diagnosed diverticular disease and given dietary advice; he ordered a barium enema, which was normal. Mrs M developed severe pain in her abdomen and was admitted to hospital with suspected appendicitis to a surgical ward. Three days after admission an ultrasound examination of her abdomen revealed a cystic and solid mass arising out of the pelvis 12 cm in diameter with associated free fluid.

Examination

On palpation, the abdomen was slightly distended with a doughy feel. There was a shifting dullness and a fluid thrill. There was the impression of a mass arising out of the right side of the pelvis, which was moderately tender, firm, and irregular, and not mobile.

Speculum examination was normal, vaginal and rectal examination revealed a fixed pelvic mass on the right side of the pelvis almost filling the pelvis and attached to the uterus.

continued

Case histories continued

Management

Chest x-ray, FBC, U&E, LFT, CA-125 and CT scans were ordered.

The patient and her husband were counselled regarding the probable diagnosis of ovarian cancer and advised as to the surgery required and the possibility of chemotherapy. They agreed to this and surgery was scheduled as soon as possible because the patient was in pain.

At laparotomy, after draining 2500 ml of ascitic fluid, a 12 cm ovarian tumour of the right ovary was found which was fixed to the side of the pelvis and invading the uterus; a loop of terminal ileum was densely adherent to the top of the tumour as was the serosa of the anterior wall of the rectum. The left ovary was normal. There were several studs of tumour 1–2 cm in the omentum and a couple of tiny nodules 3 mm diameter over the peritoneum, the bladder, and right paracolic gutter. The tumour was staged as FIGO IIIb.

A total hysterectomy, bilateral salpingo-oophorectomy and omentectomy were performed. All other tumour modules were excised including some residual tumour of the serosa of the rectum. The tumour was invading deeply into the wall of the ileum and this part was resected with primary anastomosis of the bowel.

At the end of the operation there was no visible tumour.

Mrs M made a satisfactory postoperative recovery and was referred for chemotherapy. Six cycles of cisplatin and Taxol were administered on a 4-weekly basis. At the end of treatment, Mrs M was feeling well, her serum CA-125 had fallen from 1395 U/ml preoperatively to 24 U/ml and arrangements were made for 3-monthly follow-up at the joint oncology clinic.

Further reading

Coppleson M., (1992) *Gynaecological oncology*. Churchill Livingstone, Edinburgh.

Di Saia, P. and Creasman, W. (1997) *Clinical gynaecological oncology*. Mosby, St. Louis.

Monaghan, J. (1986) *Bonney's gynaecological surgery*. Bailliere Tindall, London.

NHS Executive (1999) *Improving outcomes in gynaecological cancers*. Department of Health, Wetherby.

Novak, E. and Woodruff, D. (1979) Gynaecological and obstetric pathology. WB Saunders Company, Philadelphia.

Shepherd, J. and Monaghan, J. (1995) *Clinical gynaecological oncology*. Blackwell Scientific Publications, Oxford.

Whitfield, C. (1995) *Dewhurst's textbook of obstetrics and gynaecology for graduates*. Blackwell Scientific Publications, Oxford.

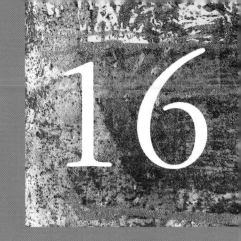

16

Gastrointestinal cancer
James J. A. McAleer

- Introduction

- Carcinoma of the stomach

- Carcinoma of the exocrine pancreas

- Hepatoma (hepatocellular cancer)

- Bile duct carcinoma (cholangiocarcinoma)

- Carcinoma of the gallbladder

- Tumours of the small bowel

- Carcinoma of the colon and rectum

- Carcinoma of the anus

Gastrointestinal cancer

Introduction

Gastrointestinal tumours are relatively common and account for almost 25% of all tumours. Since these tumours arise in a distensible hollow tube, they tend to have a relatively late presentation. Clinical vigilance and willingness to investigate patients with minimal gastrointestinal symptoms are required to detect early-stage disease and improve outcome. The tumour types occurring along the gastro-intestinal tract are quite different in terms of aetiological factors, anatomy, therapeutic options, and outcome, and accordingly they will be considered under separate headings.

Carcinoma of the oesophagus

Epidemiology

Oesophageal tumours account for approximately 7000 new cases each year in the UK. Tumours of the upper third of the oesophagus are more common in females but overall there is a male preponderance. The incidence of squamous cell cancer of the oesophagus remains stable over time. The incidence of adenocarcinoma, especially around the oesophago-gastric junction, has been increasing steadily in recent years. These tumours often extend into the stomach across the oesophago-gastric junction. There is a remarkable international variation with a very high incidence in certain provinces of China, in Iran, and in certain areas of Africa. In the USA, oesophageal cancer is much commoner in blacks than in whites.

Aetiology

The recognized risk factors for oesophageal cancer are documented in Table 16.1. Patients with Barrett's oesophagus (glandular metaplasia of the squamous cell lining of the lower third of the oesophagus, usually related to ongoing gastro-oesophageal reflux) have an increased risk of developing adenocarcinoma of the

Table 16.1 Risk factors for oesophageal cancer

- Alcohol ingestion
- Tobacco smoking
- Barrett's oesophagus
- Tylosis
- Plummer–Vinson syndrome
- Oesophageal diverticulum
- Oesophageal achalasia
- Previous oropharyngeal cancer

lower oesophagus. When this condition is identified, patients should undergo regular endoscopic surveillance.

Pathology

Less than 10% of oesophageal cancers occur in the upper third of the oesophagus and most of these are squamous cell carcinoma. About 50% of oesophageal tumours arise in the lower third and approximately half are adenocarcinoma. These may have arisen from areas of metaplasia such as Barrett's oesophagus. Tumours of the middle third are more commonly squamous carcinomas. The appearance of tumours varies from nodular exophytic tumour masses to infiltrated and ulcerating lesions. Tumours will expand circumferentially and also spread quite widely submucosally, which has implications for planning of therapy.

Tumours of the oesophagus will directly invade other mediastinal structures such as trachea, pericardium, or major vessels. Tumour also spreads through the lymphatic channels in the mediastinum and commonly involves the supraclavicular and cervical lymph nodes for the upper third of the oesophagus, mediastinal nodes for all oesophageal tumours, and coeliac nodes for the lower third of oesophagus.

Clinical presentation

Patients with oesophageal carcinoma typically present with dysphagia, which will have an insidious onset. Initially patients have difficulty with solid dry food, but later they may have difficulty even with liquids, leading to regurgitation and the possibility of aspiration pneumonia. There may also be central chest pain from mediastinal involvement and patients typically have weight loss due to inadequate food intake and to effects of advanced tumour. Patients with Plummer–Vinson's tumour may have anaemia and koilonychia. Patients with tylosis may also have palmar and plantar keratosis. Evidence of metastatic spread often includes supraclavicular lymphadenopathy or liver enlargement.

Investigations

All middle-aged or elderly patients with dysphagia must have visualization of the oesophagus. Endoscopy is the investigation of choice, allowing direct visualization of the oesophageal mucosa and biopsy of any suspicious lesion. Areas of Barrett's

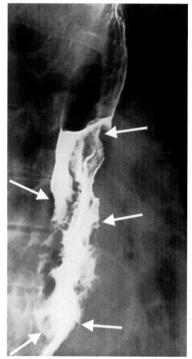

Fig. 16.1 Oesophageal cancer. Barium swallow demonstrating an extensive adenocarcinoma of the lower third of oesophagus.

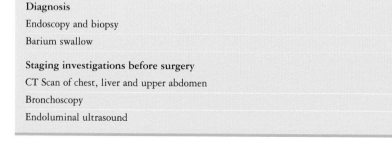

Table 16.2 Diagnostic and staging investigations for oesophageal cancer

Diagnosis
Endoscopy and biopsy
Barium swallow
Staging investigations before surgery
CT Scan of chest, liver and upper abdomen
Bronchoscopy
Endoluminal ultrasound

oesophagus can also be identified and the stomach can be examined. If tumour is identified, staging investigations will include CT scan of chest and liver. Endoluminal ultrasonography is becoming the modality of choice for determining the depth of involvement of the oesophageal wall and of the adjacent mediastinal lymph nodes. Bronchoscopy is also required to exclude a primary lung tumour and to document invasion of the trachea, which would render the tumour inoperable.

Treatment

If assessment has shown the tumour to be localized, then consideration is given to potentially curative treatment. The current standard treatment in the UK is radical surgery for tumours of the middle and lower third of the oesophagus. Contraindications to surgery include haematogenous metastases, cervical or coeliac lymph node involvement, broncho-oesophageal fistula, direct invasion of the major vessels in the mediastinum (aorta and superior vena cava), vocal cord paralysis, or invasion of pericardium.

The details of surgery are summarized in Table 16.3.

Radiotherapy is regarded as the treatment of choice for tumours of the upper third of oesophagus as surgery is technically difficult. Radiotherapy can also be used for tumours of the middle and lower third if the patient is unfit for surgery. For radical radiotherapy, the treatment volume includes a proximal and distal margin of 5 cm of clinically normal oesophagus to allow for occult submucosal spread.

There is an increasing body of evidence suggesting that the combination of chemotherapy and radiotherapy, either as a preoperative therapy, or indeed as a definitive therapy, offers benefit over surgery alone. These therapies are the subject of current clinical trials.

Patients with inoperable carcinoma of the oesophagus usually have a major problem with dysphagia and regurgitation of undigested food. They may have central chest pain or discomfort. They will also have poor energy and weight loss. Dysphagia can be improved by oesophageal dilatation or stenting. The new expanding metal stents, although expensive, are relatively easy to place at endoscopy, and will usually considerably improve swallowing. Tumours can also

Table 16.3 Surgery for oesophageal cancer

Operation name	Transthoracic (Lewis)	Transhiatal	Total thoracic	Radical *en bloc*
Incisions	Laparotomy	Laparotomy	Laparotomy	Laparotomy
	Right thoracotomy	Left neck	Left neck thoracotomy	Thoracoabdominal
Site of anastamosis	Intrathoracic	Neck	Neck	Neck
Other				*En bloc* excision with stomach, spleen, extensive nodes

be treated by radiotherapy or laser therapy to create a passage through obstructing tumour or to deal with bleeding. Where there is metastatic tumour resulting in systemic symptoms, palliative chemotherapy based on cisplatin and 5-fluorouracil can be offered to good performance status patients.

Prognosis

Overall survival for Western patients with oesophageal cancer is less than 10% at 5 years. Patients who have radical surgery do substantially better. Despite a 12% anastomotic leak rate (a complication with a mortality rate of 30–50%) with an overall in-hospital mortality rate of 11%, there is an overall 5-year survival of 21%. This can be subdivided into a survival of 40–57% for node-negative resections and 8–23% for node-positive resections.

Carcinoma of the stomach

Epidemiology

In the UK, there are around 10 000 new cases and 7600 deaths each year from stomach carcinoma. There is a slight male predominance and the tumour is most common in the 50–70 years age group. The incidence of stomach cancer is very high in Japan and Chile. In the Western world stomach cancer is commoner in lower socioeconomic groups.

Aetiology

Diets high in smoked food are associated with an increased risk of stomach cancer. Patients with a history of helicobacter pylori infection, atrophic gastritis, achlorhydria, pernicious anaemia, and blood group A all have an increased risk of stomach cancer. A previous history of a partial gastrectomy or gastroenterostomy gives an increased risk of gastric cancer, which may be related to chronic reflux of bile salts into the stomach.

Pathology

Cancers are usually seen as ulcerating lesions, often with raised edges, or as nodular polypoid tumours. Some stomach tumours are predominantly submucosal and highly infiltrative, giving rise to a greatly thickened stomach wall in a reduced capacity (leather bottle stomach, linitis plastica). Half of stomach tumours arise in the pyloric region with a majority of the remainder along the lesser curvature. Virtually all stomach tumours are adenocarcinomas and mainly associated with prior intestinal metaplasia or carcinoma in situ. Stomach cancers typically arise in the mucosal area, spreading longitudinally, submucosally, and circumferentially. Tumours will then invade the muscle wall and go directly into adjacent structures or by lymphatics to regional lymph nodes in the coeliac plexus. The adjacent organs invaded include the omentum, pancreas, spleen, left kidney, and adrenal. They can also spread across the oesophago-gastric junction and give rise to oesophageal obstruction. The transcoelomic spread of stomach cancer may give rise of peritoneal seedlings and tumour deposits in the ovaries (Krukenberg tumours) or pouch of Douglas is well recognized. Haematogenous spread can be via the portal venous circulation to the liver or via systemic circulation to the lung, brain, bone, and skin.

More than 95% of stomach cancers are adenocarcinomas (Fig. 16.2). They can be subdivided, using the Lauren system, into intestinal and diffuse subtypes. This has prognostic significance, with the intestinal variety having a better prognosis. The intestinal variety is well differentiated with gland formation and is much less likely to demonstrate submucosal spread. There is a particular pathological entity with the primary tumour invasion of the stomach wall limited to mucosa or submucosa which is classified as 'early gastric cancer' (EGC) even if lymph nodes are involved.

Clinical presentation

Patients with stomach cancer generally have a very insidious symptom pattern with minimal gastrointestinal symptoms such as nausea, vomiting, anorexia, and weight loss. They may also have epigastric discomfort or bloating. Chronic blood loss may give rise to anaemia.

Clinically, there may be a palpable epigastric mass or lymphatic spread may be palpable in the lymph nodes of the left supraclavicular fossa (Troisier's sign). Enlargement of the liver due to metastases may be palpable.

Investigations

Endoscopy is the investigation of choice, enabling visualization of oesophagus, stomach, and duodenum, with biopsy of any suspicious lesions. Barium meal will also demonstrate gastric ulcers but may not distinguish between benign and malignant disease. The barium meal may demonstrate the particular entity of linitis plastica with a small volume, non-distensible stomach, and these patients may well have no mucosal lesion at endoscopy. These investigations may also detect other conditions including peptic ulceration, gastritis, and other benign or malignant gastric tumours.

In a patient in whom a gastric carcinoma has been identified and there is no clinical evidence of metastases, further evaluation is required to exclude clinically occult metastases before considering radical therapy. This should include CT scan of liver and abdomen. Laparoscopy is a very valuable technique, allowing the surgeon to demonstrate local invasion into adjacent organs or peritoneal seedlings. At this procedure liver metastases can be visualized, or detected on laparoscopic ultrasound, and biopsied if required.

Treatment

Surgery is the definitive treatment for stomach carcinoma. Partial or total gastrectomy will be required to obtain clear margins, depending on the size and location of the tumour. Routine splenectomy, in the absence of direct splenic invasion, has not been shown to improve outcome. Palliative operations can be performed to control pain or relieve obstruction in patients with advanced disease. However, given the poor survival prospects of such patients, a balance must be struck between potential for long-term control of symptoms and morbidity and mortality of surgery. The operations include gastrojejunostomy as a bypass operation for obstruction of gastric outlet and partial gastrectomy for bleeding or pain.

In Japan, stomach cancer has high incidence and is often detected at a relatively early stage. The Japanese surgeons have developed a complex classification system for the 20 lymph node groups which they recognise. They carry out more

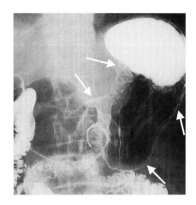

Fig. 16.2 Gastric cancer. Barium meal demonstrating a large circumferential adenocarcinoma of stomach (arrows).

extensive lymph node dissection, and have higher survival rates for their patients, than those reported in American or European patients, even when stage differences are taken into account.

There is no evidence that routine pre- or postoperative chemotherapy or radiotherapy will improve outcome in patients with surgically resectable stomach cancer, but clinical trials continue to investigate these therapeutic approaches. Endoscopic procedures such as laser or oesophageal stenting may improve haemorrhage or obstructive symptoms in patients unfit for surgery. Radiotherapy can be used for local symptoms such as dysphagia, haemorrhage, or pain.

In advanced gastric cancer, the most effective single agent chemotherapy is 5-fluorouracil and it is administered in various combinations with doxorubicin, cisplatin epirubicin or methotrexate. These combinations show response rates of around 50% and these regimens have been shown to prolong survival when compared with best supportive care.

Prognosis

In patients with stomach cancer who have had radical surgery, the involvement of lymph nodes in the resected specimen reduces predicted 5-year survival from 31% to 17%. In node-negative patients where tumour does not involve the serosa, 5-year survival is approximately 50%. The uncommon diagnosis of 'early gastric cancer', as defined above, is associated with a further improvement in outcome. For this tumour, survival at 5 years for disease confined to mucosa is 99%, involving submcosa is 91% and for EGC involving lymph nodes is 75%, 64%, and 25% for NI, N2, and N3 disease, respectively.

For patients with stage IV disease, median survival is a few months, improving to about 1 year with chemotherapy.

Carcinoma of the exocrine pancreas

Epidemiology

There are 6800 new cases of pancreatic cancer and approximately 6500 deaths each year in the UK. It tends to occur in the 60–80 years age group and there is no sex predominance.

Aetiology

The factors associated with pancreatic cancer are listed in Table 16.4.

Pathology

Tumours of the exocrine pancreas are adenocarcinoma in type. There is usually a dense stromal background and there may be evidence of pancreatitis or calcification in the non-malignant pancreas. Histological variations include ductal, mucinous cystadenocarcinoma, and acinar cell tumours, but these patterns do not have obvious prognostic significance. The tumour often stains positively for carcinoembryonic antigen (CEA). Most tumours will display a specific point mutation on the K-*ras* oncogene.

Most patients have a locally advanced tumour that obstructs the intrapancreatic portion of the common bile duct or the pancreatic duct. The tumour will often invade throughout the pancreas and spreads directly to the coeliac plexus and

---

Gastric Cancer:
Key points

- Insidious onset of symptoms
- Gastroscopy and biopsy is key to diagnosis
- Full staging avoids inappropriate surgery
- CT Liver and upper abdomen
- Chest x-ray
- Laparoscopy
- Subtotal or total gastrectomy
- Extent of nodal resection is controversial
- Chemotherapy provides effective palliation of inoperable disease

Table 16.4 Risk factors for pancreatic cancer

Tobacco smoking

Animal fats in diet

Diabetes mellitus

Chronic pancreatitis

Surgery for peptic ulcer disease

Chemicals

   2-napthylamine

   DDT

   Petrol derivatives

Occupations

   Cement workers

   Stone workers

Uncertain associations

   Caffeine

   Alcohol

Protective factors

   Citrus fruit

   Vegetables

retroperitoneal tissues. Metastatic spread to the regional lymph nodes and via the bloodstream to liver or lungs is common.

Clinical presentation

Tumours of the head of pancreas will cause progressive obstructive jaundice (dark urine, pale stools, skin itching). This occurs due to obstruction of the common bile duct and will cause dilatation of the gallbladder if the patient does not have chronic cholecystitis (Courvoisier's sign, Fig. 16.3). Prolonged bile duct obstruction may give rise to abnormalities of coagulation, due to inadequate vitamin-K-dependent clotting factors, manifested as purpura or bleeding. If the tumour causes extensive replacement of the pancreas, it may cause pancreatic insufficiency with malabsorption and steatorrhoea. In 10% of cases, diabetes mellitus will occur. Local invasion of tumour arising in body and tail of the pancreas may give rise to severe pain. The tumour may be palpable as an epigastric mass, which may be fixed due to local extension. There may be a palpable liver due to metastatic disease and the patient may have considerable weight loss and cachexia.

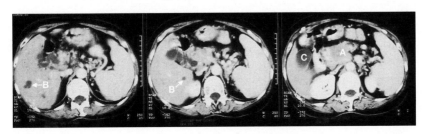

Fig. 16.3 Cancer of the head of pancreas. CT scan demonstrating (A) mass in head of pancreas, (B) dilated intrahepatic bile ducts, and (C) dilated gallbladder (clinically palpable as Courvoisier's sign).

Investigations

Liver function tests will show an obstructive pattern. The protein CA-19-9 is secreted by malignant cells from gastrointestinal tumours but very high levels are strongly suggestive of pancreatic cancer.

Definitive diagnosis of carcinoma head of pancreas can be obtained by endoscopic retrograde cholangiopancreatography (ERCP). This may show a characteristic stricture and brushings or biopsies can be taken for cytology. The stricture can be stented at this time. Percutaneous transhepatic cholangiography may also demonstrate dilated bile ducts. Ultrasound or CT of the upper abdomen may demonstrate dilated bile ducts or a pancreatic mass and guide fine needle aspiration cytology. Investigations to exclude metastases will include chest x-ray and CT of liver and abdomen. Occasionally a laparoscopy or laparotomy may be required to make a definitive diagnosis.

Treatment

After staging and investigations, only 10% of patients will be considered suitable for definitive radical surgery. The operation of pancreaticoduodenectomy (originally described by Whipple) is the operation of choice. This is a very complex and high-risk operation and should be performed by a specialist surgeon.

If the tumour is found to be inoperable at laparotomy, the surgeon can perform a biliary bypass operation to relieve the obstructive jaundice, thereby palliating the major symptoms associated with the obstructive jaundice. This will typically involve joining the hepatic duct to the jejunum (hepaticojejunostomy). If there is duodenenal obstruction due to a large periampullary mass, then a gastroenterostomy will also be performed. Patients with significant back pain may obtain relief from intraoperative or percutaneous coeliac plexus block by alcohol injection. Local radiotherapy is valuable for pain due to retroperitoneal tumour invasion.

Stenting of the bile duct across through the tumour mass may also be carried out either at ERCP or via percutaneous transhepatic procedure by an interventional radiologist. Pancreatic enzyme supplements will help malabsorption in patients with pancreatic insufficiency. Coagulation disorders can be treated with intravenous vitamin K and cholestyramine may assist with pruritis or symptoms of obstructive jaundice. Chemotherapy may have a palliative role in some patients with pancreatic carcinoma. The active agents are 5-fluorouracil and, more recently, gemcitabine has been licensed for this situation. However, benefit is limited and careful patient selection is required to optimize benefit verses toxicity.

Prognosis

Very few patients will survive 5 years; even with radical surgery, 5-year survival is less than 10%.

Hepatoma (hepatocellular cancer)

Epidemiology

Hepatoma is rare in the UK where there are approximately 100 new cases per year and approximately the same number of deaths. There is a slight male predominance. There is geographical variation with high incidence in certain areas of

Table 16.5 Risk factors for hepatoma, gallbladder cancer and bile duct cancer

Hepatoma	Gallbladder cancer	Bile duct cancer
Liver cirrhosis	Gallstones	Liver fluke infestation
Hepatitis B & C	*Salmonella typhi* carrier	Hepatolithiasis
Alcohol	Gallbladder polyp (> 1 cm)	Ulcerative colitis
Haemochromatosis	Anomalous pancreatico-biliary drainage	Sclerosing cholangitis
Chronic active hepatitis		Thorotrast
Thorotrast		Nitrosamines
?Anabolic steroids		Dioxin

Asia and Africa where hepatitis B is endemic. Hepatoma is the most common tumour worldwide with approximately one million cases occurring each year.

Aetiology

The most clearly defined predisposing factor for hepatoma is cirrhosis of the liver, which is present in 80% of cases. Cirrhosis can be due to hepatitis B or C, alcohol, haemochromatosis, chronic active hepatitis, and other less common causes. Populations with endemic hepatitis B infection have a high incidence of hepatoma. Hepatic toxins can also cause hepatoma. The mycotoxin, *Aspergillus flavus*, is found in stored cereals in tropical climates and is a significant hepatic carcinogen. Thorotrast was used as a contrast medium in radiographic studies and contains radioactive thorium. The α-radiation from the thorium is believed to be carcinogenic. The risk factors for hepatobiliary tumours are summarized in Table 16.5.

Pathology

The cells of hepatoma can vary from well-differentiated cells staining positively for bile to undifferentiated cells. The cells are often grouped around sinusoids or trabeculae lined by endothelial cells and containing blood. The tumour often arises in the regenerating nodule in the cirrhotic liver and it may be multifocal. The tumour cells characteristically secrete an oncofetal protein which serves as a tumour marker for the disease (α-fetoprotein, AFP).

Tumour cells will invade the portal venous system or ducts and therefore intrahepatic spread is common and early in this tumour. Tumour invades within the liver as described above and will also invade through the liver capsule into adjacent structures. Lymph nodes adjacent to the liver are commonly involved, and it may also spread via lymphatics and via the bloodstream. Lung and bone are common systemic sites of spread.

Clinical presentation

Patients with hepatoma often have a known diagnosis of cirrhosis and associated liver problems. The development of the hepatoma may lead to increasing anorexia and weight loss. Pain in the epigastrium may occur due to distension of the liver capsule. Haemorrhage into the capsule may cause acute pain with peritonitis or pleurisy. Most patients will have hepatomegaly with either diffuse enlargement or the presence of a sizeable mass. An arterial bruit and hepatic rub can be heard over the tumour. Compression of the inferior vena cava and liver impairment may lead to leg oedema and ascites. The patient may also notice jaundice and petechiae. The liver may be diffusely enlarged, or there may be a palpable mass due to hepatoma or cirrhosis. In the differential diagnosis of a focal mass or multiple masses in the liver, one must exclude secondary deposits. Metastases in the setting of liver cirrhosis are extremely rare and raised serum AFP supports the diagnosis of hepatoma.

A sizeable hepatoma can secrete an insulin-like peptide and give rise to hypoglycaemia. Tumour may also secrete parathormone, giving rise to hypercalcaemia, or oestrogens, giving rise to feminization. If portal vein thrombosis arises, then splenomegaly and oesophageal varices may arise. The Budd–Chiari syndrome (hepatic vein obstruction or thrombosis) will cause extensive oedema to the level of the umbilicus. Pyrexia of uncertain pathogenesis will occur in up to half of cases of hepatoma.

Investigations

Ultrasound, angiography, CT scanning, and MRI all contribute useful information regarding operability of the tumour. They will also facilitate a fine needle biopsy where the coagulation factors status permit. Chest x-ray is required to exclude lung metastases prior to definitive operation.

Treatment

If radical surgery is proposed, then angiography will demonstrate the anatomy and permit the formulation of a surgical plan. Only 10% of patients will be suitable for radical surgery.

If the tumour proves inoperable, then benefit can be obtained from ligation of the hepatic artery, which supplies a vast majority of the circulation to the hepatoma. If the portal vein is obstructed, then ischaemic necrosis of the liver is also possible. Unfortunately, collateral circulation will develop after hepatic artery embolization and this is essentially short-term palliation for a sizeable tumour mass. Hepatic artery embolization is an alternative procedure. This can be more selective, causing fewer untoward symptoms. Chemotherapeutic agents can also be infused through the hepatic artery, with increased retention in the liver if embolization is performed at the same time. Embolization can also be repeated at future dates. If significant systemic symptoms arise from metastatic disease, then anthracycline-based chemotherapy (doxorubicin) may be considered as a palliative measure.

The most important aetiological factor worldwide is hepatitis B and widespread vaccination against hepatitis B would dramatically reduce the incidence of hepatoma.

Prognosis

Overall, for hepatoma patients, median survival is less than 3 months for patients with cirrhosis and approaching 1 year in patients without cirrhosis. In the UK, only 5% of patients with cirrhosis, and 50% of patients without cirrhosis, are considered resectable.

Bile duct carcinoma (cholangiocarcinoma)

Epidemiology

These tumours are rare. There are about 1000 new cases per year in the UK. The majority of these tumours occur in the distal bile duct, the perihilar area accounts for the majority of the remainder and intrahepatic tumours are uncommon. There is a wide variation in incidence with race and geographical location. In the USA, this tumour is very common in native Americans and it is very common in eastern Asia, especially northern Thailand. The female-to-male ratio is approximately 1.3:1, in contrast to gallbladder cancer where the ratio is 3:1.

Aetiology

The recognized risk factors are listed in Table 16.5. In particular, patients with long-standing ulcerative colitis commonly develop sclerosing cholangitis leading to bile duct calculi, which predispose to cholangiocarcinoma.

Pathology

These malignant tumours involve the epithelial lining of the bile duct. More than 95% are adenocarcinoma, usually showing mucin secretion. Demonstrating malignancy is sometimes difficult in the presence of extensive inflammation and sclerosis in biopsy material. The tumours often stain positively for CEA and the antigen CA-19-9. The tumours tend to have invaded through the duct wall before detection. They invade locally into adjacent organs (liver, duodenum, and pancreas) and also to regional lymph nodes in the porta hepatis. Spread to the peritoneum with multiple seedlings is common but haematogenous spread is relatively rare.

Clinical presentation

Typically patients present with obstructive jaundice (jaundice with pale stools, dark urine, and pruritis). They may have mild pain, anorexia, and weight loss.

Investigations

The diagnosis and the potential operability can be established from a combination of transabdominal ultrasound, ERCP, percutaneous cholangiography, CT scanning, MRI, and angiography. These investigations can also provide material for cytology, usually from ERCP or percutaneous biopsy guided by CT or ultrasound. Prior to operation, CT of abdomen and chest will be used to screen for nodal or distant metastases.

Treatment

Bile duct tumours can be considered as three separate entities for treatment. Distal tumours arise in the pancreas where the surgical treatment principles follow those of pancreatic tumours with pancreaticoduodenectomy as the radical operation of choice. Intrahepatic tumours are managed as for hepatoma with segmental liver resection as the radical surgical operation. The third group of perihilar tumours represents the most challenging group, where surgical resection with restoration of biliary drainage presents a difficult challenge. This may involve resection of bile ducts together with part of the liver.

Patients with inoperable bile duct tumours may benefit from palliative radiotherapy. The limiting factor in radiation therapy is the poor tolerance of radiation by the liver. Very high doses can be delivered by brachytherapy, where radioactive wires (containing iridium-192) are threaded through the bile duct within a stent. If the tumour is bulky, this is supplemented with external beam radiotherapy. There are no randomized trials demonstrating a benefit from radiotherapy but there are impressive single institution studies.

Benefit for palliative chemotherapy has not been established. Single institution studies of combined chemoradiotherapy have demonstrated that this is tolerable but randomized trials have not yet been undertaken. Hepatic transplantation has not produced long-term survivors and is not currently considered for these patients.

Prognosis

Median survival in patients with unresectable tumours is 5–8 months. Resection of intrahepatic cholangiocarcinoma gives 5-year survival of around 40%. A similar outcome is achieved for surgery in distal tumours treated with pancreatico-duodenectomy. The outcome for perihilar tumours is poorer, where resection yields survival at 5 years in only around 20% of patients.

Carcinoma of the gallbladder

Epidemiology

There are 1400 new cases and 250 deaths registered per annum in the UK with a 3:1 female preponderance.

Aetiology

It is believed that gallstones are an important aetiological factor (found in 90% of cases) and they account for the female predominance. Gallbladder cancer is found in approximately 1% of patients coming to cholecystectomy. Gallbladder polyps are a risk factor for cancer and, if larger than 1 cm, are an indication for cholecystectomy.

Pathology

Most tumours are adenocarcinoma and there are several histological subtypes. The papillary subtype is less likely to invade through the gallbladder wall and high-grade tumour predicts for poor prognosis. There is a tendency for early spread through the wall of the gallbladder into the adjacent liver capsule and hepatic parenchyma. Lymph node and haematogenous metastases will also occur.

Clinical presentation

For 10–20% of patients with this tumour the diagnosis is made by pathological examination of a gallbladder removed routinely for gallstones. Most of the remainder present with abdominal pain indistinguishable from benign cholecystitis or biliary colic. Since disease is often advanced at diagnosis, patients may present with anorexia, weight loss, and epigastric or back pain due to lymph node or direct hepatic invasion. They may also have obstructive jaundice in up to 50% of cases.

Investigations

The diagnosis of gallbladder tumour can be established with ultrasound in about half of the cases. CT scanning will often demonstrate a mass in the gallbladder fossa with invasion of the hepatic parenchyma. It will also demonstrate enlarged involved nodes. This modality will also permit CT-guided biopsy of the mass to achieve cellular diagnosis. MRI scanning can provide detailed evidence of extent and pattern of involvement of liver parenchyma by tumour to assist with planning of resection. Cholangiography, either percutaneously or retrogradely at ERCP, will demonstrate a long stricture of hepatic duct in cases with jaundice. Prior to consideration of radical surgery, CT scan of the chest is required to exclude lung metastases.

Treatment

To achieve long-term survival, the tumour must be completely resected. This will be achieved by simple cholecystectomy in most cases of coincidental carcinoma. For more extensive tumour, segmental resection of liver and radical resection of involved nodes is attempted. If tumour cannot be resected, then palliative surgery may still be appropriate. If there is gastric outlet obstruction, this can be ameliorated by gastrojejunostomy.

Jaundice can be cleared using bypass surgery or stenting, and pain can be treated by coeliac plexus block. This is combined with opiate analgesia and with other agents suitable for treating neuropathic pain from coeliac plexus invasion. Radiotherapy can improve pain control or relieve jaundice by treatment of the primary tumour or nodal masses. Chemotherapy, using combinations of drugs based on 5-fluorouracil, has some activity and is used in the palliative setting in relatively fit patients. Given the rarity of the tumour, there are no randomized data on the efficacy of chemotherapy.

Prognosis

Coincidental gallbladder cancers found at cholecystectomy with tumour confined to the muscular layer of the gallbladder have a 5-year survival rate of better than 85%. Even if tumour invading the liver is resected with clear margins, and there are no clinically detected metastases, survival at 5 years is less than 25%. Since disease cannot be completely resected in many patients, overall survival at 5 years is less than 5%.

Tumours of the small bowel

Epidemiology

Small bowel tumours constitute less than 10% of all bowel tumours. There is a slight male predominance and approximately two-thirds are malignant. These very rare tumours are poorly documented in the literature and there are poor comparative international data.

Aetiology

Although the small bowel has 75% of the length and 90% of the absorptive surface of the entire bowel, it accounts for only 10% of all bowel tumours and

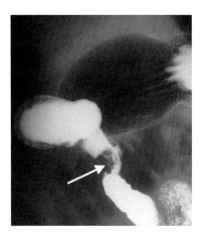

Fig. 16.4 Metastatic tumour of small bowel. Secondary tumour (from a Merkel cell primary tumour of skin) indenting the second part of duodenum.

there are several explanations offered for this paucity of tumours relative to large bowel. These include the lack of exposure to carcinogens due to rapid transit time, dilution of contents by copious secretions and an alkaline milieu which inhibits growth of bacteria that would produce toxic metabolites of ingested foodstuffs. The large number of lymphocytes in the area of the terminal ileum may also enhance immune surveillance and eliminate early clones of malignant cells. Crohn's disease, adult coeliac disease, and Peutz–Jeghers' syndrome have all been associated with increased incidence of small bowel tumours

Pathology

One-third of small bowel tumours are benign. One-third of these are leiomyomas, a further third are either adenomatous polyps or lipomas, and the remainder comprise other cell types. They are found roughly uniformly along the length of the small bowel.

Approximately two-thirds of small bowel tumours are malignant. One-quarter of all malignant small bowel tumours arise in the duodenum, one-third arise in the jejunum and over 40% in the ileum. The vast majority of tumours in the jejunum are malignant adenocarcinoma, whereas lymphomas are extremely rare. In the ileum, carcinoid tumours and lymphomas constitute more than half of all tumours. The small bowel is a recognized site for involvement by secondary spread of tumours from other sites (Fig. 16.4). Abdominal tumours can spread directly or by transcoelomic spread, the most common being ovarian cancer.

Clinical presentation

Most patients with malignant small bowel tumours have symptoms before diagnosis. The presentations can be subdivided into mass, obstruction, bleeding, and perforation. Additionally, pain without obstruction and weight loss are commonly seen with malignant tumours. In adults, small bowel intussusception is most commonly due to benign tumour. Perforation of the small bowel is most common in small bowel lymphoma and less common in sarcoma. A mass representing distended small bowel proximal to an obstruction is seen in around one-quarter of patients with malignant small bowel tumours.

Patients with metastatic tumour involving small bowel most commonly present with either bleeding from the small bowel (anaemia and melaena) or with small bowel obstruction. The most common metastatic tumour giving rise to bleeding is malignant melanoma, whereas ovarian cancer most commonly causes obstruction.

Investigations

There may be anaemia due to chronic blood loss; CEA may be raised, or liver function tests may be abnormal due to ampullary obstruction in duodenal tumour or to liver metastases. If plain x-ray films of abdomen show small bowel obstruction in the absence of previous laparotomy, this is most likely due to small bowel tumour. Upper gastrointestinal series with small bowel follow-through shows abnormality in more than half of patients and will demonstrate the tumour in about one-third of cases. Barium enema may demonstrate disease of the terminal ileum. The distinction between inflammatory disease and small bowel lymphoma in this area is difficult. Computed tomography has been increasingly recognized as very useful in identifying small bowel disease with an abnormal CT in more than three-quarters of cases.

The direct visualization of small bowel is becoming increasingly feasible. The total duodenum can be visualized with modern endoscopes. The newer enteroscopes are available in specialist centres and can visualize the entire small bowel via the upper gastrointestinal tract. Experienced operators can also perform colonoscopy with retrograde ileoscopy to visualize and biopsy lesions.

Treatment

Tumours identified in the duodenum can range from benign villous adenoma to invasive adenocarcinoma. It is possible to manage benign tumours by local excision, but ongoing endoscopic follow-up is mandatory since recurrence in this setting is very common. More extensive surgery for benign lesions depends on their location. For tumours in the first and second part, the appropriate surgery is pancreaticoduodenectomy. For benign tumours in the third and fourth part of the duodenum or remainder of small bowel, sleeve, wedge, or segmental resection is usually performed.

For malignant tumours of the duodenum the operative procedures are similar to the definitive procedures outlined for benign tumours, but the regional lymph nodes must be resected since these are commonly involved by metastatic tumour. For tumours in the remainder of the small bowel, laparotomy is performed to establish diagnosis and resectability. The malignant tumours can be surgically removed in the majority of cases. The aims of surgery are to achieve clear surgical margins and to take a wide margin of mesentery, which will clear regional nodes. In the setting of advanced disease with extensive unresectable tumour, anastomosis of small bowel to small bowel may successfully bypass obstruction and relieve distressing symptoms.

Non-surgical management of small bowel tumours is difficult. Small bowel tolerates radiation therapy poorly and this treatment is not used. Given the rarity of these tumours, there are few reports on results of chemotherapy. Some responses to chemotherapy regimens similar to those used for gastric cancer have been reported but clear evidence of benefit is lacking.

Prognosis

Outcome for tumours of the small bowel is linked to resectability. The majority of primary duodenal tumours are resectable for cure and in these patients the survival at 5 years is highly variable in published reports, averaging around 33%, but this is linked to extent of nodal involvement. If radical resection is not possible, then life expectancy is short with few 2-year survivors. For tumours of the jejunum and ileum, the survival rate at 5 years is also poor after radical resection. If lymph nodes are not involved, then 5-year survival is 45–70%, whereas, if nodes are involved, this falls to 12–14%.

Carcinoma of the colon and rectum

Epidemiology

Colorectal cancer is the third most common cancer in the UK (after breast and lung cancer), with approximately 31 000 new cases per year (13% of all new cancers) and 18 000 deaths each year. Tumours may occur at any point along the large bowel. There has been a change to a more proximal location for tumours over time. The proportion of tumours which were within reach of a sigmoidoscope (rectum and sigmoid colon), has fallen in the last two decades from over 60% to less than 50% in many studies.

Colorectal tumours have a high incidence in the USA, Canada, northern Europe and Australia. They are rare in Africa and Asia. Migration studies have demonstrated that migrant populations moving from low- to high-incidence areas adopt the incidence pattern of the host country after one to two generations, suggesting an important role for environmental factors. The outcome of colorectal tumours in Europe and North America has been improving during the last 20 years.

Aetiology

The major risk factors for colorectal cancer (Table 16.6) can be considered under the headings of:

- familial
- dietary and
- other colorectal conditions.

Colorectal cancer is the only cancer of the gastrointestinal tract where familial patterns of risk are relatively common, accounting for 6–8% of cases. Familial adenomatous polyposis (FAP) is an autosomally dominantly inherited condition. The affected individuals develop very large numbers of polyps in their colon from an early age, with malignant transformation inevitably occurring at a relatively

Table 16.6 Risk factors for colorectal cancer

Familial

Familial adenomatous polyposis

Gardner's syndrome

Hereditary non-polyposis colorectal cancer (Lynch I & II)

Dietary

High intake of red meat and animal fat

Low intake of dietary fibre

Risk reduced by ingestion of aspirin

Risk reduced by ingestion of non-steroidal anti-inflammatory agents

Colorectal disease

Previous colorectal cancer

Ulcerative colitis

Crohn's disease of colon

?Ureteric diversion to sigmoid colon

?Previous cholecystectomy

?Previous pelvic radiotherapy (rectal only)

Table 16.7 Amsterdam criteria for diagnosis of hereditary non-polyposis colorectal cancer (HNPCC)

- Colorectal cancer (histologically proven) in 3 or more relatives, one of whom is a first-degree relative of the other two
- Two successive generations affected
- One case affected by age 50 years

young age. In Gardner's syndrome, the multiple polyps are associated with specific skeletal and cutaneous findings, e.g. desmoid tumours, lipomas, sebaceous cysts and osteomas of the ilium and mandible.

Some families display an increased risk of colorectal cancer, but do not have the adenomatous polyposis of the colorectum (hereditary non-polyposis colorectal cancer, HNPCC). The actual risk of cancer is higher with stronger family history and the definition of HNPCC is somewhat arbitrary, but has been defined in the Amsterdam criteria (Table 16.7). Up to 6% of colorectal cancer cases will arise from such families and there is a predisposition for right-sided colonic tumours. The pattern of inheritance is autosomal dominant with high penetrance and this is termed the Lynch I syndrome. There is a separate pattern with a wider range of tumour types (colorectum, ovary, pancreas, breast, bile duct, ureter, endometrium, and stomach), which is also inherited in an autosomal dominant pattern and termed the Lynch II syndrome. A specific chromosomal abnormality has not been identified for the Lynch syndromes. However, there are mutations found in several DNA mismatch repair enzymes in the DNA of families with HNPCC and this leads to a chromosomal abnormality known as microsatellite instability.

A clear association between the risk of colorectal cancer and certain dietary patterns has been demonstrated in numerous studies. A high intake of animal fats and red meat and a low intake of dietary fibre are associated with increased risk. The regular consumption of non-steroidal anti-inflammatory drugs or of aspirin appears to reduce the risk of developing colorectal cancer in observational and interventional studies.

In patients with prolonged inflammatory bowel disease, the risk of colorectal cancer increases with the extent, severity and duration of the disease. The risk is more marked for ulcerative colitis than for Crohn's disease. For a patient with long-standing pancolitis due to ulcerative colitis, the relative risk may approach 20 times that of the general population.

Pathology

The development of tumours in the colorectum follows a clear progressive path from polyp to benign adenoma and on to malignant tumour. There is a clear cascade of chromosomal changes in the abnormal tissues which has been elucidated and documented (Vogelstein, 1990). When a malignant tumour arises in the mucosa, it spreads into the deeper layers of the bowel wall and will eventually penetrate the serosa. Invasion of the serosa carries a significant risk of seeding of the peritoneal cavity, which can lead to peritoneal nodules, ovarian metastases, or ascites. The tumour will invade into adjacent organs, especially if there is no seros-

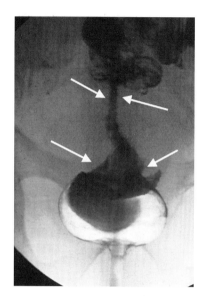

Fig. 16.5 Rectal cancer. Circumferential adenocarcinoma of mid-rectum. The rectal catheter for instilling barium can be seen at the lower edge of the figure. There is a sizeable 'apple-core' abnormality in the mid-rectum.

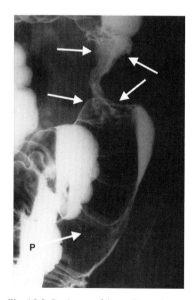

Fig. 16.6 Carcinoma of descending colon with synchronous adenomatous polyp. This patient had a tumour of proximal descending colon (four arrows) which shows as an 'apple-core' lesion. There is also a polyp in the distal descending colon (labelled 'P') which was an adenoma on histology.

al covering, as in rectal cancer. Cells may also invade lymphatic or vascular channels and spread further. There is preferential spread via the circumferential channels and most colorectal tumours will tend to encircle the lumen, giving an apple-core appearance on contrast studies (Fig. 16.5). This propensity also explains the risk of bowel obstruction with tumours, especially in left-sided tumours where the faecal content of the colon is relatively solid.

Malignant cells may also spread to lymph nodes or to liver. The pattern of spread in lymph nodes is also hierarchical, involving first the nodes adjacent to the bowel wall and spreading more proximally along the vascular pedicles of the mesentry. Systemic spread can occur directly from tumours of the lower third of rectum or from other areas without mesentry. Systemic spread can also arise in the presence of bulky liver disease. Multiple primary tumours are found in approximately 5% of patients and many will also have associated benign or adenomatous polyps (Fig. 16.6).

A tumour may be nodular, ulcerating or diffusely protruding in appearance and the vast majority are adenocarcinoma, with about 20% of these being mucinous in type. The tumour often secretes the oncofetal antigen CEA. A number of pathological features have prognostic significance (Table 16.8).

Clinical presentation

Colorectal cancer can present in several characteristic clinical patterns (Table 16.9). Around about one-fifth of patients will present as a surgical emergency with acute large bowel obstruction, usually without peritonitis. Approximately one-third of patients will present with predominantly rectal symptoms of mucus per rectum, tenesmus, and bleeding per rectum. Patients with caecal carcinoma

Table 16.8 Selected features associated with adverse prognosis on pathological evaluation of colorectal tumours

- Depth of penetration through the layers of bowel wall
- Involvement of the circumferential resection margin
- Presence and number of involved lymph nodes
- Lack of lymphocytic response to tumour
- Infiltrating rather than pushing tumour edge
- Mucinous cell type

Table 16.9 Clinical presentation of colorectal cancer

Acute large bowel obstruction (20%)	Left-sided tumour
Anaemia and palpable mass (15%)	Right-sided tumour
Rectal irritation and bleeding (33%)	Rectal tumour
Change in bowel habit (especially alternating constipation and diarrhoea)	

(10–15%) will often present insidiously with iron-deficiency anaemia (Fig. 16.7) with a palpable mass on the right side of abdomen or local pain in that area. This arises since the fluidity of the colonic contents on the right side makes obstruction mechanically less likely. Some patients will present with relatively subtle changes in bowel habit: either constipation or diarrhoea. There may be some abdominal cramping and possible blood per rectum. A pattern of alternating diarrhoea and constipation is highly suspicious of bowel cancer.

Clinical findings may include a tumour which is palpable digitally per rectum. Right-sided tumours may present as a palpable mass. A palpable liver or supra-clavicular lymph node may also be found in more advanced disease. A locally advanced rectal cancer may give rise to a fistula from rectum to bladder. This may present with recurrent urinary infection, pneumaturia, or haematuria. A fistula to the vagina may result in the appearance of faecal material in the vagina.

Investigations

Tumours of the rectum can be assessed directly by proctoscopy and sigmoidoscopy. This permits biopsy and assessment of tumour size, extent, fixation, and distance from the anal margin. Further details of extent of mural penetration can be obtained by MRI or by endorectal ultrasound. The colon can be investigated with either double-contrast barium enema, which will give excellent visualization and mucosal detail, or colonoscopy, which is more sensitive than barium enema and permits biopsy of tumour as well as therapeutic removal of any small polyps. Preoperative assessment will include full blood count to detect anaemia and ultrasound or CT scan of liver to screen for liver metastases.

The traditional staging system for colorectal tumours involves the use of the Dukes' system. In its historical form (as described by Dukes), tumour confined to the mucosa and submucosal layers is Dukes' 'A'. If the tumour had penetrated the muscularis mucosa it was Dukes' 'B', and if the regional lymph nodes were

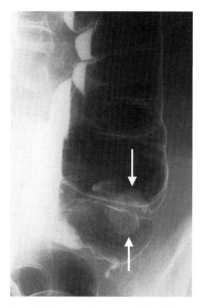

Fig. 16.7 Cancer of the caecum. This film shows a polypoid tumour in the caecum of a patient who presented with profound anaemia. The tumour is indicated by the arrow.

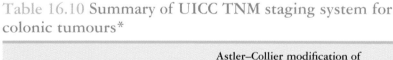

Table 16.10 **Summary of UICC TNM staging system for colonic tumours***

		Astler–Collier modification of Dukes' stage
T1	Invades submucosa	A
T2	Invades muscularis propria	B1
T3	Invades subserosa	B2
T4	Invades through serosa	B3
N0	No lymph node involvement	If lymph nodes are involved the tumour
N1	1-3 nodes involved	is classed as C1–C3 using the criteria
N2	4 or more nodes involved	used for assigning the B stage
N3	Central nodes involved	
M0	No distant metastases	
M1	Distant metastases	D

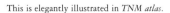

This is elegantly illustrated in *TNM atlas*.

involved this was Dukes' 'C'. Tumours were subsequently classed as Dukes' 'D' if there are distant metastases. This was modified later so that patients whose tumour penetrated the muscularis mucosae but did not extend beyond the muscularis propria were classified as B1 and the previous Dukes' B were classified as B2. Using this modification, around 5% of tumours are Dukes' A and roughly equal numbers are Dukes' B, C, and D. There have been several further modifications of the Dukes' system and this has meant that the universality of the system has been undermined. Most clinical trials and specialized clinicians now use the UICC TNM staging system to classify colorectal tumours and this is compared to the commonly used Astler–Collier modification of Dukes' stage, which is also in widespread use (Table 16.10).

Treatment

The primary management of colorectal cancer is surgical. The surgeon will resect a segment of the large bowel, which is based on the anatomy of the blood supply. This will involve a right or left hemicolectomy or sigmoid colectomy for colon tumours. In patient with obstructing left-sided tumours, a two-stage Hartmann's procedure is usually employed.

There is considerable controversy in surgical circles regarding surgery of rectal cancer. Traditional methods of abdomino-perineal resection resulted in relapse rates from 25% to 35% in the pelvis, even in clinical trials. Advocates of 'mesorectal excision' (Heald, 1988) report a local relapse rate of less than 10% following meticulous dissection along the mesorectal plane which ensures *en bloc* excision of the rectum plus the adjacent perirectal tissues.

The role of adjuvant chemotherapy and radiotherapy in colorectal cancer has been evaluated in a series of clinical trials over 20 years. It has been clearly demonstrated that postoperative chemotherapy with folinic acid and 5-fluorouracil (given over 6 months as a day patient) improves the long-term survival inpatients with Dukes' C colon cancer and this is regarded as standard therapy. For Dukes' B colon cancer, the clinical trials are not conclusive, and most practitioners will offer adjuvant therapy only as part of a clinical trial. Radiotherapy is not routinely given.

For rectal cancer, following traditional rectal surgery, survival rates can be improved and local relapse rates reduced by giving combined chemo/radiotherapy and this is currently recommended for Dukes' C rectal carcinoma. The actual role of radiotherapy is not fully clarified since there are also studies showing that a short course of radiotherapy given preoperatively to patients with operable rectal cancer will improve survival.

In more than a quarter of patients, metastatic disease is identified at initial assessment and almost as many more develop metastatic disease after initial radical therapy. Palliative bowel surgery is recommended for patients presenting with metastatic disease synchronous with their primary tumour if there is significant bleeding from tumour, or bowel obstruction, or if there is significant narrowing of the lumen (especially if the tumour is left-sided), to prevent bowel obstruction at a later date. If metastatic disease is identified in the liver, then about 5% will be suitable for surgical resection of liver disease (Fig. 16.8; Table 16.11). However, the majority of patients will have more extensive disease in the liver, or extrahepatic metastases, and will be unsuitable for surgery. Significant symptomatic

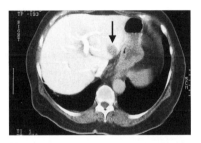

(a)

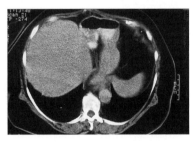

(b)

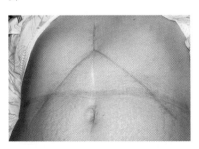

(c)

Fig. 16.8 Resection of liver metastases. (a) CT scan demonstrating a liver metastasis the left lobe of liver (arrow). This patient had had previous surgery for a carcinoma of the sigmoid colon. (b) Appearance of liver after resection of the left lobe of liver and part of the right lobe. (c) The operation scar from a partial hepatectomy.

Table 16.11 **Surgery for liver metastases from colorectal cancer**

Diagnostic investigations
Transabdominal and intra-operative ultrasound
Contrast enhanced CT scan
CT with arterial portography
Bimanual assessment at laparotomy
Indications and surgery
No extrahepatic metastatic disease
Maximum of 3 lesions
Functional liver segments are resected
2% mortality
Outcome
16–40% 5-year survival

benefit, and an increase in survival time of at least 6 months, can be achieved by the use of palliative chemotherapy. The most commonly used agent is the anti-metabolite 5-fluorouracil, modulated by folinic acid. This can be given alone, or in combination with irinotecan which is a topoisomerase-1 inhibitor. If a patient presents with advanced inoperable tumour in the pelvis, a combined chemo/radio-therapy treatment may produce excellent symptom relief.

Prognosis

Dukes' A patients have a 5-year survival better than 90%. For Dukes' B1 and B2 patients their survival is better than 80% and 50%, respectively. For Dukes' C patients, this falls to around 30–40%. Asymptomatic screening of patients for colorectal cancer can take the form of digital rectal examination, faecal occult blood testing, or colonoscopy. Faecal occult blood testing is the most applicable for population screening. Some studies have suggested that it will reduce the incidence of colorectal cancer. However, it is not yet widely adopted. Patients known to be at high risk of colonic carcinoma, i.e. those with previous polyps or of previous rectal cancer, a strong family history, or evidence of a syndrome, or an increased likelihood of the disease, may be screened with regular colonoscopy. This technique has the advantage of allowing surgical excision of the polyps which will prevent some tumours arising.

Carcinoma of the anus

Epidemiology

Anal cancer is very rare, with about 300 new cases per year registered in England and Wales. There is a slight female predominance and it is commonest in the 50–70 year age group. Tumours of the anal margin (arising in keratinized skin) are best classified and treated as skin tumours and are not further discussed here.

Table 16.12 Risk factors for anal cancer.

- Homosexual activity (anal-receptive intercourse)
- Human papilloma virus (HPV) 16 & 18
- Human immunodeficiency virus (HIV)
- Prior renal transplant
- Cigarette smoking
- Anal intraepithelial neoplasm (AIN), a pre-malignant condition associated with HPV

Aetiology

There is an association between homosexual activity (anal receptive intercourse) and anal cancer. There is increasing evidence that infection with the human papilloma viruses (types 16 and 18), which are involved in the pathogenesis of carcinoma of cervix, is also associated with the development of anal cancer. Further associated risk factors are listed in Table 16.12.

Pathology

Over 90% of anal tumours are squamous carcinomas (including the basaloid type). The remainder are adenocarcinomas, which may arise either from mucous glands or may have spread distally from the lower rectum. Tumours close to the anal margin are well differentiated and resemble squamous carcinomas of skin whereas proximal tumours are more typically poorly differentiated. Anal tumours are often present for considerable periods of time before they are diagnosed and will tend to spread out from the anal canal and invade deeper tissues, proximally into the lower rectum or laterally on to the perianal skin (Fig. 16.9a). Tumours may invade the adjacent structures such as the muscular sphincters, vagina, and urethra. Involvement of all the inguinal lymph nodes occurs in 10% of patients. Pelvic and para-aortic nodes may be involved. Haematogenous spread will eventually occur to include liver, lungs, and bone.

Anal melanoma accounts for 1% of anal tumours but has an extremely poor prognosis, with 5-year survival of around 10% regardless of therapy employed.

Clinical presentation

Patients normally present with irritative anal symptoms, which will include itching and bleeding (50%) together with discharge or tenesmus. Patients will often have a long history of symptoms treated for 'piles'. With deeper tumour invasion there may incontinence or deep pain, and a fistula may also develop. Clinically, the tumour may be visible on inspecting the external anal margin. On digital examination there will be a hard, indurated ulcer or nodule in the anal canal. Hard lymph nodes may be palpated in either groin. A differential diagnosis here includes benign anal conditions such as anal fissure or haemorrhoids, with which the symptoms are often confused. Genital warts may have a very similar appearance to anal carcinoma and patients with Crohn's disease of the anus may also have induration, inflammation, and fistulae. Other differential diagnoses include basal cell or squamous cell carcinoma of skin.

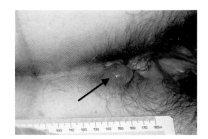

(a)

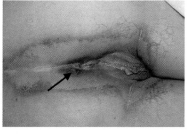

(b)

Fig. 16.9 Treatment of T4 anal cancer. This view is taken with the patient lying on her left side. The vulval area is on the right of the picture. (a) Invasion in perineal skin by a T4 anal carcinoma (arrow). (b) Acute skin reaction on completion of combined chemo/radiotherapy in same patient (note complete response of skin lesion and epilation in the treated area).

Investigations

The tumour can be palpated on digital rectal examination. Proctoscopy allows visualization and biopsy of the tumour. It may be necessary to examine the patient under anaesthesia if severe pain or spasm prevents adequate examination and biopsy. Endorectal ultrasound and MRI will provide details of depth of penetration of tumour and CT scan of abdomen and pelvis will demonstrate the extent of abdominal nodal involvement. Enlarged inguinal lymph nodes are assessed by fine needle aspiration. Tumour is generally staged using the TNM classification.

Treatment

The standard therapy for anal carcinoma has undergone significant change in the last decade. The former surgical approach of abdominoperineal resection has now been replaced by non-surgical management (achieving results as least as good as that achieved by surgery), and with surgery reserved for failure of local control. Two large European studies have demonstrated that a better outcome was achieved for treatment with concomitant chemotherapy and radiotherapy than was achieved with radiotherapy alone. The definitive therapy comprises chemotherapy with 5-fluorouracil and Mitomycin C given simultaneously with radiotherapy to the lower pelvis, including inguinal lymph nodes. A radiotherapy boost is then given to the

> ### Anal cancer: key points
> - Rare tumour
> - Presents with rectal bleeding and irritation (often with delayed diagnosis)
> - Treated with concomitant chemotherapy and radiotherapy
> - 80% survival at 5 years (most with sphincter preservation)

Case history

A 70-year-old woman reported increasing dysphagia which she localized to an area about 3 cm below her manubrium sternae. She had lost 8 kg in weight over 9 months. Dysphagia was progressive and when seen at out-patients she could swallow only fluids. Barium swallow showed a stricture extending from 5 cm below the level of the carina to just above the diaphragm. Endoscopy revealed a malignant stricture and biopsy was positive for adenocarcinoma. Staging CT scan showed no evidence of metastatic disease and she underwent total thoracic oesophagectomy with her stomach drawn up through her mediastinum and anastomosed in the neck.

She experienced considerable difficulties obtaining adequate nutrition after surgery. She had dietetic advice and consumed high-calorie food supplements. She eventually gained weight to just 2 kg less than her previous weight and is well 3 years later, having had a benign stricture at her anastomosis dilated 8 months after her surgery.

Comment

This woman's characteristic symptoms of weight loss with significant dysphagia, which resulted in weight loss due to calorie restriction, is very typical of oesophageal carcinoma. The differential diagnosis includes benign oesophageal strictures and endoscopy and biopsy is required to establish the diagnosis. Assessment of the tumour for operability is very important as surgery is the only clearly recognized therapy resulting in long-term cure. However, the majority of surgical patients will still relapse despite initially successful surgical treatment. In this case the patient required nutritional advice and support to regain weight, even after successful surgery.

anal canal, using either an implant technique or external beam radiotherapy. This is a relatively intensive regimen and produces acute toxicity with significant acute skin reaction (Fig. 16.9b), diarrhoea, and proctitis. This will settle within a few weeks of completing radiotherapy and there is some risk of longer-term proctitis.

Local relapse after combined modality therapy is treated successfully with abdominoperineal resection. Advanced anal cancer is sensitive to chemotherapy with cisplatin, 5-fluorouracil, and Mitomycin C, and worthwhile palliation can be obtained.

Prognosis

The overall outlook for patients with localized squamous carcinoma of the anus is for 80% survival at 5 years, with the majority of patients retaining sphincter function.

Further reading

Bonecamp, J. J., Songun, I., Hermans, J., *et al.* (1995) Randomised comparison of morbidity after D1 and D2 dissection for gastric cancer in 996 Dutch patients. *Lancet* **345**, 745–8.

Burris, H. A., Moore, M. J., Andersen, J., *et al.* (1997) Improvements in survival and clinical benefit with gemcitabine as first-line therapy for pancreatic cancer: a randomized trial. *J Clin Oncol* **15**, 2403–13.

Daly, J. M., Hennessy, T. P. J., and Reynolds, J. V. (eds) (1999) *Management of upper gastrointestinal cancer*. W. B. Saunders, London.

Deans, G. T., McAleer, J. J., and Spence, R. A. J. (1994) Malignant anal tumours. *Br J Surg* **81**(4), 500–8.

Heald, R. J. (1988) The holy plane of rectal surgery. *J R Soc Med* **81**, 503.

Kee, F. H., Wilson, R. H., Gilliland, R., *et al.* (1992) Changing site distribution of colorectal cancer. *Br Med J* **305**, 158.

Lynch, H. T., Smyrk, T., Watson, P., *et al.* (1991) Hereditary colorectal cancer. *Semin Oncol* **35**, 411.

UICC. (1990) *TNM atlas. Illustrated guide to the TNM/pTNM classification of malignant tumours*, 3rd edn, 2nd revision. UICC, Berlin.

Vogelstein, B. (1990) Cancer. A deadly inheritance. *Nature* **348**, 681–2.

Walsh, T. N., Noonan, N., Hollywood, D., *et al.* (1996) A comparison of multi-modal therapy and surgery for oesophageal adenocarcinoma. *N Engl J Med* **335**, 462–7.

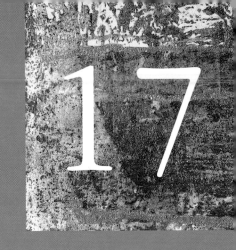

17

Genitourinary malignancy
Patrick F. Keane, John D. Kelly, and James J. A. McAleer

- Introduction

- Renal carcinoma

- Urothelial cancer

- Carcinoma of the prostate

- Cancer of the penis

- Testicular cancer

Genitourinary malignancy

Introduction

The incidence of all types of genitourinary malignancy is increasing. This is partly due to the increased numbers of elderly people in the population and improvements in diagnostic techniques, but there has been a significant real increase in the incidence of renal, prostate, and testicular cancer. Environmental exposure to carcinogens is thought to account for the increase in testicular cancer. Prostate cancer is the second biggest killer in males and will overtake lung cancer as male smoking habits change. Haematuria is the presenting sign of renal and urothelial malignancy and yet many patients delay in coming to their doctor for medical advice. Similarly, patients with testicular lumps and lesions on the penis often delay coming forward. Clearly there is a need for improved awareness in the population at large regarding the significance of these symptoms.

The outlook for patients with genitourinary malignancy is improving; testicular cancer is curable in most instances using chemotherapy or irradiation following orchidectomy. Newer techniques of urinary diversion have improved the outcome of muscle invasive bladder cancer. New surgical and radiotherapeutic techniques have improved the outcome of patients with organ-confined prostate cancer. However, new therapeutic strategies are required for patients with advanced renal, bladder, and prostate cancer and these may come from our improved understanding of the molecular control of these cancers.

Renal carcinoma

Renal carcinoma accounts for 3% of all adult malignancies. The majority of malignant tumours of the kidney are renal cell carcinoma (RCC), which is thought to arise from proximal renal tubular cells. Secondary deposits from lung and breast may involve the kidney on rare occasions. RCC is more common in males (male:female ratio 2:1), occurring in the fifth and sixth decades. The incidence of RCC has increased by 38% in the last two decades. This is in part due to the increase in the incidental detection rate resulting from the widespread use of ultrasound. At the time of diagnosis, about 20% of patients have metastatic carcinoma and 25% have locally advanced disease.

Aetiology

Smoking, obesity, exposure to carcinogens (e.g. cadmium), and hypertension contribute to the development of RCC. There is an increased incidence of RCC in patients with von Hippel–Lindau syndrome (VHL), horseshoe kidneys, adult polycystic disease, and acquired renal cystic disease from uraemia. The link between VHL and RCC suggests a genetic predisposition. The VHL syndrome is associated with chromosomal mutations, most commonly deletions, translocations, and rearrangements of the short arm of chromosome 3. The VHL gene has been mapped to chromosome 3 and structural changes of the chromosome are seen in sporadic as well as inherited forms of RCC. Patients with VHL syndrome develop bilateral RCC in their 30s and require bilateral nephrectomy. The VHL gene is involved in the regulation of vascular endothelial growth factor and may account for the neovascularity associated with these tumours.

Clinical presentation

The majority of patients present with haematuria and loin pain – with or without a mass. The classical triad of pain, haematuria, and a mass in the loin (Fig. 17.1) occurs in only 10% of patients.

RCC is detected as an asymptomatic incidental lesion in at least 20% cases. Ultrasound and CT scanning are the investigations that detect incidental RCC in the majority of cases.

Renal carcinoma may also present with a variety of paraneoplastic symptoms (Table 17.1), and pyrexia of unknown origin and for this reason it is known as the 'great imitator'.

A variety of haematological disorders may be seen, including anaemia from bleeding or marrow replacement. Polycythaemia and thrombocytosis can also occur.

Systemic malaise is associated with a very poor prognosis and 90% of patients are dead within 2 years.

Pathology of renal carcinoma

RCC accounts for 85% of renal carcinomas. RCC originates from the proximal tubular cells and develops in the cortex of the kidney. Terms for RCC, such as hypernephroma, clear cell carcinoma, and alveolar carcinoma, have been used and reflect the historical controversy over the histogenesis of the disease.

The tumour is lipid rich, which gives the cut section a characteristic orange/yellow appearance. Large tumours may contain areas of necrosis, calcification, and cyst formation.

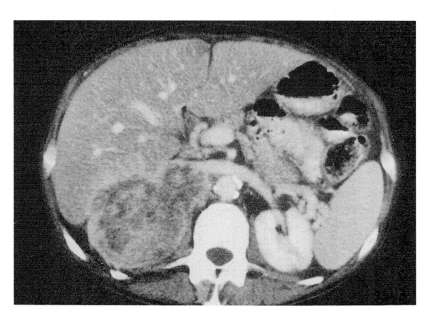

Fig. 17.1 The patient presented with loin pain, haematuria, and bilateral lower limb swelling. The CT scan demonstrates a mass in the right kidney, extending along the renal vein and obstructing the vena cava to cause bilateral lower limb lymphoedema.

Table 17.1 **Para-neoplastic effects of RCC**

Effect	Incidence
Erythrocytosis	3–10%
Hypercalcaemia	3–13%
Hypertension (increased renin secretion)	Up to 40%
Hepatic dysfunction	Uncommon
Raised alkaline phosphatase	
Hypergammaglobulinaemia	
Raised bilirubin	
Hypoalbuminaemia	
Prolonged prothrombin time	
Cushing's syndrome	Rare
Protein enteropathy	
Galactorrhoea	
Hypoglycaemia	

Histologically, tumours are mostly adenocarcinomas. The clear cell variant (25%) contains cholesterol, glycogen, and lipid-rich clear cells. Granular cells (25%) contain less lipid and abundant mitochondria and cytosomes. Tumours are often mixed clear and granular cell type. Sarcomatoid and spindle shaped cells represent a more aggressive variant.

RCC are vascular tumours and spread by direct invasion of the capsule or along the renal vein. Distant spread by blood is to lung, bone, and liver. There is also lymphatic spread to local and regional lymph nodes.

Histopathological grading for RCC

- G1 – well differentiated
- G2 – moderately differentiated
- G3–4 – poorly differentiated/undifferentiated

The TNM staging system for RCC is shown in Table 17.2.

Investigation

In addition to paraneoplastic syndromes, laboratory investigations frequently demonstrate anaemia and raised ESR. Assessment of a renal mass by CT scan or MRI is more sensitive than USS. Extension of tumour thrombus to the inferior vena cava is best assessed by MRI in addition to Doppler USS. Echocardiography may be needed if there is evidence of atrial involvement. Venography to assess thrombus is usually not necessary. Biopsy of solid lesions in the kidney is not routinely recommended, as it can be inconclusive.

Treatment

Treatment of localized RCC The mainstay of treatment of RCC is radical nephrectomy with excision of the kidney within Gerota's fascia. There is some controversy as to whether ipsilateral adrenalectomy is required, but it is recommended that the adrenal should

Table 17.2 The TNM staging system for RCC

Stage	Definition
Primary tumour (T)	
T0	No evidence of primary tumour
T1	< 7 cm, limited to kidney
T2	> 7 cm, limited to kidney
T3	
T3a	Tumour invades adrenal gland or Gerota's fascia but not beyond
T3b	Extends to renal vein or vena cava below diaphragm
T3c	Extends into vena cava above diaphragm
T4	Tumour invades beyond Gerota's fascia
Lymph node (N)	
N0	No regional lymph nodes
N1	Single regional lymph node
N2	More than one lymph node
Distant metastasis (M)	
M0	No distant metastasis
M1	Distant metastasis

be removed for all upper pole tumours. Formal regional lymphadenectomy has not been shown to improve survival; however, the presence of involved lymph nodes is a very poor prognostic indicator and is associated with a 5% 5-year survival.

Extension of the tumour into the inferior vena cava should be managed surgically by removal of the embolus from the vena cava. Occasionally the thrombus will extend beyond the liver and into the right atrium. In such cases it is necessary to perform cardiac bypass surgery to enable excision of the thrombus. Direct infiltration of the vena caval wall is associated with a poor prognosis.

Treatment of metastatic RCC Some patients will present with a solitary metastatic lesion in the lung or brain. It is recommended that a nephrectomy be performed and 3 months after nephrectomy the patient re-evaluated. If there is still a solitary lesion, then metastases at these sites should be resected. For patients with multiple metastatic lesions at presentation, there is no evidence that nephrectomy improves survival. In these cases nephrectomy is performed if symptomatic control is required, i.e. pain or bleeding. If patients are treated by immunotherapy, then nephrectomy is usually advised to reduce tumour burden.

Immunotherapy RCC exhibits multidrug resistance and at present no useful chemotherapy-only regimen exists for treatment. There have been sporadic reports of spontaneous regression of metastatic lesions in patients with RCC. This phenomenon is rare but suggests that RCC may be immunoresponsive. Presently interferon-alpha (IFN-α) and interleukin-2 (IL-2) are the two commonest forms of treatment for metastatic renal cell carcinoma. Side-effects of this include fevers, chills, malaise, nausea, and vomiting. Recent evidence does suggest that IFN-α

and IL-2 in combination with the chemotherapy agent 5-fluorouracil (5-FU) improves both progression-free interval and overall survival. High-dose immunotherapy has been given intravenously, but requires intensive care monitoring and is not used routinely. The assessment of these therapies is hampered by poorly designed, uncontrolled studies. Most patients are treated by subcutaneous injections usually three times a week. While responses in the order of 16–39% are achieved by this method, patients who are considered for such therapy should be entered into trials involving prospective controlled treatment protocols.

Nephron-sparing surgery Occasionally patients develop bilateral renal cell carcinoma or may have had a previous nephrectomy or have disease or damage to the other kidney. In these instances nephron-sparing surgery may be considered. Nephron-sparing surgery could also be considered for lesions picked up on incidental investigations if the tumour is less than 4 cm in size. The results of nephron-sparing surgery in this situation are equal to that of radical nephrectomy. For lesions at either pole of the kidney, a heminephrectomy is indicated. If there is a tumour in the mid-zone of a solitary kidney, then the kidney may be removed and perfused on the bench. The tumour is resected and the kidney reconstructed and transplanted back into the iliac fossa.

Prognosis in RCC

The survival of patients with RCC is directly related to the extent of malignancy at the time of treatment (Table 17.3). Radical nephrectomy is considered almost curative (85–95% 5-year survival) for localized disease. Overall the prognosis for patients with metastatic disease is very poor and the 5-year survival for patients presenting with metastases is less than 15%.

Other tumours of the kidney

Oncocytoma is a tumour of very low metastatic potential which presents as a solid mass in the kidney. Classically the tumour has a stellate scar, which can be picked up on imaging. These tumours sometimes present in pregnancy and can grow rapidly. Treatment is nephrectomy and the diagnosis usually established by the pathologist.

Angiomyolipoma is a hamartoma of the kidney consisting of varying amounts fat, blood vessels, and smooth muscle. CT scanning usually establishes the diagnosis and a conservative approach is adopted. Occasionally nephrectomy is required for pain and bleeding.

Urothelial cancer

The urothelium extends from the calyces of the kidney to the fossa navicularis of the penis in the male and the proximal 50% of the urethra in the female.

Table 17.3 Prognosis in RCC

Stage at presentation	5-year survival (%)
T1	90–100
T2	70–80
T3	50–80
T4	5–20

Table 17.4 **Risk factors for bladder cancer**

Recognized risk factors	
Smoking	Up to 60% of bladder cancer cases are related to smoking. Smoking reduces the age of onset of disease and increases the invasiveness of disease
Aromatic amines and azo dyes	Many diverse occupations involve exposure to chemicals (2-naphthylene, *O*-toluidine, benzidine, 4-amino-biphenyl). Occupations include textile workers, rubber workers, petroleum workers, painters, truck drivers, and hairdressers
Drugs	Cyclophosphamide therapy. Phenacetin-containing analgesics
Schistosomiasis haematobium	Schistosomiasis infection is endemic in the Middle East and parts of Africa. Infection is associated with the squamous cell variant of bladder cancer.
Stones	Chronic irritation and infection associated with squamous carcinoma
Implicated risk factors	
Coffee	A definite association has not been established
Artificial sweeteners	Induce bladder cancer in animal models but a similar link has not been demonstrated in humans

Urothelial cancer, which accounts for 1% of all cancers, can occur at any site but is 50–100 times more common in the bladder than any other area of the urothelium.

Ninety per cent of urothelial cancer is transitional cell carcinoma (TCC). TCC is more common in males (3:1 male:female ratio) and the average age at diagnosis is 65 years. TCC may occur in patients in their 20s and typically in these patients, is a more aggressive variant.

The risk factors for bladder cancer are shown in Table 17.4.

Clinical presentation

- Painless haematuria is the presenting symptom in 90% of cases. Haematuria can be either micro- or macroscopic and any patient presenting with haematuria requires investigation.

- Lower urinary tract symptoms, especially irritative symptoms (urgency and frequency of voiding).

- Symptoms of metastatic disease.

Diagnosis and staging

Patients over 40 years of age should have an intravenous urogram (IVU) and cystoscopy performed as primary investigations for haematuria. If a tumour is present at cystoscopy, a transurethral resection of bladder tumour (TURBT) is performed.

In patients under 40 years ultrasound and plain x-ray may replace the IVP but cystoscopy should be performed.

Urinary cytology, flow cytometry, and detection of tumour-associated antigens can aid the diagnosis of TCC. Retrograde pyelography and ureterorenoscopy are used to confirm the diagnosis of upper-tract tumours (Fig. 17.2). CT or MRI detects lymph nodes and metastatic disease in the investigation of invasive bladder cancer.

Staging of bladder cancer should consist of a careful bimanual examination under anaesthetic prior to endoscopic examination. The site and size and number of tumours should be recorded. The bladder tumour is resected and it is useful in most instances to send separate specimens from the tumour base and also to take random biopsies of the bladder and prostatic urethra, looking for evidence of dysplastic change in the urothelium. After resection, the bimanual examination is repeated, and if a mass is still palpable, then the patient has a minimum of T3 disease. The bimanual examination is also the most important determinant of whether a cystectomy is feasible. CT scanning and MRI scanning are simply looking for evidence of disseminated disease and have no role in the staging of the primary bladder tumour.

Pathology of bladder cancer

The urinary bladder is lined by transitional urothelium which is three to six cells in depth. The urothelial cells abut a basement membrane and are nourished by a lamina propria. The detrusor muscle (muscularis mucosa) of the bladder wall is surrounded by loose connective tissue and pelvic fat.

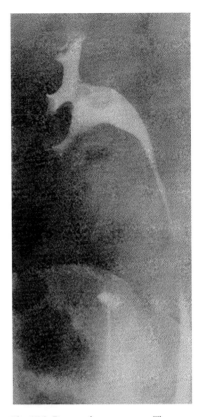

Fig. 17.2 Retrograde ureterogram. The patient presented with haematuria and a filling defect was suggested on IVP. The retrograde ureterogram confirms a filling defect in the renal pelvis.

Table 17.5 The TNM staging system for TCC

Stage	Definition
Superficial tumour	
Ta	Confined to mucosa
T1	Invasion into lamina propria
Tis	Carcinoma in situ
Invasive tumour	
T2a	Invasion of inner half of muscularis
T2b	Invades deep muscle (outer half)
T3a	Microscopic invasion of perivesical fat
T3b	Macroscopic invasion of perivesical fat
T4a	Invasion into prostate, uterus or vagina
T4b	Invasion of pelvic or abdominal wall
Lymph node (N)	
N0	No regional lymph nodes
N1	Single regional lymph node < 2 cm
N2	Single regional lymph node > 2 cm < 5 cm
N3	Node > 5 cm
Distant metastasis (M)	
M0	No distant metastasis
M1	Distant metastasis

The majority of cancers (90%) are transitional cell carcinoma (TCC). Squamous carcinoma (5–10%) and adenocarcinoma (2%) also occur. Rare tumours include melanoma, carcinoid, and carcinosarcoma and phaeochromocytoma.

TCC can be divided into superficial bladder cancer, and muscle-invasive bladder cancer. In superficial bladder cancer the tumour has not broached the muscularis mucosa of the bladder. This is a very important distinction as superficial bladder cancer (Fig. 17.3) is a curable disease whereas the 5-year survival for muscle-invasive bladder cancer drops to 40–50% on diagnosis.

The TNM classification of bladder cancer is shown in Fig. 17.4 and Table 17.5.

Tumours are graded by the World Health Organization (WHO) criteria and are categorized into three grades according to the degree of differentiation (Table 17.6).

Treatment

Treatment of superficial TCC Superficial bladder cancer is a heterogeneous group of conditions ranging from a Ta lesion, which has low invasive and metastatic potential, to the more aggressive T1 G3 TCC, which has a high risk of recurrence and progression to invasive disease. Carcinoma in situ is considered to be high grade, and although not invasive, up to 50% of cases will progress to muscle-invasive disease within 6 months.

Endoscopic resection followed by surveillance is the primary therapy for superficial disease. Up to 70% of tumours recur and so cystoscopy every 3 months is performed. For tumours which are at low risk of recurrence the surveillance period is increased from 3 months to 6 months and then yearly.

High-grade superficial bladder cancer requires careful monitoring and adjuvant therapy, which is administered intravesically. Intravesical adjuvant therapy includes chemotherapy and immunotherapy agents. The treatment is instilled into the bladder and the patient is asked to retain the solution for one hour. Contact with the urothelium is maintained by asking the patient to walk around or else to lie on either side for 15 minutes and on his/her back for half an hour. After this period the chemotherapeutic agent is voided, taking care not to the contaminate skin.

The molecular weight of the therapeutic agent is important as originally thiotepa 189 kDa was used but was found to be absorbed systemically from the bladder and caused bone marrow suppression. The two most currently used chemotherapy agents are Mitomycin C and Doxorubicin. The drugs are dissolved in saline and are usually given weekly for 6–8 weeks.

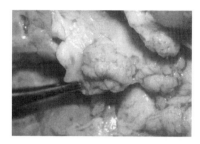

Fig. 17.3 TCC of the bladder. The papillary frond-like lesion which grows into the bladder lumen is typical of superficial disease.

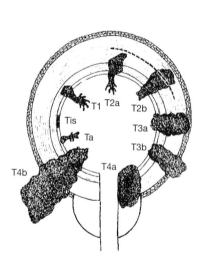

Fig. 17.4 TNM classification of bladder cancer. Carcinoma in situ (Tis), Ta and T1 disease are classified as superficial.

Table 17.6 The WHO grading system for TCC and relationship to progression

WHO grade	Differentiation	Progression (%)
Grade 1	Well	5–15
Grade 2	Moderate	20–40
Grade 3	Poor	30–70

At present there is no evidence that intravesical chemotherapy reduces progression rates, but it does prolong disease-free intervals and reduces the number of recurrences and hence the burden of the cystoscopic surveillance on these patients.

Intravesical immunotherapy – bacillus Calmette–Guérin (BCG), which is a live attenuated vaccine, has been used to treat superficial bladder cancer. BCG is thought to act by inducing a host immunological response through the activation of lymphokine activate killer cells and T lymphocytes. BCG therapy can cause haematuria and symptoms of cystitis and if systemic absorption occurs, then the patient may develop frank tuberculosis; thus these patients require careful surveillance during treatment.

BCG is the treatment of choice for carcinoma in situ and complete responses in the order of 50–70% have been reported. The treatment regimen usually consists of six weekly instillations of BCG. It is unclear whether or not maintenance therapy is effective, but many institutions use monthly instillations of BCG once the initial response has been obtained.

Phototherapy – neoplastic transitional cells concentrate haematoporphyrin derivative (HPD). This can be used to treat widespread superficial bladder cancer. Once sensitized, the tumour or bladder is treated with light of 639 nm generated from an argon laser.

Treatment of invasive TCC

The two major modalities of treatment of muscle-invasive bladder cancer are surgery in the form of radical cystectomy and radiotherapy.

Radical cystectomy with bilateral pelvic lymphadenectomy offers the best chance of cure of this disease. Five-year survivals of between 35 and 55% are achieved by surgery. Radical cystectomy is a major surgical procedure and has the disadvantage of requiring urinary diversion, which is unacceptable to many patients. Newer techniques for continent urinary diversion have made surgery more acceptable to more patients. There is no evidence that preoperative radiotherapy improves survival in the treatment of muscle-invasive bladder cancer.

Orthotopic bladder reconstruction is also possible in patients with solitary muscle-invasive bladder cancers that are well away from the internal urinary meatus. The bladder and prostate can be removed and a new bladder formed either from the ileum or an ileocolonic segment can be sutured directly onto the urethra. Advances in surgical techniques in terms of preserving potency has also made the procedure more acceptable.

Radiotherapy as a treatment modality alone is associated with 5-year survivals of between 20 and 40%, and thus surgical management is increasingly the treatment of choice for invasive bladder cancer. Local complications of bladder irritability and proctitis are common following radical radiotherapy for bladder cancer. The patients therefore need to be on continued surveillance following radiotherapy. However, radiotherapy has the single great advantage of retaining the patient's normal bladder function once the initial symptoms have settled. Good results are achieved by careful patient selection and treating small-volume, low-stage disease.

Systemic administration of chemotherapy may induce a response in up to 30% of patients with bladder cancer. Cisplatin is the most active agent against bladder cancer and is included in all current regimens. Methotrexate, vinblastine, and doxorubicin are also useful; in combination with cisplatin they are known as MVAC. Other combinations are CMV and CISCA. There is no evidence that adjuvant chemotherapy prolongs the survival in patients with bladder cancer. Chemotherapy (Cisplatin and Gemcitabine or the combinations above) provides useful palliation in fit patients with metastatic disease.

TCC of the upper urinary tract

The treatment of choice for tumours in the upper tract, i.e. ureter or kidney, is nephro-ureterectomy with excision of a cuff of bladder tissue, which helps reduce the local recurrence rate following surgery. In certain instances of low-grade disease, i.e. pTa G1 lesions, and in patients who have solitary kidneys, local excision may be attempted either in the kidney or ureter. Percutaneous renal surgery has also been used to treat upper-tract tumours. There is a risk of implantation of tumour cells along the percutaneous tract and irradiation with iridium wires has been performed. Chemotherapeutic agents and BCG can be directly instilled into the kidney when renal preservation is important.

TCC of the urethra

Urethral tumours – The absence of a muscle layer in the urethra leads to early penetration of vascular spaces and potential for metastatic spread in these cases. In the male, involvement of the urethra is best treated by cysto-urethrectomy. Isolated anterior urethral tumours are rare but may be treated by partial penectomy. Urethral cancer in the female is rare and options include urethrectomy, radiation, and chemotherapy. Radiotherapy alone gives results that seem to be equivalent to surgical excision of the tumour and brachytherapy may be employed in the treatment of urethral cancer in the female. Chemotherapy may be given as adjuvant therapy for radiosensitization.

Table 17.7 Risk factors for prostate cancer

Recognized risk factors	
Ageing	Strongest risk factor. Present in 70% of men at 80 years age
Race	High incidence in N. Europe, N. America. Low in the Far Eastern countries. Blacks are affected more than whites.
Genetic	2–3-fold increase if first-degree relative affected. About 10% of cases can be explained by the inheritance of autosomal dominant genes
Androgens	Rare in males castrated before puberty. Rare if deficient in 5α-reductase
Implicated risk factors	
Western diet	High incidence if diet rich in fat and red meat consumption. Low if rich in vitamin A
Environmental	Industrial chemicals, cadmium and nuclear industry workers may be at increased risk
Vasectomy	A slight relative risk of developing prostate cancer has been reported but the link is unproven

Carcinoma of the prostate

Prostate cancer is the most common cancer in males, comprising 32% of all cancers, and is second only to lung cancer as a cause of cancer deaths. Prostate cancer is uncommon in men under 50 years of age; the incidence increases markedly in men aged over 60 years and peaks in men around 80 years of age.

The risk factors for prostate cancer are shown in Table 17.7.

Clinical presentation

Lower urinary tract symptoms (LUTS) caused by localized prostate cancer may be indistinguishable from the symptoms caused by benign enlargement of the gland. For this reason, approximately 15% of carcinomas are diagnosed incidentally after transurethral resection of the prostate for LUTS. Approximately one-third of patients present with symptoms from locally invasive or metastatic disease. Symptoms from locally progressive disease result from invasion of neural structures, the bladder base, and perirectal tissues. Metastatic symptoms result from bone and lymph node involvement and their effect on related structures. The presenting symptoms of localized and invasive prostate cancer are shown in Table 17.8.

Pathology of prostate cancer

The prostate gland lies below the bladder neck anterior to the rectum and is traversed by the urethra. The gland is make up of four zones (Fig. 17.5).

About 70% of cancers arise in the peripheral zone, 15–20% in the transitional zone and 15–20% in the central zone of the prostate.

Prostate cancers are often multifocal. Prostate cancers are adenocarcinomas from prostatic acinar cells. Other malignancies are rare and include transitional cell carcinoma (1.5%), rhabdomyosarcoma, and leiomyosarcoma (0.25%). Prostatic intraductal neoplasia (PIN) is a form of dysplasia associated with, and may precede, some prostate cancers.

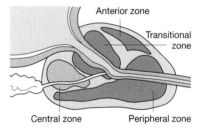

Fig. 17.5 Midline sagittal plane through the prostate. The peripheral zone, which represents 70% of the prostate volume, gives rise to 67% of adenocarcinomas. The transitional zone gives rise to benign nodular hyperplasia and about 25% of adenocarcinomas.

Table 17.8 Presenting symptoms of localized and invasive prostate cancer

Local disease	Locally invasive disease	Metastatic disease	Widespread disease
Reduced void pressure	Perineal pain	Bone pain	Anaemia
	Tenesmus	Sciatica/paraplegia	Uraemia
Hesitancy	Impotence		Weight loss
Post-micturition dribbling	Incontinence Haematospermia	Pathological fracture	Lethargy
Frequency Urgency Nocturia	Loin pain/anuria from ureteric obstruction	Lymphoedema	

Table 17.9 The Gleason grading system for prostate cancer and association with disease progression

Gleason score	Differentiation	% Likelihood of local progression by 10 years	% Likelihood of death from cancer by 15 years
2–4	Well	25	8
5–7	Moderate	50	35
8–10	Poor	70	65

Table 17.10 The TNM staging system of prostate carcinoma

Stage	Definition
Primary tumour (T)	
Tx	Cannot be assessed
T0	No evidence of primary tumour
T1	Clinically inapparent, not palpable or visible by imaging
T1a	Incidental histological finding in < 5% of tissue resected at TURP
T1b	Incidental histological finding in > 5% of tissue resected at TURP
T1c	Tumour identified by needle biopsy (because of raised PSA)
T2	Palpable tumour confined to prostate
T2a	Involves one lobe
T2b	Involves both lobes
T3	Tumour extends through the capsule
T3a	Extracapsular extension (unilateral or bilateral)
T3b	Invades seminal vesicles
T4	Tumour is fixed or invades structures other than seminal vesicles
Lymph node (N)	
Nx	Nodes cannot be assessed
N0	No regional nodes
N1	Regional lymph node metastasis
Distant metastasis (M)	
Mx	Metastasis cannot be assessed
M0	No metastasis
M1	Metastasis present

Local progression of prostate cancer occurs at sites of prostate capsular weakness, i.e. bladder neck, urethra at the apex of the prostate, and seminal vesicles. Prostate cancer has a predilection for perineural spread and this accounts for much of the microscopic extracapsular spread seen in this disease. Extension through the rectal wall is uncommon because of the relatively thick Denonvillier's fascia.

Distant metastases via the periprostatic and presacral veins are most commonly to bony sites and to lymph nodes via obturator, hypogastric, and external iliac nodes.

Diagnosis, stage, and grading for prostate cancer

The lifetime risk of developing prostate cancer is 30%, but only 10% of cancers will be clinically significant. The importance of diagnosis and accurate staging of prostate cancer is the necessity to identify patients who would benefit from the appropriate treatment. The diagnosis of prostate cancer is established by transurethral, rectal, or perineal biopsy.

Grading of prostate cancer The Gleason grading system is based on the degree of glandular differentiation (Fig. 17.6). Prostate cancers exhibit heterogeneity within tissue and so two histological areas of prostate are each scored between 1 and 5. The scores are added, to give an overall Gleason score of between 2 and 10. The score is used as an indication of the likelihood of progression (Table 17.9).

Staging of prostate cancer Prostate cancer is staged according to the tumour, node, metastasis (TNM) classification (Table 17.10). T1 disease is detected incidentally by PSA, transrectal ultrasound, or at the time of transurethral resection to relieve lower urinary tract symptoms. An assessment of stages T2–T4 can be made by digital rectal examination and transrectal ultrasound. Assessment of node status can be determined by CT scan, and metastasis by CT scan and bone scan.

Investigations for prostate cancer

Patients with raised PSA or palpable abnormalities of the prostate are usually evaluated by transrectal ultrasound (TRUS). Specific areas are biopsied or else sextant biopsies of the prostate are performed to establish the diagnosis. The diagnosis can also be incidental at the time of transurethral resection of the prostate (stage T1a and T1b).

Digital rectal examination (DRE) DRE provides information on the size of the prostate and detects changes such as induration, firmness, nodules, and extracapsular extension. The test is limited, as the accuracy of information is examiner dependent. DRE cannot detect T1 disease and it is affected by false positives such as benign prostatic hypertrophy (BPH), prostatic stones, inflammation, and granulomas of the prostate.

Prostatic specific antigen (PSA) PSA is a glycoprotein of the kallikrein family and is secreted by prostatic cells to aid the liquefaction of semen. The normal serum value is between 0 and 4 ng/ml and, although there is a modest rise in PSA with age and with increasing prostate size, it has a use in the detection and staging of prostate cancer (Tables 17.11, 17.12). PSA can also be used as a marker to monitor patients with cancer both before and after therapy.

Transrectal ultrasound (TRUS) TRUS is more accurate than DRE for staging prostate cancer, but its overall accuracy for detection of cancer is low (65%). A specially designed ultrasound probe is inserted into the rectum to image the prostate. The

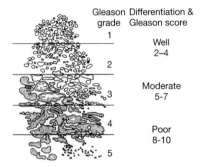

Fig. 17.6 Gleason grading system for carcinoma of the prostate.

Table 17.11 PSA and detection of prostate cancer

PSA level (ng/ml)	Cancer detection
5–10	25% of patients will have prostate cancer.
11–20	66% of patient have cancer
> 50	Associated with bone metastases

Table 17.12 PSA and staging of prostate cancer

PSA level (ng/ml)	Gleason score	Stage	Probability of positive lymph nodes (%)
≤ 6	3	T2a	0
< 20	6	T1a or T2a	10–20
> 20	6	T2b	40

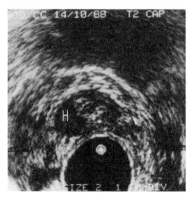

Fig. 17.7 TRUS image of prostate. Biopsy of hypoechoic regions (H) and sextant biopsy of the peripheral zone are performed.

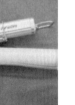

Fig. 17.8 The TRUS probe with automatic firing biopsy needle mounted.

majority (60%) of prostate cancers appear as hypoechoic areas (Fig. 17.7); the remainder are iso- or hyperechoic.

The main use of TRUS is as a guide for transrectal biopsy of the prostate (Fig. 17.8). Transrectal biopsy is usually performed as a day-case procedure and without anaesthesia. Patients require prophylactic antibiotic as there is a 1% incidence of septicaemia. Rectal bleeding, haematuria, and retention can occur following biopsy. Quadrantic or sextant biopsies of the prostate are taken to determine the Gleason grade.

Computerized tomography (CT) and magnetic resonance imaging (MRI) CT and MRI scanning can be used to identify metastatic disease involving lymph nodes. Criteria for nodal involvement are based on the size of nodes and the sensitivity and specificity of both CT and MRI are limited. The investigations are not indicated if the PSA is less than 10.

Bone scanning Radiolabelled bone scanning is a sensitive and specific method of detecting metastatic deposits (Fig. 17.9). False-positive tests due to Paget's disease and degenerative disease can be further elucidated by plain radiographs and, if necessary, MRI. As a means of staging, bone scanning is no longer considered if the PSA is less than 10.

Treatment options for localized and metastatic disease

Watchful waiting Patients with well-differentiated localized cancer who are elderly, have a life expectancy <10 years or have significant co-morbidity should be considered for conservative observation with monitoring of PSA but no treatment. Such a policy is reasonable as the cancer specific survival of patients with well-differentiated disease is 80–85%. Watchful waiting is an active process where the patient is examined regularly, reassured, and treated if there is disease progression.

Radical prostatectomy Patients with stage T1–T2 disease and who have at least a 10-year life expectancy should be considered for radical prostatectomy. The operation, which involves removal of the prostate and seminal vesicles, is associated

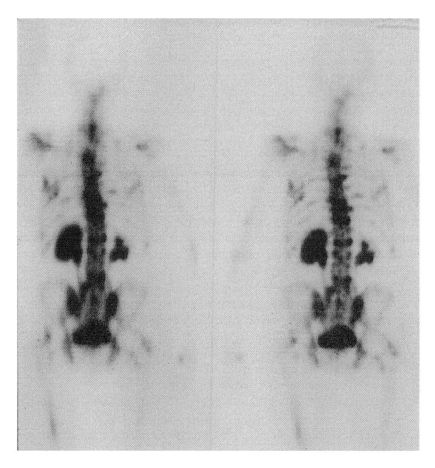

Fig. 17.9 Isotope bone scan. There is extensive infiltration of the dorsal lumbar spine, ribs, sternum, and pelvis. The radioisotope has accumulated in the left renal pelvis and less so in the right renal pelvis, suggesting bilateral ureteric obstruction secondary to advanced prostate cancer.

with significant morbidity (incontinence, impotence) and should only be performed in a potentially curative setting.

Radiotherapy Patients who would not be suitable for surgery but have good life expectancy and localized disease should be considered for radiotherapy. The side-effects of radiotherapy are similar to radical prostatectomy, but not as frequent in incidence. Radiotherapy after hormonal therapy to downsize the prostate and radiotherapy with chemotherapy to sensitize the tumour cells may in the future be of additional benefit. Prostate cancer cells are relatively resistant to radiotherapy and up to 66% of patients will have residual tumour on biopsy 1 year post-treatment. Treatment can be monitored by PSA and a consecutive rise in the PSA level indicates treatment failure. The prostate can be implanted with radioactive seeds (Iodine or Palladium) to deliver radiotherapy (brachytherapy) to a higher total dose and with less side effects than external beam radiotherapy.

Hormonal therapy Patients with locally advanced and metastatic disease may be considered for hormone therapy. Hormone therapy has been combined with both radiotherapy and radical prostatectomy in patients with locally advanced disease. At present there is insufficient evidence to show an improvement in overall survival with combination therapies. Patients with metastatic disease respond rapidly to treatment

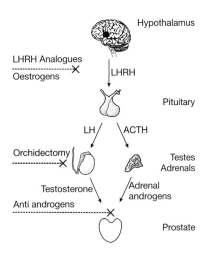

Fig. 17.10 Pituitary testicular and adrenal axis showing the major sites of hormone blockade.

but the mean duration of response is 2 years and most patients are dead within 2 years of development of hormone escape prostate cancer.

Mode of action of hormonal therapy – Hormone therapies block the androgen drive that sustains most of the prostate cancers (Fig. 17.10). There are a number of sources of circulating androgen, the majority of which is testosterone, produced by the testes. However, 5–10% of remaining androgens are of adrenal origin and must also be considered. Both testosterone and other androgens are metabolized at a cellular level, by 5α-reductase, to the active metabolite dihydrotestosterone (DHT). Testosterone from the testes is under control of luteinizing hormone (LH), which is released from the anterior pituitary when stimulated by luteinizing hormone releasing hormone (LHRH) from the hypothalamus. LHRH has a short half-life and is released in a pulsatile manner. This pulsatile release is important, as receptors for LHRH will become desensitized if permanently occupied. Androgen deprivation can be achieved in a number of ways.

- Bilateral orchidectomy (or subcapsular orchidectomy) is a simple and permanent means of stopping the testicular secretion of testosterone. Many men, however, do not opt for this treatment for psychological and cosmetic reasons.
- LHRH analogues given by monthly or 3-monthly injection disrupt the normal pulsatile release of endogenous LHRH. Initially there is a surge of LH followed by a reduction of LH and of testosterone. The initial rise in LH can cause a transient increase in tumour volume (tumour flare) which, if not blocked, can result in a worsening of symptoms. The effect of LHRH analogues is similar to castration and does not block adrenal androgen.
- Anti-androgens act to compete with DHT at the receptor level within prostate cancer cells. Pure anti-androgens can maintain some potency and spermatogenesis, but the affinity of the DHT receptor is variable and not all androgen is blocked.
- Maximal androgen blockade (combination of LHRH and anti-androgen) is being assessed but no definite benefit has been proven.
- Intermittent hormone therapy is also being assessed and withdrawal of the LHRH analogue may allow the growth of hormone-sensitive cells within the tumour, which can be treated again as the PSA or symptoms dictate.

Hormone escape prostate cancer – Once a patient's symptoms recur following full hormone therapy, treatment is limited to attempts to relieve the particular symptom. Radiotherapy is useful in treating discrete bony metastases causing pain. Hemibody radiation is also used for diffuse pain. Injection of the bone-seeking isotope strontium-90 relieves diffuse pain in 30% of patients and can be repeated. Bisphosphonates and oestrogens are used but have limited effectiveness. Steroids are useful in improving the patient's sense of well-being and proper pain management is essential in the terminal stages of the disease.

Screening for prostate cancer

The cancer detection rate using PSA is between 2 and 4% and approximately 30% of men with an elevated PSA will have prostate cancer confirmed by biopsy. Unfortunately, 20% of men with clinically significant prostate cancer will have PSA values within the normal range. There is, therefore, some controversy over the usefulness of PSA alone as a screening procedure. There are currently a number of prospective trials ongoing, which will answer the question whether or not PSA testing reduces the disease-specific mortality of prostate cancer. At present in Europe, screening is only performed within the confine of clinical trials.

Summary

Prostate cancer is the leading cancer among males and incidence increases with increasing age. The ethnic and geographical variation of the disease suggests that genetic and environmental factors are important in its development. Prostate cancers are adenocarcinomas and the majority are androgen sensitive. Hormone therapy offers a survival advantage and delays the time to onset of symptoms from disease. Hormone therapy is the mainstay for locally advanced and metastatic disease.

The advent of assays to detect and measure a tissue-specific marker, prostatic specific antigen (PSA), has revolutionized the approach to prostate cancer. With PSA testing now routinely available, the early detection of prostate cancer has prompted the development of therapies, such as radical prostatectomy, which are performed with curative intent. There is considerable morbidity associated with radical therapy for prostate cancer, which affects quality of life, and so careful assessment of stage and grade of cancer is important.

Cancer of the penis
Incidence and aetiology

Carcinoma of the penis accounts for less than 1% of cancers in men and has an incidence of l–2 cases per 100 000 per year. It is associated with lack of penile hygiene and is virtually unknown in cultures that practice routine circumcision in infancy. There may be a viral aetiology as men with the human papilloma virus and herpes simplex type-2 infections have a higher incidence of penile carcinoma. There are a number of pre-malignant dermatological conditions of the penis that predispose to carcinoma (Table 17.13). The terms erythroplasia of Queyrat and Bowen's disease are interchangeable with the term carcinoma in situ (CIS). Accurate diagnosis of CIS is important as at least 10% of men will develop invasive malignancy.

Presentation and pathology

Fear and embarrassment cause delay in presentation in many patients (Fig. 17.11). Patients present with phimosis, pain, and a lump or a discharge from the penis. All red or suspicious areas seen on clinical examination should be biopsied.

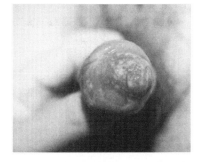

Fig. 17.11 Carcinoma of the penis. Clinical presentation was delayed until infection of the lesion resulted in the patient seeking attention.

Table 17.13 Dermatological conditions of the penis

Premalignant lesions of the penis	Benign lesions of the penis
Erythroplasia of Queyrat	Balanitis circinata (with Reiter's syndrome)
Bowen's disease	Zoon's balanitis
Buschke–Lowenstein tumour	Psoriasis of the penis
Leukoplakia	*Candida albicans*
Balanitis xerotica obliterans	Bowenoid papulosis

Table 17.14 The TNM system for staging of carcinoma of the penis

Stage	Definition
Primary tumour (T)	
T0	No evidence of primary tumour
Tis	Carcinoma in situ
Ta	Non-invasive verrucous carcinoma
T1	Invades subepithelial connective tissue
T2	Invades corpus spongiosum or cavernosum
T3	Invades urethra or prostate
T4	Invades other adjacent structures
Lymph nodes (N)	
N0	No regional nodes
N1	Single superficial node
N2	Multiple or bilateral superficial; nodes
N3	Deep inguinal or pelvic nodes unilateral or bilateral
Metastasis (M)	
M0	No metastasis
M1	Distant metastasis

Table 17.15 The Jackson staging system simplifies the TNM classification

Stage I	Confined to glans or prepuce
Stage II	Penile shaft
Stage III	Operable inguinal nodes, no metastasis
Stage IV	Beyond shaft, inoperable nodes, metastasis

The majority of tumours in the penis are squamous carcinoma (98%) and originate from the glans. Lesions may be ulcerative or papillary (verrucous carcinoma). Spread of carcinoma is via lymphatics to superficial inguinal nodes (prepuce and skin) and superficial and deep inguinal nodes (glans and corpora).

Lymphatic drainage is bilateral to the inguinal nodes, then iliac nodes. Distant metastasis are to lung, liver, bone, and brain.

Staging systems for carcinoma of the penis are shown in Tables 17.14 and 17.15.

Investigation and treatment

Initial diagnosis should be made by excision biopsy. Chest x-ray, bone scanning, and CT scanning should be performed.

Table 17.16 Prognosis in penile cancer

Stage	5-year survival
Node negative	65–95%
Inguinal nodes	30–50%
Iliac nodes	20%
Metastasis	< 3%

Carcinoma in situ (CIS) is treated by circumcision followed by ablation of the glans epithelium to a depth of 2.5 mm using either CO_2 or Nd:YAG laser.

Localized disease can be treated by partial penectomy. A 2 cm margin should be achieved and in the absence of inguinal metastases, 80% 5-year survivals are reported. For extensive lesions, total penectomy and perineal urethostomy is performed. However, amputation of the penis is associated with considerable psychological morbidity. Radiotherapy may preserve the penis and is useful in patients where there is no gross infection or the tumour is away from the urethra (which otherwise tends to stricture or fistulate).

Inguinal lymphadenopathy After excision of the primary lesion, palpable superficial inguinal nodes do not necessarily indicate malignant invasion. Infection or inflammation should be excluded by antibiotic therapy and re-examination after 6 weeks. However, there is an incidence of between 10 and 15% of lymph node involvement at the time of presentation, particularly in poorly differentiated tumours. Accordingly, surgical staging of inguinal nodes is regarded by many as an essential part of primary treatment. However, the morbidity of bilateral lymphadenectomy is considerable and sentinel node biopsy, i.e. the node in the femoral canal, and modified lymphadenectomy have been recommended by other authors to reduce morbidity.

Prognosis in penile cancer

The 5-year survival rate is dependent on the absence of node invasion (Table 17.16).

Testicular cancer

Testicular cancer represents approximately 1% of cancer in males and 90–95% are germ cell tumours derived from the germinal epithelium of the testes. Tumours are slightly more common on the right and are bilateral in 1–2% of cases. The incidence of testicular carcinoma has doubled in the last twenty years but with the development of effective chemotherapy regimens, *the overall 5-year survival is in the order of 90%.*

The classification of testicular tumours is shown in Table 17.17 and the risk factors are shown in Table 17.18.

Clinical presentation

Most commonly a painless unilateral swelling usually found incidentally by patient or partner. Scrotal pain occurs in up to one-third of patients; 10% of

Table 17.17 **Classification of testicular tumours**

Tumour type	(%)
Seminoma	35
Non-seminomotous germ cell tumours (NSGCT)	40
Teratoma differentiated	
Malignant teratoma intermediate	
Malignant teratoma undifferentiated	
Malignant teratoma trophoblastic	
Yolk sac tumour	
Mixed tumour (NSGCT and seminoma)	40
Other tumours	5
Stromal tumours	
Sertoli cell	
Leydig cell	
Lymphoma	
Leukaemia	
Cardinoma of the Rete testic	
Metastatic	

Table 17.18 **Risk factors for testicular carcinoma**

Recognized risk factors	
Cryptorchidism	Strongest risk factor. (3–14-fold increase in risk) resulting in a 3–5% chance of developing cancer in either testes
Age	Seminoma occurs, on average, ten years later than NSGT
Race	Whites are four times more likely to develop than blacks
Implicated risk factors	
Genetic	Reported in siblings and twins but no definite association

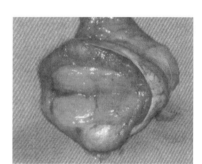

Fig. 17.12 Cut surface of testicular seminoma. The tumour surface has a grey homogenous appearance. Microscopically, there are sheets of large cells with clear cytoplasm and darkly staining nuclei. The nuclei of anaplastic seminoma (incidence 5–10%) have a pleomorphic appearance.

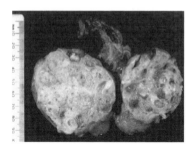

Fig. 17.13 Teratoma contains more than one germ cell layer. The macroscopic features are of a loculated mass containing gelatinous filled cysts.

patients present with acute testicular pain and 10% with symptoms from metastatic disease. These include back pain, dyspnoea, hemoptysis and gynaecomastia.

The contralateral testicle should be examined and biopsied if undescended or of small volume or if the patient is aged under thirty years.

Pathology of testicular tumours

There are two main types of germ cell testicular tumour: seminoma (Fig. 17.12) and non-seminomatous germ cell tumours (NSGCT) (Fig. 17.13). In 15% of cases elements of both tumour types are present and these cases should be treated as if they are NSGCT.

Table 17.19 Tumour markers in testicular cancer

Marker	Effect
AFP	Produced in liver, yolk sac, and gastrointestinal tract. Half-life 5–6 days, serum levels increased in 50–60% of patients with metastatic NSGCT.
β-HCG	Glycoprotein produced in placenta, half-life 24–36 hours, elevated in 50% of NSGCT, and 10–20% of patients with seminoma produced by trophoblastic elements
PLAP	Placental alkaline phosphatase isoenzyme of alkaline phosphatase, may be elevated in up to 50% of patients with metastatic seminoma
LDH	Not specific for testis cancer

AFP, α-fetoprotein; βHCG, human chorionic gonadotropin; LDH, lactate dehydrogenase; PLAP, placental alkaline phosphatase.

It is important to search for lymphovascular invasion in the excised specimen, as this features is associated with a higher risk of relapse in early stage disease.

Investigations

- Clinical examination, including examination of the spermatic cord and scrotal skin.
- Scrotal USS to confirm the presence of testicular mass.
- All patients with testicular cancer should have tumour markers estimated preoperatively. These include α-fetoprotein (AFP), β-human chorionic gonadotrophin (β-HCG) and lactate dehydrogenase (LDH) (see Table 17.19). Higher levels have an adverse prognosis.
- A pre-operative chest x-ray and CT scan of chest and abdomen and pelvis (usually done postoperatively).

Treatment of testicular cancer

Initial management of all patients
Inguinal orchidectomy with insertion of testicular prosthesis.

- Completion of staging investigations.
- Counseling regarding semen storage if further therapy required.

Seminoma

Stage I (tumour confined to testis). Occult retroperitoneal nodal metastases in 15-20% of patients. Radiotherapy to these nodes (30 Gray in 15 fractions in 3 weeks) will result in 98% cure rate.

Stage II (enlarged retroperitoneal or pelvic lymph nodes). Radiotherapy to retroperitoneal and pelvic nodes (36 Gray in 18 fractions over 3 1/2 weeks) gives 95%+ cure rate. If lymph nodes are larger than 5 cm in transverse diameter treat as stage III with chemotherapy.

Stage III + chemotherapy with 4 cycles of cisplatin and etoposide gives 90%+ cure rate.

Key points – RPLND

Primary treatment in USA and parts of Europe, but not used in the UK

Associated with retrograde ejaculation in 80% of cases but a nerve-sparing technique is now in use.

Residual mass post-chemotherapy for NSGCT should be excised:

- necrotic tissue: observe
- mature teratoma: observe
- malignant teratoma: further chemotherapy, if necessary high-dose with stem cell rescue.

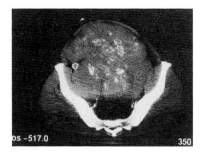

Fig. 17.14 CT scan demonstrates a large retroperitoneal mass. Biopsy confirmed seminoma in a 54-year-old man with cryptorchidism.

Table 17.20 International prognostic classification system for NSGCT

Category	5 year survival (%)
Good risk	
Testis or retroperitoneal primary	
No non-pulmonary visceral metastases	
Low serum markers*	
3 cycles BEP chemotherapy	92% 5 year survival
Intermediate risk	
Testis or retroperitoneal primary	
No non-pulmonary visceral metastases	
Intermediate serum markers*	
4 cycles BEP chemotherapy	80% 5 year survival
High risk	
Mediastinal primary	
Or Non-pulmonary visceral metastases	
Or High serum markers*	
4 cycles BEP chemotherapy	48% 5 year survival

* Low serum markers AFP < 1000, BHCG < 5,000, LDH < 1.5 times upper limit of normal
Intermediate serum markers AFP; 10000–10,000, BHCG; 5,000–50,000, LDH; 1.5–10 times upper limit of normal
High serum markers AFP > 10,000, BHCG > 50,000, LDH > 10 times upper limit of normal

NSGCT

Stage I. If pathology reveals lymphovascular invasion then risk of relapse is above 50%. Giving two cycles of chemotherapy with bleomycin, etoposide and cisplatin (BEP) will cure 98% of these patients. If no lymphovascular invasion intensive follow-up (surveillance) with regular assessments of tumour markers and CT scans will result in 90% of patients remaining disease-free, chemotherapy will salvage most patients who relapse on surveillance.

Stage II+ Give 3-4 cycles of BEP chemotherapy after assessment of prognosis (see Table 17.20). If residual masses remain in lungs or retroperitoneum after chemotherapy, these should be resected by a specialist surgeon where possible. Approximately 40% of the resected masses will contain fibrotic tissue only, 40% will contain mature teratoma (with a risk of late relapse due to malignant change over many years if not resected) and 20% will have residual active tumour. Cure rates for the recognized risk groups are included in the table.

Even patients with the most adverse prognostic features have at least a 50% chance of cure.

Case histories

Case 1 – TCC of the urethra

A 65-year-old male presented with painless haematuria on three occasions in the past 3 months. He had no other symptoms and no significant past medical history. He smoked heavily for 25 years, but had given up smoking 5 years previously. He had worked in a tyre factory for 15 years. On examination he was normotensive and systems examination was unremarkable. Urinalysis revealed 3+ of blood. An IVP showed underfilling of the pelvis with a possible lesion in the pelvis of the kidney. Endoscopy showed a normal lower urinary tract. A retrograde pyelogram demonstrated a transitional cell carcinoma of the renal pelvis on the left side. A specimen of urine from the left kidney was obtained for cytology which showed malignant grade II cells from a transitional cell carcinoma. A nephro-ureterectomy with excision of a cuff of bladder was performed and the patient made an uncomplicated recovery. Histological examination of the specimen confirmed the presence of a grade II TCC with no invasion of the lamina propria. Check cystoscopy 3 months later was normal and the patient was commenced on an annual review cystoscopy surveillance.

Case 2 – cancer of the prostate

A 69-year-old male presented with LUTS and pain in his low back. He also complained of increasing lethargy for 3 months. Physical examination was unremarkable but on DRE there was a hard suspicious nodule involving the right lobe of the prostate with obliteration of the median and lateral sulcus of the gland. Urinalysis revealed a trace of blood. His haemoglobin was 10 g/dl and creatinine was190. Serum PSA was 380 pg/ml. x-Ray of dorsal and lumbar spine revealed sclerotic changes in the D10–L1 vertebrae. Ultrasound examination of the kidneys showed mild bilateral hydronephrosis. A needle biopsy of the prostate was performed under antibiotic cover. Histology confirmed the presence of a Gleason grade 7 carcinoma. An isotope bone scan revealed multiple areas of increased uptake in the axial skeleton and ribs. The patient was commenced on cyproterone acetate 100 mg t.i.d. for 3 weeks and 5 days later was given an LHRH analogue subcutaneously. The patient was told that it would take several weeks for the treatment to take effect and that he might experience facial flushing and sweating as well as weight gain in the upper body. At review 3 months later his PSA level was 14, his pain and LUTS had settled as had his hydronephrosis. He was reassured and given a further appointment for 4 months.

Further reading

Chamberlain, J., Melia, J., Moss, S., and Brown, J. (1997) Report prepared for the health technology assessment panel of the NHS executive on the diagnosis, management, treatment and costs of prostate cancer in England and Wales. *Br J Urol* **79(Suppl 3)**, 1–32.

Chodak, G. W., Thisted, R. A., and Gerber, G. S. (1994) Results of conservative management for clinically localized prostate cancer. *N Engl J Med* 4, 242–8.

Davis, J. W. (1999) Conservative surgical therapy for penile and urethral carcinoma. *Urology* 53, 386–92.

Dearnaley, D. P. (1993) Cancer of the prostate. *Brit Med J* **308**, 780–4.

Droller, M. J. (1992) Treatment of regionally advanced bladder cancer. An overview. *Urol Clin North Am* **19**, 685–93.

Figlin, R. A. (1999) Renal cell carcinoma: management of advanced disease. *J Urol* **161**, 381–7.

Holmang, O. S., Hedelin, H., Anderstrom, C., and Johansson, S. L. (1995) The relationship among multiple recurrences, progression and prognosis of patients with stages Ta and T1 transitional cell cancer of the bladder followed for at least 20 years. *J Urol* **153**, 1823–7.

International Germ Cell Collaboratioon Group (1997) International germ cell consensus classification: a prognostic factor-based staging system for metastatic germ cell cancers. *J Clin Oncol* **15**, 594–603.

Lamm, D. L., van der Meijden, A. P., Akaza, H., *et al.* (1995) Intravesical chemotherapy and immunotherapy: how do we assess their effectiveness and what are their limitations and uses? *Int J Urol* **2(Suppl 2)**, 23–35.

McFarlane, J. P., Ellis, B. W., and Harland, S. J. (1996) The management of superficial bladder cancer: an interactive seminar. *Br J Urol* **78**, 372–8.

Moller, H. (1993) Clues to the aetiology of testicular germ cell tumours from descriptive epidemiology. *Eur Urol* **23**, 8–15.

Montie, J. E. (1994) Follow-up after penectomy for penile cancer. *Urol Clin North Am* **21**, 725–7.

Negrier, S., Escudier, B., Lasset, C. *et al.* (1998) Recombinant human interleukin-2, recombinant human interferon alfa-2a, or both in metastatic renal-cell carcinoma. Groupe Français d'Immunotherapie. *N Engl J Med* **338**, 1272–8.

Novick, A. (1998) Nephron-sparing surgery for renal cell carcinoma. *Br J Urol* **82**, 321–4.

Oesterling, J. E. (1992) Prostate specific antigen: improving its ability to diagnose early prostate cancer. *JAMA* **267**, 2236–8.

Oliver, R. T. D. (1991) A comparison of the biology and prognosis of seminoma and non-seminoma. In Horwich, A. (ed.), *Testicular cancer, investigation and management*, 51–63. Chapman and Hall Medical, London.

Smith, J. R., Freije, D., Carpten, J. D., *et al.* (1996) Major susceptibility locus for prostate cancer on chromosome 1 suggested by a genome-wide search. *Science* **271**, 1301–4.

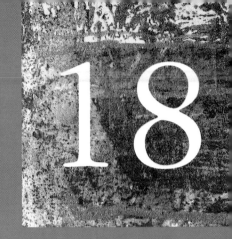

18

Thoracic tumours
Kieran McManus

- Mediastinal tumours

- Tumours of the thymus

- Neurogenic tumours of the mediastinum

- Germ cell tumours of the mediastinum

- Cardiac tumours

- Carcinoid tumours of the lung and bronchus

- Primary bronchogenic carcinoma

- Secondary lung cancers

- Malignant pleural mesothelioma

Thoracic tumours

Mediastinal tumours

Mediastinal tumours fall into three general categories, the commonest being secondary bronchogenic carcinoma. Often the primary tumour is small and asymptomatic, even being undetectable in the case of small cell carcinoma. The second group entails systemic malignancy manifesting itself in the mediastinum. Lymphomas are characteristic of this group, though metastases from breast, renal, and gastrointestinal tract cancers are also common. Primary tumours of the organs or tissues of the mediastinum make up the third group and include thymomas, neurogenic tumours, germ cell tumours, ectopic thyroid and parathyroid tumours, and the rare lipomatous, vascular, and primitive ectodermal (Askin) tumours.

Presentation

Mediastinal tumours in children are usually symptomatic with respiratory symptoms such as cough, stridor and dyspnoea. Malignant lesions are often accompanied by lethargy, fever, malaise, and chest pain. In adults many lesions are asymptomatic, found incidentally on routine chest radiographs. However, obstructive symptoms do occur when the tumour impresses on the superior vena cava (SVC), oesophagus, or tracheobronchial tree, and cardiac tamponade can be caused by large anterior compartment tumours. Invasion of phrenic, recurrent laryngeal or sympathetic chain nerves may also cause symptoms of breathlessness, hoarseness, or Horner's syndrome, respectively.

Diagnosis

Imaging of the mediastinum is crucial in distinguishing tumours from other benign cystic lesions (thymic, bronchogenic, enteric duplication, neuroenteric, mesothelial and cystic hygroma) and granulomatous lesions (sarcoidosis, histoplasmosis, and tuberculosis).

A CT scan or MRI scan will outline the exact site of the lesion and will give clues to the diagnosis. These scans will also give an indication of malignant invasion of adjacent structures.

Fine needle aspiration cytology is frequently inadequate to differentiate thymoma from lymphoma, and almost never provides enough tissue to differentiate between types of lymphoma. A core biopsy is sometimes safe and productive, though the proximity of the aorta and other great vessels dissuades some radiologists. Mediastinoscopy, mediastinotomy via anterior mini-thoracotomy, or thoracoscopy may be required to provide enough issue for the pathologist to make a full diagnosis.

Thymic tumours are unique in that they are associated with a number of paraneoplastic or parathymic' syndromes (see below). The rare paraganglionic neurogenic tumours may also be functional in that they produce biogenic amines. In this regard they resemble phaeochromocytoma. Vanillylmandelic acid or homovanillic acid may be detectable in the urine. Haematological markers of germ cell tumours (β-HCG and α-fetoprotein) should be sought. Both markers are negative in benign teratoma but both tend to be elevated in malignant non-seminomatous tumours. The β-HCG may be elevated in seminoma but the presence of an elevated α-fetoprotein suggests that there are non-seminomatous elements which need to be treated as such.

Tumours of the thymus

There are three general categories of thymic tumours: thymoma, thymic carcinoma, and tumours of other thymic elements (Table 18.1). Thymoma and thymic carcinoma are discussed in the following sections.

Thymoma

Thymomas are of particular interest because of their unusual paraneoplastic associations. The best known of these is myasthenia gravis, but the number of syndromes associated with thymoma is extensive (Table 18.2). The tumour contains both epithelial and lymphocytic elements, which can also make differentiation from lymphoma difficult.

Aetiology and epidemiology

There is no known aetiology for thymoma or thymic carcinoma. There is no relationship between thymoma and gender, sex, or race, though the peak incidence is in the fifth and sixth decades. While myasthenia gravis presenting in adolescence is usually associated with thymic hyperplasia, later onset is associated with thymic neoplasm.

Pathology

Most thymomas occur in the anterior mediastinum, though 5% occur in the neck and others in the posterior mediastinum, left hilum, and pulmonary parenchyma.

Table 18.1 Classification of thymic neoplasms

Composed of thymic epithelial elements

Thymoma

    Encapsulated (equivalent to stage T1)

    Minimally invasive (equivalent to stage T2)

    Wide local invasion including pleural or pericardial implants (stages T3 and T4)

    Metastasizing (stages N1, N2, and M1)

Thymic carcinoma

    Squamous

    Non-keratinizing

Composed of other elements

Thymic carcinoids and neuroendocrine tumours

Germ cell tumours

Hodgkin's and non-Hodgkin's lymphomas

Table 18.2 Parathymic conditions

Neuromuscular
Myasthenia gravis
Peripheral neuropathy
Polymyositis
Dermatomyositis

Haematological disorders
Red cell aplasia
Pernicious anaemia
Erythrocytosis
Pancytopenia
Autoimmune haemolytic anaemia
Leukaemia
Multiple myeloma

Immune deficiency disorders
Acquired hypogammaglobulinaemia
T-cell deficiency syndrome

Autoimmune disorders
Systemic lupus erythematosus
Rheumatoid arthritis
Sjogren's syndrome
Scleroderma

Dermatological disorders
Pemphigus
Lichen planus
Chronic mucosal candidiasis
Alopecia areata

Endocrine disorders
Multiple endocrine neoplasia
Cushing's syndrome
Thyrotoxicosis

Miscellaneous
Giant cell myocarditis
Nephrotic syndrome
Ulcerative collitis
Hypertrophic osteoarthropathy
Lymphoid interstitial pneumonitis

As benign thymoma is cured by surgery without adjuvant therapy, the twofold aim of the pathologist is to determine whether the tumour is composed of thymic epithelial elements and to assess the degree of malignancy. A diffuse lesion, invading surrounding structures, making radical clearance difficult is suggestive of malignancy. Most well defined lesions tend to follow a benign course, whereas the prognosis of thymic carcinoma is stage related.

There is a spectrum of malignant change in thymoma, which has led to a number of attempts at classification. The classification in Table 18.1 is based on that of Masoaka which categorizes thymoma purely on encapsulation and invasion of local tissues. Attempts have also been made to differentiate the malignant potential according to histological subtypes (predominantly lymphocytic, mixed lymphoepithelial, predominantly epithelial, and spindle cell). Others propose a subdivision into cortical and medullary. Whilst these classifications have been shown to correlate with survival, the differences do not become apparent until 5–10 years after diagnosis. Thus thymic carcinoma tends to run an indolent course, though most patients with stage IV tumours will eventually die of their disease.

Features of presentation specific to thymoma

Many thymomas, like other mediastinal tumours, are asymptomatic and are noticed incidentally on a chest x-ray taken for other purposes. Others present with general symptoms of malaise, lethargy, non-productive cough or dyspnoea. Fifty per cent of patients with thymic neoplasms present with myasthenia gravis. A further 10–20% will have features of other paraneoplastic syndromes, whilst a small percentage will have a combination of myasthenia and other syndromes. In some patients the parathymic syndrome does not reveal itself until after surgical thymectomy. Invasive tumours and thymic carcinomas may cause pain due to chest wall, pleural, or pericardial invasion. Superior vena caval obstruction, phrenic nerve palsy, recurrent laryngeal nerve palsy, and dysphagia can all occur.

Parathymic syndromes generally fall into the categories of neuromuscular dysfunction, haematological disorders, immune deficiencies, endocrinopathies, and autoimmune or collagen disorders. The most important are myasthenia gravis, pure red cell aplasia, acquired agammaglobulinaemia, and systemic lupus erythematosus. The other syndromes recorded in Table 18.2 are rare.

Treatment

Treatment of thymoma involves two aspects: treatment of the parathymic symptoms, and extirpation of all tumour. Frequently it is necesary to control the parathymic symptoms before surgery can be contemplated. Of importance for subsequent surgery is the development of shortness of breath on exertion as respiratory muscles become involved. Also of interest to the anaesthetist is the fact that fatiguability is often exacerbated by sedative drugs and some antibiotics.

Medical Medical treatment is only aimed at treating the parathymic conditions rather than the thymoma itself. Usually co-ordinated by a neurologist, it involves an appropriate combination of anticholinergic drugs (pyridostigmine or neostigmine), steroids, plasmapheresis, or intravenous immunoglobulin (IV Ig).

Surgery Radical surgery is the only primary treatment for thymoma, be it encapsulated or invasive. The aim of surgery is to remove all the thymic tissue and surrounding mediastinal fat including, where necessary, pericardium and pericardial fat. Care must be taken to preserve at least one phrenic nerve.

Repeat surgery for recurrent disease may be appropriate for diagnostic or cytoreductive effect as part of a multimodality approach.

Radiotherapy It is generally accepted that postoperative irradiation to the thymic bed following excision of stage II and III disease, either where there has been extracapsular invasion or where there has been gross fixation of tumour even in the absence of microscopic invasion, reduces local recurrence.

Chemotherapy Invasive thymoma is responsive to platinum-based chemotherapy, usually in combination with doxorubicin and cyclophosphamide. Its role is not well defined but it has been increasingly used for treating metastatic, locally progressive or relapsed disease.

Prognosis

Complete excision of a non-invasive stage I thymoma is curative. Recurrence of stage II tumours can be reduced from 45% to 25% by postoperative radiotherapy. For more advanced disease, multimodality therapy (cytoreductive surgery, postoperative radiotherapy, and adjuvant chemotherapy) can result in significant long-term survival.

Thymic carcinoma

Thymic carcinoma is exceedingly rare once it has been established that the tumour is not a metastasis from a tumour elsewhere. Most thymic carcinomas are of squamous histology and most have metastases at the time of diagnosis and follow an aggressive course.

Treatment consists of chemotherapy and radiotherapy appropriate to the corresponding histological type.

Neurogenic tumours of the mediastinum

Neurogenic tumours account for 20–30% of all mediastinal tumours, rising to 50–60% in children. Von Recklinghausen's neurofibromatosis is associated with an increased incidence of neurogenic tumours of all histological types.

Most tumours are benign neurilemmomas (also known as schwannomas) or ganglioneuromas (Table 18.3) and are completely cured by excision. Though benign, resection is indicated, as the benign tumours are indistinguishable from malignant tumours on imaging, and fine needle aspiration cytology is unreliable. Even when benign, these tumours may lead to compression of vital structures.

Complete resection also leads to high cure rates in the intermediate malignancy ganglioneuroblastoma and even frankly malignant neuroblastoma and paraganglionoma. Malignant schwannoma can rarely be excised completely and leads to death within a year of diagnosis; incompletely excised paraganglionoma usually proves fatal regardless of adjuvant therapy, though survival is substantially longer.

Neuroblastoma is more sensitive to chemotherapy and, when used in combination with radiotherapy, even incompletely excised tumours can achieve reasonable

Table 18.3 Classification of mediastinal neurogenic tumours

Tumour type	Frequency
Nerve sheath tumours	
Benign	60%
Neurilemmoma (schwannoma)	
Neurofibroma	
Malignant	< 5%
Malignant schwannoma	
Autonomic nerve system tumours	
Benign	12%
Ganglioneuroma	
Intermediate malignancy	18%
Ganglioneuroblastoma	
Malignant	5%
Neuroblastoma	
Paraganglionic tumours	
Aortic body tumour	< 5%
Aortico-sympathetic tumour	

long-term survival. Radiotherapy can also reduce local recurrence of incompletely excised neurilemmoma, neurofibroma, and ganglioneuroblastoma.

Germ cell tumours of the mediastinum

Twenty per cent of anterior compartment mediastinal tumours are of germ cell origin and fall into three groups: benign teratoma, malignant seminoma, and

Table 18.4 Classification of mediastinal germ cell tumours

Tumour type	Frequency
Benign	
Teratoma	60%
Malignant	
Seminoma	16%
Non-seminomatous mediastinal germ cell tumours	
Yolk sac/endodermal sinus	8%
Mixed teratocarcinoma/embryonal cell	8%
Choriocarcinoma, embryonal cell, and teratocarcinoma	8%

non-seminomatous malignant germ cell tumours (Table 18.4). The malignant germ cell tumours, which have a preponderance in males, may be associated with chromosomal abnormalities such as Klinefelter's syndrome and other blood dyscrasias.

Benign teratomas are cured by complete surgical excision. Seminomas are very radiosensitive and chemosensitive These may respond to chemotherapy with cisplatin, bleomycin, and etoposide before radiotherapy. For non-seminomatous tumours, cisplatin-based chemotherapy can produce complete remission in over 70% of cases. Surgery is indicated for residual masses in the mediastinum or for lung if serum tumour markers have reverted to normal. Where 'mature' teratoma is found, the patient can be observed with regular serum markers and chest radiographs. For residual germ cell carcinoma, salvage chemotherapy should be considered.

Cardiac tumours

Cardiac tumours are rare and most are benign. Myxomas, 90% of which occur in the left atrium, are the commonest of the benign tumours, though lipoma, fibroma, rhabdomyoma, haemangioma, and fibroelastoma also occur. The malignant tumours include the sarcomatous tumours corresponding to the above benign tumours.

Presentation

Cardiac tumours present with syncopal attacks due to obstruction of flow within cardiac chambers, valve incompetence due to impairment of valve closure, symptoms of embolization, rarely arrhythmia or constitutional symptoms such as fever, weight loss, finger clubbing, Raynaud's syndrome, or myalgia.

Investigation

Echocardiography outlines the intracardiac disease and allows planning of surgical resection. Cardiac catheterization is usually contraindicated because of the risk of inducing embolization, unless other cardiac or coronary surgery is anticipated. CT scan will outline the extent of extracardiac disease.

There is no non-invasive method of distinguishing between a benign and a malignant cardiac lesion. Therefore surgical exploration is required for any symptomatic or clinically suspicious intracardiac mass. Even histologically benign lesions can prove fatal by virtue of their location or propensity for embolization.

Treatment and prognosis

Surgical resection by open heart surgery under cardiopulmonary bypass is curative for the majority of atrial myxomas and other benign tumours. Malignant neoplasms are rarely cured with surgery alone, though patients whose tumours have been resected have a median survival of 24 months compared to 11 months for patients with unresectable tumours. Multimodality therapy has rarely been shown to change the prognosis.

Orthotopic cardiac transplantation is an alternative treatment for patients without metastatic spread but in whom complete tumour excision is not possible by standard techniques. This approach, unique in cancer surgery, has shown promising results in a number of small series, despite concerns about the immuno-suppressive effects of cardiopulmonary bypass and antirejection medication.

Carcinoid tumours of the lung and bronchus

Carcinoid tumours occur in the bronchi and lungs on an infrequent basis. They represent the less malignant end of a spectrum of lung tumours showing neuro-endocrine characteristics, which includes typical carcinoid (TC), atypical carcinoid (AC), large cell neuroendocrine carcinoma (LCNEC), and small cell carcinoma (SCLC). They range in malignant potential from benign to frankly malignant, but their main effect on the lungs is generally of an obstructive nature. Most can be cured by surgical resection with a low recurrence rate. Chemotherapy and radiotherapy are rarely required.

Aetiology and epidemiology

Typical carcinoid tumours represent 2% of lung tumours and occur equally in both sexes. The mean age of incidence is younger than that for lung cancer (50 years) with many tumours presenting in young adulthood. Carcinoid tumours are unrelated to cigarette smoking. Bronchial carcinoid can be a component of a multiple endocrine neoplasia (MEN) syndrome.

Pathology

Carcinoid tumours are a subset of neuroendocrine neoplasms of the lung. Neuroendocrine cells exist in clusters in bronchial epithelium and are responsible for the storage and release of small peptides and biogenic amines.

Bronchial carcinoid tumours make up the more benign, well-differentiated, low-grade neuroendocrine tumours. More recently the term well-differentiated neuroendocrine carcinoma has been introduced to emphasize that all these tumours have malignant potential, and therefore should be excised, and that there is a spectrum from benign behaviour to frank malignancy.

Carcinoid tumours are made up of nests, trabeculae, and mosaic patterns of polygonal cells with round uniform nuclei, granular 'salt and pepper' chromatin, and inconspicuous nucleoli. Rosettes and small acinar structures may be present. The stroma shows numerous thin-walled small blood vessels. On electron microscopy numerous membrane-bound dense core neurosecretory granules are apparent. Immunohistochemical staining can help differentiate carcinoid tumours from non-small cell lung cancer (NSCLC) but not small cell lung cancer (SCLC). It is not usually helpful in determining the level of malignancy of carcinoid tumours.

Clinical features suggestive of malignancy include peripheral location, large tumour size, and the presence of metastases. Pathological features evident on gross examination, which are commoner in atypical carcinoid, are invasion of cartilage and lung parenchyma, and necrosis or extensive haemorrhage within the tumour itself. Histological criteria of atypical carcinoid are:

- increased rate of mitotic figures (5–10 mitoses per 10 high-powered fields);
- nuclear pleomorphism, hyperchromatism, and an abnormal nuclear:cyto-plasmic ratio;

- areas of increased cellularity with disorganization of cellular architecture and a paucity of organelles;

- tumour necrosis.

Presentation

Many carcinoid tumours, particularly those occurring in the peripheral lung fields, are asymptomatic at the time of presentation, being diagnosed on a chest radiograph taken for other purposes. Central carcinoid tumours cause obstructive symptoms with recurrent 'chest infections' being treated over a period of years. Cough and pleuritic chest pain accompany such obstructive episodes.

Primary lung carcinoid tumours can release peptides into the systemic circulation. The peptides most frequently expressed are serotonin, bombesin, gastrin, leuenkephalin, and ACTH. Up to 40% of patients will on questioning report symptoms of facial flushing (independent of menopause), palpitations, heartburn, or angina-like chest pain. Whilst most 'wheezing' is actually stridor due to obstruction of a central large bronchus, a number of patients will report bronchospasm even with a peripherally located tumour. Many of these hormonally mediated symptoms are vague and only become evident when they disappear after surgery. Though they may seem of little importance to the patient, the presence of such symptoms are of concern to anaesthetists as the release of such peptides on handling of the tumour can produce catastrophic bronchospasm or cardiovascular effects.

Examination

Examination is frequently normal though unilateral stridor may be evident on auscultation. During episodes of obstruction, signs typical of a lobar pneumonia with pleuritic reaction may be evident.

Diagnosis

As for bronchogenic carcinomas, chest radiography, CT scan, fine needle aspiration (FNA), and bronchoscopy are the means used to confirm the diagnosis.

Small central tumours frequently do not appear on radiographs, though the features of obstructive pneumonitis may be apparent. Peripheral tumours appear as rounded shadows similar to carcinoma, though frequently less spiculated. A CT scan will often demonstrate a central tumour that is not apparent on the chest radiograph in addition to the parenchymal changes due to obstruction. Exfoliative sputum cytology is rarely diagnostic as these benign tumours rarely shed cells.

Bronchoscopy demonstrates most central carcinoid tumours as smooth, rounded, polypoid endobronchial masses, often covered with normal bronchial mucosa.

Staging

The staging system for carcinoid tumours of the lung is the same as that for carcinoma. Staging procedures such as mediastinoscopy, anterior mediastinotomy, and thoracoscopy are directed by CT findings but are usually not required in the more benign typical carcinoid tumours. The frequent pneumonitis found with carcinoid tumours that obstruct pulmonary lobes is associated with hilar and mediastinal lymhadenopathy. CT findings should not be over-interpreted without histological confirmation. Somatostatin receptor scintigraphy using the labelled somatostatin analogue, octreotide, may illuminate secondary disease, which may not be apparent on CT, or rule out metastases in otherwise enlarged nodes. Hepatic metastases may need ultrasound evaluation and FNA for cytological examination.

Treatment

The main treatment is aimed at ablating the primary disease and preventing obstructive damage to lung tissue. Where secondary disease is present, there is the added aim of controlling any symptoms due to peptide release. Such peptide release can occur during surgical handling of a primary tumour and there exist anecdotal reports of severe bronchospasm, hypertension, arrhythmias, and even cardiac arrest during surgery for carcinoid. Perioperative treatment with somatostatin has been used to reduce such incidents. Whilst radiation has also been used to 'deactivate' hormonally active tumours, reports on its use for this purpose are scanty.

Endoscopic treatments Where surgical resection is deemed to be impossible or the patient is unfit for the required resection, endoscopic ablation is a useful palliative modality. It may also be used as a precursor to resection in an attempt to reduce the amount of lung parenchyma that needs to be resected. Nd:YAG laser via flexible bronchoscopy is probably to be preferred to mechanical debridement due to the vascularity of carcinoid tumours. Endoscopic ablation is rarely curative as much of the tumour is extrabronchial, often forming a 'dumb-bell tumour'.

Surgery Surgery should aim to remove all the primary tumour and draining lymph nodes as for malignant carcinoma. As many tumours arise near the origin of major bronchi, most procedures will entail lobectomy, removing the tumour, and the destroyed distal lung. For tumours of major bronchi, bronchotomy and wedge resection of the bronchial wall or sleeve resection in association with lobectomy will preserve maximal lung parenchyma.

Radiotherapy Carcinoid tumours are relatively insensitive to radiotherapy. However, radiotherapy has been used in the postoperative setting where lymph nodes have been involved and for symptomatic relief in inoperable tumours.

Chemotherapy Some atypical carcinoid tumours, particularly those which tend towards the malignant end of the neuroendocrine carcinoma spectrum, may respond to chemotherapy.

Hormonal therapy Bronchial carcinoid tumours, like other neuroendocrine tumours, have somatostatin receptors which not only aid diagnosis and staging but can be used for therapeutic intervention. Subcutaneous injection of somatostatin analogues (octreotide, lanreotide, and pentetreotide) can induce rapid, marked symptomatic relief.

Prognosis

The prognosis of typical carcinoid tumours which have not metastasized is excellent if all tumour has been excised with clear margins. Even when complete tumour excision has not been possible, prolonged survival can be obtained as these are slow-growing tumours. Atypical carcinoid tumours or well-differentiated neuroendocrine carcinomas have a worse prognosis with complete resection being less common.

Primary bronchogenic carcinoma

Though primary bronchogenic lung cancer is the major cancer killer in the western world, most tumours occurring in the lung are secondary.

Epidemiology

In the UK, the deaths among the male population from lung cancer reached 150 per 100 000 in the late 1980s. However, there is an epidemic of lung cancer occurring in women in the late twentieth century. The epidemic in the female population lags behind that in the male by approximately 30 years. The postulated reason for this is that the modern habit of chain-smoking cigarettes was taken up by men after World War I, whereas women did not take up smoking in large numbers until after the World War II. Lung cancer now kills more women in western Europe and the USA than does breast cancer.

Lung cancer is highest in areas where smoking is most prevalent. It is therefore more common in inner city urban areas and in social classes 4 and 5. Clusters of increased incidence also occur in areas where there is high environmental exposure to other carcinogens. This may explain some cases in inner cities. Shipyards, naval installations, power stations, and other sites where asbestos exposure is common may also have an increased risk to their personnel.

The peak in incidence is in the sixth and seventh decades of life as the risk is proportional to the total exposure to carcinogens in inhaled smoke. However, with more smokers starting the habit earlier in their teen years, cancers are being found in younger patients. The true incidence may be underestimated as many elderly patients unfit for any radical therapy have not in the past been referred for full diagnostic procedures.

Aetiology

Lung cancer is mainly a disease of cigarette smokers. Though there are a number of other recognized causes, the number of cases of lung cancer wholly due to other carcinogens is uncommon (Table 18.5). While asbestos can cause carcinoma of the

Table 18.5 Environmental factors associated with lung cancer

- Active smoking of tobacco
- Passive smoking
- Urban pollution
- Uranium mining
- Asbestos exposure
- Arsenic
- Chromates
- Nickel
- Radon gas
- Lung fibrosis – 'scar carcinoma'

upper aerodigestive tract in non-smokers, the combination of cigarette smoke and asbestos fibres is particularly carcinogenic, with the risks multiplied rather than being additive.

Cigarette smoke contains at least 40 known carcinogens. It is thought that the major carcinogen is 3,4-benzpyrene. This may induce changes such as deletions in the short arm of chromosome 3 found in 50% of non-small lung cell cancer (NSCLC) and 100% of small cell lung cancer (SCLC). It is suggested that there is a tumour supressor gene in the 3p chromosomal region. Other common genetic changes found in lung cancer include mutations of the tumour suppressor gene p53 and over-expression of the tumour promoters K-*ras* (present in 33% of adeno-carcinomas in smokers and suggested to be associated with poor prognosis), c-*myc*, *bcl-2* and c-*erbB2* (also known as the *HER2/neu* gene).

Prevention

Nicotine is a physically and psychologically addictive drug. Most smokers are hooked in their teenage years. Therefore, prevention campaigns need to be directed at early teenagers. Education programmes need to be designed in such a way that the children of smokers, who have learned by observation of their parents that smoking is normal and has no harmful effects, can learn the true dangers of smoking before they too become addicted.

Legislation has already started to reduce exposure to other carcinogens, especially asbestos, air pollution and ionizing radiation, but governments have been slow to legislate for a reduction in the promotion and availability of tobacco products.

Screening

Mass screening of at-risk, middle-aged smokers has not been successful at detecting lung cancers at an early curable stage. Attempts using both sputum cytology and chest radiographs have been tried but have not proved cost-effective. Early cancers are often not visible on chest radiographs. Morphological examination of cells exfoliated into sputum is too coarse a method of detecting the early changes of neoplasia. More promising is the possibility of staining exfoliated cells for genetic changes, which long precede changes that can be detected on cytological examination. Genetic probes have been developed for a number of the common oncogenes seen in lung cancer. The exfoliation of cells into sputum gives a ready vehicle for detecting changes deep within the bronchial tree. Unfortunately, once abnormal cells are found in sputum, finding their exact source is more difficult. Laser light can illuminate areas of metaplasia, but frequently this is so widespread throughout the bronchial tree that determining the segment likely to develop an invasive tumour is not possible.

Chemoprevention

Chemoprevention usually using retinoic acid (vitamin A) compounds has shown promise in a number of cancers of the upper aerodigestive tract. However, at this stage the regular use of chemoprevention has not proved effective in lung cancer.

Pathology

Lung cancers are divided into two readily identified subgroups, small cell and non-small cell lung cancer, upon which treatment strategies are based, though further

Table 18.6 Cellular classification of bronchogenic carcinomas (1999 WHO/IASLC revision)

Preinvasive lesions

Squamous dysplasia/carcinoma in situ

Atypical adenomatous hyperplasia

Diffuse idiopathic pulmonary neuroendocrine cell hyperplasia

Invasive malignant

Non-small cell carcinoma

  Squamous cell carcinoma

    Papillary variant

    Clear cell variant

    Small cell variant

    Basaloid variant

  Adenocarcinoma

    Acinar

    Papillary

    Bronchoalveolar carcinoma

    Solid adenocarcinoma with mucin formation

    Mixed

  Large cell carcinoma

    Large cell neuroendocrine carcinoma

    Basaloid carcinoma

    Lymphoepithelioma-like carcinoma

    Clear cell carcinoma

    Large cell carcinoma with rhabdoid phenotype

  Adenosquamous carcinoma

  Carcinomas with pleomorphic, sarcomatoid, or sarcomatous elements

    Carcinomas with spindle and/or giant cells

    Carcinosarcoma

    Blastoma (pulmonary blastoma)

Small cell

  Small cell carcinoma

    Variant: combined small cell carcinoma (SCLC with squamous and/or glandular elements)

subgroups are also identified (Table 18.6). NSCLC is further subdivided into squamous, adenocarcinoma, and large cell carcinoma, each of which has different clinical and morphological appearances. Their behaviour is generally similar, though a primary squamous cell carcinoma frequently grows to quite a size before metastasizing, whereas adenocarcinoma may metastasize while the primary tumour is still relatively small.

An interesting subgroup of adenocarcinomas spreads along alveolar walls in a 'bronchoalveolar' pattern. When small, these have a particularly good prognosis. However, if they have consolidated a complete lobe, resembling a lobar pneumonia, they tend to continue to spread like a pneumonic process, exfoliating cells to other lobes. This stage is rarely curable. The bronchoalveolar spread may also resemble interstitial lung fibrosis, leading to a delay in diagnosis, which is often eventually made on thoracoscopic or open lung biopsy.

Small cell lung cancer is believed to be the malignant end of a spectrum of tumours showing neuroendocrine differentiation. These tumours consist of highly anaplastic small cells with a high nuclear:cytoplasmic ratio. They are highly malignant and virtually all have metastasized by the time of diagnosis. Small cell tumours make up approximately 25% of lung cancers. Many tumours have mixed components resembling both small cell and non-small cell components. These in general behave as small cell carcinoma. Frequently, after chemotherapy small cell components have responded well, leaving residual non-small cell tumour. For this reason consolidation radiotherapy should be considered for residual tumour after standard small cell chemotherapy.

Presentation

Symptoms from a lung cancer are produced by local bronchial irritation and invasion, bronchial obstruction with distal pneumonitis, invasion of local chest wall and mediastinal structures. Metastatic disease and paraneoplastic symptoms can mimic the symptoms of a plethora of other diseases. Therefore lung cancer, the modern 'great imitator', should always be kept in mind when treating any medical condition in the at-risk group.

The classic symptoms of lung cancer are haemoptysis, cough, dyspnoea, chest pain, and recurrent or persistent chest infections. Unfortunately, lung cancers tend to occur in elderly smokers, all of whom have a 'smoker's cough' and frequent bouts of 'bronchitis' with associated sputum production and frequently haemoptysis. Many have breathlessness due to emphysema, and chest pain due to ischaemic heart disease. The difficulty for the primary care physician is to determine which of these exacerbations is due to lung cancer. Furthermore, by the time a lung cancer has become symptomatic with the above symptoms, it is frequently incurable. Most patients who have curable tumours at the time of presentation have had an incidental chest x-ray for preoperative assessment for another condition or an insurance medical examination, or have had one of the above danger symptoms during a chest infection unrelated to the tumour. Therefore it is important to emphasize and encourage such 'pseudo-screening', particularly in the high-risk group: the middle-aged smoker.

Locally advanced lung cancer can present with a number of symptoms due to invasion on other organs in the chest. Superior vena caval obstruction is due to mediastinal nodes encompassing the SVC and usually the azygos vein. The patient is plethoric with enlarged subcutaneous veins in the upper trunk and a persistently raised, non-fluctuating jugular venous pressure. When advanced, the patient cannot lie flat because of a breathless 'drowning sensation'. Subcarinal or inferior mediastinal nodes can also impinge on the oesophagus, causing dysphagia and aspiration pneumonitis. Hoarseness is a sign of recurrent laryngeal nerve palsy. It is more common on the left due to tracheobronchial and aortopulmonary window nodes invading the nerve as it loops under the ligamentum arteriosum. Hoarseness may also be due to direct invasion of the vagal nerves by an apical tumour or cervical node metastases. Similarly, the phrenic nerve may be involved with mediastinal tumour invasion, particularly as the nerve crosses the pericardium. A raised hemi-diaphragm is the sign on chest x-ray, though this can be produced by lobar atelectasis. Confirmation of nerve palsy can be made by fluoroscopic examination of the diaphragm on inspiration. The brachial plexus, when invaded by a tumour of the superior sulcus in the apex of the chest, produces the 'Pancoast syndrome' with pain radiating to the shoulder and inner aspect of the arm, a Horner's syndrome due to sympathetic chain invasion, and subclavian vascular compression or thrombosis. Like other nerve invasion signs, this syndrome usually indicates inoperability, though the use of pre-operative radiotherapy followed by surgery can result in long-term survival.

As lung cancers can be present for many years and grow to a considerable size before they become symptomatic, many actually present with metastatic disease. The adrenal, liver, bone, brain and contralateral lung are the common sites of metastases.

Non-metastatic paraneoplastic syndromes Of particular interest are the non-metastatic paraneoplastic syndromes associated with lung cancer. These are particularly well documented for small cell carcinoma and large cell undifferentiated carcinoma, both of which tend to have many neuroendocrine features. However, they do occur to a lesser degree with squamous and adenocarcinoma. Many of these syndromes are mediated by peptides, which mimic active portions of known hormones. The common paraneoplastic syndromes are listed in the Table 18.7.

Table 18.7 Common paraneoplastic syndromes associated with lung cancer

Endocrine
Syndrome of inappropriate antidiuretic hormone (SIADH)
Atrial natriuretic peptide
Ectopic adrenocorticotropic hormone
Hypercalcaemia (non-metastatic)

Neurological
Eaton–Lambert myasthenic syndrome
Paraneoplastic cerebellar degeneration
Encephalomyelitis
Sensory neuropathy
Retinopathy
Intestinal pseudo-obstruction
Autonomic dysfunction

Other
Hypercoagulability
Nephrotic syndrome

While they are often no more than clinical curiosities, it is important that when the syndromes are diagnosed that an underlying carcinoma must be suspected. It is also important to realize that these are not symptoms of metastatic disease and the tumour itself may be curable with appropriate therapy to the primary site. Frequently it is necessary to control the paraneoplastic symptom in order to make the patient fit enough to undergo radical therapy.

Examination

Examination can be remarkably normal despite a sizeable tumour. The patient will frequently show signs of weight loss and have the habitus of a patient suffering from chronic obstructive airways disease, with a ruddied face, cyanosis, and pursed lip breathing. The fingers will often be tobacco stained and clubbing may be evident.

Examination of the chest frequently reveals the hyperinflated chest of the chronic bronchitic. A central tumour may invoke stridor on auscultation or signs of distal lung atelectasis with sympathetic effusion. A more peripheral tumour may show signs of pleural irritation. An apical tumour which has begun to invade the brachial plexus will cause a Pancoast syndrome. This initially involves painful paraesthesia of the inner aspects of the upper arm and of the ulnar aspect of the hands. Thromboembolic phenomena may develop as the subclavian artery is encased in tumour. A tumour invading the sympathetic chain and stellate ganglion in the apex will cause a Horner's syndrome, with sweating on the affected side, ptosis of the eyelid, and constriction of the pupil. Other clinical signs would be those of a paraneoplastic or metastatic lesion.

Diagnosis

The diagnosis may be made on sputum cytology and is more successful if taken as early morning specimens on successive days. Chest x-ray will usually show a hilar mass in the presence of a central tumour or a spiculated peripheral mass. Obstructive pneumonitis and a pleural effusion may also be evident.

Bronchoscopy is essential to biopsy any central tumour, take bronchial washings from the site of a peripheral lesion, and to exclude other endobronchial disease.

Staging

In NSCLC, treatment and prognosis are entirely dependent on accurate staging (Fig. 18.8 and 18.9). Stage I tumours are small and readily resectable with good prognosis. The standard treatment is surgery though radical radiotherapy is an

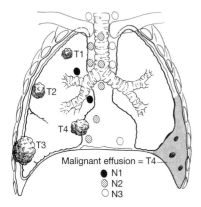

Fig. 18.1 Non-small cell lung cancer, tumour and node staging.

Table 18.8 NSCLC Stage groupings (1997 update)

	N0	N1	N2	N3	M1
T1	Ia	IIa	IIIa	IIIb	IV
T2	Ib	IIb	IIIa	IIIb	IV
T3	IIb	IIIa	IIIa	IIIb	IV
T4	IIIb	IIIb	IIIb	IIIb	IV
M1	IV	IV	IV	IV	IV

Table 18.9 Non-small cell lung cancer TNM definitions (UICC update 1997)

Primary tumour (T)

Tx	Primary tumour cannot be assessed, or tumour proven by the presence of malignant cells in sputum or bronchial washings but not visualized by imaging or bronchoscopy
T0	No evidence of primary tumour
Tis	Carcinoma in situ
T1	A tumour that is 3 cm or less in greatest dimension, surrounded by lung or visceral pleura, and without bronchoscopic evidence of invasion more proximal than the lobar bronchus (i.e. not in a main bronchus)*
T2	A tumour with any of the following features of size or extent:

- more than 3 cm in greatest dimension
- involves a main bronchus, 2 cm or more distal to the carina
- invades the visceral pleura
- associated with atelectasis or obstructive pneumonitis that extends to the hilar region but does not involve the entire lung

T3	A tumour of any size that directly invades any of the following:

- chest wall (including superior sulcus tumours), diaphragm, mediastinal pleura (or phrenic nerve), parietal pericardium; or
- tumour in the main bronchus less than 2 cm distal to the carina but without involvement of the carina; or
- associated atelectasis or obstructive pneumonitis of the entire lung

T3a	Atelectasis or obstructive pneumonitis of one entire lung without other criterion for T3
T3b	Other criterion present for T3
T4	A tumour of any size that invades any of the following:

- mediastinum, heart, great vessels, trachea, oesophagus, recurrent laryngeal nerve, vertebral body, carina; or
- separate tumour nodules in the same lobe; or
- tumour with a malignant pleural effusion**

T4a	All T4 except T4b
T4b	Invasion of the carina or presence of a malignant pleural effusion

Regional lymph nodes (N)

Nx	Regional lymph nodes cannot be assessed
N0	No regional lymph node metastasis
N1	Metastasis to ipsilateral peribronchial and/or ipsilateral hilar lymph nodes, and intrapulmonary nodes including involvement by direct extension of the primary tumour
N2	Metastasis to ipsilateral mediastinal and/or subcarinal lymph node(s)
N2a	Metastases in ipsilateral mediastinal nodes other than the paratracheal or para-oesophageal nodes
N2b	Metastases in the paratracheal and para-oesophageal nodes

Table 18.9 *contd.*

N3	Metastasis to contralateral mediastinal, contralateral hilar, ipsilateral or contralateral scalene, or supraclavicular lymph node(s)
N3a	Metastases in the contralateral (hilar or mediastinal) nodes
N3b	Metastases in the supra-clavicular fossae or scalene nodes

Distant metastasis (M)

Mx	Distant metastasis cannot be assessed
M0	No distant metastasis
M1	Distant metastasis present***

*The uncommon superficial tumour of any size with its invasive component limited to the bronchial wall, which may extend proximal to the main bronchus, is also classified as T1.

**Most pleural effusions associated with lung cancer are due to tumour. However, there are a few patients in whom multiple cytopathological examinations of pleural fluid are negative for tumour. In these cases, fluid is non-bloody and is not an exudate. When these elements and clinical judgement dictate that the effusion is not related to the tumour, the effusion should be excluded as a staging element and the patient should be staged as T1, T2, or T3.

***M1 includes separate tumour nodule(s) in a different lobe (ipsilateral or contralateral).

Specify sites according to the following notations: BRA, brain; EYE, eye; HEP, hepatic; LYM, lymph nodes; MAR, bone marrow; OSS, osseous; OTH, other; OVR, ovary; PER, peritoneal; PLE, pleura; PUL, pulmonary, SKI, skin.

option in those who are unfit for a surgical procedure. Stage II tumours have local lymph node metastases. They are readily resectable but because of the node metastases they have a reduced prognosis. Stage III tumours are locally advanced and cure is uncommon with surgery alone. They fall into two general categories: either invading structures which compromise surgical resection, or metastatic to mediastinal lymph nodes. Unlike stage IV tumours (disseminated), they may be encapsulated in a therapeutic radiation field. Recent advances in neoadjuvant chemotherapy and radiotherapy have changed the approach to these tumours and the prognosis has been improved, especially where a good response to induction therapy has allowed complete surgical resection.

The staging of NSCLC is based on the TNM classification (Table 18.8). A Revised International System for Staging Lung Cancer was adopted in 1997 by the American Joint Committee on Cancer and the Union Internationale Contre le Cancer (Table 18.9). The major changes were the division of stage I into A and B depending on the T stage of the tumour and the reallocation of T3N0 tumours to stage IIB in line with their better prognosis than those tumours that have N2 node metastases.

CT scan has become the main tool for assessment of the site and size of tumour, chest wall invasion, mediastinal lymphadenopathy and metastases to liver, adrenal, and dorsal spine. MRI may clarify chest wall or mediastinal invasion.

Fitness for radical therapy

Virtually all lung cancer sufferers have cardiovascular, respiratory, and cerebrovascular co-morbidity on the basis of their age, smoking, and other occupational exposure.

The most useful test is that of exercise tolerance with the ability to walk a mile on flat ground or climb six flights of stairs without prolonged rest usually indicating fitness for lung resection. The forced expiratory volume in one second (FEV_1) has been a useful guide to respiratory fitness for resection, with a figure of 40% of the normal value indicating the ability to survive lobectomy without being left postoperatively as a 'respiratory cripple'. For pneumonectomy an FEV_1 of 60% is usually required.

Treatment of non-small cell lung cancer

Best supportive care As most patients are unfit or unsuitable for curative therapies, the main emphasis of care is on symptom control. Pain is the great fear of the cancer patient and has secondary effects of debilitation, loss of appetite, depression, and even breathlessness. Judicious use of oral and topical NSAIDs and narcotics in slow release or transdermal preparations, dosed to prevent pain rather than treat it, will maintain the patient's feeling of well-being. At later stages subcutaneous infusions may be required. These analgesic medications can be combined with antidepressant and anticonvulsant therapies or transcutaneous nerve stimulation (TENS) to treat difficult neuralgia.

Cough is difficult to treat as cough suppressants are frequently inadequate and radiotherapy, which is very effective in treating pain and haemoptyis, tends to exacerbate cough. Chemotherapy can provide good relief of cough, haemoptysis, and pain but nausea and malaise with each course can counteract the benefits. Chemotherapy may be cost-effective in allowing patients to live with their disease at home rather than needing admission to hospital for expensive treatment of symptoms.

Breathlessness is usually due to bronchial obstruction but may be due to anaemia of chronic disease or to bone marrow infiltration. Blood transfusion may be needed for symptomatic relief. Malignant pleural effusion is a remediable cause of breathlessness (see below).

Surgery Surgery remains the mainstay of treatment for lung cancer. Though responses are seen following chemotherapy in NSCLC and good remission is common in small cell, cures are the exception. Similarly, radical radiotherapy is possible in only a small percentage of patients and when surgery is an option the results are superior to radiotherapy.

The aim of surgery is to resect the primary tumour with clear lateral and bronchial resection margins, the peribronchial lymphatic drainage of the tumour and the hilar lymph nodes. Mediastinal lymph node dissection performed at the time of lung resection provides vital staging and prognostic information, which will determine the need for further therapies and may in itself contribute to local tumour control or cure.

Lobectomy is the most commonly performed operation for lung cancer, fulfilling the above criteria for complete oncological resection. Bilobectomy is the term for removing the middle lobe of the right lung in conjunction with either the upper or lower lobe. When the tumour crosses a major fissure involving all lobes of a lung, encroaches close to a main bronchus, either on the mucosal surface or with extrinsic compression by lymph nodes, or involves a main pulmonary artery, pneumonectomy, the removal of a whole lung, is necessary. This operation has a substantially higher mortality and incidence of long-term debility and should only be performed when tumour clearance cannot be obtained by a lung-preserving procedure.

Lung resection is major surgery, requiring not only particular surgical skill but specialist anaesthesia and postoperative care. Ideal operative conditions require maintaining the patient's respiration on the contralateral lung while the affected lung is deflated for surgery. Cardiac instability is a frequent consequence. Postoperatively the patient spends 24–48 hours in a high-dependency nursing unit and will spend a further week to 10 days in hospital, depending on the severity of complications or the persistence of an air leak from the operated lung. Because of co-morbidity, major complications occur in 30% of patients undergoing lung cancer surgery and the quoted perioperative mortality is 3% for lobectomy and 8–10% for pneumonectomy.

When adjuvant therapy is indicated, it can usually be commenced 3–6 weeks after surgery, allowing time for wounds to heal and for the patient to pass the postoperative catabolic phase. There is at present no agreement on the indications or effects of postoperative radiotherapy or chemotherapy. It is common to irradiate areas where macroscopic tumour has been left at the time of surgery or where the surgeon feels he has not been able to achieve satisfactory margins. Similarly, postoperative radiation to the mediastinum when microscopic deposits have been found in mediastinal nodes decreases local recurrence but may also have a small but relevant survival benefit. As most life-threatening recurrence is outside the chest cavity, only systemic therapy can be expected to prolong life. Platinum-based chemotherapy regimens provide an improvement in survival following surgery.

Chemotherapy Experience has shown that the drugs which have served so well in the treatment of small cell lung cancer, such as the alkylating agents, have actually had an adverse effect on survival in non-small cell cancer. It is only recently that the possibility of effective chemotherapy has emerged (meta-analysis by NSCLC Collaborative Group 52 trials, 9387 patients, *BMJ* 1995; **311**, 899–909). The regimens that have shown the most response have been those containing cisplatin, particularly in combination with one or two other effective drugs. MIC (Mitomycin C, Ifosfamide, Cisplatin) and MVP (Mitomycin C, vinblastine, cisplatin) have shown response rates in the vicinity of 50% with acceptable toxicity. The effects, whilst being very useful in terms of palliation, have not translated into long-term survival. Newer drugs such as paclitaxel, doxetaxel, gemcitabine, and vinorelbine have all shown responses as single agents and trials are ongoing to determine the most effective combinations.

Radiotherapy Both small cell and non-small lung cancer are sensitive to radiotherapy with the effect being more dependent on the dose that is able to be delivered than on the histology of the tumour. The thorax contains many vital organs, which are themselves sensitive to radiation. This limits the doses of radiotherapy that can be delivered to tumours. Many tumours, particularly unresectable tumours, are sited near the hilum, making it difficult to plan effective irradiation while avoiding the heart, spinal cord, and parenchymal lung tissue.

Radical radiotherapy – A tumoricidal dose of radiation is approximately 60 Gy (delivered in 18–30 fractions) for NSCLC. In addition to the tumour itself, it is necessary to deliver this dose to a margin of 2 cm. This limits the size of tumours that can be treated with curative intent to approximately 3 cm in maximum diameter. Therefore only a small percentage of tumours in patients unfit for resection or who refuse surgery can be treated radically. Five-year survival has been reported in 15–20% of this highly selected group.

Newer techniques for delivering radiotherapy have been developed. The latest spiral CT scanners allow more accurate three-dimensional planning. Delivery of conformal radiation fields, which follow the contour of the tumour more closely and avoid irradiating contiguous radiosensitive structures, translates into a tumorocidal dose as high as 80 Gy to tumours which at present can only be palliated. Continuous hyperfractionated radiotherapy (CHART) has been shown to increase the response rate of tumours treated radically. There is also early evidence of increased survival.

Palliative radiotherapy – In patients unfit for radical radiotherapy, single fractions of 5–10 Gy are effective for specific symptoms such as haemoptysis or pain.

Special situations

Bronchial obstruction – An obstructed bronchus results in symptoms out of proportion to the size of the tumour. It results in an atelectatic, infected lobe or lung through which unoxygenated blood is shunted. Effective doses of radiation and chemotherapy are not possible because of the associated sepsis. One of the aims of external beam radiation is to reduce such obstruction. However, post-radiation fibrosis and protracted pre-treatment atelectasis make such a desirable effect less common.

Intraluminal brachytherapy with sources delivered by bronchoscopy can relieve obstructed bronchi and can lead to complete resolution of superficial tumours. The effect is enhanced by external beam radiotherapy. Nd:YAG laser delivered by flexible fibreoptic bronchoscopy can also be used to reopen obstructed major bronchi. The CO_2 laser is effective in a straight line for laryngeal and tracheal tumours. Recently, self-expanding metal sens stents, deliverable over a guidewire under radiological control, have been successfully used to recanalize bronchi. Relief of obstructive pneumonitis by intraluminal brachytherapy, Nd:YAG laser, or sens can relieve otherwise untreatable sepsis and allow the use of radiation and chemotherapy.

Massive haemoptysis – Haemoptysis is one of the primary alert signs for bronchogenic carcinoma. It is ironic that in many cases of lung cancer the haemoptysis arises from another lesion such as an area of bronchitis. Similarly, massive haemoptysis is more common with benign diseases such as TB, cystic fibrosis, or terminal congenital heart disease than with malignancy.

Flexible bronchoscopy is usually impractical in the face of massive blood loss as a good view cannot be obtained. Rigid bronchoscopy may allow better control of the airway and allow larger suction catheters to be used but at the expense of allowing contamination of the contralateral lung as the cough reflex is temporarily abolished. Often the only useful bronchoscopic manoeuvre is to pass a balloon catheter as a bronchial blocker. This tamponades the affected lung until other treatment such as embolization or radiotherapy can be commenced.

SVC obstruction – Facial and upper limb oedema with distension of veins on the upper torso are the immediate signs of superior vena caval obstruction. The commonest cause in Western societies is malignant mediastinal lymphadenopathy. In young patients, lymphoma is frequently the culprit but in the ageing smoker, bronchogenic carcinoma must be suspected. The presence of the syndrome of SVC obstruction is an indicator of advanced local disease, usually indicating that the azygos system has also been blocked. It is an indication for urgent treatment as cardiac decompensation due to impaired venous return can develop rapidly.

Dysphagia – Mediastinal metastases from lung cancer, particularly those in sub-carinal nodes, may compress the oesophagus, causing dysphagia. This may be treatable with chemotherapy or radiotherapy, but such treatment may be compromised by aspiration pneumonitis. Self-expanding metal endo-oesophageal stents can be passed endoscopically under fluoroscopic control to immediately relieve the dysphagia and the danger of aspiration.

Hypercalcaemia – Hypercalcaemia in lung cancer may be the result of multiple bone metastases. However, it may also be a paraneoplastic effect of a peptide resembling parathyroid hormone. It is commoner in small cell carcinoma and when it does occur in NSCLC it is frequently an indication of a poorly differentiated tumour with poor prognosis. Initial treatment involves rehydration with normal saline accompanied by a frusemide-induced diuresis. Bisphosphonate drugs such as palmidronate or etidronate may also be effective in the acute phase. Further treatment is that which is appropriate to the underlying malignancy.

Spinal cord compression – Vertebral metastasis compromising the spinal cord is not uncommon in lung cancer. If it leads to paralysis it is a disastrous complication as a patient living with his cancer, able to carry on the activities of daily living, is transformed into a bedbound cripple requiring total care for the remainder of his/her short life. Once neurological signs are present, there is rarely any return of function. Therefore anticipation and early recognition are essential. Any suggestion of back pain, loss of bowel or bladder function, or limb signs should be treated as an oncological emergency and urgent CT, myelogram, or MRI obtained. Some patients are suitable for neurosurgical spinal decompression but most will be treated with radiotherapy.

Malignant pleural effusion – See secondary lung cancers.

Treatment of small cell lung cancer

Despite treatment, most patients with small cell lung cancer die of their disease. Treatment is generally aimed at palliating symptoms, though significant prolongation of life can be obtained with relatively non-toxic chemotherapy.

Treatment and prognosis in small cell cancer are not as dependent on loco-regional tumour as is the case with non-small cell cancer, as most patients have systemic metastatic disease at the time of diagnosis. Indeed, the patients' performance status has more relevance to the treatment modality to which they are most suited. Disease is therefore classified as limited or extensive (Table 18.10).

However, non-surgical staging procedures allow an improved assessment of prognosis and identify sites of tumour that can be evaluated for response. They may also have treatment implications when chest irradiation is being considered. In those uncommon instances when surgery is an option as part of a combined modality programme, staging is performed in accordance with the TNM staging system for NSCLC (American Joint Committee on Cancer/UICC/IASCLC).

Table 18.10 Small cell lung cancer staging

Limited stage

Tumour confined to the hemithorax of origin,

the mediastinum, and

the supraclavicular nodes,

which can be encompassed within a 'tolerable' radiotherapy port

Differences arise in the classification of patients with pleural effusion, massive pulmonary tumour, and contralateral supraclavicular nodes.

Extensive stage

Tumour too widespread to be included within the definition of limited stage disease.

Source: Veterans' Administration Lung Cancer Study Group.

In addition to the procedures in Table 18.11, a mediastinoscopy is virtually mandatory in this setting.

Standard regimens for treatment of small cell lung cancer include CAV (cyclophosphamide, doxorubicin and vincristine) and ECMV (Etoposide, Cyclophosphaside, Methotrexate, Vincristine). These are well tolerated and have response rates in the region of 70%. They are administerd as out-patient regimens on a day case basis. Side-effects are usually moderate bone marrow toxicity. The combination of a platin drug with etoposide (EP) has become the treatment of choice. Increasing the dose and intensity of the standard drugs has not shown an improvement in survival. However, more intensive three- and four-drug combinations such as ICE (Ifosfamide, Carboplatin, Etoposide) or VICE (Vincristine, Ifosfamide, Carboplatin, Etoposide) are currently undergoing trials. Other new drugs to show response include toptecan and the taxanes, paclitaxel and docetaxel.

As most patients present with metastatic disease, locoregional treatments play little part in treatment and systemic therapy is necessary. A small number of patients are suitable for surgery usually followed by chemotherapy. Local radiation may be indicated for emergency situations such as SVC obstruction or to areas less likely to respond to chemotherapy such as brain, epidural or bone metastases.

Radiation to residual primary tumour is also used to consolidate chemotherapy. Improved survival has been reported in series investigating this approach. Interestingly, the residual tumour may contain non-small cell elements not responsive to chemotherapy but sensitive to radiotherapy.

Table 18.11 Staging procedures for small cell cancer

Bone marrow examination

Computed tomographic or magnetic resonance imaging scans of the brain

Computerized tomographic scans of the chest and the abdomen

Radionuclide bone scans

(If surgery is to be considered, mediastinoscopy is mandatory)

As the brain acts as a 'sanctuary' site for metastatic disease, cerebral metastases are common despite a good response of the main tumour to chemotherapy. Prophylactic cranial irradiation (PCI) is often administered to those who have survived their chemotherapy and remain in good performance status. This reduces the incidence of brain metastases, but there is debate over whether it improves survival. There is concern that cerebral irradiation may lead to brain damage. Neuropsychological deficit is not uncommon in small cell patients and there is no evidence that PCI adds to its severity.

Treatment success rates and prognosis

NSCLC The prognosis in NSCLC is dependent on the stage of the tumour and the completeness of surgical resection. When tumour is completely excised, the 5-year survival rates of stages I and II are 80% and 40%, respectively. For some subgroups of stage IIIA NSCLC which are resected, the survival can approach 20%, but for most the survival is in the region of 8%. When, either due to stage IIIB disease or for medical reasons, surgery is not possible but radical radiotherapy can be delivered, long-term survival can be achieved in 15% of patients. This can be increased by giving adjuvant chemotherapy. For patients with metastatic disease, the median survival is 6–9 months and is rarely influenced by therapy.

SCLC Seventy per cent of small cell lung cancer patients will show a response to chemotherapy and up to 30% will have a complete response. However, only 10% will survive 2 years after commencement of treatment. Survival is not prolonged by maintenance chemotherapy and second-line therapies have not been shown to be successsful.

Conclusion

Future strategies to reduce the mortality rates for lung cancer may include chemoprevention with improved dietary agents and improved screening based on molecular biological techniques to determine early genetic changes in exfoliated bronchial cells. New chemotherapeutic approaches will see the introduction of the taxane drugs and the use of liposomal coatings to improve the delivery of drugs and the targeting of tumour cells. Anti-angiogenesis agents may also reduce tumour growth without actually being tumoricidal. However, above all, lung cancer is a smoking-related disease and any major reduction in mortality from this disease will be from a reduction in cigarette smoking.

Secondary lung cancers

Most tumours occurring in the lung and pleura are secondary tumours. Usually this is obvious, as a primary tumour has been previously diagnosed. Lung infiltration frequently heralds the onset of the terminal phase of the disease. However, whenever certain tumours, particularly adenocarcinomas, are diagnosed in the lung, the question must be asked whether it is a primary or secondary tumour. The question is important as resection may be curative for a primary tumour but the occurrence of a secondary may indicate the necessity of further chemotherapy or radiotherapy.

Key points

- Most NSCLC is inoperable by the time it becomes symptomatic.
- Some NSCLC respond to chemotherapy.
- Induction therapy may render a tumour operable.
- Those showing complete response to chemotherapy have the longest survival in neoadjuvant trials.
- Induction chemotherapy can increase postoperative complications, especially after pneumonectomy and mediastinal node clearance.

Primary or secondary?

A bronchial origin or an origin in a background field of metaplasia is helpful in making the decision whether a tumour is a primary or a secondary. This is useful when differentiating from laryngeal, oesophageal, or other squamous primary tumours.

However, adenocarcinomas, be they primary or secondary, tend to occur in the lung periphery and often have no bronchial origin identifiable in the resection specimen. A smoking history, endobronchial position, bronchoalveolar pattern of spread, or nodal metastases are all suggestive of a primary tumour but do not exclude secondary disease.

Second primary tumours

Second primary tumours are not uncommon in patients who have previously had an upper aerodigestive tract cancer. In fact, in patients who have survived 5 years from their first lung cancer and are therefore regarded as cured of that cancer, the incidence of a second primary lung cancer, pharyngeal, laryngeal, or oesophageal cancer, reaches nearly 10%, particularly in those who continue to smoke. If the cell type is the same as the first tumour, it can be difficult to tell whether it is indeed a second primary. Again the presence of a definite bronchial origin or epithelial metaplasia, may suggest that it is, indeed, a second primary. The prognosis is dependent on the stage of the new primary. Frequently it is not possible to determine preoperatively whether a tumour is secondary or a new primary. If the patient is otherwise fit, it is probably wisest to treat the tumour as a new primary. If it turns out to be secondary, any operation may be regarded as a metastasectomy (see below).

Pulmonary metastasectomy

The presence of lung metastases need not be seen as a sign for despair. Many patients can achieve prolongation of good quality life by undergoing metastasectomy, the removal of lung metastases. This has now been well documented, particularly when the primary tumour is of germ cell, colorectal, renal, bone, or soft tissue origin. It is important when selecting patients for metastasectomy that primary tumour control has been achieved, that there are no extrathoracic metastases, and that the patient has enough cardiopulmonary reserve to enable complete resection of all metastases. Though better long-term success is more likely with a solitary metastasis and a long disease-free interval, these should not be regarded as absolute criteria as survival is more dependent on tumour histology and predicted tumour doubling time.

Metastasectomy can be performed unilaterally via thoracotomy or bilaterally via median sternotomy. Surgeons stress the importance of being able to bimanually palpate the lung to detect metastases that may not appear on CT scan. Therefore the benefit of minimal access metastasectomy is questionable.

Notable exceptions to the above policy are breast and melanoma metastases. Excision in these circumstances should only be reserved for diagnostic purposes, a positive diagnosis being an indication for further systemic therapy. Similarly, whilst metastasectomy may be indicated for sarcomas and some germ cell metastases, the finding of persistent viable disease is usually an indication for further radiotherapy or chemotherapy.

Malignant pleural effusion

The pleura is a common site for metastatic disease. A malignant pleural effusion can produce breathlessness out of proportion to the amount of disease present. As patients can live for extended periods even in the presence of metastatic pleural disease, effective palliation should be undertaken.

A malignant effusion will virtually always recur after an initial diagnostic pleural aspirate. Attempts at repeated aspiration will result in a trapped, collapsed lung due to a loculated effusion that can no longer be drained. Early pleurodesis is a more effective strategy. This can be achieved by insertion of sclerosant substances into the pleural cavity, though there are circumstances when surgical pleurectomy, or mechanical pleural abrasion, is indicated. The most effective sclerosant is sterile talc, which can be introduced by insufflation at thoracosopy when pleural and lung biopsies may also be obtained and pleural loculations broken down. When the diagnosis has already been established, it is often easier to drain the pleura to dryness with a chest drain and insert the talc through the drain as a slurry.

Malignant pericardial effusion

Malignant pericardial effusion presents with the more acute clinical picture of pericardial tamponade. Acute decompression can be achieved by pericardiocentesis under echocardiographic control. To prevent recurrent tamponade, a pericardial window can be fashioned either at thoracoscopy or via a subxiphoid laparotomy. The latter can be performed even in debilitated patients under local anaesthetic without the need for special anaesthetic techniques such as double lumen endotracheal intubation.

Malignant pleural mesothelioma (MPM)
Epidemiology

Mesothelioma is a malignant tumour of the pleural surface, usually beginning on the parietal surface but eventually covering the visceral pleura, trapping the lung. Cases of pleural mesothelioma tended to cluster around certain industrial sites, particularly those where asbestos was frequently used (Table 18.12). The use of asbestos was banned gradually from the mid-1960s. As there is a lag time of approximately 30–40 years from the time of first exposure until the diagnosis of mesothelioma, the incidence can expect to rise for a further 15 years in Western Europe, peaking in 2015.

Ninety per cent of cases are males with the mean age at diagnosis being 64 years. The mean lag time from first asbestos contact to diagnosis is 40 years, though it is shorter for insulation workers, suggesting a dose–reponse relationship.

Aetiology

Long fibre asbestos has been identified as the cause of most cases of mesothelioma. The length of the fibres is critical to their ability to enter the respiratory tract,

Table 18.12 Occupations associated with mesothelioma

Asbestos miners

Asbestos cement workers – Emilia Romagna region of Italy

Insulation workers – a high incidence of mesothelioma occurred where asbestos was sprayed onto pipes and boilers; less so when applied in a paste form; the powdered form removed during relining of pipes was particularly damaging to the respiratory tract

- Shipyard workers – pipes and boilers heavily insulated with asbestos
- Merchant navy personnel, particularly boiler room workers
- Power-station workers – pipes and boilers heavily insulated with asbestos
- Railway workers – carriages were frequently lined by asbestos leading to exposure of construction, maintenance and demolition workers.
- Sugar refineries
- Wood and pulp industry

Production and usage of asbestos textiles – asbestos was used to make hard wearing and heat resistance fabrics

Farmers – many farm buildings were made of asbestos sheeting. Farmers who frequently built their own outbuildings were exposed to powdered fibres on cutting the sheets

Spouses and families of asbestos workers – fibres often found their way into households on the clothing of families. Wives who washed their husbands contaminated work clothes. Children living in the environs of asbestos industries or using asbestos dumps as playgrounds are also at risk

Builders and building maintenance personnel – since the banning of asbestos in industry it is now the removal of asbestos which provides a greater risk than its installation. The environmental asbestos fibre count remains very low till removal is attempted. For at least 5 years after removal of asbestos sheeting or insulation the atmospheric fibre count remains elevated

Friction-products industry – while mesothelioma has been reported in automobile brake lining workers the incidence is very low

setting up a florid reaction in the larynx, trachea, and bronchi, which can ultimately lead to squamous metaplasia and bronchogenic cancer, particularly in association with tobacco smoke. Passing into the lung parenchyma, the fibres cause fibrosis referred to as asbestosis. This fibrosis is pre-malignant for bronchogenic carcinoma. Those fibres long and thin enough pass onto the parietal pleural surface. There they accumulate in anthracotic 'black spots' where they are phagocytosed by macrophages, and develop a characteristic inflammatory reaction, eventually forming calcified pleural plaques. It is not yet certain whether mesothelioma arise in these plaques or in non-plaque mesothelium.

There are different forms of asbestos (Table 18.13), each causing different pathologies. It is thought that the amphibole fibres cause mesothelioma. However, different types of fibres frequently occur together, making it difficult to specifically assign causation to individual fibre types. It would be prudent therefore to treat chrysotile with the same caution as the amphibole forms. Other

Table 18.13 Types of asbestos

Chrysotile

'White'

Curled serpentine fibres

Cleared from lungs by lymphatics

Not thought to cause mesothelioma

May have a role in causing bronchogenic carcinoma

Amphibole

Rod-like

Not cleared by lymphatics

Accumulate in macrophages

Associated with mesothelioma

Subtypes of amphibole asbestos

Crocidolite 'blue' – particularly carcinogenic

Amosite – 'brown' asbestos

Anthrophylite – mines with pure anthrophylite have a low reported incidence mesothelioma

Actinolite

Tremolite

organic fibres have also been implicated as causes for mesothelioma. Fibrous zeolite (erionite) is a common cause in rural Turkey and Greece.

Evidence of asbestos exposure is found in 80% of mesothelioma cases. However, the history may be difficult to elicit. Unlike asbestosis and lung cancer, which are related to the dose of asbestos and length of exposure, MPM can be more idiosyncratic, with brief exposure up to 40 years before the diagnosis is made.

The genetic changes include aneuploidy and specific chromosomal changes including deletions, inversions, or translocations most commonly found on chromosomes 1, 3, and 9. p53 abnormalities seem to play only a minor role in MPM. The c-*sis* gene, which codes for PDGF, implicated in proliferative mesenchymal disease, is sited on chromosome 22, abnormalities of which are frequently seen in MPM. Also implicated are the growth promoters insulin-like growth factor 1 (IGF-1), transforming growth factor beta (TGF-β), and epidermal growth factor (EGF), and the cytokines IL-6 and granulocyte-macrophage colony-stimulating factor (GM-CSF).

Prevention

Control of exposure to amphibole asbestos will prevent most cases of mesothelioma. Legislation in most countries has reduced the incidence of new exposure. The incidence of new cases of mesothelioma, however, will continue until at least 2015 as amphibole asbestos was widely used in many European countries up to 1975.

Screening for mesothelioma is not practical as early disease is often not apparent on chest x-ray. Even when early disease is detected there is no treatment proven to change the course of the disease.

Pathology

Mesothelioma generally arises in the parietal pleura, spreading diffusely along the pleura before invading chest wall or diaphragmatic muscle, fissural pleura, and lung. Mediastinal node metastasis is late. The tumour gradually 'strangles' the lung and eventually encases it. Transdiaphragmatic spread can lead to peritoneal involvement. Contralateral pleura and pericardial encasement are common in advanced cases. Mesothelioma has a propensity to spread along needle tracks, chest drain incisions, thoracoscopic port sites, and operative incisions.

Macroscopically the tumour consists of thickened pleura with nodularity. On microscopy, sheets of spindle-shaped cells admixed with a fibrotic stroma are the main feature.

Three types of mesothelioma are commonly described: sarcomatous, epithelial, and mixed. Sarcomatous mesothelioma, the less common, is more obviously malignant with a poor prognosis. It can occur as a discrete, but invasive, chest wall mass. Microscopically it can be difficult to differentiate from secondary sarcoma elsewhere in the body. The epithelial type resembles adenocarcinoma with complex acinar spaces lined by mesothelial cells, with frond-like papillary projections. Electron microscopy and immunohistochemistry can aid differentiation of mesothelioma from other tumours and pleural conditions.

Electron microscopy Electron microscopical ultrastructural evaluation shows multiple long, thin, sinuous microvilli covering the cell surface. In contrast to adenocarcinoma cells, these are not covered by glycocalyx.

Presentation

The onset of mesothelioma is insidious. A 'herald' effusion may predate the diagnosis by up to 5 years. Non-mesotheliomatous effusions that do not proceed to mesothelioma also occur in conjunction with benign asbestos-related conditions such asbestosis, pleural plaque, and asbestos pseudo-tumour.

Breathlessness is common due to pleural effusion or entrapment of the lung by tumour. It is important to differentiate from parapneumonic effusion or infected empyema. Pain at this stage is pleuritic, making such differentiation difficult. Pulmonary embolism is often suspected. More persistent neuralgia-type pain is usually a sign of chest wall invasion and in an asbestos worker is almost pathognomonic of mesothelioma.

Vague symptoms of lethargy, malaise, and weight loss are common. Pyrexia and night sweats may be due to infection in an atelectatic lung, secondary empyema after pleural instrumentation, or due to a direct effect of the tumour itself.

Examination

Decreased chest wall movement is a feature as the thickened pleura crowds the ribs. Dullness to percussion may be due to the thick pleura or the associated effusion. Breath sounds would be decreased on the affected side. Differentiation from a simple effusion may be difficult. The development of tumour nodules at the biopsy or surgical sites is strongly suggestive of mesothelioma.

Diagnosis

A strong index of suspicion in those who have been exposed to asbestos will expedite the diagnosis. Chest x-ray may show non-specific volume loss in the affected hemithorax with pleural effusion and pleural thickening. CT scan, however, will often give more distinct clues, such as nodularity of the pleura and mediastinal pleural thickening, which are uncommon in benign pleural conditions. Associated calcified pleural plaques will confirm the asbestos exposure. Pleural fluid may show overt signs of malignancy with blood staining. High viscosity, low pH (7.0), low glucose (< 40 mg/dl), low WBC (< 5000 cells/μl) and raised LDH (> 1000 IU/dl) are all suggestive of pleural malignancy. The presence of abnormal mesothelial cells is not diagnostic as such cells are shed in many pathological pleural processes.

Cytology may show malignant mesothelioma cells but frequently reactive mesothelial cells are reported. Percutaneous biopsy using an Abrams' needle is frequently successful but false-negative biopsies are common. Thoracoscopy not only allows directed biopsies but also enables drainage of fluid, breakdown of adhesions and loculations, and chemical pleurodesis with talc or other agents. Unfortunately, even a negative thoracoscopy does not rule out the diagnosis.

Staging

Therapeutic interventions are usually decided on the patient's performance status more than the pathology disease stage. Staging does, however, give useful information as to expected median survival. There is currently no accepted staging system for malignant pleural mesothelioma, with at least six attempts in the last 20 years. The International Mesothelioma Interest Group has suggested the system in Table 18.14 based on a TNM classification. This system has yet to be tested clinically. It is heavily surgically orientated with lung parenchymal invasion and chest wall invasion usually only being apparent after surgical resection. Mediastinoscopy rarely changes the therapeutic approach, but there is a case to be made for it before any attempt at surgical resection.

CT scan will show the extent of local intrathoracic and mediastinal disease as well as showing the extent of any peritoneal disease. MRI has as yet not shown much advantage over CT, except that chest wall invasion may be more accurately diagnosed.

Treatment

As yet no therapeutic intervention has been shown to change survival in malignant pleural mesothelioma. Therefore, all patients should be considered for clinical trials.

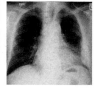

A   B

Fig. 18.2 Pleurectomy with decortication of the lung for pleural mesothelioma, (a) before and (b) after surgery.

Table 18.14 Staging of malignant pleural mesothelioma

Stage I	Disease confined within the capsule of the parietal pleura: ipsilateral pleura, lung, pericardium, and diaphragm
Stage II	All of stage I with positive intrathoracic (N1 or N2) lymph nodes
Stage III	Local extension of disease into the following: chest wall or mediastinum; heart or through the diaphragm, peritoneum; with or without extrathoracic or contralateral (N3) lymph node involvement
Stage IV	Distant metastatic disease

Surgery The effectiveness of radical surgical (extrapleural pneumonectomy or pleuropneumonectomy) intervention is questionable. Mortality approaches 20% and there are only a small number of long-term survivors reported. These data must be compared to a series of lesser interventions and supportive care, many of which have anecdotal evidence of survivors greater than 5 years.

Less radical, but nevertheless extensive surgery, considering the aim is palliation, consists of parietal pleurectomy and decortication of the lung (Fig. 18.2). Good symptomatic relief can be obtained with a mortality of less than 5%.

For those not fit for major surgery a thoracoscopic biopsy and talc pleurodesis is effective in preventing recurrent of effusion.

Radiotherapy Mesothelial cells are at least as radiosensitive as non-small cell lung cancer. However, because of the large volumes that need to be treated, namely all pleural surfaces, diaphragm, mediastinum with a boost to surgical incision sites, it is not possible to deliver tumoricidal doses. More recent techniques involving three-dimensional, conformational planning may allow better radiation delivery in malignant mesothelioma, especially in conjunction with tumour reduction surgery or induction chemotherapy.

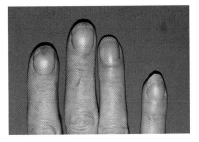

Fig. 18.3   Finger clubbing.

Case history

NSCLC

A 45-year-old asymptomatic lady accompanied her sister to a consultation with her GP. The doctor noticed that her fingers were 'clubbed' (Fig. 18.3) and arranged a chest x-ray. This showed a right upper lobe tumour occupying nearly half the right lung (Fig. 18.4). On bronchoscopy, tumour was seen protruding from the right upper lobe orifice into the right main bronchus (Fig. 18.5); biopsy showed this to be poorly differentiated squamous carcinoma. CT scan showed a bulky tumour with maximum diameter 15 cm, abutting the chest wall laterally and the mediastinum medially, surrounding the hilum on a broad front (Fig. 18.6).

Surgical opinion was that the tumour was inoperable but would be considered if there was significant tumour shrinkage after induction therapy. After two courses of uncomplicated 'MIC' chemotherapy (Mitomycin C 6 mg/m^2, Ifosamide 3 g/m^2 and Cisplatin 50 mg/m^2), there was noticeable tumour shrinkage. After the fourth course (the Mitomycin was witheld from the last course to reduce effects on the lung), there remained a 5 cm necrotic mass well clear of the chest wall and mediastinum.

At surgery there was a 5 cm mass restricted to the upper lobe but thickened tissue around the main bronchus and in the ower paratracheal nodes. Right pneumonectomy was performed with clearance of ipsilateral mediastinal lymph nodes (Fig. 18.7); 24 hours later there was evidence of acute post-pneumonectomy lung injury in the remaining lung. This was successfully treated with diuretics, imipenem, intensive chest physiotherapy and a minitracheostomy (cricothyroidotomy to remove secretions).

Four and a half years later the patient is alive with no evidence of recurrent disease. She lives independently and provides day care for her new grand-daughter. The finger clubbing remains; it may have been congenital.

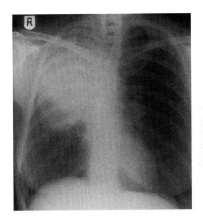

Fig. 18.4   Pre-chemotherapy chest radiograph.

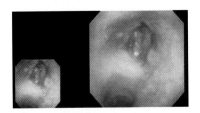

Fig. 18.5 Bronchoscopy. The right upper lobe bronchus is occluded by tumour.

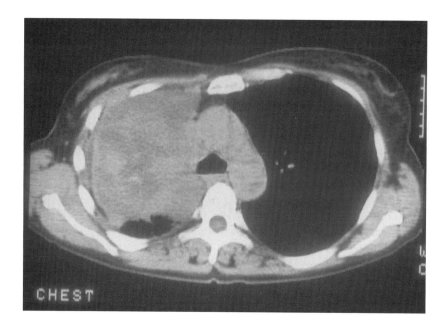

Fig. 18.6 Pre-chemotherapy CT scan.

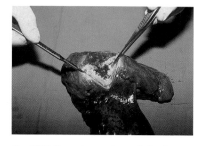

Fig. 18.7 Operative specimen. Following pneumonectomy, a 5 cm necrotic tumour is seen in the right upper lobe.

Chemotherapy Mesothelioma has until recently been regarded as a chemoresistant tumour. However, recent studies have shown that up to 20% of these tumours are sensitive to platinum-based chemotherapy. Like non-small cell lung cancer, the response rates are better when used in conjunction with other drugs. Both MVP and MIC have been used with some success.

Prognosis

The natural history of mesothelioma varies greatly from patient to patient. Mean survival is 18 months from first symptoms and 12 months from diagnosis regardless of therapy. However, all series, be they radical surgery or best supportive care, report 5-year survivors. Such variability in the natural course of the disease makes conclusions difficult when assessing therapeutic options.

Further reading

Books

Rosai, J. (1996) *Ackerman's surgical pathology*, 8th edn. Mosby, Springfield.

De Vita, V. T., Rosenberg, S. A. and Hellman, S. (eds) (1995) *Cancer: principles and practice of oncology*, 5th edn. Lippincott, Philadelphia.

Fischer, D. S., Knobf, M. T., and Durivage, H. J. (1997) *The cancer chemotherapy handbook*. Mosby Handbook. Mosby-Year Book, Springfield.

Perez, C. A. and Brady, L. W. (eds) (1997) *Principles and practice of radiation oncology*, 3rd edn. Lippincott, Philadelphia.

Shields, T. W. (ed.) (1994) *General thoracic surgery*, 4th edn. Williams & Wilkins, Baltimore.

Journals

Annals of Thoracic Surgery

Cancer

Chest Surgery Clinics of North America

European Journal of Thoracic and Cardiovascular Surgery

International Journal of Radiation Oncology, Biology, Physics

Journal of Clinical Oncology

Journal of the National Cancer Institute

Journal of Thoracic and Cardiovascular Surgery

Lung Cancer

Proceedings of the American Society of Clinical Oncology

Websites

http://www.oncolink.upenn.edu/disease/lung1

http://www.oncolink.upenn.edu/pdq_html

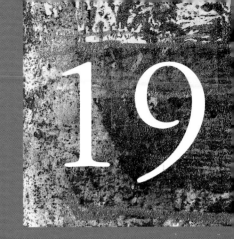

Haematological and lymphoid tumours T. C. M. (Curly) Morris

- Haematological malignancy

- Leukaemia

- Lymphoma

- Myeloma

- Myeloproliferative disorders

- Myelodysplastic syndromes (myelodysplasia; MDS)

Haematological and lymphoid tumours

Haematological malignancy

The malignant haematological conditions considered individually (see Box 19.1) are relatively uncommon conditions. However, acute lymphatic leukaemia is the commonest cancer of childhood, and taken together, the haematological malignancies, because of a relatively high incidence in younger patients, are the most common cause of cancer in the working population. Modern therapeutic techniques, including improved supportive measures, dose intensification, and bone marrow transplant procedures, have produced a significant cure rate in many of these conditions over the past four decades.

Pathogenesis

The malignant cell populations in the haematological malignancies probably result from clonal proliferation by successive divisions from a single transformed stem cell. Some conditions are associated with a specific chromosome abnormality, e.g. the Philadelphia chromosome t(9;22) in chronic myeloid leukaemia, t(15;17) in acute promyelocytic leukaemia, and t(14;18) in follicular lymphoma, whilst in

---

Box 19.1 *Haematological malignancies*

- Leukaemia
- Lymphoma
- Myeloma
- Myelodysplastic syndromes
- Myeloproliferative disorders

Simple definitions
- Leukaemia – cancer of the blood-forming cells of the bone marrow
- Lymphoma – cancer of the various cells of the lymph glands
- Myeloma – cancer of the plasma cells of the bone marrow
- Myelodysplastic syndromes – malformation of the haemopoietic cells frequently progressing to acute leukaemia
- Myeloproliferative disorders – low-grade malignancy of multipotent bone marrow precursor cells

This is an oversimplification, hiding multiple subtypes and variants. In addition, these conditions are in many respects a spectrum so that the differentiation of certain lymphomas and acute lymphatic leukaemia may be extremely difficult whereas other lymphomas may closely resemble myeloma. Many of the relatively benign conditions may undergo change into more aggressive forms of leukaemia.

other conditions numerous chromosomal abnormalities are possible, some of which may infer favourable or poor prognosis. As many malignant haemopoietic cells share the ability of normal haemopoietic stem cells to circulate freely in the bloodstream, the leukaemias, myelodysplastic conditions, and myeloproliferative disorders are always widespread at diagnosis, whereas the lymphomas may be localized to one set of glands or more often be widespread. Ultimately, non-haemopoietic organs will become involved, either from the blood or as a result of direct invasion.

Table 19.1 Aetiology of leukaemia

Proven factors	Examples
Genetic abnormalities	Down's syndrome
	Klinefelter's syndrome
Ionizing radiation (except CLL)	Atomic bombs
	Accidental release from nuclear power plants
	Therapeutic irradiation
	Occupational exposure
	Diagnostic irradiation
Chemicals	Benzene & other industrial chemicals
	Cytotoxic chemotherapy
Viruses	HTLV-1 – adult TLL
	EBV, HIV – mainly lymphomas

Possible factors	Not proven
Non-ionizing radiation	Electricity transformers
	Mobile phones
Agrichemicals	Pesticides & others
Cigarette smoking	Mainly myeloid – small statistical increase
Lack of infection in childhood	Increase incidence in childhood ALL in remote communities
Radon gas	

Table 19.2. A simple classification of the leukaemias

Leukaemia
    Acute
        Myeloid – AML
        Lymphatic – ALL
    Chronic
        Myeloid – CML
        Lymphatic – CLL

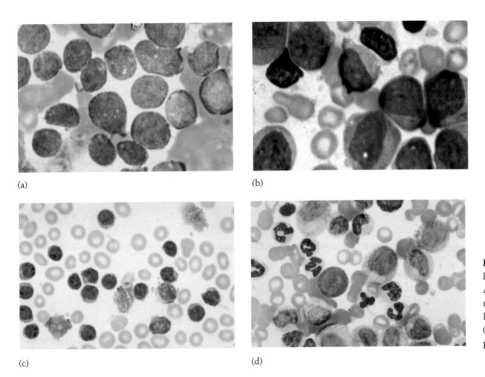

Fig. 19.1 (a) Acute lymphatic leukaemia – bone marrow. (b) Acute myeloid leukaemia – bone marrow. (c) Chronic lymphatic leukaemia – peripheral blood. (d) Chronic myeloid leukaemia – peripheral blood.

Leukaemia

Aetiology

The majority of cases of leukaemia have no recognizable aetiological factors; opportunities for prevention are therefore limited. Table 19.1 summarizes the current state of knowledge on known and suspected aetiological factors. Continued vigilance is required with regard to exposure to high-level irradiation from whatever source and the risks of therapeutic or diagnostic exposure should be carefully weighed against the benefits and risks at all times.

Pathology

Leukaemias may be subdivided into acute and chronic, myeloid and lymphatic as shown in Table 19.2. Morphological examples are shown in Fig. 19.1. The acute leukaemias are characterized by the accumulation of blast (primitive) cells in the bone marrow. These cells are usually also present in the peripheral blood, sometimes in high number. Blast cells are characterized by high nuclear to cytoplasmic ratio and the relative similarity of cells. Normal precursors are generally greatly reduced. By contrast, in chronic myeloid leukaemia there is an excessive production of cells of the myeloid line from blast cells through to mature granulocytes although an increase in the relative proportion of primitive precursors is common. In addition, the white cell count is invariably raised with all stages of myeloid maturation also present in the peripheral blood. Chronic lymphatic leukaemia presents a relatively monotonous picture with mature lymphocytes in excessive numbers in both peripheral blood and bone marrow. The diagnosis of each of these conditions requires confirmation by cytochemical, immunocytochemical, cyto-genetic, and occasionally molecular techniques. Some cases with specific features (such as Auer rods in acute myeloid leukaemia) make the diagnosis firm at an early stage.

Presentation

Patients with leukaemia are likely to present with one of three groups of symptoms; anaemia, infection, and bleeding, or any combination of these. Common features of these are shown in Table 19.3. However, as leukaemia is by its nature widespread at the time of diagnosis, almost any organ may from time to time be involved. Table 19.4 summarizes some of the more common ways which specific organs may be affected. Attention should also be paid to the metabolic problems associated with leukaemia. These problems require urgent and intensive management and close co-operation between haematologists, nephrologists, intensive care, etc.

Examination

A thorough clinical examination may help to reveal the features of anaemia, infection, or bleeding. If purpura is not widespread it may sometimes be found over the abdomen or the shoulders, on the hard or soft palate or the retina. Patients with acute myeloid leukaemia rarely have lymphadenopathy but enlarged lymph glands may be present in up to 50% of cases with acute lymphatic leukaemia and be even

Table 19.3 **Results of bone marrow failure in acute leukaemia**

Anaemia	Failure of production
	Bleeding
	Excessive breakdown (DIC, haemolysis)
Infection	Septicaemia
	Respiratory
	Skin
	UTI
Bleeding	Thrombocytopenia
	purpura
	bruising (spontaneous)
	epistaxis
	menorrhagia
	gum bleeding
	DIC
	acute promyelocytic leukaemia (M_3)
	infection

DIC, disseminated intravascular coagulation; UTI, urinary tract infection.

Table 19.4 Effect of leukaemia on other organs

GI tract	Mouth	Candida infection (thrush)
		Petechiae
		Ulceration
		Infiltration
	Gums	Bleeding
		Hypertrophy (esp. M_5)
	Oesophagus	Candida
Skin	Infiltration	(esp. M_4 & M_5)
	Infection	Bacterial, e.g. staphylococcal
		Viral, e.g. herpes zoster
CNS	Meningeal leukaemia	Headache
		Vomiting
		Lassitude
		Photophobia
		Cranial nerve palsies
Lymph glands	Gland enlargement	Mediastinal enlargement (esp. T-cell ALL)
Metabolic problems	Tumour lysis syndrome	Hyperuricaemia
		Renal failure
		Hyperkalaemia
	Electrolytes	Hyponatraemia
		Hypokalaemia
		Hypercalcaemia
Leucostasis	Myeloid leukaemias	Very high white cell count affects lungs & brain
Skeletal system	Bone pain	Infiltration
		Infarction

more common in patients with chronic lymphatic leukaemia. The spleen is not commonly enlarged in acute leukaemia, whereas patients with chronic myeloid leukaemia may present with massive enlargement of the spleen, which is also a feature of more advanced cases of chronic lymphatic leukaemia. In individual patients the systematic manifestations outlined in Table 19.4 may contribute to diagnosis and/or management.

Diagnosis

In cases where leukaemia is suspected, a peripheral blood count with a blood film should be performed. Although there is frequently anaemia and thrombocytopenia, the white cell count may be normal, low, or raised. However, examination of the peripheral blood film will usually demonstrate the presence of some abnormal cells. Confirmation of the diagnosis is made by examining a bone marrow smear and performing appropriate cytochemical, immunocytochemical, and cytogenetic examinations. Bone marrow samples are usually taken from the posterior illac crest, anaesthetizing the patient using local anaesthetic (short-acting benzo-diazepine may also be used). It is usual to take a core of bone (trephine biopsy) in addition to aspirating marrow. The trephine biopsy is particularly useful in those cases where there is a dry tap (no marrow can be sucked out) or a blood tap (what is sucked out is the same as blood). Touch preparations made from the core of bone on to individual slides may help to make a diagnosis rapidly. Very haemorrhagic patients may require platelet transfusion to prevent excessive bruising and bleeding from the procedure.

As leukaemia is normally widespread at the time of diagnosis, staging is usually inappropriate (chronic lymphatic leukaemia is an exception).

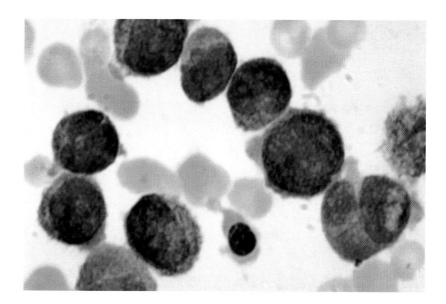

Fig. 19.2 Acute promyelocytic leukaemia, bone marrow aspirate, showing hypergranulation and frequent Auer rods.

Table 19.5 Acute myeloid leukaemia subtypes

M_0	Undifferentiated
M_1	Minimal myeloid differentiation
M_2	Clear-cut myeloid differentiation
M_3	Promyelocytic [t(15;17)]
M_4	Myelomonocytic
M_5	Monocytic
	(a) blastic
	(b) differentiated
M_6	Erythroid
M7	Megakaryocytic

The French-American-British (FAB) classification of acute myeloid leukaemia.

Acute myeloid leukaemia

Morphological, cytochemical, and immunocytochemical examination of the blood and marrow from patients with acute myeloid leukaemia allows categorization into one of eight subgroups, depending on the presence to a greater or lesser degree of myeloid, monocytic, erythroid, or megakaryocytic features (Table 19.5). Of particular importance is the M_3 (promyelocytic/progranulocytic) variant. Patients with this condition comprise one of the most acute medical emergencies as the granules in the promyelocytes (see Fig. 19.2) release thromboplastin, causing disseminated intravascular coagulation which can lead to life-threatening haemorrhage. Progranulocytic leukaemia and its hypogranular variant are both associated with a specific chromosomal translocation t; 15:17, occasionally t; 11:17 involving the retinoic acid receptor on chromosome 17 which appears to have a role in differentiation of myeloid cells, explaining the arrest at the promyelocytic stage. Other chromosomal abnormalities are also of significance; the t(8;21) and inversion 16 abnormalities are associated with a favourable prognosis whereas translocations involving chromosomes 5 and 7 are associated with a poor prognosis. Also of significance is the presence of dysplastic features involving red cell, white cell, and platelet precursor cells, which may be found more commonly in older patients and implies a progression from myelodysplasia.

Treatment

The most effective treatment for acute myeloid leukaemia consists of a combination of an anthracycline, e.g. daunorubicin, together with cytarabine. Additional or alternative drugs may be used both in remission induction and consolidation treatment. Given that the blood count is frequently abnormal with neutropenia and thrombocytopenia at the start of antileukaemic treatment, the 2–3 weeks after completing the first treatment is often a stormy time with infection, particularly septicaemia, requiring broad-spectrum intravenous antibiotics, and bleeding requiring the transfusion of red cells, platelets, and plasma products. Depending on age, 50–80% of patients will achieve a remission with younger patients faring better. With a total of four or five courses of intensive chemotherapy, about 20% of patients in the under 65 age group will be apparently cured with younger patients again faring better. However, for young patients with unfavourable characteristics at diagnosis (this includes high white cell count at diagnosis and adverse chromosomal abnormalities), bone marrow transplantation from an HLA-matched sibling is the treatment of choice, giving cure rates as high as 50%, although there is a significant procedure-related mortality due to acute graft-versus-host disease. Similar regimens may be tried in older patients but concomitant disease and frailty, together with more common adverse chromosomal abnormalities, means treatment is much less frequently successful. In the very old patient there is an argument in favour of supportive treatment, particularly when the white cell count is not excessively high, as median survival is in the order of 6–8 weeks.

Prognosis

The advent of modern chemotherapeutic techniques and supportive therapies has improved the average prognosis for patients with acute myeloid leukaemia from

6 weeks to 15 months with a significant proportion of patients having long-term remissions, i.e. cures. These figures are based on patients with an age of over 1 year and decline with age.

Quality of life

Successful treatment of acute leukaemia is a highly specialized task as patients may be extremely susceptible to infection, bleeding, and many other complications. Prompt and vigorous management of complications should be undertaken in specialist units. Part of the improved prognosis in these patients is due not only to the chemotherapy but better support and management with broad-spectrum antibiotics, antifungals and antivirals, blood-product support, and intensive care standard management. In the initial stages with prolonged periods of hospitalization, chemotherapy-induced nausea and vomiting (which can now be relatively well controlled with HT_3 antagonists), neutropenia, thrombocytopenia, and hair loss, the patient may be severely tested. However, the advent of remission signals a possible return to the premorbid state of health, and following the completion of treatment hair will re-grow and normal life may be resumed. In younger patients, particularly women, fertility may be retained.

Acute lymphatic (lymphoblastic) leukaemia

Acute lymphatic leukaemia (ALL) is the common form of leukaemia in children and has an age peak under 5 years of age. It is subdivided into types L1, commonly found in children; L2, which is the usual form in adults; and L3, in which the cytoplasm is intensely basophilic and the cells are similar to those in patients with Burkitt's lymphoma. Immunophenotyping has shown that ALL may be of either B- or T-cell precursor types. 'Common' ALL, which accounts for the majority of cases, shows an early pre-B phenotype (positive for CD10 and terminal deoxynucleotidal transerrase (tdT) but negative for cytoplasmic and cell surface immunoglobulin) – see Table 19.6. Central nervous system (CNS) leukaemia is common in patients with ALL and cerebrospinal fluid should be examined at an early stage to exclude this possibility.

Table 19.6 Classification of ALL

Category	FAB morphology	Immunology
B-cell types		
Early B-precursor ALL	L1, L2	TdT+ CD19+ CD10–
Common ALL	L1, L2	TdT+ CD19+ CD10+
Pre-B ALL	L1	TdT+ CD19+ Cy Ig
B-cell ALL	L3	TdT– CD19+ 5 m Ig+
T-cell types		
Early T-precursor ALL	L1, L2	TdT+ CD2– CD7+
T-cell ALL	L1, L2	TdT+ CD2+ CD7+

Table 19.7. Favourable prognostic features in ALL

- Young (but not < 2 years)
- Female
- Caucasian race
- Low WBC at diagnosis ($< 20 \times 10^9$/l)
- 'Common' type
- No CNS disease at presentation
- < 4 weeks to remission

Treatment

Although the combination of prednisone and vincristine can induce remissions in up to 90% of patients with ALL, a series of studies have shown that the long-term survival is improved with the addition of more drugs, such as daunorubicin and asparaginase, in the induction period. Remission induction is therefore nearly as hazardous as in acute myeloid leukaemia, although the remission rate, particularly in children, is higher. Because of the frequency of the development of meningeal leukaemia (up to 75% of cases not given prophylaxis), 'prophylactic' treatment is started after the first consolidation therapy and normally consists of cranial irradiation and intrathecal methotrexate. Patients normally receive up to 6 months of intensive therapy (including the cranial prophylaxis) before progressing to maintenance therapy. This usually consists of continuous mercaptopurine, weekly methotrexate (both oral) and monthly IV injections of vincristine with short courses of prednisolone. This type of therapy has been shown to improve remission duration and to reduce relapse rates. This form of therapy is capable of giving 'cure' rates of 75–80% in children under the age of 16. Unfortunately, the cure rate drop rapidly with age and only a small proportion of older patients will be cured by conventional chemotherapy. In the older age group, consideration must therefore be given to bone marrow transplantation, whereas in children, apart from those with adverse prognostic features, transplantation is normally only used after relapse occurs and a second remission has been induced.

Prognosis

Factors predicting more favourable outcomes are shown in Table 19.7. In good prognosis patients, long-term survival rates are in excess of 80% with rates falling as adverse factors are accumulated. In general, patients achieving long-term remission will lead normal lives; the majority of patients treated as children will retain reproduction function. CNS irradiation has been shown to affect some aspects of intelligence, particularly in the very young, and for this reason it is normally delayed until the patient is aged at least 2 years. Some trials have tried to eliminate the use of CNS irradiation by substituting intrathecal and systemic high-dose methotrexate. Isolated relapses in sanctuary sites, e.g. testes, may be treated by local radiotherapy followed by further induction and maintenance therapy.

Quality of life

The majority of children cope well with the side-effects and complications of treatment during the induction, consolidation, and maintenance phases. They will be relatively susceptible to infection and appropriate measures must be taken if they encounter viral infections such as chickenpox. However, after the cessation of therapy, normal life can be resumed. The duration of hospitalization in the initial stages of treatment generally means that most children may drop back by 1 year at school. In older patients quality of life is largely determined by remission duration.

Chronic myeloid leukaemia

Chronic myeloid leukaemia (CML) is invariably characterized by a raised white cell count and the presence in the peripheral blood of all stages of immature cells, from blast cells to mature granulocytes (see Fig. 19.1). There is normally splenic enlargement – this may often be the presenting feature. The platelet count is frequently normal but may be elevated and the patient is usually anaemic. The condition can normally be differentiated from a 'leukaemoid' reaction by the leucocyte alkaline phosphatase stain. This is strongly positive in leukaemoid reactions and negative or low in CML. In addition, the vast majority of cases of CML possess the Philadelphia chromosome t(9;22). This translocation was the first to be associated with a specific malignant disease. The resulting hybrid gene, *bcr/abl*, its messenger RNA, and resulting protein have been extensively studied. Rare cases of Philadelphia-negative CML and chronic neutrophilic leukaemia should be differentiated from CML.

CML may also first present in its transformed state (blastic transformation). Blast cells, which may be either myeloid or lymphatic, are those which dominate. The Philadelphia chromosome is, however, retained but additional chromosomal changes are frequent.

Treatment

Although CML will respond to a wide variety of cytotoxic agents, it remains an essentially incurable disease unless exceptional measures are instituted. Essentially, patients up to the age of 50–55 years should be treated, following remission induction with hydroxyurea, by allogenic transplantation from a sibling donor whenever such a donor is available. If no sibling donor is available, then bone marrow registers should be searched for an unrelated matched donor in patients up to the age of 30. Where a match cannot be found or in patients above these age limits, interferon α (IFN-α) should be given an adequate trial. A considerable proportion of patients will respond to this agent and a small proportion will become Philadelphia-chromosome negative. Survival in this latter group of patients is exceptionally good. Alternative approaches involve the harvesting of Philadelphia-negative stem cells, which may sometimes be induced after early intensive chemotherapy. For oral therapy, hydroxyurea is the drug of choice, having fewer long-term side-effects than busulphan, an otherwise equally effective drug. The *all* tyrosine tunase inhibitor ST1 S71 (*glivec*) is also proving to be an effective form of therapy.

Prognosis

Any form of treatment which reduces the leucocyte count and the size of the spleen will produce clinical benefit. However, at random time intervals patients may develop 'accelerated disease', when the patient becomes relatively resistant to treatment with conventional agents, or 'blastic transformation', where there is a progression to an acute leukaemia (usually myeloid) with further chromosomal changes. Except for relatively rare transformations to acute lymphatic leukaemia, the response to intensive chemotherapy is poor. Median survival for chronic-phase patients not being transplanted is in the order of 4 years.

Quality of life

Simple drug treatment significantly improves quality of life but with little benefit to overall survival. On the other hand, those measures which may offer improved survival and indeed 'cure' are high-risk procedures with significant sequelae such as chronic graft-versus-host disease. Patients receiving long-term interferon may also tend to have ongoing side-effects of varying types, with fatigue and nausea particularly common.

Chronic lymphatic leukaemia

Chronic lymphatic leukaemia (CLL) is a relatively indolent disease mainly of the elderly; some patients may never require treatment. However, modern immunophenotypic methods have revealed the relatively monotonous lymphocytes (see Fig. 19.1) hide a wide range of disorders (Table 19.8), many of which are associated with an adverse prognosis compared to 'classical' CLL. Thus T-cell variants, prolymphocytic variants, and other abnormalities which indicate the lymphocytes are an 'overflow' of a lymphomatous process (blood spill), tend to indicate an adverse prognosis.

Table 19.8 Variants of CLL

Variant	Features
'Classic'	Often stage A / asymptomatic
	May not require therapy
'Aggressive'	Seen in younger patients
	Symptomatic & progressive disease
Prolymphocytic	High count, splenic enlargement, increased prolymphocytes
T-cell variants (T-CLL, T PLL)	Tend to have high counts, poor prognosis, may respond well to purine analogues
Large granular lymphocyte leukaemia	Associated with neutropenia. Predominant cells are large granular lymphocytes
Hairy cell leukaemia	Splenic enlargement, pancytopenia, good response with nucleotides Variant form with ↑ WBC
Lymphomas with blood spill	Features depend on underlying lymphoma variant

Table 19.9 Usual haematological findings in the leukaemias

	Acute	Chronic myeloid	Chronic lymphatic
Haemoglobin	↓ or N	Usually ↓	N or ↓
Leucocytes	↓ N or ↑	↑	↑ occ. N
Platelets	↓ or N	N or ↑	N or ↓
Blast cells	0–100%	2–10%	0%
Neutrophils	↓ or N	↑	N or ↓
Neutrophil alkaline phosphatase	N or ↑	↓	N or ↑
Lymphocytes	N or ↓	N or ↓	↑ (> 5 × 10^9/l)
Smear cells	Rare	Rare	Common
Basophils	↓	N or ↑	↓
Chromosomes	Various inc Ph$_1$	Ph$_1$ in > 95%	Not usually performed
Bone marrow	Blast cells > 30%	All stages myeloid maturation, blast cells usually < 10%	Variable lymphocytosis, blast cells < 5%

Table 19.10 Staging system for CLL

Stage	Gland/organ enlargement	Haemoglobin (g/dl)	Platelets (× 10^9/l)
A	0, 1, or 2 areas	≥10	≥ 100
B	3, 4, or 5	≥ 10	≥ 100
C	Not considered	< 10 and/or	< 100

Table 19.9 compares the laboratory findings of cases of acute leukaemia, chronic myeloid leukaemia, and chronic lymphatic leukaemia.

Staging

An international working party classification of CLL is shown in Table 19.10. Secondary causes of anaemia (e.g. iron deficiency), or autoimmune haemolytic anaemia, or thrombocytopenia must be treated before staging. For organ enlargement one area equals lymph nodes > 1 cm in the neck, axilla, groin, or spleen, or liver enlargement.

Treatment

Asymptomatic stage A patients do not require treatment. Patients with stage B or C may need treatment, particularly if there is evidence of bone marrow failure, symptomatic involvement of lymph nodes or skin, splenomegaly or hypersplenism. Symptoms and signs of immune haemolytic anaemia and/or thrombocytopenia are common in CLL and are a further indication for treatment.

Patients with bone marrow failure, autoimmune haemolytic anaemia, or thrombocytopenia should receive corticosteriods. For other patients, alkylating agents such as chlorambucil are the usual initial therapy and may be combined with corticosteroids. Patients becoming resistant to these agents may be treated with combination chemotherapy, e.g. CHOP (see section on non-Hodgkin's lymphoma) or newer reagents such as fludarabine, alone or in combination. Radiotherapy is useful for treatment of areas of bulky disease, including lymph nodes and/or spleen. Patients with CLL have impaired immune systems and will require active antibiotic treatment for infections and possibly prophylaxis with antibacterial, antifungal or antiviral drugs.

Prognosis

'Classic' CLL presenting in the elderly, especially when it is found from a routine blood count rather than as the result of symptoms, may not require immediate therapy or indeed any therapy. Patients may continue to lead a relatively normal life and some may never require treatment; for others, treatment may ultimately become necessary. In younger patients and those with more advanced disease, i.e. stage C, treatment will be required and median survivals are significantly reduced. If remissions can be induced, prognosis is significantly improved. However, except for some patients who have successful bone marrow transplants, long-term cures are rare.

Quality of life

For patients with indolent disease presenting in the elderly, quality of life may be little affected. However, when more aggressive forms are present and more intensive therapy required, this will affect quality of life along with survival.

Lymphoma

The lymphomas are the malignant manifestations of the cells of the lymph glands. Their wide diversity reflects the complexity of these organs. They are normally considered in two major groups – Hodgkin's disease and the non-Hodgkin's lymphomas – and together account for approximately 4% of all cancers. They are significant in that they occur with a higher frequency in young adults than many other malignancies and that they are treatable and in some instances curable.

Hodgkin's disease

Hodgkin's disease is a group of related disorders sharing some common pathological features and clinical behaviour. The disease is named after Thomas Hodgkin who described the first cases at Guy's Hospital in 1832. Subsequent review of the pathological material still available more than 150 years later confirms some of the cases he described are what we know today as Hodgkin's disease.

Epidemiology

Hodgkin's disease has a bimodal age distribution with the first peak occurring in young adults between the ages of 15 and 34 and the second peak in older patients. As with most haematological disorders, there is a slight male preponderance of cases.

Aetiology

A number of factors point to a possible viral aetiology in at least some cases of Hodgkin's disease. Epstein–Barr (EB) virus has been demonstrated in a significant proportion of Hodgkin's disease lymph nodes and studies have shown that Reed–Sternberg cells (the presumed tumour cell in Hodgkin's disease) can be infected with EB virus. In some studies, a seasonal incidence has been shown. As with other haematological malignancies, no preventative measures or screening techniques have been developed.

Presentation

Patients may present with isolated or multiple swellings of the lymph glands or symptoms arising from enlargement of the lymph nodes. For example, enlargement of the glands of the mediastinum may cause obstruction to the return of blood from the head and upper limbs, superior vena cava syndrome. Other manifestations include generalized symptoms such as weakness, lassitude, loss of appetite, weight loss, abnormal sweating (particularly at night) which may be severe, itch, and very occasionally pain on swallowing alcoholic beverages.

Examination

Where Hodgkin's disease is suspected, physical examination should include palpation of neck, axilla, and groins. In addition, occipital and epitrochlear glands may occasionally be present. Mediastinal widening may be suspected on chest examination and abdominal palpation may reveal central abdominal masses or enlargement of spleen and/or liver. Involvement of other organs at diagnosis is rare but may occur with disease progression.

Diagnosis

Gland biopsy is necessary for diagnosis; fine needle aspirates are rarely diagnostic and needle biopsy is usually inadequate for the full diagnosis. Occasionally laparotomy or thoracotomy may be necessary to obtain a gland for diagnostic morphology.

Pathology

One of the most remarkable features of Hodgkin's disease is that the malignant cells constitute only a minority of abnormal cells in the gland. Indeed, sometimes it may be difficult to find the binucleate mirror image Reed–Sternberg cells without which it is difficult to make a firm diagnosis. The affected glands contain a variety of cells including lymphocytes, plasma cells, mononuclear cells, and eosinophils. In some instances, bands of fibrous tissue are seen (nodular sclerosing variant). The identity and nature of the malignant cell has been the subject of debate for many years. Current opinion favours the concept that the malignant cells are the Reed–Sternberg cells which may represent transformed B lymphocytes. The pathological classification of Hodgkin's disease is shown in Table 19.11 along with its relationship to prognosis and response to therapy.

Table 19.11 Relationship of pathological classification in Hodgkin's disease to prognosis

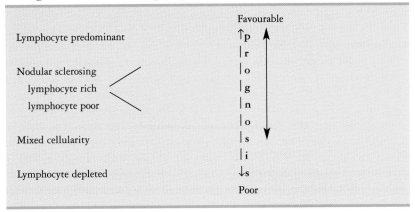

	Favourable
Lymphocyte predominant	↑p
	│r
Nodular sclerosing	│o
lymphocyte rich	│g
lymphocyte poor	│n
	│o
Mixed cellularity	│s
	│i
Lymphocyte depleted	↓s
	Poor

Staging

Clinical staging is of importance with regard to both prognosis and choice of treatment. The Ann Arbor scheme devised in the 1960s and shown in Table 19.12 is universally accepted. Staging requires not only careful clinical examination but chest x-ray, CT scan of chest, abdomen, and pelvis, and preferably one more imaging technique for abdominal glands such as ultrasound or gallium scanning. Staging laparotomy is no longer necessary. The presence or absence of constitutional symptoms (B symptoms) has been demonstrated in clinical trials to be of greatest significance. These symptoms are present if there has been weight loss equal or greater than 10% of total body weight in the past 6 months or if there are significant night sweats – usually sufficient to require the patient to change night

Table 19.12 Ann Arbor staging system (simplified)

Stage	
I	Involvement of single lymph node region or lymphoid structure (e.g. spleen, Waldeyer's ring)
II	Involvement of 2 or more lymph node regions or structures on same side of the diaphragm
III	Involvement of lymph node structures or regions on both sides of the diaphragm
IV	Involvement of extra nodal site(s), e.g. liver, bone marrow
A	No symptoms
B	Fever, drenching sweats, weight loss
E	Involvement of a single extranodal site from known nodal site

clothes/sheets. Itch is no longer considered sufficiently reliable to rank as a B symptom.

Treatment

Stages IA and IIA are suitable for treatment with local (involved field) or extended field radiotherapy. If patients are staged correctly, this will be curative in approximately 90% of cases. Patients relapsing after radiotherapy may be salvaged by chemotherapy and patients with more advanced disease, i.e. stages III and IV and all patients with B symptoms, should receive chemotherapy. The four-drug regimen devised by Vincent de Vita in the late 1950s, known as MOPP and consisting of mustine, Oncovin (vincristine), procarbazine, and prednisone given in short courses followed by time for marrow recovery, represented one of the great strides forward in the treatment of malignant disease, with more than 50% of patients with advanced disease being cured of their illness. MOPP and its variants such as LOPP [Leukeran (chlorambucil)] remained the gold standard treatment for more than two decades with augmentation of treatment by using radiotherapy to the area of bulk disease. However, current trials are evaluating the new gold standard four-drug regimen, ABVD (Adriamycin, bleomycin, vinblastine and dacarbazine), against alternating four-drug regimens and hybrid seven- or eight-drug regimens. Five-year survivals are expected to be in the order of 80% or better and the majority of patients will have long-term cures. Patients relapsing after conventional chemotherapy may achieve second remissions with the same drugs, but remission duration is usually shorter than the previous remission. However, high-dose therapy with autologous peripheral blood or bone marrow transplantation has been found to give high remission rates in relapsed patients and long-term disease-free survival in the order of 50%.

Prognosis

Subtle alterations in immune function may remain in patients with Hodgkin's disease for many years and patients should be warned to be on guard for serious and opportunist pathogens. Although late relapses following therapy may occur, the majority of patients who are disease free 5 years following the cessation of treatment are cured. Long-term sequelae include increased risk of malignant disease, including therapy-related acute myeloid leukaemia, lung and other solid malignancies. These may be treated in the normal way, although the majority of therapy-related acute leukaemias are relatively resistant to conventional chemotherapy. Patients with hyposplenism or who have had the spleen removed for staging laparotomy (a procedure no longer necessary for evaluation with modern imaging techniques and the knowledge that all patients with B symptoms require chemotherapy) are at risk from septicaemia, particularly with encapsulated organisms such as *Pneumococcus*, *Meningococcus*, and *Haemophilus* species.

Quality of life

Most of the above chemotherapies can be given on a day-patient/out-patient basis. Side-effects with modern anti-emetics are tolerable and leucopenia is only rarely of sufficient severity to require in-patient treatment for sepsis, etc. If patients are young enough, gonadal function may be retained and for many patients there are few long-term sequelae.

Table 19.13 **The REAL classification of non-Hodgkin's lymphoma***

B-cell neoplasms

Precursor B-cell neoplasms

    Precursor B-lymphoblastic leukaemia/lymphoma

    Peripheral B-cell neoplasms

    B-cell chronic lymphocytic leukaemia/prolymphocytic leukaemia/small lymphocytic lymphoma

    Immunocytoma/lymphoplasmacytic lymphoma

    Mantle cell lymphoma

    Follicle centre lymphoma

    Marginal zone B-cell lymphoma

    Hairy cell leukaemia

    Plasmacytoma/plasma cell myeloma

    Diffuse large B-cell lymphoma

    Burkitt's lymphoma

T-cell and natural killer cell neoplasms

Precursor T-cell neoplasm

    Precursor T-lymphoblastic leukaemia/lymphoma

Peripheral T-cell and NK cell neoplasms

    T-cell chronic lymphocytic leukaemia/prolymphocytic leukaemia

    Large granular lymphocyte leukaemia (LGL)

    Mycosis fungoides/Sézary syndrome

    Peripheral T-cell lymphomas, unspecified

    Angioimmunoblastic T-cell lymphoma (AILD)

    Angiocentric lymphoma

    Intestinal T-cell lymphoma

    Adult T-cell lymphoma/leukaemia (ATL/L)

    Anaplastic large cell lymphoma (ALCL)

---

*Revised European-American classification of lymphoid neoplasms.

Non-Hodgkin's lymphoma

The histopathological classification of non-Hodgkin's lymphoma (NHL) has been an area of great confusion, with numerous schemes containing overlapping nomenclature, often complicated by the fact that the histopathological nomenclature often failed to give helpful information to the clinician. With regard to the correct management strategy, the REAL scheme for classifying NHL has gained wider acceptance. This scheme makes use not only of morphological appearance but also immunocytochemical, cytogenetic, and molecular data to help identify meaningful subgroups which are of some prognostic significance. A simplified version of the REAL scheme for NHL is shown in Table 19.13. Ten B-cell and ten T-cell neoplasms are shown; provisional and rare diagnoses have been excluded for simplicity. (Note, the B-cell neoplasms include chronic lymphocytic leukaemia and myeloma which are considered in greater detail elsewhere.)

It is not necessary to consider each of these lymphomas individually, but rather in groups, depending on whether they are highly proliferative and rapidly fatal diseases or much more low-grade and chronic. Lymphomas may therefore be considered as low, intermediate or high grade. Low-grade lymphomas run a chronic course, they frequently respond to simple chemotherapy, and may have remissions lasting from a month to many years, but for the most part will eventually relapse with progressive disease. As a general rule, it has been found to be impossible to achieve a significant cure rate even when the most intensive of chemotherapies is used. By contrast, intermediate- and high-grade lymphomas have a more aggressive course with some of the high-grade lymphomas being potentially rapidly fatal. However, a significant proportion will respond to multidrug chemotherapy and enduring remissions are possible for a proportion of patients.

Aetiology

Although non-Hodgkin's lymphoma is one of the tumours with the fastest rate of increase in the 1990s, its aetiology remains unknown. Some predisposing conditions and their associated types of lymphoma are shown in Table 19.14.

Pathogenesis

Enlargement of the lymph glands is a predominant feature of NHL. The disease is presumed to arise in one site, although it is frequently widely disseminated by the time diagnosis is made. The superficial glands are often involved but this is not invariable since involvement of the mediastinum/abdomen or pelvis without superficial lymphadenopathy is not uncommon and may provide a diagnostic challenge. Bone marrow involvement may lead to anaemia, neutropenia, with infections or thrombocytopenia. The gastrointestinal tract is the most commonly

Table 19.14 Predisposing disease in non-Hodgkin's lymphoma

Immune dysfunction	
AIDS	Usually B-cell high or intermediate grade
Inherited	
Therapeutic immunosuppression, e.g. chemotherapy, radiotherapy	
Coeliac disease	Usually T-cell lymphomas
Dermatitis herpetiformis	
Angoimmunoblastic lymphadenopathy	
Intestinal infections	Marginal zone B-cell lymphoma
Autoimmune diseases, e.g. RA, SLE	

involved extranodal site after the bone marrow and may be particularly involved in some types of T-cell lymphomas and marginal zone lymphoma of B-cell origin. Other organs such as skin, brain, testes, or thyroid may be involved and CNS lymphoma is relatively frequent in AIDS patients.

Clinical findings

Presentation will depend on the glands and other organs involved. Constitutional symptoms such as fever, night sweats, and weight loss occur less frequently than in Hodgkin's disease and usually indicate a disseminated disease. Peripheral blood spill (see Table 19.8) may sometimes be seen. Lymph node biopsy is usually required for diagnosis; fine needle aspiration and True-cut biopsies are indicative but unreliable techniques. Misdiagnosis may lead to the introduction of inappropriate therapy.

Staging

The Ann Arbor staging scheme (see Table 19.12) is generally applicable to NHL, although NHL is more frequently widely disseminated at diagnosis than Hodgkin's disease. Bone marrow aspirate and trephine biopsies are required for the exclusion of marrow disease; two methods for radiological examination of the abdomen should be used to show the presence or absence of intra-abdominal involvement.

Treatment

Treatment varies significantly with the type of lymphoma diagnosed (Table 19.15), hence the important of accurate diagnosis. In general, isolated disease may be treated with radiotherapy, although microscopic spread may result in disease relapse elsewhere. Low-grade lymphomas are treated with simple out-patient therapies which do not cause too great a fall of the peripheral white cell and platelet counts. For intermediate and high grade lymphomas, the CHOP regimen (Table 19.15) remains the gold standard treatment. The second and third generation regimens incorporating

Table 19.15 Chemotherapy in non-Hodgkin's lymphoma

Low grade	Chlorambucil ± prednisolone
	COP
	Fludarabine
	High grade therapy
Intermediate & high grade	CHOP
	Salvage regimens
	High dose therapy with PBSC rescue
Precursor B/T lymphoblastic lymphoma	ALL-type regimens
Hairy cell leukaemia	Interferon, purine analogues e.g. pentostatin, cladribine
Mycosis fungoides/Sézary syndrome	Chemotherapy e.g. CHOP
	Photopheresis, electron beam therapy

C, cyclophosphamide; H, Adriamycin (hydroxydaunorubicin); O, vincristine (Oncovin); P, prednisone.

extra drugs such as bleomycin and intermediate or high dose methotrexate have failed to improve on the remission and long-term survival rates of properly administered CHOP. In patients who fail or relapse after first-line chemotherapy, salvage regimens, which include drugs such as cisplatin, ifosfamide, and etoposide, are available. The role of high dose therapy with bone marrow or peripheral blood stem cell rescue (which has been shown to produce a significant cure rate in chemosensitive relapsed patients) is currently being evaluated as first line therapy in poor prognosis high-grade patients.

A number of conditions require more specific treatment. The precursor B- and T-cell lymphoblastic lymphomas, which merge into the spectrum of acute lymphatic leukaemia, should have leukaemia-type treatment with CNS prophylaxis. CNS prophylaxis with methotrexate may also be indicated in younger patients with high grade lymphomas. Hairy cell leukaemia, a very indolent malignancy that usually presents with cytopenias and splenomegaly, responds poorly to conventional therapy; splenectomy is useful but does not produce bone marrow remission. Subcutaneous interferon improved the outlook in this condition and now excellent remission rates with long-term survival have been produced by both pentostatin and cladribine. These are given on weekly or biweekly outpatient schedules. These agents may also be of value in treating some of the other T-cell lymphomas, but have little activity in the B-cell lymphomas.

Cutaneous T-cell lymphomas, which include the Sézary syndrome and mycosis fungoides, differ from most lymphomas in that they are essentially diseases of the skin with bone marrow and other organs being involved relatively late in the pathogenesis of the disease. Multilobed Sézary cells may be seen circulating in the peripheral blood and are useful in making a diagnosis in erythrodermic patients. The effects of conventional chemotherapy are disappointing and remissions are not usually long lived. Alternative therapies, including the immune-modulating photopheresis and topical treatments, which can include certain cytotoxics, may be beneficial.

Prognosis

Prognosis varies greatly depending on the precise diagnosis. As a general rule, low grade lymphomas run an indolent course; in some patients repeated remissions can be obtained with relatively simple therapies and a proportion of patients may live 15 or 20 years, although few patients are ever cured. For the majority of intermediate grade lymphomas, the disease behaves in a more aggressive fashion and response to simple chemotherapy is disappointing. More intensive chemotherapies such as the CHOP regimen produce significant remission rates and long-term disease survival in 30–50% of patients. Some subgroups with particularly poor prognosis can be identified, these include the mantle cell lymphomas, with t(11;14) translocation) and the adult T-lymphoblastic leukaemia most usually seen in Japanese and West Indian populations. By contrast, anaplastic large cell lymphoma [sometimes referred to as Ki-1 lymphoma and characterized by the t(2;5) translocation] has a relatively high cure rate. Prognosis is also adversely affected by a number of other factors including patient age (older than 60–65 years), poor performance status, multiple sites of extranodal disease, raised serum LDH, areas of bulk disease, and a prior history of low grade disease or AIDS.

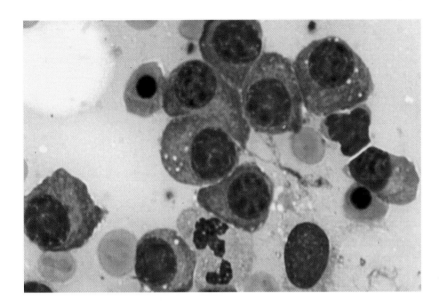

Fig. 19.3 Myeloma – bone marrow aspirate showing excessive plasma cells.

Myeloma

Myeloma (also called multiple myeloma or myelomatosis) is a neoplastic mono-clonal proliferation of bone marrow plasma cells. The disease may typically affect bone, kidneys, and the immune system or any combination of these. The treatment is relatively unsatisfactory and since the introduction of simple chemotherapy it has been difficult to make significant progress in this difficult disorder.

Aetiology

The aetiology of myeloma is unknown; there are variable chromosomal abnormal-ities demonstrable. The disease affects older patients, being rare under the age of 40 and reaching a peak in the seventh decade. The incidence is approximately 4 per 100 000 cases per year.

Pathology

The disease is characterized by the presence of increased numbers of plasma cells in the bone marrow (Fig. 19.3). These plasma cells may often appear normal. Morphology is not a reliable guide to malignancy, although an excess of mitotic figures and multinucleate forms is suggestive. Myeloma is generally a widespread patchy disease. Occasionally only a single lesion may be present – this is known as a plasmacytoma. Long-term follow up of these patients show that classical myeloma is a frequent development.

The course of the disease is related to the presence in the bone marrow of ma-lignant plasma cells and the distant effect of their products. Plasma cells are responsible for immunoglobulin production. In myeloma the plasma cells may secrete a single monoclonal, immunoglobulin (M-protein), either on its own or with the additional excretion of light chains. Heavy chain excretion alone is rare; occasionally little or no M-protein is produced. The frequency of these para-

Table 19.16 **Relative frequency of M-proteins**

IgG	56%
IgA	27%
IgM	< 1%
IgD	1%
IgE	Rare
Light chain only	15%
Non-secretory	1%

proteins is shown in Table 19.16 and a typical protein electrophoresis strip shows a characteristic monoclonal spike. In about 15% of cases this paraprotein will be absent, with the production of light chains only which are excreted in the urine and may be missed if the urine is tested for albumin and not for protein. The presence of light chains in the urine is known as Bence Jones proteinuria. The characteristic feature is precipitation on heating at approximately 65°C with the precipitate disappearing if the urine is heated to boiling point.

In addition, a number of cytokines are secreted which may have local and distant effects, contributing significantly to the production of lytic lesions of the bone. Immunoglobulin light chains may precipitate in the renal tubules, leading to renal failure, which is associated with poor survival. The various effects of myeloma cells and their products are summarized in Table 19.17.

Presentation

Clinical findings relate to the effect of the myeloma cells on the other organs (see Table 19.17). Lytic lesions of bone may give rise to pain; in some cases the only

Table 19.17 **How malignant plasma cells may affect other organs**

Organ	Effect of myeloma	End result
Bones	Local expansion with bone destruction (aided by cytokine excretion)	Lytic lesions Pathological fractures Collapsed vertebrae Hypercalcaemia
Kidney	Light chain deposition in tubules	Renal failure
Bone marrow	Marrow replacement	Marrow failure (anaemia, etc.)
Immune system	Suppression of normal immunoglobulin production	Immunosuppression infections
Blood	Excess protein	Hyperviscosity
Other organs	Amyloid deposition Local invasion Non-metastatic distant effects	Dysfunction Neuropathy, etc.

radiological change that may be seen is osteoporosis as many patients have no bone changes in the early stages. Plasma protein electrophoresis and a urine sample for Bence Jones protein should be an integral part of investigation of any patient aged over 40 with persistent back pain (patients may sometimes show a significant loss of height over the course of their disease due to multiple vertebral fractures and collapse). Patients may have features of renal failure, frequently with hypercalcaemia leading to polydipsia, polyuria, anorexia, and vomiting, constipation, and mental disturbances. There may be clinical findings of anaemia and repeated infections, which are usually related to deficient antibody production, although in advanced disease neutropenia may also be present. Excessive protein production may produce an hyperviscosity syndrome and in some instances interfere with platelet function, leading to abnormal bleeding. In some cases, amyloid features may be present or develop, such as macroglossia, carpal tunnel syndrome, diarrhoea, or cardiac dysfunction. A significant number of cases are diagnosed as a result of laboratory investigations of other complaints.

Laboratory findings include raised erythrocyte sedimentation rate (ESR), raised total protein (except in Bence Jones and non-secretory myeloma), abnormal protein electrophoresis, and reduced immunoglobulin levels. Anaemia is a frequent finding; hypercalcaemia may occur on its own or with raised urea and creatinine, indicating renal failure.

Diagnosis

Diagnosis usually requires a demonstration of two of the features shown in Table 19.18. However, particularly in non-secretory myeloma, the diagnosis may be made on the bone marrow appearances only.

Staging

Myeloma may be staged into groups I, II, or III according to the Salmon–Durie staging system, shown in Table 19.19.

Treatment

Except for a very few cases cured by allogenic bone marrow transplantation (most cases present an age group that is too old for this form of treatment), myeloma remains incurable. Progress in treatment has been slow since the introduction of melphalan and prednisone 40 years ago, which significantly improved survival. A wide variety of melphalan-based regimens have shown only marginal (if any) superiority over melphalan and prednisone alone, although Adriamycin has also proved to be an effective agent with good responses in combination with

Table 19.18 Diagnosis of myeloma

1. Excess monoclonal plasma cells usually > 30% in bone marrow
   Note: trephine biopsy may be more accurate than aspirate
2. Significant monoclonal paraproteinaemia and/or Bence Jones proteinuria
3. Radiological evidence of lytic lesions (osteoporosis is non-specific)

The diagnosis may be made by 1 alone. If there are fewer than 30% plasma cells, then 2 and/or 3 is required for confirmation.

Table 19.19 Myeloma staging system (Salmon–Durie)

Stage	
I	All of
	• Hb > 10 g/dl
	• normal serum calcium
	• no x-ray lytic lesions (or solitary plasmacytoma only)
	• Low M-protein production rates
	(a) IgG < 50 g/l
	(b) IgA < 30 g/l
	(c) urinary light chain excretion < 4 g/24 hours
II	Fitting neither stage I nor III
III	One or more of the following:
	• Hb < 8.5 g/dl
	• Raised serum calcium
	• Advanced lytic bone lesions
	• (a) IgG > 70 g/l
	• (b) IgA > 50 g/l
	• (c) urinary light chain excretion > 12 g/24 hours
A	Relatively normal renal function
B	Abnormal renal function

vincristine and dexamethasone. Incorporation of Adriamycin into melphalan-based regimens has only produced a small beneficial increment. Recent trials have focused on the benefit of high-dose melphalan, usually given with peripheral blood stem cell rescue, which has significantly increased the complete remission rate. This, unfortunately, has not translated into the hoped-for survival benefit due to a continuous relapse rate. Interferon may improve remission duration but has not been shown to affect overall survival significantly. Bisphosphonates have been shown to reduce the incidence of pathological fracture and bone pain and are now a standard component of therapy. New therapeutic approaches are urgently needed in this condition.

Prognosis

Median survival is 30–36 months, but a proportion of patients with indolent myeloma or who respond well to treatment may have significantly greater survivals. Patients presenting with advanced disease, particularly with renal failure, have much worse survival figures. High-dose therapy may prolong survival.

Quality of life

If pathological fractures and vertebral collapse can be prevented and renal disease avoided, patients may maintain a reasonable quality of life. However, disease progression leads to a downhill course with many of the problems outlined above.

Table 19.20 Diseases associated with M Proteins in serum

M-protein usually present
Myeloma
MGUS
Waldenström's macroglobulinaemia (IgM)
Heavy chain disease
Plasma cell leukaemia (blood spill of myeloma cells)
M-protein occasionally present
Chronic lymphatic leukaemia
Non-Hodgkin's lymphoma
Primary amyloid
Chronic cold haemagglutinin disease
Transient M-proteins
AIDS
Carcinomas (rare)

MGUS, Monoclonal Gammopathy of Uncertain Significance.

Related conditions – other causes of paraproteins

Not all paraproteins are necessarily myeloma (Table 19.20). There is a condition formerly termed benign paraproteinaemia, now known as monoclonal gammopathy of uncertain significance (MGUS), in which the M-protein is usually relatively small, no lytic lesions are seen, and with insufficient plasma cells in the marrow for a diagnosis of myeloma. These patients' M-proteins may remain unchanged for many years or slowly progress to frank myeloma. IgM paraproteins are usually due to a lymphoplasmacytoid proliferation known as Waldenström's macroglobulinaemia. Other B-cell lymphomas may also from time to time produce paraproteins, including chronic lymphatic leukaemia and hairy cell leukaemia.

Myeloproliferative disorders

The myeloproliferative disorders are a group of conditions characterized by proliferation of one or more of the haemopoietic components of the bone marrow. The close inter-relationships of these disorders are shown in Fig. 19.4 and the conditions may evolve into each other, although such evolutions generally signify a worsening of prognosis. Chronic myeloid leukaemia has already been considered among the leukaemias; polycythaemia vera, essential thrombocythaemia, and myelofibrosis are considered as the non-leukaemic myeloproliferative disorders.

Aetiology

Myeloproliferative conditions may occur in young people, but are more common in elderly. The cause is largely unknown, but platelet-derived cytokines can be

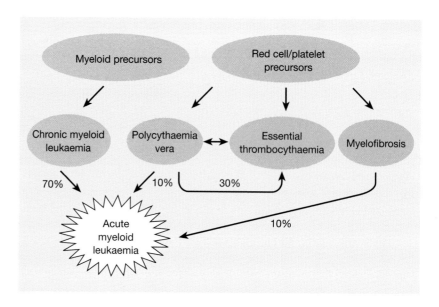

Fig. 19.4 Inter-relationships of the myeloproliferative disorders.

responsible for the fibrosis seen in myelofibrosis. Spleen and liver may frequently be involved and enlarged in these conditions.

Presentation

Patients may present with features specific to the disease, e.g. plethora due to high haemoglobin in polycythaemia vera or massive splenomegaly in myelofibrosis. Patients may also present with non-specific constitutional symptoms including lethargy, weakness, and weight loss.

Pathology

There is a clonal proliferation of one or more of the components in the bone marrow; in many cases the liver and spleen may also be involved. There is a close inter-relationship between these conditions, transitional forms may occur, and there may be evolution from one entity into another. A progressive transition to acute leukaemia may also occur.

Polycythaemia (rubra) vera (PV)

Polycythaemia (also called erythrocytosis) is a syndrome in which there are a number of changes with an increase in the haemoglobin above 17.5 g/dl in adult males and 14.5 g/dl in females; there will be a corresponding rise in red cell count and haematocrit. The causes of polycythaemia are shown in Table 19.21. Polycythaemia vera refers to a condition in which the increase in red blood cells is caused by endogenous myeloproliferation. There is frequently an increase in granulocytes and platelets, indicating the stem cell nature of the disorder. Chromosome changes are non-specific. The condition is often suggested by the ruddy features and the high colour of the patient. The clinical features are related to the overproduction of cells with resulting increase in blood viscosity, blood

Table 19.21 **Causes of polycythaemia**

Primary

Polycythaemia vera

Secondary

Compensatory erythropoietin increase

    High altitude living

    Cardiovascular disease (congential ± cyanosis)

    Pulmonary disease

    Heavy cigarette smoking

    Haemoglobinopathies with increased O_2 affinity

    Methaemoglobinaemia

Inappropriate erythropoietin increase

    Renal diseases

    Massive uterine fibromyoma

    Carcinomas – hepatocellular, renal (all rare)

    Cerebellar haemangioblastoma

    Stress or pseudo-polycythaemia

    Cigarette smoking

    Dehydration

    Plasma loss (burns, enteropathy)

volume, and metabolic activity. Clinical features are summarized in Table 19.22 and the diagnostic criteria in Table 19.23.

Treatment

The object of treatment is to maintain the blood count, particularly haemoglobin and red cell volume, within normal limits. Where thrombocytosis also features, the platelet count should also be kept within normal limits. When the

Table 19.22 **Clinical features of polycythaemia vera**

- General – headaches, pruritis (especially after hot baths), dyspnoea, blurred vision, night sweats
- Plethoric appearance – ruddy cyanosis, conjunctival suffusion, retinal venous engorgement
- Splenomegaly (two-thirds of patients)
- Haemorrhage (GI, uterine, cerebral)
- Thrombosis, arterial or venous
- Hypertension (one-third of patients)
- Gout (due to raised uric acid production)
- Peptic ulceration (5–10% of patients)

Table 19.23 **Diagnosis of polycythaemia vera**

1	Red cell mass > 25% above patients' predicted value
2	No evident cause of secondary polycythaemia (arterial oxygen saturation > 92%)
3	Palpable splenomegaly
4	Evidence of clonal disorder, e.g. abnormal karyotype
	For diagnosis 1 + 2 obligatory + 3 or 4
	If neither 3 nor 4 present, then 2 of a–d
a	Platelet count > $400 \times 10^9/l$
b	Neutrophils > $10 \times 10^9/l$
c	Splenomegaly on ultrasound in absence of liver pathology
d	Spontaneous erythroid colony growth or low serum erythropoietin

haemoglobin and platelet count are maintained at these levels there is a significant reduction in symptoms and complications, and long survival is possible. Treatment should therefore avoid, where possible, therapeutic agents with leukaemogenic effects, in view of the inherent risk of leukaemic transformation. The treatment of choice is therefore venesection. Newly diagnosed cases with very high haemoglobin and haematocrit represent a medical emergency due to the risk of thrombosis. Daily or alternate-day venesection may be used until the haemoglobin approaches normal levels. Generally, venesection is used to keep the haemoglobin/haematocrit within normal levels. Chemotherapy, using hydroxyurea or other agents, is indicated when the platelet count is also elevated.

Prognosis

Once the haematocrit and platelet count are controlled the risk of complications (which are similar to the presenting features) is greatly reduced. Many patients with polycythaemia vera may live a relatively normal lifespan; however, the risk of transformation to myelofibrosis or acute leukaemia is always present and will clearly modify the prognosis.

Quality of life

Whilst the condition remains as simple polycythaemia vera, and serious complications such as thrombosis reduced by venesection, the quality of life is largely related to the degree of itch experienced by the patient. This is often aggravated by exposure to water, e.g. baths and showers. Some patients may require skin cleansing with baby oil or other means of avoiding water. Occasionally, antihistamines are useful in controlling itch, and in some cases cytotoxic therapies are also helpful. Thrombosis and haemorrhage remain more common and affect both prognosis and quality of life.

Essential thrombocythaemia (ET)

Essential thrombocythaemia (ET) is a rare condition characterized by persistent overproduction of platelets. The patient's platelet count at diagnosis may frequently exceed $1000 \times 10^9/l$; there is an associated megakaryocytic proliferation in

Table 19.24 Causes of thrombocythaemia

Reactive

Haemorrhage (any cause)

Chronic iron deficiency

Malignancy

Chronic infections

Connective tissues diseases, e.g. rheumatoid arthritis

Post-splenectomy

Endogenous

Essential thrombocythaemia

Other myeloproliferative conditions (PV, CML & myelofibrosis − not in all cases)

the marrow. For diagnosis it is necessary to show a persistently elevated platelet count ($> 600 \times 10^9/l$) in the absence of any of the known causes of thrombocytosis (Table 19.24). A moderate degree of splenic enlargement is frequent but some patients may develop splenic atrophy, due to platelets blocking the splenic microcirculation. There is no specific diagnostic test for ET. Bone marrow appearances with megakaryocytic hyperplasia, sometimes accompanied by fibrosis (but essentially similar to polycythaemia vera) is suggestive and tests for platelet aggregation are consistently abnormal but non-specific.

Treatment

Patients with grossly elevated platelet counts may require platelet apheresis to bring about an initial reduction in platelet count. The optimal treatment for ET remains to be established. Hydroxyurea has the virtue of being cheap and relatively straightforward, although regular blood counts are required. Interferon and anagrelide will also reduce the platelet count and may in the long run carry a lesser risk of leukaemic transformation than hydroxyurea. Busulphan and radioactive phosphorus-32 are less favoured due to the higher risk of leukaemic transformation.

Prognosis

Essential thrombocythaemia is a chronic condition providing death does not occur as a result of bleeding or thrombotic events. Patients may transform after a number of years to polycythaemia vera, myelofibrosis, or acute leukaemia.

Myelofibrosis

Myelofibrosis is characterized by varying degrees of marrow fibrosis associated with circulating primitive cells. There is a characteristic blood picture with a leuco-erythroblastic anaemia and characteristic teardrop-shaped red cells (poikilocytes). Laboratory findings in this condition are summarized in Table 19.25. Marrow fibrosis is thought to be due to platelet-derived growth factors produced by the excessive number of megakaryocytes and in some instances the disease will develop from polycythaemia vera or essential thrombocythaemia. Splenomegaly is frequent and may be massive; constitutional symptoms may also occur.

Table 19.25 **Laboratory findings in myelofibrosis**

- Anaemia (occasionally Hb may be N or ↑ usually early in disease
- Leucocytosis, early in disease, leucopenia in later stages
- Thrombocytosis, early in disease, thrombocytopenia in later stages
- Leuco-erythroblastic blood film
- 'Teardrop' poikilocytic red blood cells
- Bone marrow difficult to aspirate
- Trephine biopsy
   hypercellular
   excessive fibrosis
   increased megakaryocytes
   occasionally increased bone formation
- Low serum and RBC folate, raised vitamin B_{12} & vitamin B_{12} binding capacity
- Increased leucocyte alkaline phosphatase score
- Raised serum urate
- Raised serum lactic dehydrogenase
- Extramedullary haemopoiesis (radioactive iron studies, liver biopsy, splenectomy)
- Transformation to acute leukaemia 10–20%

Treatment

The treatment of myelofibrosis is in general unsatisfactory as no satisfactory means have been found to alter the progressive nature of the disease. Possible treatments are summarized in Table 19.26. Splenectomy may seem an attractive option to alleviate symptoms and reduce transfusion requirements, but is a relatively high-risk strategy with a significant postoperative mortality and morbidity. Progression to acute leukaemia is not uncommon.

Table 19.26 **Treatment of myelofibrosis**

- Blood transfusion (for anaemic patients)
- Regular folic acid supplementation
- Allopurinol – prevent gout and urate neuropathy
- Hydroxyurea controls hypermetabolism – counts may fall
- Splenic irradiation – reduces splenic size and symptoms due to hypermetabolism
- Splenectomy (possible indications):
   for large spleens producing symptoms, not controlled by other means
   unacceptably high transfusion requirements (most of transfused cell pooled and broken down in spleen)
   if thrombocytopenia severe and causing bleeding

Table 19.27 Myelodysplastic syndromes

Syndrome	Synonym	Features	Median survival
Refractory anaemia	RA	pb blasts < 1%, BM blasts < 5%	50 months
RA with ring sideroblasts	RARS	As RA but ring sideroblasts > 15% of total erythroblasts	50 months
RA with excess blasts	RAEB	pb blasts < 5%, BM blasts 5–20%	11 months
RAEB in transformation	RAEB-t	pb blasts > 5%, BM blasts 20–30% or Auer rods present	5 months
Chronic myelomonocytic leukaemia	CMML	pb > 5 × 109/l monocytes, BM blasts variable and monocytes	18 months

BM, bone marrow; pb, peripheral blood.

Prognosis and quality of life

As patients tend to have progressive disease, life expectancy is poorer than the other non-leukaemic myeloproliferative disorders. Quality of life tends to be more adversely affected, due to the splenomegaly, anaemia, and requirement for blood transfusion.

Myelodysplastic syndromes (myelodysplasia; MDS)

This is a group of clonal neoplastic disorders, producing qualitative and quantitative changes in the cells of the bone marrow and peripheral blood. The French-American-British (FAB) classification (Table 19.27) has replaced earlier terminology such as pre-leukaemia or smouldering leukaemia and has helped to

Table 19.28 Additional laboratory findings in myelodysplastic syndromes

Anaemia	Common
Macrocytosis	Common
Microcytosis or dimorphic picture	Occasional
Reticulocytes	Usually reduced
Leucopenia	Common (but may be ↑↑ in CMML)
Neutropenia	Common
Neutrophils without granules	Common
Pelger abnormality of neutrophils (reduced lobes in nucleus)	Fairly common
Thrombocytopenia	Fairly common (but ↑ in 10%, esp. RARS)

identify factors with prognostic significance. Essentially all of the myelodysplastic syndromes may develop to frank leukaemia; progression may sometimes be seen such as RA → RAEB → RAEB-t; in other instances, the disease may remain unchanged for many years. For the remainder of the patient's lifespan, clinical problems may arise from anaemia, thrombocytopenia, or neutropenia or any combination of these.

Pathology

The bone marrow is often but not invariably hypercellular and morphological changes in the precursor cells may range from subtle to the bizarre. Anaemia, leucopenia, and thrombocytopenia may occur in any combination. In the more leukaemic forms (RAEB, RAEB-t), blast cells may be present in the peripheral blood. Additional laboratory findings are shown in Table 19.28.

Aetiology

The aetiology of MDS is unclear but may be similar to that of acute leukaemia. Secondary cases, particularly related to prior chemotherapy, are identified and tend to have a poor response to treatment.

Treatment

Treatment tends to be largely supportive with red blood cell transfusion given as necessary. The majority of cases do not respond to cytokines such as erythropoietin or the white cell stimulating hormone, granulocyte colony-stimulating factor (G-CSF). Chemotherapy may have a role to play in younger patients with bad prognosis disease (RAEB, RAEB-t), but remission, if achieved, tends to be short lived. There may be a role for bone marrow transplantation in patients who are sufficiently young and with a donor available.

Quality of life

Patients with RA or RARS may live relatively normal lives for many years, or can be transfusion dependent; however, the other diagnostic categories tend to be more symptomatic. Symptoms may relate to blood cell deficiency or may be more generalized and can include lassitude, fevers, sweats, and weight loss.

Bone marrow transplantation

The dose-limiting factor with most forms of chemotherapy is the ability of the marrow cells to recover their function before the patient dies through lack of immune defence mechanisms. Short periods of profound neutropenia can generally be managed by means of vigorous treatment of infection with broad-spectrum antibiotics, antifungals, and antiviral agents as appropriate. However, over the longer term, the use of these agents will select resistant strains (frequently present as normal flora although pathogenic in the immune suppressed patient). These may prove difficult to treat and are potentially ultimately fatal without granulocytes to combat the problem organisms. A number of mechanisms are available to augment the host defence in this situation. They include transfusion of neutrophils – due to their short half-life it has been difficult to prove any benefit for this approach. The white cell hormones G-CSF or GM-CSF may be given to speed neutrophil recovery after conventional chemotherapy, and are effective in

Table 19.29 Types of blood cell transfusion

	Source of stem cells	Donor
Autologous	PBSC BM	Patient
Syngenic	PBSC BM	HLA identical twin
Allogenic	PBSC BM	HLA matched sibling, partially matched relative
Volunteer unrelated donor	PBSC BM	HLA matched unrelated
Cord blood	Cord & placenta following delivery	Occasionally sibling, otherwise cord blood bank

BM, bone marrow; PBSC, peripheral blood stem cell.

allowing small increments in the dose of chemotherapy, or reduction in time between courses of chemotherapy. They are, however, unable to play much role in recovering marrow function if patients are given mega doses of chemotherapy.

The alternative approach is to provide the patient with a new source of haemopoietic stem cells following the delivery of high-dose chemotherapy. The sources are outlined in Table 19.29. Each type of transplant has advantages and disadvantages. These relate to the development of graft-versus-host disease and graft-versus-leukaemia effect. These conditions will not occur in autologous or syngenic transplants, making these transplants easier to perform, but the relapse rate is higher in these transplantations. Graft-versus-host disease may occur even in apparently perfectly HLA-, B-, and DR-matched sibling allogenic transplantation; the development is variable and relates to other as yet undiscovered tissue compatibility systems or minor variation in the identified systems. Acute graft-versus-host disease is characterized principally by skin rashes, intractable diarrhoea, and abnormal liver function, and occurs in the first 100 days post-transplant. Chronic graft-versus-host disease occurs after this time. Immuno-suppressive agents are routinely used to try to prevent graft-versus-host disease, although a minor degree is welcomed by some clinicians as heralding the promise of graft-versus-leukaemia effect. Graft-versus-host disease is a potentially fatal condition; it also predisposes patients to opportunist infections as do the agents used to suppress it. These problems bring about a relatively high death rate in the period immediately following transplantation; despite this, long-term results are superior to conventional treatment in a number of situations. The concept of a graft-versus-leukaemia effect, which may help to destroy residual leukaemia cells, is now accepted and research is directed at exploiting this phenomenon without excessive manifestation of graft-versus-host disease.

Peripheral blood stem cell transplantation is gaining in popularity over bone marrow transplantation because of the shorter time to recovery of neutrophil and platelet numbers following transplantation. However, ethical issues with regard to giving donors the white cell hormones necessary for mobilization of the peripheral blood stem cells remain to be resolved. Umbilical cord blood transplants are only suitable for patients under 60 kg because of the numbers of stem cells normally available in cord blood donations. The longer time from transplantation to cellular recovery makes this form of treatment more difficult. Despite this, there is now a significant number of cord blood donations stored for potential transplant.

There is no set chemotherapy regimen for treating the patients (conditioning) prior to transplantation. Common regimens include the use of total body irradiation with cyclophosphamide bulsulphan, and cyclophosphamide and regimens including melphalan at very high dosage. The stem cells, from whatever source,

Case history

Young man with lymphadenopathy

Dear Doctor

This young man is unwell and has glands in his neck. Please advise.

History

Mr H is aged 35 years and has been unwell for the past 3 months with loss of appetite, weight loss of 1 stone and night sweats, for which he has to change his night clothes usually once per night. For the past 2–3 weeks he has been getting short of breath and has poor exercise tolerance.

On examination he had multiple hard glands on both sides of his neck and in his axillae and groins. Spleen and liver were not palpable and other systems were unremarkable.

Investigations
- Haemoglobin 12.1 g/dl
- Leucocytes 15.9×10^9/l
- Platelets 460×10^9/l
- ESR 6 mm in the first hour
- LDH 1024 (N=360–720)
- Remainder of the biochemical screening within normal limits
- Chest X-ray showed significant widening of the mediastinum
- CT scan showed involvement of mediastinal, para-aortic and iliac glands
- Ultrasound of abdomen confirmed normal liver; spleen was slightly bulky, multiple gland masses seen in the para-aortic area
- Axillary lymph node biopsy showed Hodgkin's disease (nodular sclerosing, type II)

Treatment

Patient received six courses of ABDV (Adriamycin, bleomycin, vinblastine and dacarbazine) with a resolution of all glands and symptoms.

Physical examination showed complete resolution of all gland masses. CT scan confirmed this impression but there were some residual slightly enlarged glands in the mediastinum.

are given back to the patient by infusion into a vein following the completion of therapy and with enough time allowed for the drugs to be cleared from the system. The stem cells find their own way to the bone marrow micro-environment where they proliferate to form blood cells.

Further reading

Canellos, G. P., Lister, T. A., and Sklar, J. L. (1998) *The lymphomas*. W. B. Saunders Company, London.

Degos, L., Linch, D. C., and Löwenberg, B. (1999) *Textbook of malignant haematology*. Martin Dunitz, London.

George, J. N., Woolf, S. H., and Raskob, G. E. (1999) The evidence-based analysis of treatment for chronic myeloid leukaemia: an introduction to its methods and clinical implications. *Blood* 94(5), 1515–17.

Henderson, E. S., Lister, T. A., and Greaves, M. F. (1996) *Leukemia*, 6th edn. W. B. Saunders Company, Philadelphia.

Laurence, A. D. J. and Goldstone, A. H. (1999) High-dose therapy with hematopoietic transplantation for Hodgkin's lymphoma. *Semin Hematol* 36(3), 303–12.

Lee, G. R., Foerster, J., Lukens, J., Paraskevas, F., Greer, J. P., and Rodgers, G. M. (1999) *Wintrobe's clinical hematology*, 10th edn, Vol. 1. Williams & Wilkins, London.

Löwenberg, B., Downing, J. R., and Burnett, A. (1999). Acute myeloid leukemia. *N Engl J Med* 341(14), 1051–62.

Thomas, E. D., Blume, K. G., and Forman, S. J. (1999) *Hematopoietic cell transplantation*, 2nd edn. Blackwell Science, London.

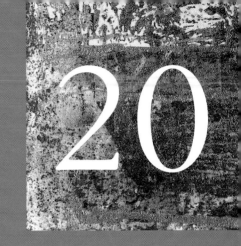

20

Bone tumours and soft tissue sarcomas *Angus J. Patterson and David C. Harmon*

- Malignant primary bone tumours

- Osteosarcoma

- Ewing's sarcoma

- Chondrosarcoma

- Malignant fibrous histiocytoma

- Giant cell tumour

- Adult soft tissue sarcomas

- Rhabdomyosarcoma (RMS)

- Kaposi's sarcoma (KS)

- Desmoid tumours

Bone tumours and soft tissue sarcomas

Malignant primary bone tumours

The commonest malignant primary bone tumours are the matrix-producing tumours, osteosarcoma and chondrosarcoma. Less frequently seen is the small round cell tumour, Ewing's sarcoma. Malignant fibrous histiocytomas, primary bone lymphomas, and malignant giant cell tumours are rare but well recognized.

Aetiology

The exact aetiology of most malignant primary bone tumours is unknown but there is strong evidence to suggest that the fundamental process is one of genetic mutation. An increased preponderance of bone and soft tissue sarcomas has been documented with two well recognized genetic cancer-associated syndromes. Hereditary or familial retinoblastoma involves the inheritance of a germline mutation of the retinoblastoma gene, which encodes a protein involved in controlling the cell cycle. The mutated gene can no longer function as a tumour supressor gene; the condition has been associated with a 400-fold increase in the frequency of osteosarcoma. A similar situation is observed in Li–Fraumeni syndrome with excess malignancy including sarcomas and breast cancers often arising before mid-40s. It involves a mutation in the p53 gene, which encodes a nuclear phosphoprotein responsible for checking the progress of the cell cycle. Mutated p53-produced protein is no longer able to control the cell cycle. Both conditions are inherited in the heterozygous state and deletion of the other allele is required, creating homozygosity, before tumour development is seen.

Exposure to ionizing radiation has also been clearly linked with an increased incidence of bone and soft tissue sarcomas. Some of the first evidence came after the First World War when an increased frequency of bone sarcomas was observed in young women working in the factories using dials containing radium and mesothorium.

External beam radiotherapy both in paediatric and adult oncology practice has been associated with an increased chance of developing a sarcoma in the irradiated area. The carcinogenic effect of radiation may be increased by additional chemotherapy. The risks of a radiation-induced sarcoma are much greater in children than adults, representing one reason for the decline in the use of this treatment modality in paediatric practice. The absolute risk in adult radiation therapy is small and not enough to mitigate against its beneficial use.

Osteosarcoma has long been recognized as a complication of Paget's disease of bone where bone turnover rates may approximate those in the growing long bones of teenagers who have the highest incidence of osteosarcoma.

Bone infarction, chronic osteomyelitis, and the presence of metal prostheses have also been linked to bone sarcoma development, but in the vast majority of cases the aetiology is unclear.

Table 20.1 AJCC classification of primary malignant bone tumours

Bone forming
  Osteosarcoma
Cartilage forming
  Chondrosarcoma
  Mesenchymal chondrosarcoma
Giant cell tumour, malignant
Ewing's sarcoma
Vascular tumours
  Haemangioendothelioma
  Haemangiopericytoma
  Angiosarcoma
Connective tissue tumours
  Fibrosarcoma
  Liposarcoma
  Malignant mesenchymoma
  Undifferentiated sarcoma
Other tumours
  Chordoma
  Adamantinoma of long bones

Classification

The American Joint Comission on Cancer (AJCC) staging classification of bone sarcomas, shown in Table 20.1, is widely accepted (AJCC, 1997).

Clinical presentation

Most patients with malignant bone tumours present with symptoms of local pain and/or the development of a slow-growing mass. Occasionally the first sign may be a pathological fracture through the tumour. Osteosarcomas may produce systemic symptoms mimicking osteomyelitis, creating diagnostic difficulties and delays.

Investigations

In most cases, the investigation begins with plain x-rays of the affected bone. These may show varying changes, from bone destruction to new bone formation and associated soft tissue swelling. The exact extent of the lesion and the presence of vascular or neurological invasion must be clarified by CT and MRI scanning, which have now become standard. Definitive diagnosis requires biopsy and this must take place before any treatment is considered. An excision biopsy may be appropriate for small, easily accessible and benign-looking lesions, but in most cases a core needle biopsy is performed. Incisional biopsies run the risk of spreading tumour cells within the field of the incision and are avoided if possible. Conventional histopathological techniques using light microscopy are usually sufficient but immunohistochemistry, electron microscopy, and cytogenetics may occasionally be needed to distinguish certain tumour types, particularly small round cell tumours. Defining the histological grade is also of vital importance as it is this feature that most closely predicts the behaviour of the tumour and is incorporated into most major staging systems.

An isotope bone scan is performed to search for skip lesions within the affected bone and distant bone metastases. CT scanning of the chest must be carried out to exclude pulmonary metastases, which represent the commonest site of metastatic spread. Some of the most commonly used cytotoxic drugs, particularly doxorubicin (Adriamycin) can be cardiotoxic at high cumulative doses and patients likely to receive these must have a baseline assessment of cardiac function by echocardiogram. Accurate assessment of ejection fraction is recorded for future comparative purposes.

Staging

The most frequently used staging system is that proposed by Enneking (1980). It considers the histological grade, the local extent of the tumour, and the presence or absence of distant metastases (Table 20.2).

Table 20.2 **Enneking staging system for primary bone tumours**

Stage	Grade	Site	Metastases
IA	Low	Intracompartmental	Absent
IB	Low	Extracompartmental	Absent
IIA	High	Intracompartmental	Absent
IIB	High	Extracompartmental	Absent
IIIA	Low or high	Intra- or Extracompartmental	Single site
IIIB	Low or high	Intra- or Extracompartmental	Multiple metastases

Table 20.3 **Principles of limb-sparing surgery**

- Wide resection of involved bone. A 3–4 cm margin is taken beyond radiologically discernible abnormal bone
- A cuff of normal muscle tissue is removed in all directions
- Adjacent joint and capsule are resected
- No major neurovascular involvement
- All sites of previous biopsies and potentially contaminated tissue are resected *en bloc*
- Adequate soft tissue coverage
- Regional muscle transfers must be sufficient to allow adequate motor function

Management

Most patients will require treatment involving a combination of surgery, radiotherapy, and/or chemotherapy. The principles of limb-sparing sarcoma surgery (Table 20.3) are now well established (Malawer, 1997). Surgery may be the first therapeutic procedure undertaken or it may be preceded by chemotherapy in an effort to improve the resectability of the tumour. Surgery is planned using the most recent MRI scans and if preoperative chemotherapy has been given, scans must be repeated after chemotherapy. Blood vessel involvement with extraosseus tumour need not be a contraindication if vessels can be dissected clear of the tumour or excised and replaced. Interestingly, bone sarcomas infrequently involve nerves so these rarely need to be resected.

The placement of bone allografts or of reconstructive endoprostheses is planned using preoperative MRI scans. Unfortunately, many bone tumours arise near joints, which may need to be excised and replaced by artificial ones.

Most sarcomas are considered relatively radioresistant tumours and their control requires the use of high doses of radiation. Radiotherapy is used to treat unresectable tumours or to reduce the risk of recurrence postoperatively in certain circumstances. The risk of local recurrence is increased in three main situations:

- postoperative residual microscopic disease;
- preoperative pathological fracture;
- open biopsy tracks which can not be adequately excised at surgery.

As with surgery, a number of well defined principles underlie the safe and effective delivery of radiotherapy in this setting (Table 20.4).

Although important in the treatment of primary bone tumours, radiotherapy is not without toxicity. Most patients will experience acute radiation skin reactions, which will subside over a period of days or weeks. Long-term abnormalities of growth and limb function are seen in younger patients if growth in the irradiated limb is not complete. Normal tissues lying near the radiation field are also at risk of long-term damage and irradiated bone itself undergoes cortical destruction, weakening it and increasing the likelihood of pathological fracture. The high doses of radiation needed in this setting are associated with a two- to threefold increase in second malignancies at the irradiated site. Most patients, however, have minimal compromise of limb function.

Table 20.4 **Principles of radiotherapy**

- Radiation fields are planned on pre-chemotherapy CT or MRI scans
- The irradiated limb is immobilized to ensure accurate delivery of radiation
- Joint spaces and critical normal tissues are shielded or excluded from radiation fields
- A strip of unirradiated tissue is left to allow lymphatic drainage
- Scars from open biopsies, not excised at surgery, are included in the radiation field
- Treatment is usually delivered in two phases. The first volume of tissue treated involves a 5–7 cm margin on the postoperative site or tumour. The second phase of treatment is delivered to a tighter field with a margin of 2 cm

Osteosarcoma

Osteosarcoma is a bone tumour occurring predominantly in adolescents and young adults. It accounts for approximately 20% of primary bone cancers and 5% of childhood tumours. All age groups may be affected but a bimodal age distribution is observed. Seventy-five per cent of tumours are seen in patients younger than 20 years of age. The second peak in incidence is seen in the elderly who are more likely to have Paget's disease, bone infarcts, or have had prior radiotherapy. The tumour arises more frequently in males and in younger patients usually originates in the metaphysis of long bones, particularly the distal femur, proximal tibia, proximal femur, and humerus in order of frequency (Fig. 20.1). Between 60 and 80% arise around the knee in younger patients (Huvos, 1979). It may also arise within flat bones and, in older patients, occurs as commonly there as in long bones. It is a malignant mesenchymal tumour in which the neoplastic cells produce bone matrix and is the commonest malignant bone tumour excluding multiple myeloma and lymphoma.

Pain and swelling are the usual presenting symptoms. Pain usually precedes swelling and is typically worse at night. The relative frequency of musculoskeletal symptoms in this age group often gives rise to diagnostic delays. Particularly aggressive tumours may produce constitutional symptoms of weight loss, fever, malaise, and anaemia. Unfortunately, this is often indicative of metastatic disease.

Localized tumours are limited to the bone of origin, although skip lesions may be present, worsening the prognosis. The disease most commonly metastasizes to the lungs, but may also spread to other bones (the second most frequent site), skin, and brain. Disseminated metastases are found in 10–20% of patients at diagnosis.

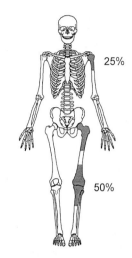

Fig. 20.1 Osteosarcoma: common sites of origin.

Investigations

Enlarging tumour causes expansion within the bone, until finally the cortex is breached and the periosteum is elevated. This gives rise to the classic x-ray appearance of Codman's triangle (Fig. 20.2). The tumour appears as a lytic lesion without a clearly defined boundary, and varying degrees of tumour bone formation produce dense sclerosis. Spicules of bone may form at right angles to the long axis of the bone, so called 'sun-ray spiculation'. Radiosotope bone, CT, and MRI scanning help accurately delineate the tumour, define any local invasion into nearby structures and may reveal the presence of skip lesions within the same bone or metastases to other bones. Chest CT scanning is performed on all patients to exclude pulmonary metastases. Alkaline phosphatase can be a useful tumour marker.

Pathological classification

The tumour is characterized by the formation of osteoid tissue by the malignant cells. The World Health Organization's classification (Table 20.5) separates the tumours into central and surface tumours (Schajowicz, 1995). A number of different subtypes are recognized. High-grade central osteosarcoma is the commonest accounting for more than 70% of the disease. Histopathological examination reveals spindle cell formation and variable amounts of tumour bone formation.

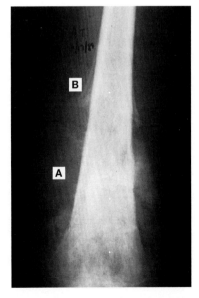

Fig. 20.2 Osteosarcoma: radiograph showing tumour of the lower femur with sun-ray spiculation (A) and bilateral periosteal elevation producing Codman's triangles (B).

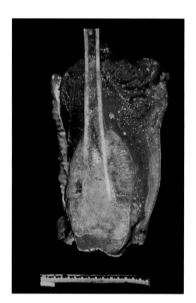

Fig. 20.3 Osteosarcoma: resection specimen from same patient as in Fig. 20.2.

Table 20.5 WHO classification of osteosarcoma

Central (medullary)

Conventional central osteosarcoma

Telangiectatic osteosarcoma

Intraosseus well-differentiated (low-grade) osteosarcoma

Small, round cell osteosarcoma

Surface (peripheral)

Parosteal (juxtacortical) well-differentiated (low-grade) osteosarcoma

Periosteal osteosarcoma (low to intermediate grade)

High-grade surface osteosarcoma

There are usually areas of necrosis and numerous atypical mitoses. The malignant osteoblasts make alkaline phosphatase. Stains to detect this assist in diagnosis. Parosteal and intraosseus well-differentiated osteosarcoma are associated with a more favourable prognosis and can often be successfully treated by radical resection of the primary tumour. High-grade central osteosarcomas typically arise in the epiphyseal or metaphyseal regions whereas surface tumours are more usually diaphyseal in origin.

Treatment

For most patients with localized high-grade central osteosarcoma, treatment will involve a combination of chemotherapy and surgery. Randomized clinical trials have clearly established the benefit of adjuvant chemotherapy (Link, 1986; Eilber, 1987). Treatment may be administered following surgery alone or both pre- and postoperatively. There is no survival benefit with preoperative chemotherapy, but it does increase the number of patients with locally advanced tumours who become suitable for limb-sparing surgery and has the additional advantage of creating more time for the manufacture of an appropriate endoprosthesis. Currently 70–90% of patients with extremity osteosarcoma are able to avoid amputation.

Fewer than 20% of patients were cured prior to the advent of effective chemotherapy. Cure rates of 50–80% have become typical over the past 20 years as chemotherapy has involved combinations of cytotoxic drugs including high-dose methotrexate, doxorubicin, bleomycin, cyclophosphamide, dactinomycin (actinomycin D), cisplatin, carboplatin, etoposide, and ifosfamide. Studies have compared intra-arterial and intravenous administration and shown little difference. The commonest regimen in current use involves the combination of doxorubicin and cisplatin.

If a tumour is clearly easily resectable at diagnosis, then surgery is sometimes performed first and chemotherapy administered postoperatively. Most patients, however, receive two or three cycles of chemotherapy preoperatively, especially if there is any doubt regarding the feasibility of limb-preserving surgery. The response to chemotherapy indicated by the degree of necrosis found in the resected tumour is highly predictive of overall survival. A poor response raises the question of whether or not the postoperative chemotherapy regimen should be changed. Whilst this seems intuitively appropriate, it has not been tested in a randomized trial.

Whilst every effort is made to avoid amputation, it is still necessary if the risk of local tumour recurrence is unacceptably high. This is the case if there is a large soft tissue mass invading the neurovascular bundle, or diffuse soft tissue or skin infiltration. Patients with displaced pathological fractures also have a high risk of recurrence and amputation is usually advised in this setting.

Osteosarcomas are relatively radioresistant. Treatment with radiation therefore requires a high dose. It is used as the primary modality of therapy when the tumour is unresectable or delivered as adjuvant postoperative therapy when microscopic residual disease is found in the surgical resection specimen. Radiotherapy has been reported as having a local control rate of 20–25% when used alone in cases of unresectable disease.

Intraosseus well-differentiated osteosarcoma and parosteal osteosarcoma carry a much more favourable prognosis and can usually be managed by radical surgical excision alone. Periosteal osteosarcomas have a more intermediate prognosis and are treated in the same way as high-grade central osteosarcomas as are small cell and telangiectatic osteosarcoma.

Metastatic osteosarcoma

The prognosis for patients with metastatic osteosarcoma has improved over the past two decades but it is still a grave situation. The outcome is very much dependent on the sites of metastases and their amenity to surgical resection (Table 20.6). Pulmonary metastases are by far the commonest and account for 85% of metastases. In the past less than 20% of such patients survived but this has improved to more than 40% in recent years for those with small numbers of lung metastases. Patients with bone metastases rarely survive. Improved outcome has resulted from the aggressive management of such patients and treatment involves surgical resection of the metastases along with the primary tumour, if presenting synchronously, in addition to several cycles of intensive multi-agent chemotherapy. Regimens involve various combinations of the cytotoxic compounds previously outlined. Pulmonary metastases presenting metachronously are treated in the same way and multiple thoracotomies may be performed to resect recurrent disease. Even patients with unresectable, or multiple sites of, metastatic disease should receive intensive chemotherapy as they may have prolonged and durable responses. The

Table 20.6 Good prognostic indicators for pulmonary metastatectomy

- Fewer than 5 metastases
- Long disease-free interval since resection of the primary tumour
- Peripherally sited, easily resected lesions
- Unilateral pulmonary metastases

After Ward *et al.* (1994).

presence of a malignant pleural effusion indicates intrapleural spread of tumour and is usually incurable.

Prognosis

Historical data prior to the 1970s suggests a survival rate of 20% in patients with non-metastatic, resectable disease treated with a combination of surgery and radiotherapy. A number of prognostic factors are well recognized. The most important of these are histological subtype and site of the tumour. Distal tumours have a better prognosis compared with axial skeleton lesions and lesions of the flat bones also appear to have a better outcome. Radiation-induced osteosarcoma or tumours complicating Paget's disease have a particularly poor outlook. Other factors associated with a poor outcome include age, size of tumour, presence of skip lesions, lactate dehydrogenase and alkaline phosphatase levels, tumour cell ploidy, duration of symptoms, and loss of heterozygosity of the Rb gene. For the 20% of patients with pulmonary metastases at diagnosis, aggressive therapy provides long-term survival for 20–40%. Since the advent of effective chemotherapy, degree of necrosis in the resected primary tumour, indicating response to chemotherapy, has become a powerful indicator of which patients will enjoy the modern expectation of up to 80% curability.

Ewing's sarcoma

Ewing's sarcoma is a primary malignant small round cell tumour of bone and is closely related to a group of tumours known as primitive neuroectodermal tumours (PNET), which exhibit neuroectodermal differentiation and are probably derived from neural crest cells. Differentiation between the two depends on demonstrating neural differentiation histologically. Absence, by convention, indicates Ewing's sarcoma.

It accounts for 6–10% of primary malignant bone tumours and is the second commonest bone tumour in children. Most patients are between 10 and 15 years old and the vast majority are under 20 years old. It affects males more commonly than females and Africans are rarely affected. The tumour typically originates in the axial skeleton and the commonest sites are the pelvic bones, femur, humerus, and ribs but it may also arise in the skull, jaw, and the small bones of the hands and feet (Fig. 20.4) (Green, 1985). Less commonly, the tumour develops outside bone when historically it has been termed 'extraosseus Ewing's sarcoma'. Its appearance and behaviour in this situation is, however, the same.

More than 90% of tumours are associated with a characteristic translocation t(11;22) and less commonly with t(21;22). These are also found in PNET, confirming their likely common origin. The 11;22 and 21;22 translocations result in the production of the fusion genes *EWS-FLI1* and *EWS-ERG*, respectively.

The tumour may be localized to the primary site but the majority have metastases in lung or bone at diagnosis. These, however, are often microscopic and not radiologically discernible.

Investigations

The tumour permeates widely within the medullary cavity of the diaphysis and usually invades the periosteum. The frequently associated periosteal reaction pro-

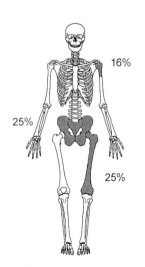

16%

25%

25%

Fig. 20.4 Ewing's sarcoma: common sites of origin.

Table 20.7 Round cell tumours

- Ewing's sarcoma/PNET
- Neuroblastoma
- Rhabdomyosarcoma
- Lymphoma
- Small cell osteosarcoma

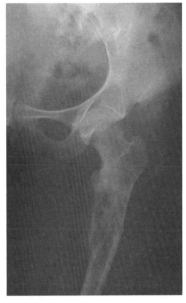

Fig. 20.5 Ewing's sarcoma: radiograph showing tumour of the femur with evidence of pathological fracture.

duces layers of reactive new bone formation, giving rise to the 'onion-skin' appearance often seen on plain x-rays. Once again the local extent of the tumour and degree of local soft tissue invasion may be clarified by CT and MRI scanning. Isotope bone scanning helps exclude evaluable distant bone metastases or skip lesions within the bone of origin. A core biopsy of the primary lesion is required to confirm the diagnosis. Lactate dehydrogenase (LDH) can be a useful marker.

Pathology

Diagnosis again requires skilled histopathological confirmation. Microscopy reveals small, round, densely packed cells with nuclei free of nucleoli and scant glycogen-rich cytoplasm which may appear clear. Differentiation between other primitive round cell tumours of childhood is vital (Table 20.7).

Immunocytochemistry and electron microscopy help in this process. The future definitive diagnosis of Ewing's sarcoma may be simplified by direct assays for the *EWS-FLI1* and *EWS-ERG* genes; currently these tests are only available in a research setting. Mic 2 is usually positive.

Treatment

Effective combination chemotherapy regimens have significantly improved the outlook for patients with Ewing's sarcoma and PNET. It is a particularly crucial part of the management as disseminated micrometastases are present in more than 90% of patients with apparently localized disease. If the primary tumour is easily resectable and arising in an expendable bone (or accessible soft tissue), then the lesion is usually surgically resected. Improving surgical techniques and allograft or endoprosthetic replacement mean this is increasingly possible with a satisfactory functional outcome.

Radiation treatment, particularly in children and adolescents, is associated with disruption of normal growth and also with an increased incidence of second, radiation-induced malignancy. This risk can be minimized by close attention to radiation dose. Radiotherapy, however, provides a useful adjunct to surgery in the presence of residual macroscopic or microscopic disease. For unresectable tumours, radiation to 40–60 Gy in combination with chemotherapy gives a high rate of local control.

Chemotherapy is indicated in all cases and is administered both before and after local therapy. Typically, patients will receive two or more cycles of induction therapy before surgery or radiotherapy and further cycles afterwards. Regimens have traditionally included vincristine, doxorubicin (Adriamycin), dactinomycin, and

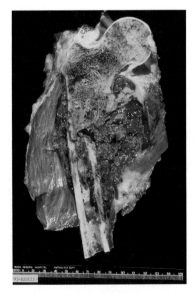

Fig. 20.6 Ewing's sarcoma: resected tumour from the same patient as in Fig. 20.5.

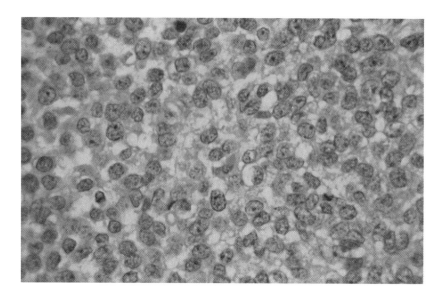

Fig. 20.7 Ewing's sarcoma: multiple, round, small, darkly staining cells.

cyclophosphamide (V Adria C or VAC). A large randomized trial showed improved outcome when patients received cycles of ifosfamide and etoposide alternating with vincristine, doxorubicin or dactinomycin, and cyclophosphamide. Treatment is protracted and patients receive chemotherapy for a year. Diminishing marrow reserves and intense chemotherapy mean that significant supportive care is needed for the inevitable myelotoxicity.

Tumours arising in the pelvis, ribs or proximal extremity have a poorer prognosis and this has led to attempts to intensify therapy in these patients. Similarly, patients with metastatic disease at presentation have a poor outlook. High-dose chemotherapy induction regimens, combined with autologous bone marrow transplantation (ABMT), or peripheral blood stem cell (PBSC) rescue have produced long-term survival in approximately 15% of cases. If pulmonary metastases are the only site of distant disease, then those that fail to show a complete response to chemotherapy, are irradiated or surgically resected. Generally, the outlook is better if relapse occurs after primary therapy. Management depends on the nature of previous treatment and may involve further chemotherapy with cytotoxic agents not previously used or aggressive treatment with myeloablative chemotherapy.

Table 20.8 Ewing's sarcoma indicators of poor prognosis

- Site – tumours of the pelvis, ribs, and upper extremity
- Size – tumours > 100 cm^3
- Presence of metastatic disease
- Extensive local soft tissue extension
- Failure of histological response to chemotherapy
- Type of *EWS-FLI 1* transcript

Prognosis

Prior to the development of effective chemotherapy, the 5-year survival rate for Ewing's sarcoma was only 5–15%. Now more than 50% of patients with localized Ewing's sarcoma are cured of their disease. This figure, however, drops to only 20–30% if identifiable metastases are present (Table 20.8).

Chondrosarcoma

Chondrosarcomas are malignant tumours of cartilage. Next to osteosarcoma, they are the second commonest matrix-producing bone tumour. They typically arise in mid- to later life and are rare before the age of 30 years. Men are affected twice as commonly as women. They have been associated with Paget's disease and fibrous dysplasia and may also arise within pre-existing bone disease such as osteochondromata or, more typically, within enchondromata.

They arise most frequently in the central portion of the skeleton, particularly the shoulder, pelvis and ribs (Fig. 20.8). When long bones are affected the tumour is almost always proximal. They usually present as slow growing, painful, progressively enlarging masses.

Chondrosarcomas vary in malignant appearance and are graded I–IV. The majority are well-differentiated lesions (grades I and II) which are associated with a low risk of metastatic spread. That risk increases significantly with grade III and high-grade, dedifferentiated (grade IV) lesions. Interestingly, 1 in 10 low-grade chondrosarcomas may have a second focus of high-grade, poorly differentiated sarcoma within them.

Plain x-ray films show scalloping of the endosteum (Fig. 20.9). The cortical appearance helps identify the likely grade. High-grade lesions cause cortical destruction and rapidly form a soft tissue mass, whereas low-grade tumours produce reactive cortical thickening. High-grade tumours are therefore more radiolucent. Once the diagnosis has been confirmed by needle biopsy, high-quality imaging of the tumour, with CT and MRI, is particularly important as most chondrosarcomas do not respond to chemotherapy or radiotherapy, making complete surgical excision particularly crucial if progressive locally recurrent disease is to be avoided. These tumours rarely invade nerves and can usually be safely resected even when they have reached a significant size and are awkwardly sited. Dedifferentiated tumours are more sensitive to radiotherapy and chemotherapy and may respond to combinations of doxorubicin (Adriamycin), cisplatin, and ifosfamide. Typical of bone sarcomas, the main sites of metastases are the lungs and other areas within bone.

Most chondrosarcomas are well-differentiated grade I and II lesions which carry 5-year survival rates of approximately 90% and 80%, respectively. Survival falls to around only 40% for grade III tumours and further still for high-grade, dedifferentiated, disease. Metastatic disease is rarely found in low-grade tumours but may exceed 70% in higher-grade chondrosarcoma.

Malignant fibrous histiocytoma

Malignant fibrous histiocytoma is a fibroblastic, collagen-producing, bone sarcoma making up approximately 5% of primary malignant bone tumours. It may

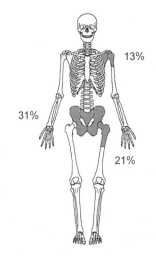

Fig. 20.8 Chondrosarcoma: common sites of origin.

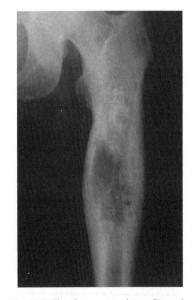

Fig. 20.9 Chondrosarcoma: plain radiograph.

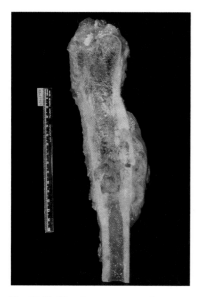

Fig. 20.10 Chondrosarcoma: resection specimen from same patient as in Fig. 20.9.

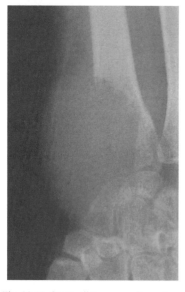

Fig. 20.11 Giant cell tumour: radiograph showing large giant cell tumour of the lower ulna, causing extensive bone destruction and an associated soft tissue mass.

affect any age but most commonly arises in the middle-aged and elderly and has a male preponderance. The majority arise in previously normal bone but one in five develop in areas of fibrous dysplasia, Paget's disease, bone infarction, or in association with previous therapeutic irradiation. The lesion usually develops in the metaphysis of the femur, tibia, humerus, or the flat bones of the pelvis. They are typically permeating, lytic tumours with prominent local extension into soft tissue and pathological fracture is not uncommon. Poor outcomes with surgery alone or in combination with radiotherapy have led to more intensive therapy with the addition of pre- and postoperative chemotherapy and current treatment is similar to that of osteosarcoma. It is anticipated that this approach will increase 5-year survival rates beyond the previous figure of approximately 30%.

Giant cell tumour

Giant cell tumours (Fig. 20.11) are uncommon, benign, but locally aggressive neoplasms. Histological examination reveals multinucleated giant cells, giving rise to the name. They typically arise in early to middle adult life. The majority develop around the knee but any bone may be affected. Radiologically, they are large lytic lesions which are eccentric and often destroy overlying bone cortex. A soft tissue mass may form surrounded by a shell of reactive bone. Although appearing histologically benign, occasionally they may metastasize to the lungs. Generally, their management involves complete surgical excision. Anything less is associated with a high local recurrence rate.

Adult soft tissue sarcomas

Soft tissue sarcomas are rare, malignant tumours, generally arising from mesenchymal tissue. They make up less than 1% of all invasive malignancy. Although bone and lymphoid tissue are mesenchymal in origin, primary tumours developing in these sites are considered separately and malignant tumours of peripheral nerve sheaths are included, despite their ectodermal origin, as they share a similar clinical pattern of disease. It is important to note that benign tumours of the soft tissues are many times more common (Suit, 1995).

Soft tissue sarcomas may arise in any location. The lower limb (40%) and the trunk, including the retroperitoneum (30%), are the commonest sites of origin. The remainder arise in the upper limb (20%) and head and neck (10%). Any age group may be affected, but 40% arise in patients over the age of 55 years. Fifteen per cent of tumours arise in children and they are the fourth commonest type of childhood malignancy (Cotran *et al.*, 1989). Rhabdomyosarcomas show a particular predilection for children and young adults, synovial sarcomas typically arise in late adolescence or young adulthood and malignant fibrous histiocytomas and liposarcomas arise in mid- to late adult life.

Histologically soft tissue sarcomas are markedly heterogeneous and accurate diagnosis requires an adequate tissue sample in the hands of an experienced sarcoma pathologist. Developments in immunohistochemistry and, to a lesser extent, cytogenetics, have assisted the pathologist in this regard. The principal determinant of treatment approach is tumour grade. Involvement or contamination of local, adjacent tissues governs planes of surgical resection and radiation fields, so the biopsy path of any suspicious lesion should be considered carefully.

Soft tissue sarcomas are often highly treatable, given appropriate management within a multidisciplinary team. In the past, radical surgery alone was considered the only approach likely to achieve cure. For sarcomas of the upper or lower limb this often meant amputation, as the risk of local recurrence was unacceptably high with simple local excision. The cosmetic, psychological, and functional effects were often devastating. Combining radiotherapy with more limited, conservative, non-amputative resection has produced similar local control and overall survival rates in high-grade sarcomas with greatly reduced functional and psychological morbidity. No clear benefit for adjuvant chemotherapy has been demonstrated, although a meta analysis of several studies suggests there may be some modest benefit for patients with extremity sarcomas (Sarcoma Meta analysis Collaboration, 1997). As with some primary malignant bone tumours, patients with pulmonary metastases may still be potentially curable through metastatectomy.

Aetiology

Most soft tissue sarcomas occur sporadically and aetiological factors behind the disease are unknown. There are, however, a number of well-recognized associations. The fundamental process once again is one of genetic mutation. The previously described hereditary syndromes of Li–Fraumeni and familial retinoblastoma are also associated with an increased incidence of soft tissue sarcomas. Loss or mutations of the relevant p53 and Rb tumour suppressor genes are also seen in some cases of apparently sporadic sarcomas. Gardner's syndrome is associated with an increased incidence of fibromatosis. Neurofibromas and neurofibrosarcomas arise with increased frequency in neruofibromatosis type 1 (von Recklinghausen's disease); malignant schwannomas are also more common in this condition and in multiple endocrine neoplasia (MEN). A high proportion of patients with malignant fibrous histiocytoma and liposarcomas show amplification of the *SAS* gene and overexpression of c-*erbB2* and EGF is a feature of a significant proportion of patients with soft tissue sarcomas.

Some chromosomal aberrations show a well-established association with certain sarcomas; one of the best examples of this is the translocation t(x;18) found in synovial sarcomas. The association is strong enough that a cytogenetic search for this can assist in making the definitive diagnosis (Suit *et al.*, 1995).

Radiation is well described as an aetiological factor in sarcomas. A dose–response relationship exists and the tumour usually only develops as a complication of high-dose therapy (> 40 Gy). The risk is small and is typically greatly outweighed by the indication for radiotherapy. In one large study of patients receiving radiotherapy for breast carcinoma, the incidence was 0.2%. Malignant fibrous histiocytoma is the commonest histological type in this setting. Cytotoxic chemotherapy may also increase the risk of sarcoma development as can exposure to certain industrial chemicals such as phenoxy herbicides, vinyl chloride, chlorophenols, arsenic, and phenoxyacetic acid. Patients with long-standing chronic lymphoedema show an increased risk of lymphosarcoma and angiosarcoma, a well-recognized complication of post-radical mastectomy upper limb lymphoedema. There is evidence that trauma and thermal or chemical burns may also precipitate sarcoma development.

There is also evidence that viruses may induce sarcoma development. The Rous sarcoma virus causes sarcomas in avians and human herpes virus 8 has been closely linked to the development of AIDS-related Kaposi's sarcoma.

Clinical presentation

These lesions typically present as a painless lump, which may have been present for weeks or months. Other local symptoms depend on pressure or infiltration of adjacent structures. Systemic symptoms such as fatigue, weight loss, and anaemia are usually indicative of metastatic disease but some soft tissue sarcomas, particularly malignant fibrous histiocytomas, may be associated with histamine-like reactions. Careful clinical examination should include a close assessment of the primary tumour with particular attention to site of origin, fixation to adjacent structures (including skin), muscular function, and status of nearby nerves and blood vessels. Regional lymph nodes should be assessed; the incidence of regional lymph nodal metastases is proportionally related to both the size and the grade of the tumour. Generally, they are only found with any frequency in association with tumours > 5 cm and/or of grade III histology. They are also more frequent in patients with rhabdomyosarcoma or epithelioid sarcoma.

Investigations

Investigations are aimed at assessing the primary lesion and also excluding metastatic disease. Lesions lying close to bone require plain radiographs looking for the cortical bone destruction that suggests bone involvement. CT and MRI are crucial in evaluating the local extent and any tumour invasion into adjacent structures. MRI scanning is now generally considered the imaging modality of choice. T2-weighted images particularly demonstrate the best contrast between tissues. All patients should

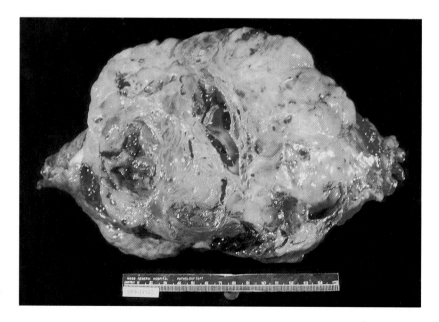

Fig. 20.12 Malignant fibrous histiocytoma: a large tumour resected from a patient's thigh.

have a whole lung CT scan to exclude lung metastases. Pulmonary metastases may not be clearly visible on plain chest radiographs. Biopsy of the suspicious lesion should be undertaken carefully using the CT or MRI images to plan a track that can easily be removed at definitive surgery and included in the radiation field if required. Biopsies of upper or lower limb lesions should be longitudinal and kept as short as possible whilst allowing the retrieval of an adequate and representative sample of tumour tissue. In general, a needle biopsy is considered only sufficient to diagnose recurrent or metastatic sarcoma, but in some cases it may be considered satisfactory to make the initial diagnosis if incisional biopsy would be a major surgical undertaking.

Pathological classification

Soft tissue sarcomas are classified according to their histological appearance and their similarity to a normal tissue counterpart. Current opinion suggests they develop from the neoplastic transformation of a primitive or stem-like mesenchymal cell that differentiates along one or several cell lines, depending on its contained genetic code. The final diagnosis may involve immunohistochemistry, cytogenetics studies, flow cytometry, electron microscopy, and molecular studies. Although histological classification carries prognostic relevance, the principal determinant of tumour behaviour, outcome, and hence management is tumour grade.

Pathological analysis will record the histological classification of the tumour, its grade, proximity to nearby normal structures, vascular invasion, the effect of any previous chemotherapy, expressed as percentage necrosis, and, finally, the width of normal tissue margins surrounding tumour and the presence or absence of tumour at those margins.

The best predictor of aggressiveness representing the potential for locoregional and distant metastases is tumour grade. Grading is based principally on a number of features (Cotran *et al.*, 1989) shown in Table 20.9. The first three are the most important. Sarcomas are described as low-, intermediate- or high-grade tumours. The designation of grade requires the opinion of an experienced pathologist.

A widely used classification of soft tissue sarcomas is the AJCC classification (Table 20.10). Light microscopy remains the modality of choice in assigning the

Table 20.9 Histological features considered when ascribing tumour grade

- Degree of differentiation
- Number of mitoses per high power field
- Extent of necrosis
- Pleomorphism
- Cellularity
- Vascularity
- Haemorrhage
- Vascular invasion
- Quantity of matrix

Table 20.10 AJCC classification of soft tissue sarcomas

- Alveolar soft-part sarcoma
- Angiosarcoma
- Dermatofibrosarcoma protuberans
- Epithelioid sarcoma
- Extraskeletal chondrosarcoma
- Extraskeletal osteosarcoma
- Fibrosarcoma
- Leiomyosarcoma
- Liposarcoma
- Malignant fibrous histiocytoma
- Malignant haemangiopericytoma
- Malignant mesenchymoma
- Malignant schwannoma
- Malignant peripheral nerve sheath tumours
- Peripheral neuroectodermal tumours
- Rhabdomyosarcoma
- Synovial sarcoma

Table 20.11 Immunohistochemical markers of soft tissue sarcomas

Antibody	Distribution
Vimentin	Most sarcomas and some carcinomas
Keratin	Most carcinomas and some sarcomas
Desmin	Leiomyosarcoma, rhabdomyosarcoma, and occasionally MFH
Neurofilament	PNET and neuroblastoma
Leucocyte common antigen	Lymphoma
S-100 protein	Malignant schwannoma, melanoma, clear cell, chondrosarcoma, leiomyosarcoma, rhabdomyosarcoma, liposarcoma
Myoglobin	Rhabdomyosarcoma
Factor VIII related antigen	Angiosarcoma, Kaposi's sarcoma
Actin	Leiomyosarcoma, rhabdomyosarcoma (MFH)
EMA	Carcinomas, synovial sarcoma, meningioma
Leu 7	Malignant schwannoma, leiomyosarcoma, synovial sarcoma, rhabdomyosarcoma

Table 20.12 **AJCC staging system for soft tissue sarcomas (TNMG)**

Grade and TNM definitions	
Histological tumour grade (G)	
Gx	Grade cannot be assessed
G1	Well differentiated
G2	Moderately differentiated
G3	Poorly differentiated
G4	Undifferentiated
Primary tumour (T)	
Tx	Primary tumour cannot be assessed
T0	No evidence of primary tumour
T1	Tumour 5 cm or less in greatest dimension
T1a	Superficial tumour
T1b	Deep tumour
T2	Tumour more than 5 cm in greatest dimension
T2a	Superficial tumour
T2b	Deep tumour
Regional lymph nodes (N)	
Nx	Regional lymph nodes cannot be assessed
N0	No regional lymph node metastases
N1	Regional lymph node metastases
Distant metastases (M)	
Mx	Distant metastases cannot be assessed
M0	No distant metastases
M1	Distant metastases
Stages	
Stage IA	Low-grade, small, superficial and deep tumours (G1/2, T1a/b, N0, M0)
Stage IB	Low-grade, large and superficial tumours (G1/2, T2a, N0, M0)
Stage IIA	Low-grade, large and deep tumours (G1/2, T2b, N0, M0)
Stage IIB	High-grade, small, superficial and deep tumours (G3/4, T1a/b, N0, M0)
Stage IIC	High-grade, large and superficial tumours (G3/4, T2a, N0, M0)
Stage III	High-grade, large and deep tumours (G3/4, T2b, N0, M0)
Stage IVA	Regional lymph node metastases but no distant metastases present (any G, any T, N1, M0)
Stage IVB	Distant metastases present (any G, any T, any N, M1)

cellular classification of a soft tissue tumour. However, advances in immuno-histochemistry, electron microscopy, DNA flow cytometry, cytogenetics, and molecular analysis often provide important supplemental information.

Immunohistochemical analysis involves the use of visually tagged monoclonal or polyclonal antibodies directed against specific proteins. Some examples are shown in Table 20.11 (Suit *et al.*, 1995). The detection of certain proteins may help identify a line of differentiation. Unfortunately, there is significant overlap and deviations from the expected distribution of antigens are not uncommon. Immunohistochemical analysis may also provide additional information on proliferative rate, the expression of growth factors, and some assessment of degree of drug resistance.

Staging

Staging has a crucial role in determining optimal therapy. The principal consider-ations are the size and grade of the primary tumour and the presence or absence of lymph node and distant metastases. The currently used scheme is an extension of the TNM system. Histopathological grade determines stage and tumour size determines substage (Table 20.12) (AJCC,1997). It applies to all soft tissue sarco-mas except Kaposi's sarcoma and rhabdomyosarcoma, the later has its own special system.

Management

Foremost amongst the changes that have taken place in the management of soft tissue sarcomas is the discovery that combining conservative surgery with radio-therapy produces equivalent local control rates and overall survival to more radical surgical procedures like amputation. The situation is analogous to that in breast cancer where, in certain circumstances, partial mastectomy together with radio-therapy is an equally viable option to radical mastectomy alone. High-grade soft tissue sarcomas of the extremities can now often be successfully treated while preserving the limb. There are obvious functional and psychological benefits to limb-conserving therapy.

Surgery

Before improvements in our understanding of the local biological behaviour of sarcomas, surgery involved simple resection without any real attention to wide surrounding margins of normal tissue. This approach was associated with unacceptable rates of local recurrence, as high as 75–90%. With a greater appre-ciation that microscopic disease extended beyond the limits of gross tumour, the recurrence rates dropped to 10–30% when more radical resections were employed, typically involving amputation for extremity tumours. Improvements in radio-logical imaging have further enhanced our appreciation of patterns of local tumour extension. Ideally any surgical procedure should involve resection of the pri-mary tumour with a wide margin of normal tissue; the track of any previous biopsy should also be removed as this is a well-recognized site of potential local recurrence. If the margins are histologically free of tumour, the rates of local recurrence are usually low (approximately 5%). Unfortunately, it is often not possible to remove tumours with a satisfactory margin of surrounding tissue whilst preserving function and sparing adjacent vital structures. When all patients are considered, the recurrence rates for surgery alone are in the region of 10–20%.

When small well-differentiated sarcomas arise in areas of the body where the cosmetic result of surgery is important, Moh's surgical technique may be an alternative. Tissue margins free of tumour can be assured with minimal normal tissue removal. This technique was originally devised for the excision of skin tumours by Frederick Moh who observed that injecting 20% zinc chloride into tissues resulted in the fixation and preservation of histological structure when later viewed under a microscope. When used *in situ*, the tumour could be excised and divided into segments and examined histologically. With careful orientation of specimens, the procedure can be repeated until all margins are free of disease and the entire tumour has been removed. Frozen sectioning has taken the place of the fixed tissue technique, now renamed Moh's micrographic surgery (Safai, 1997).

Radiotherapy

In the past sarcomas were thought to be largely resistant to radiotherapy. Clinical and laboratory research has shown them to be as radiosensitive as epithelial tumours. They do, however, require high doses of radiation for disease control. Radiotherapy has been used as the only treatment modality for patients who are unsuitable for surgery by virtue of tumour location, medical frailty, or patient choice.

Combined radiotherapy and surgery

The combination is based on the rationale that radiation can eradicate the small number of tumour cells left behind after conservative surgery that would other-wise have been removed by more extensive surgery. This combined modality approach produces local control rates and overall survival similar to those obtained by radical surgery alone, but with improved functional and cosmetic results (Table 20.13).

Table 20.13 Treatment overview

Grade I tumours	
• Easily resected with generous margins and good functional and cosmetic result, margins microscopically free of tumour	Surgery alone
Grade II and III tumours	
• Diagnosis known preoperatively	Preoperative radiotherapy followed by surgery. Postoperative radiotherapy (if positive margins in the resection specimen)
• Small lesions found unexpectedly to be sarcomatous after resection	Postoperative radiotherapy

Table 20.14 **Common regimens**

IA	Ifosphamide and Adriamycin
MAID	Adriamycin, Ifosphamide with Mesna (a urothelial protective agent) and Dacarbazine. Administered on a 21 day cycle

Chemotherapy

A number of agents have shown activity in soft tissue sarcoma. The most active of these are doxorubicin (Adriamycin), ifosphamide, dacarbazine, cisplatin, and methotrexate. Of these, the most commonly used agent is doxorubicin and most combination regimens contain this drug (Table 20.14). Many patients with disseminated metastatic disease may derive symptomatic benefit from such palliative chemotherapy and response rates of 25–40% can be expected.

Adjuvant chemotherapy

Whilst a combination of surgery and radiotherapy can locally control most primary tumours, unfortunately, a significant number of patients with grade II or III tumours will subsequently develop, and die of, metastatic disease. Despite the fact that chemotherapy produces significant responses in patients with metastatic disease, studies using it in an adjuvant setting (to treat occult micrometastases) have generally failed to produce any improvement in overall survival. They have, however, consistently shown an increase in the disease-free interval. A recent meta analysis of 14 trials involving 1568 patients again showed that chemotherapy increases the time to local and distant relapse and overall recurrence-free survival. A trend towards improved overall survival was observed, but this did not reach significance; the best evidence of survival benefit was seen in patients with sarcomas of the extremities (Sarcoma Meta analysis Collaboration, 1997). Adjuvant chemotherapy in rhabdomyosarcoma, osteosarcoma, and Ewing's/PNET is now standard and its efficacy is beyond doubt.

Pulmonary metastatectomy

The resection of pulmonary metastases can result in cure for significant numbers of patients. With careful patient selection, 5-year survival figures of between 26% and 34% have been recorded. Clearly this is only appropriate to consider when lung metastases are the only site of disease (Table 20.15). The prognosis relates primarily to the biological behaviour of the tumour. Some indication of this is

Table 20.15 **Guidelines for pulmonary metastatectomy**

- Primary tumour is controlled
- No evidence of extrapulmonary metastases
- Metastases technically resectable
- General condition and respiratory status good enough for surgery
- Tumour doubling time of at least 40 days

Table 20.16.   Overall and disease-free survival in soft tissue sarcoma

Stage	Freedom from local recurrence	Disease-free survival	Overall survival
I	79.09%	77.91%	98.79%
II	75.16%	63.63%	81.80%
III	74.46%	36.27%	51.65%

given by the disease-free interval (i.e. length of time from resection of the primary tumour to the appearance of metastases) and the tumour doubling time, which can be estimated by measurements from serial radiographs. The same guidelines apply to pulmonary metastatectomy in soft tissue sarcoma as do in bone sarcoma patients (Joseph, 1974). Multiple metastases can be resected, but the success rate of the procedure falls if multiple resections are necessary.

Prognosis

The outcome for patients with soft tissue sarcomas is adversely affected by a number of factors. Large (> 5 cm), high-grade tumours with spread to regional lymph nodes or distant sites carry a poorer outlook as does disease arising in older patients (> 60 years). Figures for local control, disease-free and overall survivals are shown in Table 20.16 (AJCC, 1997).

Rhabdomyosarcoma (RMS)

Rhabdomyosarcomas are worthy of specific reference as, unlike most other soft tissue sarcomas, they have a particular predilection for occurrence in childhood and their treatment has been the subject of intensive investigation. They represent the commonest soft tissue malignancy in children and infants with a median age at diagnosis of 4 years. It is a curable disease in the majority who receive optimal therapy, with more than 60% alive 5 years after diagnosis. The commonest sites of origin in order of frequency are the head and neck, the genitourinary tract, the extremities, and thorax. There are three main histological subtypes: embryonal, alveolar, and pleomorphic rhabdomyosarcoma.

Embryonal RMS makes up 60–70% of childhood RMS and typically arise in the orbit or genitourinary tract. They are composed of small, round cells. The botryoid subtype develops as a polypoid tumour, arising from the mucosal surfaces of visceral organs or body orifices such as vagina and bladder. When appearing in adults, they unfortunately carry a poorer outcome despite responding to paediatric chemotherapy regimens. A consistent cytogenetic finding is the loss of genetic material from the short arm of chromosome 11 (11p15 region), suggesting that tumour development involves the loss of a tumour suppressor gene at that location.

Alveolar RMS typically develops on the extremities or trunk of adolescents or young adults. It is composed of aggregates of poorly defined, round or oval cells and loss of cellular adhesion may produce irregular spaces. Most cases are associated with one of two characteristic translocations between the *FKHR* gene on chromosome 13 and either the *PAX* gene on chromosome 2 (70%) or the *PAX* gene on chromosome 1 (20%). They carry a poorer prognosis in children than embryonal RMS.

Pleomorphic RMS is the commonest form of the tumour in adults, where it behaves much like any other high-grade sarcoma.

Unlike other soft tissue sarcomas, rhabdomyosarcomas more commonly metastasize to bone, bone marrow, and lymph nodes, so staging investigations will involve assessment of regional lymph nodes and careful radiological bone evaluation and bone marrow aspirate and trephine in addition to CT scan of the lungs. Treatment involves a multidisciplinary approach. All children should receive chemotherapy, the composition and duration of which depends on appropriate risk factor analysis. If possible, surgical resection is performed. The original extent of the tumour and the results of surgical resection govern decisions regarding radiotherapy. In an attempt to maximize survival rates whilst minimizing the long-term consequences of chemotherapy, children with favourable prognostic disease usually require treatment with only two cytotoxic agents, vincristine and dactinomycin. Cyclophosphamide (or ifosfamide) is added (VAC) if the disease involves the orbit or has less favourable prognostic features. Other regimens that are also in use involve the sequencing of differing cycles of combination chemotherapy in an attempt to minimize the effects of drug resistance.

Kaposi's sarcoma (KS)

First described in 1872 by Moritz Kaposi, an Austro-Hungarian dermatologist, this dermal tumour warrants specific mention because of its association with AIDS. Prior to the HIV epidemic the tumour was rare.

Four types of Kaposi's sarcoma are recognized which, although of similar histopathological appearance, show different clinical features and course of disease. Classic KS is mainly seen in elderly men of Italian/Eastern European Jewish ancestry and appears as single or multiple purple-red skin lesions on the lower limbs, especially around the ankles. It typically shows a slow, indolent course over many years, but metastases finally develop. Such patients also have an increased risk of second malignancy, typically non-Hodgkin's lymphoma. African KS is more common and endemic in the native population of equatorial Africa. Its behaviour varies from relative indolence to aggressive, locally invasive disease. As with classic KS, it shows a strong predilection for males, although of a younger age. KS is also associated with the use of immunosuppressant therapy, particularly in patients with transplanted organs. Discontinuation or modulation of immunosuppressant treatment, if possible, may produce disease regression and should always be considered when KS arises in this setting.

Epidemic KS is a fulminant and often widely disseminated form of the disease, which was first described in young homosexual and bisexual men in 1981. We now know this to be associated with the disease AIDS (Fig. 20.13). The presence of human herpes virus 8 has been clearly linked to KS, but the virus has not been shown to transform or immortalize cells, which would more strongly suggest

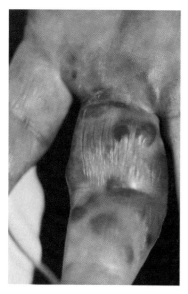

Fig. 20.13 Kaposi's sarcoma in a patient with AIDS.

causation. The incidence of KS within the AIDS population is linked to the mode of disease acquisition. Heterosexual and intravenous drug users with HIV have a much lower risk of KS compared with homosexually acquired disease. The incidence of KS in AIDS patients is falling. The lesions may affect skin, oral mucosa, lymph nodes, or visceral organs. It usually becomes disseminated in these patients, although typically opportunistic infection is the cause of death. Homosexual men without any evidence of HIV infection are also at increased risk of KS, although this form of the disease is more typically indolent and affects the genitalia and extremities.

Treatment depends on the extent of disease. Single or small numbers of cutaneous lesions may best be treated with local therapy. Relatively low-dose radiotherapy in single or small numbers of fractions often provides good local control. Intra-lesional chemotherapy with such agents as vinblastine can also be effective, especially in the case of intraoral lesions where radiotherapy may be difficult. Surgical excision or cryotherapy may be used, but recurrence is relatively common. Sometimes simple cosmetic camouflage may be sufficient, but this often does not conceal the full thickness of the lesion or its nodularity.

Severe oro-cutaneous or symptomatic visceral disease requires systemic therapy. High-dose interferon has been successfully used, but patients with visceral disease or a history of opportunistic infection are less likely to respond. Single agent or combinations of cytotoxic drugs have been investigated. Doxorubicin, bleomycin, vinblastine, and etoposide have all shown activity. Bleomycin and vinblastine alone (BV) or with doxorubicin (Adriamycin) (ABV) have been used effectively, giving response rates of approximately 25%. Recent studies suggest that single-agent liposomal-encapsulated anthracyclines, particularly pegylated liposomal doxorubicin (PLD), are more effective, with response rates between 45 and 60%, but at the expense of myelosuppression. Taxanes have also shown activity.

Desmoid tumours

These uncommon tumours are benign but locally aggressive, with a propensity for local recurrence following apparently complete resection. They are also known as aggressive fibromatoses. Their aetiology is unclear, but they are found in association with some genetic diseases such as Gardner's syndrome. An association with trauma has also been suggested as they may arise in the anterior abdominal wall of postpartum women or in surgical wounds.

Although they do not metastasize, they may be locally destructive and progress relentlessly, possibly with fatal consequences, depending on their location. Microscopic projections of tumour often extend well beyond the visible extent of the main tumour, hence optimum management involves surgical resection with a wide margin. Patients with unresectable lesions, or who are unfit for, or, decline surgery, may be treated with radiotherapy. Local control of the tumour is possible in most cases. The majority will be cured with a radiation dose of 60 Gy in 6–8 weeks. Radiation can also be used to control postoperative local recurrence. Interestingly, the majority of patients who have microscopically positive margins after surgery will never develop recurrence. For this reason postoperative radiotherapy is not routinely recommended in these patients, provided they comply

Case history

Four years ago a 13-year-old boy presented to his GP with a 2-month history of pain in the left knee. The pain had been increasing, was particularly noticeable at night, and the boy had begun to limp. The attendance at the GP was precipitated when swelling developed just proximal to the knee joint. Plain radiographs of the lower femur showed a large, poorly delineated sclerotic and destructive lesion in the metaphyseal region. The lesion had breached the cortex and the periosteum was elevated, giving rise to the classical appearance of Codman's triangle. Bone spicules were visible at right angles to the long axis of the femur. CT and MRI scanning showed a destructive tumour without any evidence of neurovascular invasion.

A core needle biopsy confirmed the presence of osteosarcoma. Staging CT scans of the lungs showed no evidence of lung metastases and an isotope bone scan showed only the tumour at the lower end of the femur; there were no skip lesions or distant bone metastases. An echocardiograph was normal.

Treatment commenced with two cycles of chemotherapy with cisplatin and doxorubicin. This was well tolerated with the exception of a lower respiratory tract infection associated with mild neutropenia, midway through the second cycle. This responded quickly to broad-spectrum antibiotics. Repeat MRI scanning after two cycles of chemotherapy showed significant reduction in tumour size and changes in the signal, in keeping with marked tumour necrosis. Resection of the lower femur, upper tibia, and fibula was performed 5 weeks after the second cycle of chemotherapy and an endoprosthesis and artificial joint were inserted. Histopathology confirmed almost 95% tumour necrosis with only a little viable osteosarcoma remaining. The margins of excision were all clear of disease. A further four cycles of cisplatin and doxorubicin were delivered.

The boy remained well until 2 years later, when a routine chest radiograph revealed a solitary lung metastasis. CT scanning confirmed the solitary nature of the lesion; examination and radiological imaging of the site of previous surgery showed no evidence of locally recurrent tumour. An isotope bone scan was unremarkable. The metastatic lesion was surgically resected. The young man, now 18 years old, remains alive and well and free of disease.

with a strict surveillance policy of close follow-up for several years. Recurrent tumour should be treated aggressively. Occasional reports of spontaneous disease resolution or regression with oestrogens or indomethacin have been recorded. Chemotherapy with vinblastine and methotrexate or with doxorubicin has also helped control this low-grade tumour.

Acknowledgements

The authors would like to thank Andrew E. Rosenberg MD, Department of Pathology, Massachusetts General Hospital, for supplying the photographs and Simonne Longerich MSc, Department of Hematology/Oncology, Massachusetts General Hospital, for her helpful advice with the graphics.

Further reading

American Joint Committee on Cancer (AJCC) (1997) *Cancer staging manual*, 5th edn, pp. 144, 149–56. Lippincott-Raven, Philadelphia.

Cotran, R. S., Kumar, V., and Robbins, S. L. (1989) *Robbins pathologic basis of disease*, 4th edn, pp. 1315–84. W. B. Saunders, Philadelphia and London.

Eilber, F., Giuliano, A., Eckardt, J., *et al.* (1987) Adjuvant chemotherapy for osteosarcoma: a randomized prospective trial. *J Clin Oncol* 5(1), 21–6.

Enneking, W. F., Spanier, S. S., and Goodman, M. A. (1980) A system for the surgical staging of musculo-skeletal sarcomata. *Clin Orthop* 153,106–20.

Green, D. M. (1985) *Diagnosis and management of solid tumors in infants and children*. Martinus Nijhoff, Boston.

Huvos, A. G. (1979) *Bone tumors. Diagnosis, treatment and prognosis*. W. B. Saunders, Philadelphia and London.

Joseph, W. L. (1974) Criteria for resection of sarcoma metastatic to the lung. *Cancer Chemother Rep* 58, 285–90.

Link, M. P., Goorin, A. M., Miser, A. W., *et al.* (1986) The effect of adjuvant chemotherapy on relapse-free survival in patients with osteosarcoma of the extremity. *N Engl J Med* 314(25), 1600–6.

Malawer, M. M., Link, M. P., and Donaldson, S. S. (1997) Sarcomas of bone. In De Vita, V. T., Hellman, S., and Rosenberg, S. T. (eds), *Cancer: principles and practice of oncology*, 5th edn, pp. 1789–52. Lippincott-Raven, Philadelphia.

Moore, K. L. (1992) *Clinically orientated anatomy*, 3rd edn. Williams & Wilkins, Baltimore.

Price, P. and Sikora, K. (eds) (1995) *Treatment of cancer*, 3rd edn, pp. 775–823. Chapman & Hall Medical, London.

Safai, B. (1997) Management of skin cancer. In De Vita, V. T., Hellman, S., and Rosenberg, S. T. (eds), *Cancer: principles and practice of oncology*, 5th edn, pp. 1789–52. Lippincott-Raven, Philadelphia.

Sarcoma Meta analysis Collaboration (1997) Adjuvant chemotherapy for localised resectable soft-tissue sarcoma of adults: meta analysis of individual data. *Lancet* 350, 1647–54.

Schajowicz, F., Sissons, H. A., and Sobin, L. H. (1995) The World Health Organization's histologic classification of bone tumors: a commentary on the second edition. *Cancer* 75(5), 1208–14.

Souhami, R. L., Cassoni, A. M., and Cobb, J. P. (1995) Bone. In Price, P. and Sikora, K. (eds), *Treatment of cancer*, 3rd edn, pp. 775–94. Chapman & Hall Medical, London.

Suit, H. D., Rosenberg, A. E., Harmon, D. C., Mankin, H. J., Spiro, I. J., and Rosenthal, D. (1995) Soft tissue sarcomas. In Price, P. and Sikora, K. (eds), *Treatment of cancer*, 3rd edn, pp. 795–823. Chapman & Hall Medical, London.

Ward, W. G., Mikaelian, K., Dorey, F., *et al.* (1994) Pulmonary metastases of stage IIB extremity osteosarcoma and subsequent pulmonary metastases. *J Clin Oncol* 12(9), 1849–58.

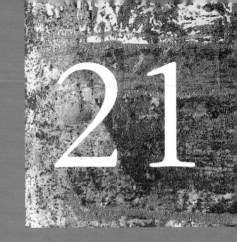

Paediatric solid tumours
Peter C. Adamson and Brigitte C. Widemann

- Introduction
- Neuroblastoma
- Nephroblastoma (Wilms' tumour)
- Rhabdomyosarcoma
- Retinoblastoma
- Hepatic tumours
- Germ cell tumours

Paediatric solid tumours

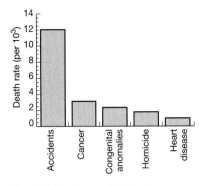

Introduction

Remarkable progress in the treatment of childhood cancer has been made over the past 40 years, such that today more than 70% of children diagnosed with cancer can be expected to be cured of their disease. Cancer remains, however, the second leading cause of death in children younger than 15 years, and the leading cause of death from disease (Fig. 21.1).

In contrast to adult cancers, which are predominantly of epithelial origin (Table 21.1), most childhood solid tumours are of mesenchymal or embryonal origin. The annual incidence of childhood cancers is shown in Fig. 21.2. Acute lymphoblastic leukemia (ALL), the most common childhood malignancy, accounts for nearly one-quarter of all childhood cancers. With the use of multi-agent chemotherapy, the prognosis for children with ALL has improved dramatically (see Chapter 19). The outcome of children with brain tumours, the most frequent solid tumour of childhood, varies considerably depending on histology and extent of disease. Childhood brain tumours are presented in Chapter 23.

This chapter reviews the common non-central nervous system solid tumours of childhood, which include neuroblastoma, Wilms' tumour, rhabdomyosarcoma, retinoblastoma, malignant hepatic tumours, and germ cell tumours. Solid tumours arising from bone, which include Ewing's sarcoma and osteosarcoma, are presented in Chapter 20.

Fig. 21.1 Significance of childhood cancers: leading causes of death in children younger than 15 years.

Neuroblastoma

Neuroblastoma is a malignant embryonal tumour derived from primordial neural crest cells, which ultimately populate the sympathetic ganglia, adrenal medulla, and other sites. The clinical behaviour of neuroblastoma is diverse. In addition to forms that may undergo spontaneous regression and differentiation, neuroblastoma often exhibits extremely malignant behaviour. Neuroblastoma in infants

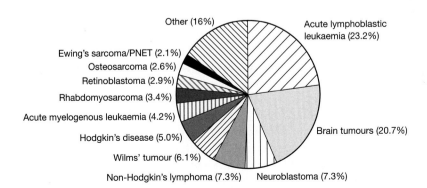

Fig. 21.2 Annual incidence of cancer in children younger than 15 years by diagnosis.

Table 21.1 Features of cancer in adults and children

	Adults	Children
Incidence	Common	Rare
Origin	Epithelial	Embryonal/mesenchymal
Aetiology	Environmental	Developmental
Kinetics	Slow growing	Rapid growing
Chemosensitivity	Low	High
Curability	Low	High

< 1 year of age tends to have a good prognosis, even in the presence of metastatic disease, with minimal or no treatment. The outcome for children diagnosed after the first year of life is significantly worse.

Epidemiology

Following brain tumours, neuroblastoma is the most commonly occurring solid tumour of childhood, with an incidence of approximately 8.0 per million per year in children younger than 15 years of age. Neuroblastoma accounts for 8–10% of all childhood cancers. It is predominantly a tumour of young children, with 80% of cases occurring before the age of 4 years.

Aetiology, genetics, and molecular biology

Neuroblastomas are characterized cytogenetically by deletion of the short arm of chromosome 1, potentially resulting in deletion of a tumour suppressor gene. Amplification of the N-*myc* proto-oncogene, which occurs in about 35% of newly diagnosed patients, is associated with advanced disease, rapid tumour progression, and a poor prognosis. The DNA index (DI), which represents the DNA content of tumour cells and correlates with the modal chromosome number, is also an important prognostic factor in neuroblastomas. Tumours that are hyperdiploid (DI > 1) are associated with lower stage disease and a better response to therapy.

Other neurotropic factors and their receptors may play a role in the pathogenesis and biology of neuroblastoma. Expression of the *trkA* gene, a tyrosine kinase receptor which encodes the primary receptor for neurotrophin-3, has been associated with good prognosis neuroblastoma.

Pathology

Histologically, neuroblastomas are heterogeneous, displaying a pathological spectrum ranging from the malignant, undifferentiated neuroblastoma to the mature, benign ganglioneuroma. The two predominant cell types comprising neuroblastoma are the neuroblast, which can differentiate into a ganglion cell, and the Schwann cell, which is responsible for the stromal element of the tumour. Undifferentiated neuroblastoma belongs to the group of small, round, blue cell tumours of childhood, with uniformly sized cells containing dense, hyperchromatic nucleoli and scant cytoplasm. Undifferentiated neuroblastoma can be differentiated histologically from other small, round, blue cell tumours of childhood (rhabdomyosarcoma, Ewing's sarcoma, non-Hodgkin's lymphoma) by the presence of Homer–Wright pseudo-rosettes, which are composed of neuroblasts surrounding areas of eosinophilic neutrophils (neuritic processes). Electron microscopy and immunohistochemistry are helpful adjuncts to light microscopy. Neuroblastoma stains with monoclonal antibodies recognizing neurofilaments, synaptophysin, and neuron-specific enolase (NSE).

The pathological classification of neuroblastoma, developed by Shimada, divides tumours into favourable and unfavourable histological groups. It is based on the degree of differentiation of neuroblasts, the presence/absence of Schwann cells, and the proliferative index of the tumour.

Clinical presentation

Neuroblastoma can arise anywhere along the sympathetic chain, from the neck to the pelvis, and from the adrenal glands. The site of the primary tumour is correlated with the age of the child, with abdominal primaries occurring more often in children > 1 year of age. Presenting signs and symptoms are a function of the primary site, presence and location of metastases, and presence of paraneoplastic syndromes (Table 21.2). Horner's syndrome, with unilateral ptosis, miosis, and absence of sweating, may occur with cervical or thoracic primaries. Invasion of paraspinal lesions through the neural foramina may lead to epidural lesions (termed 'dumb-bell' lesions because of their characteristic radiographic appearance), which may result in nerve root or spinal cord compression. The presence of back pain, radicular pain, paraplegia, or bladder and bowel symptoms should result in prompt evaluation for potential cord compression.

A typical case presentation for metastatic neuroblastoma is a 3–4-year-old pale, irritable child with a limp as a result of bony metastases, and periorbital ecchymoses as a result of orbital and retrobulbar tumour invasion (Fig. 21.3). The latter finding may be confused with child abuse. Typical findings for neuroblastoma in an infant are the presence of subcutaneous tumour nodules and an enlarged liver, which can result in respiratory distress.

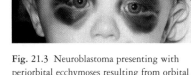

Fig. 21.3 Neuroblastoma presenting with periorbital ecchymoses resulting from orbital metastases. (Courtesy Nita L. Seibel, George Washington School of Medicine, Washington, DC).

Table 21.2 Neuroblastoma: symptoms and signs

Tumour site	Symptoms/signs
Abdominal	Abdominal distension, mass, pain
Thoracic	Silent (detection on routine chest radiograph), cough, Horner's syndrome
Paraspinal	Neurological symptoms (paralysis, pain)
Cervical	Horner's syndrome, mass
Metastatic	Bone pain, proptosis, periorbital ecchymosis, fever, weight loss, irritability, pancytopenia
Paraneoplastic	
Opsomyoclonus	Myoclonic jerking, random eye movement
Verner–Morrison syndrome	Secretory diarrhoea, dehydration, hypokalaemia

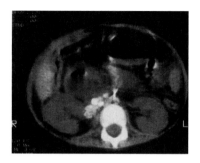

Fig. 21.4 Computed tomographic scan of the abdomen in a patient with neuroblastoma. The tumour arises from the adrenal gland. (Courtesy Nita L. Seibel, George Washington School of Medicine, Washington, DC).

Table 21.3 Neuroblastoma diagnostic work-up

Primary tumour	CT/MRI, MIBG scan or ^{99m}Tc bone scan
Metastases	Bilateral bone marrow aspirate and biopsy
	Chest radiograph
	MIBG scan or ^{99m}Tc bone scan
	Spine MRI (paraspinal disease)
	CT/MRI scan of head and orbits, abdomen
Tumour markers	Urinary catecholamine metabolites (VMA, HVA)
	Serum markers: NSE, LDH, ferritin

Diagnosis

The diagnostic work-up for neuroblastoma includes radiographic imaging of the primary tumour and assessment for metastatic disease spread (Table 21.3). Abdominal CT is helpful in differentiating neuroblastoma from other childhood intra-abdominal masses (Fig. 21.4). Stippled calcifications are seen in 50% of abdominal tumours on plain x-ray. MIBG (meta-iodobenzylguanidine) scans are particularly useful in the diagnosis and work-up of patients with neuroblastoma, as this tracer is selectively taken up by catecholaminergic cells. Urinary catecholamine metabolites – homovanillic acid (HVA) and vanillylmandelic acid (VMA) – are increased in more than 90% of patients, and are helpful in confirming the diagnosis of neuroblastoma and in following disease activity. Serum lactate dehydrogenase (LDH), ferritin, and NSE are non-specific tumour markers, and significant elevations are associated with a poorer outcome.

The diagnosis of neuroblastoma is confirmed by pathological diagnosis from a tumour biopsy. If at all possible, the biopsy specimen should be sufficiently large to allow for the analysis of genetic and biological markers. In absence of a biopsy, the finding of typical tumour cells in the bone marrow in the presence of elevated urinary catecholamine metabolites allows for the diagnosis.

Staging

The age of a patient with neuroblastoma correlates with the extent of disease, with children over 1 year more likely to present with disseminated disease. Neuroblastoma tends to spread to regional lymph nodes and haematogenously to bone marrow, bone, liver, and skin. Disease spread to the lung and brain parenchyma is uncommon. The International Neuroblastoma Staging System (INSS) is now the preferred staging system (Table 21.4).

One subgroup of patients present with a clinically and prognostically distinct pattern of disease. These children, who are younger than 1 year, present with a localized, unilateral primary tumour and dissemination to the liver, bone marrow (not bone), and skin, a stage of disease termed IV-S. Children with stage IV-S neuroblastoma do well, with minimal or no therapy, despite the presence of metastatic disease. This is in contrast to children older than 1 year with metastatic disease who are rarely cured even with aggressive treatment approaches.

Table 21.4 **International Neuroblastoma Staging System (INSS)**

Stage	Description
1	Localized tumour confined to area of origin, complete gross excision, positive or negative microscopic residual disease; identifiable ipsilateral and contralateral lymph nodes negative
2A	Unilateral tumour with incomplete gross excision; identifiable ipsilateral and contralateral lymph nodes negative microscopically
2B	Unilateral tumour with complete or incomplete gross excision; identifiable ipsilateral lymph nodes positive, and contralateral lymph nodes negative microscopically
3	Tumour infiltrating across the midline; or unilateral tumour with positive contralateral lymph nodes; or midline tumour with bilateral lymph node involvement
4	Tumour dissemination to distant lymph nodes, bone, bone marrow, liver or other organs (except 4S)
4S	Localized primary tumour (stage 1 or 2) with dissemination limited to skin, liver or bone marrow

Treatment

The current treatment of neuroblastoma is based on the INSS tumour stage and other clinical and biological variables. Treatment approaches for neuroblastoma range from observation alone to intensive chemotherapy followed by bone marrow transplantation. Treatment components include surgery, chemotherapy, and radiation therapy. Neuroblastoma at diagnosis is a chemosensitive tumour, but metastatic disease is rarely cured with chemotherapy. Active agents include cyclophosphamide, platinum analogues, doxorubicin, epidophyllotoxins, and vincristine. Radiation therapy has a role in local control for primary unresectable tumours, regional lymph node spread, epidural spread, and in cases of massive hepatomegaly from hepatic tumour. Because of the poor long-term results with chemotherapy for stage IV neuroblastoma, myelo-ablative chemotherapy with total body irradiation followed by autologous bone marrow transplantation has been evaluated as front-line consolidation therapy and may improve the outcome for these patients.

Prognosis

The disease-free survival of neuroblastoma varies from > 85% for children with localized, low-risk disease to < 20% for older children with disseminated disease.

Nephroblastoma (Wilms' tumour)

Wilms' tumour, an embryonal tumour, is the most common renal tumour of childhood, comprising 90% of the renal tumours observed in this age group. The combined use of surgery, chemotherapy, and radiation therapy has led to high cure rates even for children who present with metastatic disease.

Table 21.5 Wilms' tumour: Associated congenital syndromes

Syndrome	Description	Genetics	Incidence Wilms' tumour
WAGR	Wilms' tumour, aniridia, genitourinary malformations, mental retardation	Constitutional deletion at 11p13	30–50%
Dennys–Drash	Pseudohermaphroditism, nephrotic syndrome, Wilms' tumour	*WT1* mutation	> 30%
Beckwith–Wiedemann	Macroglossia, organomegaly, hemihypertrophy, neonatal hypoglycaemia, embryonal tumours	11p15; loss of maternal IGF2 allele or loss of imprinting	< 5%

Epidemiology

The mean age at diagnosis for patients with unilateral disease is 44 months, and for patients with bilateral disease 31 months. More than 80% of patients present before the age of 5 years. Wilms' tumour is strongly associated with several congenital syndromes (Table 21.5). These syndromes account for less than 1% of all children with Wilms' tumour, but identify patients with a high risk for the development of Wilms' tumour and have helped in the identification of Wilms' tumour suppressor genes.

Genetics and molecular biology

The development of Wilms' tumour has been described by Knudson's 'two-event hypothesis', which was originally applied to retinoblastoma (see page 398). The model suggests that Wilms' tumour is due to loss of two copies of a tumour suppressor gene. Children with a genetic susceptibility have a constitutional (germline) genetic change leading to loss of one allele, either inherited from one parent or resulting from a spontaneous mutation. Only one additional genetic event (mutation) is required for tumour formation. By contrast, in sporadic cases of Wilms' tumour, two rare independent somatic mutations are required for tumour development. The younger mean age of presentation in patients with bilateral Wilms' tumour is consistent with this two-hit hypothesis.

A tumour suppressor gene, Wilms' tumour 1 gene (*WT1*), has been identified and is located on the short arm of chromosome 11 (11p13). A second putative Wilms' tumour gene (*WT2*) has been localized to the short arm of chromosome 11 (11p15), the locus of the Beckwith–Wiedemann syndrome (*BWS*) gene. The candidate genes for the *WT2* gene include the insulin-like growth factor type 2 (*IGF2*) gene and the *H19* gene. Both genes are imprinted (expression of each allele of a gene depends on its parental origin). *IGF2* is imprinted from the paternal allele and *H19* from the maternal allele. The presence of two paternal copies of the

11p15 region has been associated with *BWS* and the development of Wilms' tumour. Loss of imprinting of *IGF2* and loss of heterozygosity by mitotic recombination can both lead to a doubling *IGF2* dose and silencing of *H19*.

Pathology

Most Wilms' tumours are unilateral and unicentric. In contrast to neuroblastoma, tumour calcifications are observed in only 10% of cases. The classic histology of Wilms' tumour involves a triphasic pattern of blastemal, stromal, and epithelial elements. Anaplasia is found in 5% of Wilms' tumours and is associated with a poor outcome (Fig. 21.5). Wilms' tumour must be differentiated from clear cell sarcoma and rhabdoid tumour of the kidney. These are highly malignant tumours, have a higher frequency of metastasis to the brain and bone, and carry a poor prognosis. Congenital mesoblastic nephroma, a rare, distinctive tumour of the kidney, occurs predominantly in males, presents during infancy, and is characterized by a benign outcome, curable by nephrectomy alone. Nephrogenic rests, precursor lesions of Wilms' tumour, are found in 25–40% of kidneys with unilateral and in all patients with bilateral Wilms' tumour.

Clinical presentation

The typical presentation (Table 21.6) is that of a rapidly enlarging abdominal mass in an otherwise healthy appearing child, which is often noticed by a parent. Palpation of the abdomen should be performed gently to avoid rupture of the tumour capsule. Associated congenital malformations are present in over 12% of the patients. Paraneoplastic syndromes are uncommon. Wilms' tumour spreads locally into the renal capsule, resulting in the formation of an inflammatory pseudocapsule, and into intrarenal blood and lymphatic vessels. Distant spread is most common to the lungs, followed by liver and lymph nodes. For other renal tumours of childhood, spread to bone (clear cell sarcoma) and brain (rhabdoid tumour) commonly occur.

Diagnosis

The primary renal tumour, including the renal vein and inferior vena cava, as well as the contralateral kidney, must be imaged appropriately. Modalities commonly employed include ultrasound, CT, and MRI. An intravenous pyelogram (IVP) is also performed. The IVP in Wilms' tumour usually shows distortion of the collecting system of the affected side, whereas the collecting system is typically displaced in neuroblastoma. Unlike neuroblastoma, Wilms' tumour is less frequently disseminated at the time of diagnosis. The performance of a chest CT to

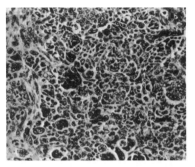

(a)

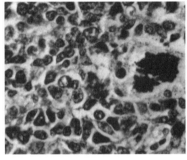

(b)

Fig. 21.5 Histology of Wilms' tumour. (a) Favourable histology with well-defined tubules surrounded by blastemal cells and zones of pale staining stromal differentiation. (b) Unfavourable (anaplastic) histology with several enlarged, hyperchromatic, bizarre nuclei. (Reproduced with permission from Green, D. M. (1993) Chapter 30. In Pizzo, P. and Poplack, D. (eds), *Principles and practice of pediatric oncology*, J. B. Lippincott, Philadelphia)

Table 21.6 Wilms' tumour: clinical presentation

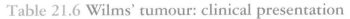

Symptoms/signs	Common: asymptomatic abdominal mass
	Less common: haematuria, pain, fever, anaemia
Associated anomalies	Aniridia, genitourinary anomalies, hemihypertrophy
Paraneoplastic	Hypertension (renin), erythrocytosis, hypercalcaemia (rhabdoid tumour)

rule out pulmonary metastases has shown no advantage over a plain chest radiograph in terms of treatment outcome, but is performed by many institutions as a baseline staging study.

Staging

Two staging systems exist. The National Wilms' Tumour Study Group (NWTSG) bases the staging on the extent of disease at the time of diagnosis prior to treatment (Table 21.7), whereas the International Society of Paediatric Oncology (SIOP) bases the staging on the outcome of nephrectomy following preoperative chemotherapy.

Treatment

Combined-modality treatment using surgery, radiotherapy, and chemotherapy results in an overall cure rate of > 85%. Surgical treatment consists of nephrectomy, and most tumours are amenable to complete resection despite their large size. Meticulous care has to be taken to avoid tumour spillage. The NWTS recommends surgery prior to administration of chemotherapy, whereas SIOP recommends surgery only after administration of neoadjuvant chemotherapy. At the time of surgery, lymph nodes, renal vein, and the inferior vena cava are assessed for tumour involvement. The surgical management for patients with synchronous, bilateral Wilms' tumours (5% of all children with WT) aims at preservation of normal renal tissue, and includes bilateral partial nephrectomies, nephrectomy on the more affected side, and partial nephrectomy of the less affected side.

Wilms' tumour is radiosensitive, but radiation treatment to the tumour bed is reserved for stage III and extensive stage IV tumours, stage I–IV clear cell sarcoma, and stage II–IV diffusely anaplastic Wilms' tumours. Lung irradiation is

Table 21.7 National Wilms' Tumour Study Group staging system for Wilms' tumour

Stage I	Completely excised tumour with intact tumour capsule, no involvement of the vessels of the renal sinus, no evidence of tumour at or beyond the margins of the resection
Stage II	Completely excised tumour which extended beyond the kidney. Blood vessels outside the renal parenchyma may contain tumour. Status post-biopsy or tumour spillage limited to the flank and not involving the peritoneal surface, no evidence of tumour at the margins of the resection
Stage III	Residual non-haematogenous tumour confined to the abdomen with any of the following: (1) positive lymph node involvement within the abdomen or pelvis; (2) penetration of the tumour to the peritoneal surface; (3) peritoneal tumour implants; (4) positive tumour margins; (5) incompletely resectable tumour; (6) tumour spillage outside the flank
Stage IV	Haematogenous metastases (lung, liver, bone, brain, etc.) or lymph node metastases outside the abdomen or pelvis
Stage V	Bilateral renal involvement at diagnosis

Table 21.8 Wilms' tumour survival (NWTS3)

Stage/histology	Survival
Favourable	
I	97%
II	92%
III	87%
IV	83%
Unfavourable	
I–III	69%
IV	56%

reserved for patients with pulmonary metastases on plain chest radiographs. Chemotherapy based on the NWTSG includes vincristine and dactinomycin (actinomycin D) for patients with stages I, II favourable histology, and stage I unfavourable histology. Doxorubicin is added for stages III and IV favourable histology, for stages I–IV clear cell sarcoma, and for unfavourable histology stage II–IV with the addition of cyclophosphamide.

Prognosis

Overall, Wilms' tumour is highly curable with overall survival exceeding 85%. Less favourable results are achieved for patients with unfavourable histology (Table 21.8).

Rhabdomyosarcoma

Sarcomas arise from mesenchymal tissue (bone, cartilage, connective tissue, muscle) and usually manifest at an older age than embryonal tumours. The most common sarcomas of childhood are rhabdomyosarcoma, osteosarcoma, and Ewing's sarcoma (see Chapter 20).

Epidemiology

Rhabdomyosarcoma is the most common soft tissue sarcoma of childhood with an annual incidence of four to seven per million children 15 years of age or younger. It arises from striated muscle but can arise in a variety of sites throughout the body, including tissues or organs where striated muscle is not ordinarily found (e.g. bladder, prostate).

Pathology and genetics

There are two subtypes of rhabdomyosarcoma in children that have distinct genetic, pathological, prognostic, and clinical features (Table 21.9, Fig. 21.6). Embryonal rhabdomyosarcoma is a stroma-rich spindle cell tumour with abundant myoid stroma that occurs primarily in the head and neck or genitourinary tract of younger patients. Characteristic genetic changes for embryonal rhabdomyosarcoma are loss of heterozygosity (LOH) on the short arm of chromosome 11. Alveolar rhabdomyosarcoma is a small, round, blue cell tumour with fibrovascular

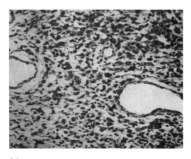

(a)

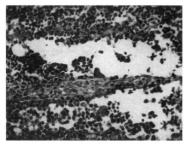

(b)

Fig. 21.6 Histology of rhabdomyosarcoma (RMS). (a) Embryonal RMS: spindle-shaped cells with abundant myoid stroma. Alveolar RMS (b): small, round cells lined up along spaces resembling pulmonary alveoli. (Reproduced with permission from Raney, R. B. (1993) Chapter 32. In Pizzo, P. and Poplack, D. (eds), *Principles and practice of pediatric oncology*, J. B. Lippincott, Philadelphia)

Table 21.9 Rhabdomyosarcoma subtypes

	Embryonal	Alveolar
Histology	Spindle-cell, stroma-rich	Small, round, blue cell tumour
Cytogenetics	Loss of heterozygosity at 11p15	t(2;13)
Location	Head and neck	Extremities, trunk
Age group	Young child 4–6 years	Older child > 10 years

septa that form alveolar-like spaces with tumour cells lining the septa. It is found most frequently in the trunk and extremities of adolescents. Alveolar rhabdomyosarcoma is characterized by a translocation between chromosome 2 and 13 that results in a fusion protein from the *PAX3* and *FKHD* genes, which are transcription factors.

Most cases of rhabdomyosarcoma are sporadic in nature, but the disease has been associated with familial syndromes such as neurofibromatosis and the Li–Fraumeni syndrome, a familial cancer syndrome where families have an increased incidence of soft tissue sarcomas, breast, lung, brain, bone and adrenocortical cancers, and acute leukaemias. Families with Li–Fraumeni syndrome have a germline mutation of the p53 tumour suppressor gene.

Clinical presentation

Presentation of rhabdomyosarcoma depends on the location of the tumour (Table 21.10). Approximately 40% arise in the head and neck, 20% in genitourinary tract, and 30% in the trunk and extremities. Orbital tumours present with proptosis and double vision. Parameningeal tumours arise in the sinuses, nasopharynx, middle ear, or mastoid region, and present with nasal, aural, or sinus obstruction. Seizures may occur in the presence of intracranial extension. Genitourinary tumours may present with haematuria, obstruction, or a palpable

Table 21.10 Rhabdomyosarcoma: presenting features

Tumour location	Symptoms and signs
Head and neck	Asymptomatic mass
Orbit	Proptosis, ocular paralysis, eyelid mass
Parameningeal	Nasal- aural- sinus obstruction, sinusitis, pain, cranial nerve palsies
Nasopharynx	Airway obstruction, nasal voice, epistaxis, dysphagia, cranial nerve palsies, local pain
Genitourinary tract	Haematuria, urinary retention, polypoid vaginal extrusion of mucosanguineous tissue, vaginal or scrotal mass
Trunk	Mass, pain
Extremity	Mass, pain

mass. Rhabdomyosarcoma metastasises to regional lymph nodes, lung, bone, and bone marrow. Spread to the liver is rare.

Diagnosis

Evaluation includes determining the extent of the primary tumour and surveying for metastatic disease (Table 21.11). The physical examination should give attention to regional lymphatic structures. The primary tumour should be evaluated with CT or MRI, including imaging of draining lymph nodes. Bilateral bone marrow biopsies, bone scan, and chest CT are performed as part of the routine metastatic evaluation. Patients with parameningeal disease should undergo

Table 21.11 Diagnostic work-up for rhabdomyosarcoma

Primary tumour	Plain radiograph
	CT/MRI
	Gadolinium-enhanced head and spine MRI (parameningeal rhabdomyosarcoma)
Metastases	Bilateral bone marrow aspirate and biopsy
	^{99m}Tc bone scan
	Chest radiograph, chest CT
	Gadolinium-enhanced head MRI and lumbar puncture (parameningeal rhabdomyosarcoma)
	Abdominal CT (paratesticular tumour)
Tumour markers	None

Table 21.12 Clinical Group staging system for rhabdomyosarcoma

Clinical Group	Extent of disease, surgical result
I	
A	Localized tumour, confined to site of origin, completely resected
B	Localized tumour, infiltrating beyond site of origin, completely resected
II	
A	Localized tumour, gross total resection, microscopic residual disease
B	Locally extensive tumour (spread to regional lymph nodes), completely resected
C	Locally extensive tumour (spread to regional lymph nodes), gross total resection, but microscopic residual disease
III	
A	Localized or locally extensive tumour, gross residual disease after biopsy only
B	Localized or locally extensive tumour, gross residual disease after 'major' resection (> 50% debulking)
IV	Distant metastases

gadolinium-enhanced MRI and lumbar puncture to evaluate for leptomeningeal spread. Adequate tissue for routine pathology, cytogenetic analysis, and molecular genetic studies needs to be obtained.

Staging

Two staging systems exist for rhabdomyosarcoma: the tumour–node–metastasis (TNM) system and the surgico-pathological Clinical Group system (Table 21.12). The TNM system stages tumours preoperatively based on tumour size and spread of disease. The Clinical Group system is based on the outcome of the surgical resection and the extent of residual tumour.

Treatment

Complete surgical resection of the tumour should be attempted if it is neither mutilating nor cosmetically damaging. In cases where complete resection is not feasible, initial biopsy followed by neoadjuvant chemotherapy and definitive local control measures are appropriate.

Similar to most childhood solid tumours, rhabdomyosarcoma is associated with the presence of micrometastatic disease at the time of diagnosis, necessitating administration of chemotherapy to all children with the disease. Active agents include vincristine, dactinomycin, cyclophosphamide, etoposide, ifosfamide, and doxorubicin.

Radiation therapy plays an important role in the treatment of rhabdomyosarcoma. It is used to eradicate tumour and achieve local control in cases where microscopic residual disease is present after surgery, or in cases of primary unresectable tumours such as orbital or many pelvic tumours. Doses of 4000–4500 cGy are used for microscopic disease, and 4500–5000 cGy for gross residual disease and tumours > 5 cm.

Prognosis

Of newly diagnosed patients with non-metastatic disease, 60–70% can be cured with combined modality treatment. Less than 20% of patients with metastatic rhabdomyosarcoma are currently cured from their disease. Sites of tumours associated with a better outcome include orbital tumours, head and neck tumours (excluding parameningeal tumours), and most genitourinary tumours. Outcome of children with embryonal histology is better than for children with alveolar rhabdomyosarcoma.

Retinoblastoma

Retinoblastoma is a malignant endo-ocular tumour of childhood arising in the embryonic neural retina.

Epidemiology

Retinoblastoma occurs with a frequency of 1 in 15 000–18 000 live births in developed countries. Retinoblastoma can occur in a sporadic and a familial form (6–10%). Retinoblastoma is often present at birth. The median age at diagnosis is 2 years, with 80% of cases being diagnosed before age 3–4 years. The estimated frequency of bilaterality ranges from 20 to 30%, with bilateral cases being diagnosed earlier than unilateral cases. Inherited retinoblastoma is transmitted as an autosomal dominant trait with nearly complete penetrance. Of all cases, 60% are non-heritable and unilateral, and 40% are heritable (15% unilateral, 25% bilateral).

Genetics and molecular biology

The retinoblastoma gene (*RB1*), a tumour suppressor gene, is instrumental in cell cycle regulation. It was isolated on chromosome 13q14 and cloned in 1987. Knudson developed the two-event hypothesis (see Wilms' tumour) for retinoblastoma, and thereby developed the concept of a tumour suppressor gene. The first step in tumourigenesis in hereditary cases involves a germline mutation or deletion at the *RB1* locus, whereas in non-hereditary cases the somatic genetic alteration at the *RB1* locus occurs in a single retinal cell. The second step in heritable and non-hereditary cases involves a somatic alteration of the remaining normal allele at the *RB1* locus. Molecular diagnosis has important implications for patients with retinoblastoma: detection of a germline mutation in a family member allows for testing of the other family members. Regular fundoscopic examination need only be performed in children with a germline mutation.

Pathology

Retinoblastoma is of neuroepithelial origin and consists of small, undifferentiated, anaplastic cells with scant cytoplasm, large nuclei, and multiple mitotic figures. Calcification occurs in necrotic areas of tumour. Retinoblastomas display various degrees of differentiation and may lead to the formation of Flexner–Wintersteiner rosettes, which are characteristic for the disease. Retinoblastoma may either grow in an endophytic (into the vitreous cavity) or exophytic (into the subretinal space) fashion (Fig. 21.7). Retinoblastoma can disseminate outside the eye and involve the brain and meninges. Haematogenous metastases may occur to the bone, bone marrow, and, less frequently, to the liver, lungs, or other organs.

Clinical presentation

In developed countries most cases of retinoblastoma are diagnosed while the tumour is intraocular (Table 21.13). In developing countries, late diagnosis is the rule after an enlarged eye or gross orbital extension is apparent. The most common sign leading to the diagnosis of retinoblastoma is leukocoria (Fig. 21.8), a white reflex seen through the pupil, often noticed initially by the parents. Strabismus is

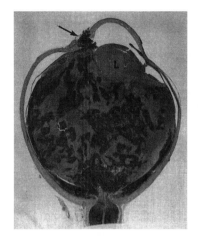

Fig. 21.7 An eye filled with retinoblastoma. Light staining areas of necrosis are interspersed between darker areas of viable tumour. Extra-ocular tumour extension through the limbus (arrow), and invasion of the choroid (C) and optic nerve (ON). Compression of the lens (L). (Reproduced with permission from Donaldson, S. S. (1993) Chapter 28. In Pizzo, P. and Poplack, D. (eds), *Principles and practice of pediatric oncology*, J. B. Lippincott, Philadelphia)

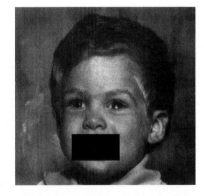

Fig. 21.8 Child exhibiting leukocoria of the left eye, the most common presenting sign of retinoblastoma. (Reproduced with permission from Donaldson, S. S. (1993) Chapter 28. In Pizzo, P. and Poplack, D. (eds), *Principles and practice of pediatric oncology*, J. B. Lippincott, Philadelphia)

Table 21.13 Retinoblastoma: symptoms and signs

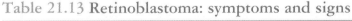

Intraorbital disease	Leukocoria
	Strabismus
	Vision loss (older child)
	Fixed pupil
	Heterochromia iridis
	Pain (orbital inflammation, secondary glaucoma)
	Extraocular tumour extension
Metastatic disease	Anorexia, weight loss, headache

the second most common presenting sign. Other signs are decreased visual acuity, especially in older children, and a red, painful eye.

Diagnosis

Eye examination under anaesthesia with fully dilated pupils by an experienced ophthalmologist is the most important examination. Ultrasound is helpful in delineating the tumour, and CT and MRI to evaluate the optic nerve, orbit, and central nervous system. Tumour calcifications are frequently observed. In patients with extraocular disease, bone marrow and cerebrospinal fluid should be examined to rule out tumour involvement. A bone scan can demonstrate metastases to the bone.

Staging

The Reese and Ellsworth staging system is used to stage intraocular retinoblastomas (Table 21.14).

Treatment

For patients presenting with intraocular disease, the treatment aims at preservation of vision without compromising local control or survival. In addition, attempts are made to minimize late effects of therapy. Cryosurgery or photocoagulation is used to achieve local control in tumours of limited extent. External beam radiation is used for local control as an adjunct to cryosurgery and photocoagulation. Local control rates with radiation therapy range from 60 to 80%. In view of the undesirable side-effects of radiotherapy (retardation of bone growth

Table 21.14 Reese–Ellsworth staging classification of retinoblastoma

Group I: very favourable	
A	Solitary tumour smaller than 4 disk diameters, * at or behind the equator
B	Multiple tumours smaller than 4 disk diameters, all at or behind the equator
Group II: favourable	
A	Solitary tumour 4–10 disk diameters in size, at or behind the equator
B	Multiple tumours 4–10 disk diameters, behind the equator
Group III: doubtful	
A	Any lesion anterior to the equator
B	Solitary tumours larger than 10 disk diameters behind the equator
Group IV: unfavourable	
A	Multiple tumours, some larger than 10 disk diameters
B	Any lesion extending anteriorly to the ora serrata
Group V: very unfavourable	
A	Tumours involving more than half the retina
B	Vitreous seeding

*1 disk diameter = 1.5 mm.

leading to facial asymmetry, dry eye syndrome, second malignancies), attempts are made to avoid external beam radiotherapy unless it is the only therapeutic option that can preserve vision.

Enucleation of the affected eye is reserved for very large tumours or for patients with glaucoma, irreversible vision loss, or when local therapy cannot be evaluated due to cataract. Enucleation performed in the first 2 years of life results in facial asymmetry because of inhibition of orbital growth. Preoperative chemotherapy may shrink very large orbital tumours and allow enucleation of the eye as opposed to orbital exenteration. Similar to enucleation, radiation causes growth inhibition of the orbital bone.

The use of adjuvant chemotherapy for patients with localized disease is being increasingly explored as a treatment option. The intraocular penetration of systemic drugs, however, may be poor, and thus chemotherapy has historically been reserved for patients with extraocular disease and with regional or distant metastases. For patients with overt extraocular disease, preoperative chemotherapy is administered, with carboplatin, cisplatin, etoposide, teniposide, cyclophosphamide, vincristine and Adriamycin being active agents. For most of the patients with orbital invasion, long-term survival can be achieved with the combined use of chemotherapy, surgery, and radiation therapy. Complete remission can be achieved for patients with central nervous system or haematogenous metastases, but long-term survival is infrequent.

Prognosis

Event-free survival is high (> 90%) for patients with localized disease, and poor for patients with CNS or haematogenous metastases. Patients with heritable retinoblastoma are at high risk for second malignancies. Radiotherapy, and to a lesser extent chemotherapy, increase this risk. Most secondary cancers in children with retinoblastomas are sarcomas, usually osteosarcomas, and arise within the radiation field. The incidence of second malignancies increases with time and reaches 30–50% at 20 years in patients who received radiation therapy. For non-irradiated patients, the cumulative incidence of second malignant tumours reaches 4% at 18 years (8% among patients with hereditable retinoblastoma).

Hepatic tumours

Approximately 60% of all hepatic tumours are malignant with an annual incidence of 1.6 per million children. Hepatoblastoma and hepatocellular carcinoma are the most frequent malignant hepatic tumours of childhood.

Hepatoblastoma

Epidemiology

Hepatoblastoma, an embryonal tumour, is the most common malignant hepatic tumour of childhood. It occurs with an incidence of less than 0.9 cases per one million children less than 15 years of age in North America. More than 80% of tumours are diagnosed in children under 3 years of age, with 45% of patients being diagnosed during the first year of life.

Genetics

Hepatoblastoma occurs with increased incidence in children with Beckwith–Wiedemann syndrome (see Wilms' tumour). Abnormalities of the short arm of chromosome 11 (11p15.5) have been found in children with Beckwith–Wiedemann syndrome and hepatoblastoma. Over-expression of the paternally derived allele at this locus may have a causal role in the development of hepatoblastoma. Hepatoblastoma also occurs with increased incidence in children of families with familial adenomatous polyposis, a dominantly inherited disorder predisposing to multiple colonic adenomas and early-onset carcinoma. The gene for this syndrome maps to chromosome 5q.

Pathology

Hepatoblastoma is usually solitary, with the right lobe of the liver more commonly involved than the left. Twenty per cent of tumours are multifocal or diffusely infiltrating the liver. Two morphological subtypes of hepatoblastoma have been described. The epithelial type contains either fetal or embryonal cells or admixtures of the two. The mixed hepatoblastoma contains mesenchymal tissue in addition to epithelial cells. Fetal cells are slightly smaller than normal hepatocytes and have a low nucleo-cytoplasmatic ratio and infrequent mitoses. Embryonal cells have a much higher nucleo-cytoplasmatic ratio, and mitoses are more frequent than in fetal cells. The configuration of cells may resemble ducts of the embryonal liver.

Clinical presentation

Hepatoblastoma most commonly presents as an asymptomatic abdominal mass. Children with advanced disease may present with anorexia, weight loss, or anaemia. Isosexual precocious puberty may develop in patients with tumours secreting human chorionic gonadotropin (β-HCG).

Diagnosis

Hepatoblastoma has to be differentiated from hepatocellular carcinoma (Table 21.15), other malignant and non-malignant hepatic tumours, non-neoplastic hepatomegaly and other abdominal masses. The diagnostic work-up is outlined in Table 21.16. Plain abdominal radiography, ultrasound of the abdomen, and CT or MRI of the abdomen are performed to delineate the location and extent of tumour. An angiogram may be required preoperatively to delineate the relationship of the tumour to hepatic vessels. Chest x-ray or CT and bone scan are performed to rule out distant metastases. The diagnosis is made based on a tumour biopsy with the typical histological appearance.

α-Fetoprotein (AFP), a glycoprotein synthesized in the yolk sac and liver at an early stage of fetal life, is a sensitive tumour marker in hepatoblastoma. Embryologically, production of AFP stops at birth, and levels drop until 6–8 months of age. The biological half-life of AFP is 5–7 days. The vast majority of patients with hepatoblastoma (98%) present with an elevated AFP, which decreases after tumour reduction by surgery or chemotherapy, and increases in case of tumour recurrence.

Table 21.15 **Distinctive presenting features of hepatoblastoma and hepatocellular carcinoma**

Feature	Hepatoblastoma	Hepatocellular
Age at presentation (years)	0–3	5–18
Associated congenital anomalies	Hemihypertrophy Beckwith–Wiedemann syndrome	Glycogen storage disease, lipid storage disease tyrosinaemia
	Family history of familial adenomatous polyposis	
Advanced disease at presentation	40%	70%
Usual site of origin	Right lobe, solitary	Right lobe, multifocal
Abnormal liver function test	15–30%	30–50%
Jaundice	5%	25%
Elevated α-fetoprotein	80–90%	50%
Positive hepatitis B serology	Absent	Present in some

Table 21.16 **Diagnostic work-up for children with suspected liver tumour**

Primary tumour	Plain film of the abdomen, ultrasound, CT/MRI, angiography (not routinely)
Metastases	Plain chest radiograph, CT
Tumour markers	α-Fetoprotein, β-HCG if precocious puberty
Other tests	Complete blood count, liver function tests, hepatitis B serology (child older 5 years), vitamin B_{12}-binding protein (child older 5 years)

Staging

The Children's Cancer Study Group in the USA stages tumours based on the extent of the tumour and the completeness of the surgical resection (Table 21.17).

Treatment

Complete surgical resection is the treatment of choice and required for cure. However, only 50% of tumours are amenable to complete resection at the time of diagnosis. Tumours involving both liver lobes or invading the porta hepatis are usually unresectable. Chemotherapy plays an important role in the treatment of hepatoblastoma. Active agents include cisplatin, doxorubicin, vincristine, cyclophosphamide, 5-fluorouracil, carboplatin, and etoposide. The benefit of chemotherapy has been documented in the adjuvant setting after complete surgical resection to prevent distant recurrent disease. Neoadjuvant administration of cisplatin and doxorubicin has been documented to allow complete resection of

Table 21.17 Grouping of malignant hepatic tumours

Group	Criteria
I	Complete resection of tumour
IIA	Tumour rendered completely resectable by initial irradiation or chemotherapy
IIB	Residual disease confined to one lobe
III	Disease involving both liver lobes
IIIB	Regional node involvement
IV	Distant metastases, irrespective of the extent of liver involvement

previously unresectable tumours. Radiation therapy has a limited role in the treatment of hepatoblastoma. It has been used to achieve local control in the setting of residual disease after surgery, and as an adjunct to surgery and chemotherapy in patients with pulmonary metastases. Recurrent disease often manifests in the lungs, and a cure may still be possible with a combination of surgery and chemotherapy.

Prognosis

Overall survival for hepatoblastoma is > 60%, and for completely resected tumours > 80%.

Hepatocellular carcinoma

Epidemiology

Hepatocellular carcinoma occurs with an incidence of 0.7 cases per one million children less than 15 years of age in North America. Hepatocellular carcinoma accounts for 10–30% of primary malignant hepatic tumours in Western countries, but is more common in areas where hepatitis B virus infection is endemic. The tumour is usually diagnosed in children older than 5 years of age and more frequent in males than females. Hepatitis B infection is causally related with hepatocellular carcinoma. Hepatocellular carcinoma is also associated with tyrosinaemia, biliary atresia, idiopathic neonatal hepatitis and α1-antitrypsin deficiency (Table 21.15).

Pathology

Underlying cirrhosis is present in 5–30% of children. The tumour has a nodular appearance, and is often multicentric or extensively invasive. Hepatocellular carcinoma is differentiated from hepatoblastoma by the presence of larger cells, nuclear pleomorphism, nucleolar prominence, and giant cells. In contrast to hepatoblastoma, no extramedullary haematopoiesis is observed. A variant of the hepatocellular carcinoma is the fibrolammellar carcinoma, which is associated with a specific abnormality of the vitamin B_{12} binding protein, and has a more favourable prognosis. It is characterized by plump, deeply eosinophilic hepatocytes encompassed by abundant fibrous stroma. Metastatic spread is to the lungs, regional lymph nodes, and rarely to the bone.

Clinical presentation

Abdominal distension, a palpable right upper quadrant mass, and pain are the most common initial manifestations. They may be superimposed on symptoms of underlying disease such as cirrhosis or tyrosinaemia. Patients may present with jaundice and systemic manifestations of fever and weight loss.

Diagnosis

Laboratory abnormalities include anaemia, hyperbilirubinaemia, and elevated serum AFP in 50–80% of cases (Table 21.15). Hepatitis B serology should be performed. Ultrasound and CT or MRI of the primary tumour, and chest CT to rule out pulmonary metastases, should be performed. Spread to bone is rare.

Staging

The staging system is shown in Table 21.17.

Treatment and prognosis

Complete surgical resection is the treatment of choice, but unfortunately an option only for 10–20% of the patients with hepatocellular carcinoma. Aggressive chemotherapy, mainly with cisplatin and Adriamycin, has not resulted in a significant improval in outcome. Most children with hepatocellular carcinoma die within 12 months of diagnosis. Liver transplantation is experimental, and overall 2-year survival rates for patients undergoing liver transplantation range from 20 to 30%.

Germ cell tumours

Pathogenesis and epidemiology

Gonadal and extragonadal germ cell tumours occur infrequently during childhood, with a yearly incidence rate of 2.4 cases per million children, and represent 1% of cancers diagnosed in children younger than 15 years of age. Germ cell and non-germ cell tumours arise from primordial germ cells and coelomic epithelium, respectively. Tumours arising from the unipotential germ cell are dysgerminoma and seminoma. The multipotential germ cell gives rise to embryonal carcinoma, teratoma and, through extra-embryonal differentiation, endodermal sinus tumour (yolk sac tumour) and choriocarcinoma. Tumours arising from the stromal epithelium are sex cord-stromal tumours and epithelial tumours.

Germ cells can be identified at approximately 4 weeks in the extra-embryonal yolk sac of the human embryo. From here cells migrate through the middle and dorsal mesentery and can be found in the germinal epithelium of the gonadal ridge at 6 weeks. These cells then populate the developing ovaries or testes.

In children, 70% of germ cell tumours arise in extragonadal sites, including the sacrococcygeal region, the retroperitoneum, the mediastinum, the neck, and the pineal region of the brain. Germ cell tumours commonly arise in two age groups: infants and adolescents. Maldescent of the testis and disorders of sexual differentiation (e.g. testicular feminization, Turner syndrome) predispose to germ cell tumours, possibly due to associated gonadal atrophy. Germ cell tumours are among the tumours observed in patients with Li–Fraumeni syndrome (see rhabdomyosarcoma). The most frequent cytogenetic finding in adolescent germ cell tumours is an isochrome 12 formed by duplication of a single arm of the chromosome. There may be duplication or deletion of the short arm of chromosome 1.

Pathology

Germ cell tumours may be composed of benign and malignant tissue. The most malignant component determines the clinical behaviour and treatment, and extensive sectioning of the tumour is therefore necessary. The histological differentiation based on site and cellular origins is shown in Table 21.18.

Teratomas are classified as mature, immature, and malignant. The mature teratoma is benign, highly differentiated and contains components derived from

Table 21.18 Histological classification of paediatric gonadal and extragonadal tumours

Ovarian
Germ cell
Dysgerminoma
Endodermal sinus tumour (yolk sac tumour)
Teratoma (mature, immature, malignant)
Embryonal carcinoma
Polyembryoma
Choriocarcinoma
Gonadoblastoma
Non-germ cell
Epithelial
Sex cord-stromal (granulosa, Sertoli/Leydig, mixed)
Testicular
Germ cell
Endodermal sinus tumour
Embryonal carcinoma
Teratoma
Teratocarcinoma
Gonadoblastoma
Seminoma
Choriocarcinoma
Non-germ cell
Sex cord-stromal (Leydig cell, Sertoli cell)
Extragonadal germ cell
Teratoma (sacrum, mediastinal, retroperitoneal, pineal, other)
± Endodermal sinus tumour
± Embryonal carcinoma

ectoderm, endoderm, and mesoderm. The sacrococcygeal teratoma, for example, is a predominantly cystic tumour with mucoid or keratinous content. Histologically there may be mature neuroglia, hair, bone, or cartilage. The immature teratoma in childhood usually behaves as a benign tumour, and contains some fully mature tissues but also embryonal tissues at varying degrees of differentiation. The malignant teratoma, which contains malignant elements such as yolk sac tumour, germinoma or embryonal carcinoma, often has elevated serum markers.

Germinomas develop in the undifferentiated germ cell and show no differentiation towards embryonal or extra-embryonal differentiation. The tumour is called germinoma when it occurs at an extragonadal site, seminoma when it occurs in the testis, and dysgerminoma when it occurs in the ovary. Seminomas are the most common malignant germ cell tumours in the adult male, but rarely occur in infants or young boys. In contrast (dys)germinomas are the most common pure malignant germ cell tumour occurring in the ovary and CNS in children. Germinoma is the most common tumour found in the dysgenetic gonad or undescended testis. Histologically the tumour contains monotonous, large cells with abundant cytoplasm. There may be fibrous septa and lymphoid infiltrate with necrosis and granulomatous reaction.

Embryonal carcinomas rarely occur in the pure form in children, and are more commonly a component of mixed malignant germ cell tumours in the testis and mediastinum. In the pure form, tumours are well circumscribed, have a friable, pale grey appearance, and contain areas of haemorrhage and necrosis. Tumour cells are large with large nuclei and nucleoli. Tumour cell nests contain central necrosis. The pure embryonal carcinoma is negative for tumour markers.

Yolk sac tumours (endodermal sinus tumours) are the most common pure malignant germ cell tumours in children, and, with the exception of the rare malignant neural component, the only malignant germ cell tumour to occur in the sacrococcygeum. Pseudopapillary, reticular, polyvesicular (vitelline and solid) have been described. The pseudopapillary type is the most common. Papillary projections associated with characteristic perivascular sheets of cells give rise to the term endodermal sinus and are also known as Schiller–Duval bodies. Intra- and extracellular hyaline droplets are para-aminosalicylic acid and α-fetoprotein positive.

Choriocarcinoma in its pure form is rare in childhood but is more commonly a feature of mixed histology subtypes. Microscopically choriocarcinomas consist of syncytiotrophoblasts, which contain HCG, and cytotrophoblasts. The tumours are usually very friable, haemorrhagic and contain areas of necrosis.

Polyembryoma is a rare tumour. It occurs in the mediastinum and ovary, and microscopically may resemble amniotic cavity and yolk sac. HCG and α-fetoprotein may be demonstrable.

Gonadoblastomas are also rare tumours. They are found in dysgenetic gonads, sometimes in association with malignant germinomas, and are benign tumours. Microscopically they are composed of a mixture of immature germ cells and gonadal sex cord cells, usually granulosa or Sertoli cell type, and frequent calcifications.

Clinical presentation

Many germ cell tumours present as asymptomatic masses. Clinical symptoms depend on the location of the germ cell tumours (Table 21.19). AFP and the β-subunit of human chorionic gonadotropin (β-HCG) are often elevated at the time of diagnosis and serve as a marker of disease status. AFP, an α1-globulin, is the earliest and predominant serum-binding protein found in the fetus. It is produced in the yolk sac, hepatocytes, and gastrointestinal tract, reaches its peak concentration at 12–14 weeks of gestation and gradually falls to adult levels of 10 ng/dl at approximately 1 year of age. Elevated AFP is found in children with yolk sac tumours or embryonal carcinomas. Elevation of AFP can occur after chemotherapy-induced tumour lysis, in viral hepatitis, cirrhosis of the liver, hepatoblastoma, and other epithelial malignancies. HCG is a glycoprotein synthesized by syncytiotrophoblasts of the placenta during pregnancy to maintain viability of the corpus luteum. Elevation of the β-subunit of HCG is found in patients with choriocarcinoma and germinomas. Precocious puberty may be the presenting feature of ovarian tumours.

Table 21.19 Germ cell tumours: site-related symptoms, age at presentation, and histology

Site	Symptom	Age	Histology
Testis	Painless testicular mass	0–5 years, adolescence, post-puberty	Yolk sac/teratoma (85% stage I) mixed germ cell tumour/teratoma
Ovary	Abdominal pain, distension, palpable mass, vaginal bleeding, amenorrhoea, precocious puberty, ascites, constipation	Infancy Adolescence	Mature, benign, cystic teratoma Mature and immature teratoma, dysgerminoma, malignant mixed germ cell tumour, gonadoblastoma in streak or dysgenetic ovaries
Anterior mediastinum	Asymptomatic, cough, dyspnoea, chest pain	Males	Teratoma mature, mixed cell, yolk sac
Sacrum/coccyx	Prenatal ultrasound, obstructed labour, dermal pit, mass, constipation	Young age (= better prognosis)	Mature teratoma (80%), immature teratoma, yolk sac tumour
Intracranial			
Pineal gland (62%)	Elevated intracranial pressure, Perinaud syndrome		Mixed cell, teratoma, yolk sac tumour, embryonal carcinoma
Suprasellar	Diabetes insipidus, vision changes, hypopituitarism	Adolescence	Predominantly germinoma Mixed cell tumours
Basal ganglia	Hemiparesis, precocious puberty, oculomotor palsy, hemianopsia, speech disturbance		

Diagnosis

Imaging studies include plain x-ray, ultrasound and CT of the primary tumour and regional lymph nodes. For gonadal tumours, bone scan, chest CT, and bone marrow examination should be performed to rule out distant metastatic spread. Table 21.20 shows the differential diagnosis for sacrococcygeal, testicular and anterior mediastinal tumours. The final diagnosis is based on microscopical examination of the resected tumour or tumour biopsy.

Table 21.20 Differential diagnosis of masses in the sacrococcyx, testis, and anterior mediastinum

Sacrococcygeal	Testicular	Anterior mediastinum
Myelomeningocele	Torsion	Thymus
Imperforate anus	Infarct	Thyroid enlargement
Pilonidal cyst	Epidydimo-orchitis	Bronchogenic cyst
Lipoma	Haematoma	Enteric cyst
Lymphangioma	Hernia	Lipoma
Chondroma	Hydrocele	Lymphangioma
Giant cell tumour	Leukaemia/lymphoma	Thymoma
Neurogenic tumour	Paratesticular rhabdomyosarcoma	T-cell lymphoma
Soft tissue sarcoma		

Table 21.21 CCG/POG staging system for germ cell tumours of the ovary and testis

Stage	Testis	Ovary
I	Confined to testis, completely resected; normal tumour marker after surgery	Confined to ovaries; normal tumour marker after surgery
II	Gross tumour spill after transcrotal orchidectomy; microscopic disease in scrotum or high in spermatic core; positive retroperitoneal lymph nodes (≤ 2 cm); increased tumour markers after surgery	Microscopic residual or positive lymph nodes (< 2 cm); tumour markers positive or negative
III	Positive retroperitoneal lymph nodes (> 2 cm)	Gross tumour residual or biopsy only; positive lymph nodes (≥ 2 cm); contiguous visceral involvement (omentum, intestine, bladder); peritoneal washings positive for tumour cells
IV	Distant metastases, including liver	Distant metastases, including liver

CCG, Children's Cancer Group; POG, Paediatric Oncology Group.

Staging

The staging for testicular and ovarian tumours is shown in Table 21.21. For tumours at other sites, stage I represents completely resected tumour and stage IV distant metastatic disease.

Therapy

Treatment depends on the tumour location, histology and stage (Table 21.22). Complete surgical resection is curative for mature (benign) and for immature, teratomas of low grade, and for stage I testicular and ovarian tumours, provided tumour markers decrease to normal levels and remain normal after surgery. For testicular tumours, orchidectomy is carried out after high cord ligation through an inguinal approach. For ovarian tumours, sampling of the contralateral ovary and lymph nodes may be considered at the time of oophorectomy. For sacrococcygeal tumours, excision must include the coccyx to prevent local recurrence. Surgical removal is also indicated for malignant lesions. However, because of the availability of effective chemotherapy, resections should not sacrifice vital structures or be mutilating.

Chemotherapy has an important role in the treatment of germ cell tumours, and is employed for stages II–IV. Active agents include cisplatin, carboplatin, vinblastine, bleomycin, dactinomycin, doxorubicin, methotrexate, ifosfamide, and etoposide.

Table 21.22 Treatment of germ cell tumours

Stage	Histology and site	Treatment
Any	Mature teratoma (any site)	Surgical excision
I	Any malignant germ cell tumour	Surgical excision
I, poor risk	Any malignant germ cell tumour	Surgical excision followed by chemotherapy
II–IV	Malignant teratoma gonads, mediastinum, retroperitoneum	Chemotherapy, surgical excision of residual disease
II–IV	Dysgerminoma	Chemotherapy, radiotherapy for residual disease
Intracranial germ cell tumour	Mature, immature low-grade	Biopsy and excision
	Malignant teratoma and yolk sac tumour, immature, high grade	Biopsy, chemotherapy, radiation to tumour bed, craniospinal radiation for cerebrospinal fluid spread
	Germinoma	Craniospinal radiation plus chemotherapy and focal radiation to tumour bed
	Gonadoblastoma	Surgical excision
	Sacrococcygeal	
	benign	Surgical excision including coccyx
	malignant	Chemotherapy followed by surgical excision

Most of these agents are used in a combination of three to four drugs (e.g. cisplatin, etoposidec and bleomycin) and are administered for four to six courses, depending on the stage of disease. Radiotherapy plays almost no part in the treatment of germ cell tumours in childhood with the exception of intracranial germinomas. Dysgerminoma is a highly radiosensitive tumour and high cure rates of 80–95% can be achieved for intracranial dysgerminomas with craniospinal radiation. For intracranial malignant teratomas and yolk sac tumours, the combination of surgery, chemotherapy, and radiation is used with the goal to eradicate disease (see Chapter 23).

Prognosis

The introduction of combination chemotherapy for patients with moderate- and high-risk germ cell tumours has resulted in a significant improval of survival, and disease-free survival rates ranging from 60% to 100% have been reported.

Case histories

A 2-year-old boy with neuroblastoma

A 2-year-old boy was brought to a GP by his mother who was concerned about his poor appetite and failure to grow over the past 2 months. His mother was also concerned that the child's abdomen had become distended. On examination, the GP noted a large mass palpable in the left flank.

The GP referred the child to the paediatric surgeon who repeated the clinical examination and found no abnormalities other than the abdominal mass. A full blood picture revealed a normochromic, normocytic anaemia with raised serum ferritin. An ultrasound of the abdomen was arranged and demonstrated a solid tumour with cystic areas arising from the left adrenal gland. The liver appeared normal. A urine sample demonstrated elevated catecholamines. The child underwent a CT scan of chest and abdomen that confirmed a mass arising from the left adrenal gland that crossed the midline and surrounded the aorta and coeliac vessels. The chest appeared normal. An isotope bone scan was reported as normal.

A presumptive diagnosis of locally advanced neuroblastoma was made but required further histological confirmation and diagnosis. The surgeon performed a diagnostic laparotomy at which he found a 10 cm by 10 cm semicystic mass arising from the left adrenal gland. The tumour was not resectable as it surrounded the aorta and coeliac vessels. A biopsy was taken for a histopathological diagnosis and confirmed the presence of a moderately differentiated neuroblastoma.

The child was referred to a medical oncologist who recommended a combination of three cycles of platinum-based chemotherapy and local radiotherapy as a neoadjuvant treatment. The first cycle of chemotherapy was complicated by severe nausea and vomiting, which were not adequately controlled with ondansetron alone. This was attributed to the platinum part of the chemotherapy and the addition of dexamethasone as an anti-emetic allowed the following cycles to be given uneventfully. Following completion of chemotherapy and radiotherapy, a repeat CT scan of the abdomen demonstrated a > 50% reduction in tumour size. *continued*

Case histories continued

The paediatric surgeon performed a repeat laparotomy and was now able to resect the remaining tumour. Histopathology revealed necrotic tissue and areas of mature tumour.

Since the tumour became resectable after combination radiotherapy and chemotherapy, this child has a 60% chance of long-term survival.

A 4-year-old girl with a Wilms' tumour

A 4-year-old girl attended the local paediatric clinic with a 1-month history of abdominal pain and night sweats. On examination the paediatrician noted a mass palpable in the right abdominal flank. The child's blood pressure was elevated at 130/100 mmHg. Urinalysis identified moderate haematuria. No organisms were detected on direct microscopy or culture. A full blood picture revealed a normochromic, normocytic anaemia. The platelet count and white cell count were both normal.

The paediatrician organized an ultrasound scan of the patient's abdomen that identified a solid mass arising from the right kidney. The liver and left kidney appeared normal. A CT scan of chest and abdomen confirmed a tumour arising from the right kidney with no evidence of distant metastases.

The child was referred to a paediatric surgeon who performed a laparotomy. At surgery a solid tumour was seen to penetrate through the right renal capsule. The surgeon was able to completely resect the mass. Histopathology of the resected specimen revealed an anaplastic Wilms' tumour with uninvolved resection margins.

The patient was referred to an oncologist for 11 weeks of vincristine and dactinomycin chemotherapy following surgery. A central venous line was inserted to allow administration of chemotherapy. She did not require local radiotherapy, as resection margins were clear of disease following surgery.

After 6 weeks of chemotherapy she developed an infection in her central line which required admission to hospital. She was managed with wide-spectrum, intravenous antibiotics for 10 days after which she was discharged.

On completion of chemotherapy she complained of 'coldness' affecting her fingers and toes, although she had no difficulty with using her hands or walking. The consultant oncologist noted that her deep tendon reflexes were diminished. A diagnosis of grade I vincristine neurotoxicity was made and the patient's mother was reassured that the symptoms should resolve over the next few months.

With surgery and adjuvant chemotherapy this child has a greater than 90% chance of long-term survival.

Further reading

Bleyer, W. A. (1992) Magnitude of the childhood cancer problem. *Cancer Bull* 44, 444.

DeVita, V. T., Hellman, S., and Rosenberg, A. (1997) *Cancer: principles and practice of ncology*, 5th edn. Lippincott-Raven, Philadelphia.

Gree, D. M. and D'Angio, G. J. (eds) (1992) *Late effects of treatment for childhood*. Wiley-Liss, New York.

Hammond, D. (1982) Multidisciplinary management of childhood cancers. A model for the future. In Willoughby, M., and Siegel, S. (eds), *Butterworth's international medical reviews. Paediatrics (haematology and oncology)*. Butterworth, London.

Holland, J. F., Bast, R. C., Morton, D. L., Frei, E., Kufe, D. W., and Weichselbaum, R. C. (eds) (1997) Section XLI. Neoplasms in children. In *Cancer medicine*, 4th edn. Williams & Wilkins, Baltimore.

Pizzo, P. and Poplack, D. (eds) (1993) *Principles and practice of pediatric oncology*, 2nd edn. Lippincott, Philadelphia.

Rubin, P. (1992) *Clinical oncology – a multidisciplinary approach for physicians and students*, 7th edn. W. B. Saunders, Philadelphia.

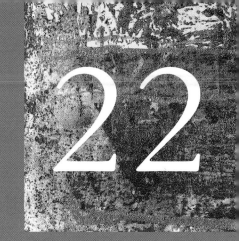

22

Breast cancer
William Odling-Smee

- Risk factors
- Diagnosis
- Screening
- Pathology
- Staging
- Treatment
- Follow-up of the breast cancer patient
- Breast cancer and pregnancy
- Breast cancer and the elderly
- Paget's disease of the nipple
- Support for the breast cancer patient
- Prevention of breast cancer
- Male breast cancer

Breast cancer

Cancer of the breast is the most common cancer in women with the UK having a high incidence. It is highest in the USA and Western Europe and lowest among the Japanese. It also causes great anxiety amongst women, and breast clinics are flooded with symptomatic women who need reassurance that they do not have breast cancer. Despite this anxiety, the results of early, adequate treatment are good in comparison to treatment of other cancers.

History

Breast cancer in women has been known for as long as history has been recorded. The Edwin Smyth papyrus dating from 3000–2500 BC, which is a medical treatise discovered in Egypt, describes the treatment of women with breast cancer. Subsequent Egyptian papyri also describe it, suggesting that it was quite common amongst rich women in Egypt from 3000 BC.

Herodotus in his *History* described Atossa, wife of Darius, King of Persia, as having a ulcerating lesion of the breast from which she died. Hippocrates (c. 460–370 BC) described the symptoms of the disease and advocated treatment with herbs and applications. The Romans in the first century AD, was the first to practise surgery for breast cancer, but breast cancer was normally treated by applications until Scultetus introduced the mastectomy, in AD 1620. Because this was usually performed in women with advanced disease, it was generally unsuccessful, and not popular. However, records show that it was done sporadically for the next

Table 22.1 Risk factors for breast cancer

Factor	Estimated relative risk
Age	15
Geographical location	6
Early age at menarche	2
Late age of menopause	3
Age at first birth greater than 32 years	4
Nulliparity	4
Obesity	3
Alcohol intake	1.2
Irradiation	5
Oral contraceptive (young age before 1st pregnancy)	1.84
Hormone replacement therapy	1.36
Benign disease:	
atypical ductal hyperplasia,	5
Sclerosing adenosis	1.5
Family history of 1st degree relatives	8

400 years. The advent of aseptic surgery and anaesthetics made it a much more acceptable operation, and in 1895 Halsted introduced the radical mastectomy as the standard operative procedure for breast cancer.

Risk factors

Table 22.1 shows the risk factors associated with breast cancer, and the changes that they make to the relative risk of the patient developing breast cancer.

Age

The incidence of breast cancer increases with the age of the patient. The woman aged 80 is 20 times as likely to develop breast cancer as the woman aged 30. There is a steep rise in incidence from the age of 40 to 50, and then a plateau between 50 and 60, followed by a slower, but steady rise (Fig. 22.1).

Geographical location

The pattern of incidence shows a remarkable variation between different countries. The rates are six times higher in the UK than in Asia, with Japan having a particularly low incidence. The risk of developing breast cancer is significantly influenced by geography (Fig. 22.2).

There is also a distinct difference in incidence between the regions within one country. Table 22.2 shows the internal variation within the UK. There is a higher incidence in urban areas, and an increase in incidence with rising social class.

Age at menarche and menopause

Women who start menstruating early in life (less than 12 years of age) have an increased risk of developing breast cancer, and women who have a late menopause also have an increased risk. Women whose menopause occurs before the age of 45 have a relative risk which is 50% lower than those who continue menstruating until 55 years of age. This applies to women undergoing either a spontaneous or artificial menopause.

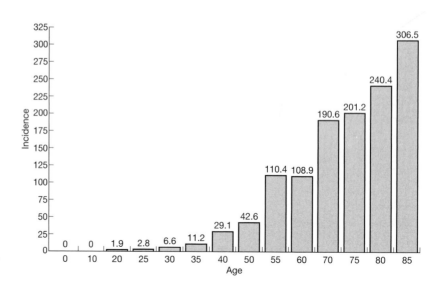

Fig. 22.1 Breast cancer incidence by age per 100 000 population.

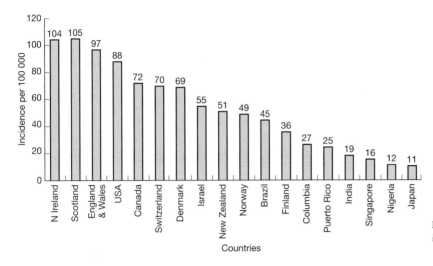

Fig. 22.2 Geographical variation in incidence of breast cancer.

Table 22.2 Breast cancer in the British Isles

Country	Cases	Mortality per 100 000
Scotland	3168	105.6
Northern Ireland	866	104.2
England & Wales	29 200	96.9
Republic of Ireland	1555	94.7

Age at first full-term pregnancy

Women who have their first full-term pregnancy before the age of 20 have a lower risk.

There is an inverse relationship between parity and risk. However, the protective effect of having more children depends entirely on an early age of the first full-term birth. Incomplete pregnancies do not have a comparable effect, and in order for the first birth to be protective it must have occurred before the age of 32.

Lactation

It has always been assumed that lactation confers a protective effect on the subsequent risk of breast cancer. Several studies have dismissed this as an independent factor, but more recent investigations have shown that if breast-feeding continues longer than 6 months there may be a protective effect. This protection may lower the rate of breast cancer in premenopausal women.

Weight

There is a strong relationship between weight and breast cancer risk, which is dependent on age. Women under the age of 50 years have little or no increased risk associated with increased weight, but by the age of 60 a 10 kg increment in weight results in an 80% increase in relative risk.

Diet

Increased dietary fat has been indicted as responsible for increased breast cancer rates. This hypothesis was based on international correlation studies, but results from more recent prospective studies do not support this hypothesis. However it is thought that increased fat in the diet may increase breast cancer risk.

Alcohol

Substantial evidence has accumulated to support a positive association between breast cancer risk and the intake of alcohol. The relative risk as compared to those who never drink is 1.2, and this seems to apply equally to beer, wine, or spirits.

Radiation

From studies of women exposed to the atomic bombs in Japan and women who have been exposed to repeated medical radiation, it is well established that ionizing radiation to the chest before the age of 40 years increases the breast cancer risk. The higher the radiation dose, the higher the breast cancer risk.

The oral contraceptive

Women who use oral contraception between the age of 25 and 40 years would appear to have no increased risk of breast cancer. However, the use of oral contraception for more than 4 years before the age of 25 years and before first full-term pregnancy does increase the risk of premenopausal breast cancer. Women who used diethylstilboestrol whilst pregnant during the 1940s and 1950s had an increased risk of breast cancer which did not appear until 20 years after exposure. Therefore, it may be that women taking the oral contraceptive have an increased risk, which will not become apparent until many years after use.

Hormone replacement therapy

Meta-analysis of population-based studies of the effect of hormone replacement therapy (HRT) in postmenopausal women show that after 10 years of use the relative risk is 1.36. However, the benefits of HRT, in relieving menopausal symptoms and reducing ischaemic heart disease and osteoporosis may well outweigh the increase in relative risk of breast cancer, and suggest that a risk–benefit analysis may prove positive. Unfortunately, HRT increases the density of breast tissue on mammography, which can make detection of breast cancer more difficult.

Previous benign breast disease

Women with atypical ductal hyperplasia have a four to five times higher risk of developing breast cancer than women who do not have any proliferative change in their breast. In women with gross cysts, papilloma, and sclerosing adenosis there is a slight increase in risk (1.5–2 times). Tamoxifen may lower the risk in women with atypical ductal hyperplasia.

Family history

About 10% of women who develop breast cancer have a genetic disposition. This means that the majority of women who develop breast cancer (90%) do not have a genetic disposition. The genetic mutation is autosomal dominant with a limited penetrance, meaning that the mutation may skip a generation. Recently, genes that appear to be tumour suppressor genes for breast cancer have been discovered. The gene *BRCA1*, which is on the long arm of chromosome 17, appears to be mutated in up to 30% of all familial breast cancer. It is a large gene, and so may have several mutations. The gene *BRCA2*, on the short arm of chromosome 13 and the p53 gene on the short arm of chromosome 17 are mutated in a small proportion of familial

Table 22.3 The risk of breast cancer

Family history	Expected breast cancer cases between 40 and 50 years	Lifetime risk	Mammography
1 relative over 50 years	< 1 in 75 (1.3%)	< 1 in 10 (10%)	NHS BSP at age 50
1 relative 40–50 years	1 in 50 (2%)	1 in 7.5 (13.3%)	NHS BSP at age 50
1 relative below 40 years	1 in 25 (4%)	1 in 5.6 (18%)	Baseline mammogram at referral. NHS BSP at age 50
2 relatives over 60	< 1 in 45 (2.2%)	< 1 in 7 (14%)	NHS BSP at age 50
2 relatives 50–60 years	< 1 in 25 (4%)	1 in 4 (25%)	2-yearly until age 50
2 relatives average age below 50	1 in 17 (6%)	1 in 3 (33%)	2 yearly until age 50
2 relatives average age below 40	1 in 12 (8.4%)	1 in 2.5 (40%)	Annually
3 relatives average age below 60	1 in 10 (10%)	1 in 2 (50%)	Annually
1 or more relatives over 50 + 1 or more relatives with ovarian cancer	< 1 in 7 (6%)	1 in 3 (33%)	Annually
1 or more relatives < 40 + relative with childhood malignancy			Await genetics review

Notes: a relative means mother, sister, daughter, maternal or paternal aunt, grandmother. A male relative with breast cancer counts as a female < 40. A relative with bilateral breast cancer counts as two.
Population risk for breast cancer age 40–50 years is 1 in 100 (1%). Population lifetime risk (aged 20–80) is 1 in 12 (8.4%).

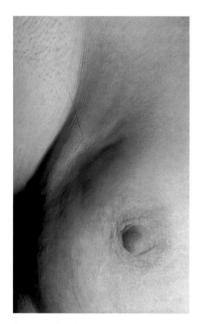

Fig. 22.3 Skin dimpling, indicating carcinoma of the breast.

breast cancers. Almost certainly there are other genes that are also mutated in some familial cases. These genes are linked to the genes that cause ovarian cancer, and linkage studies show links with other cancers, such as colon and prostate. Li–Fraumeni, Cowden's syndrome, Muir's syndrome, and ataxia telangiectasia are all genetic syndromes with a high incidence of breast cancer. Table 22.3 shows the likely increase of risk in those who have a family history, and shows those who ought to have genetic advice.

Diagnosis of breast cancer

History

Patients with breast cancer present with a lump in the breast, with breast pain, or with nipple discharge in over 90% of cases. There are few other symptoms of breast cancer, unless it is advanced, when it may present with symptoms referable to the site of the metastases (i.e. bone pain, shortness of breath, nausea, etc.) (Table 22.4).

Examination

The breast should be examined in a good light, with the patient sitting upright so that the breast is dependent. The arm should be raised to allow access to the axilla. The breast should be observed, and in particular skin dimpling should be sought (Fig. 22.3). This is usually associated with an underlying lump. Although it can be associated with previous surgery, or trauma, it is a sign that is highly suspicious of a cancer.

Breast palpation is performed in a systematic manner, using the fingertips only, with the hand held parallel to the chest wall. It is important to be sure that all areas of the breast have been covered (Fig. 22.4).

Once the breast has been palpated, the axillae and the supraclavicular fossae must be checked. Finding palpable lymph nodes does not mean that they contain metastases. Palpable lymph nodes occur in 30% of patients with benign breast disease and 40% of breast cancer patients who have clinically normal lymph nodes have nodal metastases.

Table 22.4 Frequency of symptoms of patients attending a symptomatic breast clinic

Symptom	Frequency (%)
Lump in the breast	36
'Lumpiness' and pain	30
Pain alone	18
Nipple discharging	5
Nipple retraction	1
Strong family history of breast cancer	8
Swelling and inflammation	2

Mammography

A mammogram is a soft tissue x-ray of the breasts. It is taken in two planes: oblique and craniocaudal. The breast is compressed between two plates during exposure, and this is uncomfortable. With modern film screens the dose of radiation is less than 1.5 mGy. Mammography will not show up all breast cancers, because lobular breast carcinoma does not absorb x-rays well.

Therefore, 10–15% of cases will not appear on mammography. Mammography allows detection of mass lesions with or without spiculation, microcalcification, and parenchymal distortions, which are typical of breast cancer (Fig. 22.5).

Ultrasonography

This investigation is not as good as mammography for diagnosing breast cancer. It shows whether a lesion is a cyst or is solid. Cysts usually have clearly demarcated edges whereas cancers have indistinct outlines.

Fine needle aspiration cytology (FNAC)

If a lump is palpable in the breast, a needle ought to be inserted into it, even though clinically it is definitely benign. If the lump is a cyst it can be aspirated (Fig. 22.6), but if it is solid cells can be aspirated, spread on to a slide, and processed and examined by the cytopathologist. If the cytopathologist is present in the clinic, a result can be available within 30 minutes. The cytopathologist will be able to indicate whether it is definitely malignant, suspicious, definitely benign, or

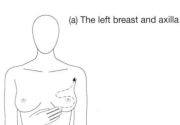

(a) The left breast and axilla

1. Uncover the left breast
2. Look at the breast
3. Ask the patient to put her left hand on your right shoulder
4. Look at the breast again
5. Palpate the breast
   (i) with the fingertips of the right hand
   (ii) systematically, going right up into the axilla

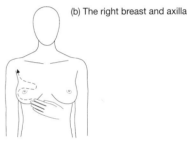

(b) The right breast and axilla

1. Walk round to the left side of the patient
   Repeat the above process with the left hand examining the right breast

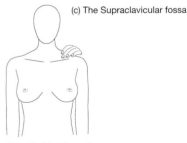

(c) The Supraclavicular fossa

Stand behind the patient
Palpate the supraclavicular fossa with the fingertips

Fig. 22.4 Examination of the breast. The patient should be seated on the examination couch, facing you.

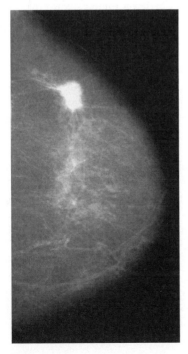

Fig. 22.5 Mammogram showing breast cancer.

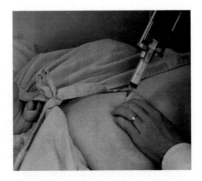

Fig. 22.6 Fine needle aspiration.

that there are insufficient cells for a diagnosis. The accuracy of this procedure depends on the needle entering the lesion under investigation, and depends on the experience of the operator (Fig. 22.7). FNAC can be ultrasound guided.

Core biopsy

If a lump is suspicious and the FNAC does not give a definitive answer, a core biopsy may give a definitive diagnosis. A small core is removed by a special needle with a recess for the specimen. It is usually attached to a mechanical device to make localization in the lesion more accurate.

Open biopsy

Open biopsy is performed in women in whom, after clinical examination, mammography, fine needle aspiration cytology, and core biopsy, have still not given a diagnosis. Women who are told that their lesion is benign are usually satisfied with this information, but some of them continue to be anxious and request excision of the lesion.

Open biopsy is not without morbidity, and patients may develop a further lump under the scar, or pain specifically related to the biopsy site. Frozen section is no longer used in breast surgery (Table 22.5).

Screening for breast cancer

If a tumour is small, the prognosis is good, and the smaller the tumour the better the survival. Clinical examination can detect a carcinoma of about 1.5 cm in diameter and the hands of an experienced clinician can detect tumours down to about 1.0 cm in diameter. However, mammography can detect tumours down to about 0.5 cm (Fig. 22.8).

Screening tests should be simple to perform, cheap, easy, and unambiguous to interpret, and able to identify women with cancer and to exclude those without cancer. Mammography is expensive. It requires high-technology equipment, special film and dedicated processing, and highly trained radiologists to interpret the films, and it only detects about 95% of cancers. It is, however, the best screening tool that is available for detecting breast cancer, and it has been shown to lower mortality in randomized trials.

There have been several randomized studies looking at the effect of regular mammography on the mortality of breast cancer. The summary of these studies is shown in Fig. 22.9. There is a reduced mortality of 30%. Population screening was introduced in the UK in 1988. All women between the ages of 50 and 64 are invited to have a mammogram at 3-yearly intervals. If a woman has a significant abnormality, she is asked to come for further assessment.

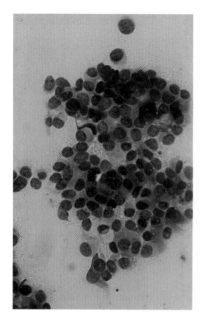

Fig. 22.7 Fine needle aspirate of a breast cancer, showing nuclei and cells breaking off at the edge.

Table 22.5 Indications for open biopsy of a breast lump

- Clinical suspicion of malignancy even when FNAC and mammogram are normal
- Suspicion of malignancy on FNAC or mammography, even though clinically normal
- Atypical cells on FNAC
- Request by the patient for excision biopsy

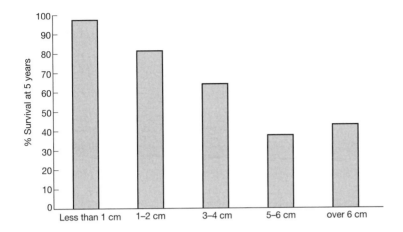

Fig. 22.8 The effect of size on survival.

At assessment, further imaging and clinical examination are performed. If there is a composite shadow that is not seen on subsequent mammography, and if there are no clinical abnormalities, the women are returned to the normal screening round. If there is any doubt, a stereotactic FNAC and/or core biopsy are performed.

An experienced radiologist, surgeon, and pathologist are present at assessment, and the patient is supported by a breast care nurse.

If there is doubt about the diagnosis, then an open biopsy may have to be performed. If the suspect lesion is impalpable, a marker wire is inserted stereotactically to guide the surgeon to the suspicious area. A specimen x-ray of the removed tissue is compared with the mammogram to make sure that the suspicious area has been removed. If this procedure is being carried out to establish a diagnosis, care is taken to remove a small amount of tissue (< 20 g).

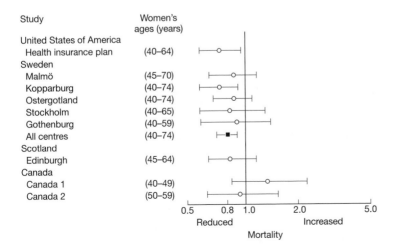

Fig. 22.9 Summary of the randomized trials comparing the mortality of women who received regular mammography with those who did not.

Pathology of breast cancer

Carcinoma of the breast develops in the terminal duct/lobular unit, from the epithelial cells. If the malignant cells have not breached the basement membrane, it is called an '*in situ*' cancer, and if the basement membrane is breached, the cancer is called 'invasive'.

Classification

Classically, breast cancers have been divided into ductal and lobular types, because it was believed that the morphological type known as ductal arose from the terminal duct, and the type known as lobular arose from the lobule. However, we now know that both types arise from the terminal duct/lobular unit, and so the terminology is outdated, but still commonly used. Some cancers show particular morphological patterns and are called 'special types' (Table 22.6). The remainder are called 'no special type' (NST), and constitute the majority.

In situ cancers

These are tumours that have not breached the basement membrane and, in theory, have not metastasised. The labels 'ductal carcinoma *in situ*' (DCIS) and 'lobular

Table 22.6 Histological classification of invasive breast cancer

Special types
Tubular
Mucoid
Cribriform
Papillary
Medullary
Classic lobular
No special type
Grade I
Good tubular formation
Little nuclear pleomorphism
Few mitotic figures
Grade II
A little tubule formation
Moderate nuclear pleomorphism
Some mitotic figures
Grade III
Little or no tubule formation
Massive nuclear pleomorphism
Many mitotic figures

Table 22.7 Classification of ductal carcinoma *in situ*

Prognosis	Nuclear grade	Necrosis	Calcification	Size (mm)
Good	Low	Absent	Microfoci	<15
Intermediate	Intermediate	Present	Microfoci	14–40
Poor	High	Present	Branched	>41

carcinoma *in situ*' (LCIS) are regularly used but probably have no more relevance than in invasive cancer.

There are classifications of DCIS which indicate which type has the better prognosis (Table 22.7).

Tumour differentiation

It is possible to grade tumour differentiation according to a scale known as the Bloom and Richardson scale, which is an important predictor of both disease-free and overall survival. The degree of tubular formation, the nuclear pleomorphism, and the frequency of mitotic figures are scored from 1 to 3. A tumour with many well-formed glands would score 1, whereas a tumour with no glands would score 3. These values are combined and converted into three groups: grade I (score 3–5), grade II (score 6–7), and grade III (score 8–9) (Fig. 22.10).

Lymphovascular invasion

The presence of malignant cells in blood vessels or lymphatics is a marker of more aggressive disease, and there is an increased risk of local recurrence, especially in the premenopausal woman.

Extensive in situ disease

This designation is applied when more than 25% of the main tumour mass contains *in situ* disease, and when the latter is present in the surrounding breast tissue. This is another marker for an increased risk of developing a local recurrence.

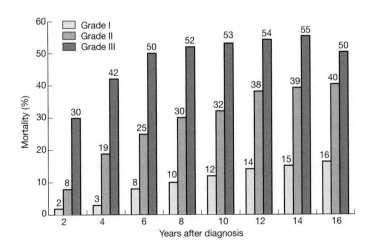

Fig. 22.10 The effect of grade on mortality.

Staging of breast cancer

Primary tumour

T staging is dependent on tumour size and the presence or absence of fixation to surrounding structures. Primary tumours should be described as precisely as possible with accurate measurement of diameters in centimetres and characterization of the shape, consistency, location, and involvement of skin, pectoral fascia, or ribs.

Regional lymph nodes

Clinically negative axillae associated with T1 or T2 breast tumours will contain histologically positive nodes in approximately 39% of cases, while clinically N1 axillae will be pathologically negative about 24% of the time. In general, larger tumours have more axillary nodal involvement. Internal mammary node involvement varies in frequency with the location of the primary breast cancer; it is more common with central and internal quadrant cancers and when there are axillary nodal metastases.

The characteristics of the primary tumour and the presence or absence of axillary lymph node metastases are strongly correlated with survival. The TNM system of staging has been extensively used in breast cancer.

A prognostic index

Although individual factors are useful, combining three independent prognostic variables in the form of an index allows identification of groups of patients with

Table 22.8 TNM classification and stage grouping for breast tumours

TNM classification		Stage grouping			
Tis	In Situ	Stage 0	Tis	N0	M0
T1	≤2 cm	Stage I	T1	N0	M0
		Stage IIA	T0	N1	M0
			T1	N1	M0
			T2	N0	M0
T2	>2 to 5 cm	Stage IIB	T2	N1	M0
T3	>5 cm		T3	N0	M0
T4	Chest wall/skin	Stage IIIA	T0	N2	M0
			T1	N2	M0
			T2	N2	M0
			T3	N1,N2	M0
		Stage IIIB	T4	Any N	M0
			Any T	N3	M0
N1	Movable axillary nodes involved	Stage IV	Any T	Any N	M1
N2	Fixed axillary				
N3	Internal axillary				
M1	Distant metastases				

T = tumour; N = node; M = metastasis

different prognosis, and allows a numerical prognosis to be applied to an individual woman. The Nottingham Prognostic Index is the most widely used, and has been independently validated in several centres (Table 22.9).

Oestrogen and progesterone receptors

A number of studies have shown that patients with a positive oestrogen receptor (ER) status have a better survival than those who are ER negative. There is definite evidence that women whose tumours are ER negative do not respond to hormonal manipulation. This is particularly true in premenopausal women. In these women if their tumour is ER +ve they will respond to ovarian oblation, and if the tumour is ER −ve they will respond to chemotherapy. To a lesser degree, this is true of the progesterone receptor.

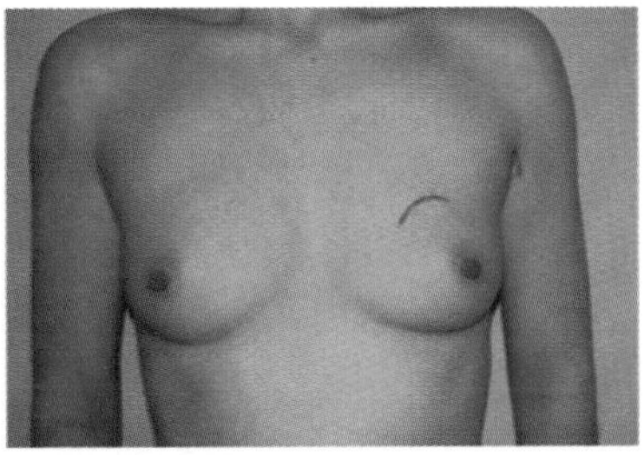

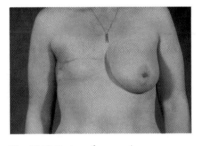

Fig. 22.11 Patient after partial mastectomy.

Treatment of breast cancer

The treatment of breast cancer can be divided into the treatment of early breast cancer, and the treatment of advanced disease. The objective of treating early disease is to effect a cure, if possible, whereas the treatment of advanced disease is palliative, for a cure is extremely unlikely.

Early breast cancer ($T_{0,1,2}$; $N_{0,1}$; M_0)

Treatment of early disease can be divided into primary treatment, which is surgical, and adjuvant treatment, which is radiotherapy, hormone therapy, and chemotherapy.

Fig. 22.12 Patient after a total mastectomy.

Primary treatment

Although there are potentially many operations for breast cancer, only a partial mastectomy and a total mastectomy are commonly undertaken. A **partial mastectomy** is the removal of the tumour with a margin of normal breast tissue of about 1 cm in diameter on all sides of the tumour (Fig. 22.11).

Partial mastectomy can only be offered to the patient if the tumour is less than 3 cm in diameter, or if the tumour is not behind the nipple. A partial mastectomy under these circumstances would leave a very distorted breast. Sometimes in a very small breast, removal of a tumour and a 1 cm margin of normal breast tissue will leave so little normal breast tissue that a total mastectomy must be performed. A partial mastectomy should always be supplemented by radiotherapy as part of the primary treatment.

A **total mastectomy** is the removal of all the breast tissue on the affected side (Fig. 22.12). The incision on the breast is normally split to include the nipple in the specimen. Flaps are then raised and the breast dissected off the pectoralis major muscle.

If patients are selected carefully, there is no difference in survival between those treated with partial mastectomy and those treated with total mastectomy.

Axillary node clearance or axillary node sampling is done at the same time as a partial or total mastectomy. There are two reasons for this:

- if there are metastases in the axillary nodes
- to prevent recurrence in the axilla, which is very difficult to treat.

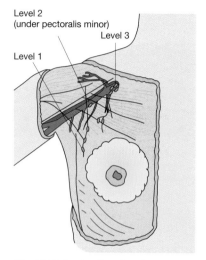

Level 2
(under pectoralis minor)
Level 3

Level 1

Fig. 22.13 Levels of lymph nodes in the axilla.

The axillary node clearance consists of removing as many nodes as possible below the upper border of the pectoralis minor muscle, and medial to the axillary vein. Axillary node sampling consists of removing the lower four nodes in the axilla. The latter procedure gives as good prognostic information as 'clearance', but does not stop recurrence in the axilla (Fig. 22.13).

Which operation should be done?

All women should be offered the choice of a total mastectomy or partial mastectomy and radiotherapy unless the cancer is greater than 3 cm on clinical or mammographic measurement, or the lump is directly behind the nipple, when they should be offered a total mastectomy only. If a woman chooses a partial mastectomy, she should be warned that if the tumour is at the margin, or if there is

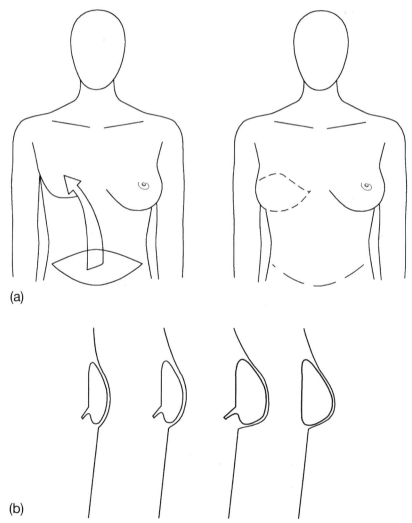

(a)

(b)

Fig. 22.14 Reconstruction of the breast. (a) TRAM flap. (b) A tissue expander in situ. See text.

extensive DCIS, she will be recommended to have a mastectomy. If the tumour is between 0 and 5 mm from the margin, a re-excision of the wound is usually recommended. If the margins are at least 5 mm clear of tumour, as measured pathologically, the patient should be referred for radiotherapy.

Women who have to have a total mastectomy after a partial mastectomy because the tumour is at the margin, or for some other reason, usually feel satisfied that they have at least tried the lesser procedure.

Reconstruction after mastectomy

For most women, the loss of a breast in a total mastectomy affects their body image. The majority of women first want to be sure that the cancer is removed, and only secondly are concerned with their shape. However, there are those to whom body shape is as important as eradicating the cancer, and who request an operation to reconstruct the breast.

Does reconstruction of the breast mask recurrence? There is no evidence that reconstruction of the breast masks recurrence. Local relapse after mastectomy occurs in the skin flaps, and these flaps are still easily visible and palpable. There is no reason why the operation should make metastatic disease more common.

Is it better to do an immediate reconstruction or a delayed reconstruction? An immediate reconstruction is no better and no worse than a delayed reconstruction. However, for the patient, the immediate reconstruction involves one major operation, where as the delayed reconstruction involves two less major operations. Most women who have the opportunity to choose will choose an immediate operation.

What operations are available for reconstruction? (Fig. 22.14) The choice of operation for an individual patient depends on how much fat the patient has and whether she smokes. The operations available are as follows.

- **Insertion of a silicone prosthesis.** These are suitable for patients with small breasts. They are inserted under the pectoralis major muscle. Before they are inserted a tissue expander is inserted and slowly expanded with injections of saline. When the skin is sufficiently stretched to allow for ptosis of the expanded breast, the expander is removed and a silicone gel prosthesis inserted.
- **Latissimus dorsi myocutaneous flap (LD flap).** The lateral half of the latissimus dorsi muscle together with an area of skin over it is raised as a pedicle flap based on the thoracodorsal neurovascular bundle. It can then be brought forward to make a breast, using the skin on the chest wall. This flap may require a prosthesis to make a big enough breast.
- **Transverse rectus abdominus myocutaneous flap (TRAM flap).** This flap is taken from one of the rectus abdominus muscles and based on the superior epigastric artery. The superior epigastric artery can be used as a pedicle or can be a free flap using a microvascular anastomosis. TRAM flaps are bulkier than LD flaps and do not require the insertion of a prosthesis.

All these are major operations. However, when done by experienced surgeons, they can give an excellent result. After the breast shape has been restored, a nipple can be fashioned to sit on the top of the mound, giving a very realistic breast (Fig. 22.15).

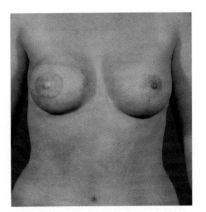

Fig. 22.15 A patient who had a TRAM flap and a contralateral reduction mammoplasty following a mastectomy for breast cancer.

- **Fibrous capsule.** A fibrous capsule forms around a prosthesis and contracts, leaving a hard mass on the chest wall. The use of textured prostheses has reduced this occurrence to less than 10%.
- **Infection.** About 3% have to have a prosthesis removed because of infection.
- **Implant rupture.** About 1% of all implants will rupture, either through trauma or silicone fatigue. All silicone implants 'bleed' a small amount of silicone gel, but there is no evidence that this is carcinogenic, or causes problems in other organs. Women with silicone implants do not have a higher risk of connective tissue disorders and the Ministry of Health in London has recently summarized the evidence.
- **Flap necrosis.** This is a major hazard in TRAM flaps but the edges can usually be revised. It is very rare in LD flaps.

It is not always possible to reconstruct a breast mound that matches the other breast. Where there is a substantial difference in size and symmetry, a reduction mammoplasty on the contralateral side can achieve a good cosmetic result.

Histological assessment

The histopathologist coats the edges of the specimen with alcan blue before cutting, and so is able to measure distance of the tumour from the alcan blue (the margin). A search is also made for lymphovascular invasion. If it is found in women under the age of 50 years, then a total mastectomy would be recommended, as there is a high risk of local recurrence, except in very small tumours (under 1 cm in diameter).

Primary chemotherapy

The role of chemotherapy before surgery remains to be defined, and this cannot be recommended as standard management. Patients with locally advanced disease (T3/4, N0–2, M0) may be treated with chemotherapy before surgery, or with radiotherapy. The choice of regimen will depend on tumour and patient characteristics and if chemotherapy is chosen the regimen is normally anthracycline based.

Table 22.9 Nottingham Prognostic Index (NPI)

NPI = (size of tumour in cm × 0.2) + grade + axillary node score
Axillary node score
0 +ve nodes = 1
1–3 +ve nodes = 2
4 or more +ve nodes = 3
Interpretation
Below 3.5 – prognosis very good
3.6–5.5 – prognosis fair
Over 5.6 – prognosis poor

Adjuvant therapy

Adjuvant therapy is treatment added to surgery. Since its introduction in the late 1960s it has been shown to improve the results of treatment (Table 22.9).

Radiotherapy All patients who have had a partial mastectomy must have radiotherapy to the breast as this reduces the local recurrence rate. Patients who have had a total mastectomy, and who have a high risk of local recurrence, should have radiotherapy. A high risk of local recurrence occurs in tumours which are histologically grade III, in which there are more than three axillary nodes involved, or when the tumour is over 3 cm in diameter. The premenopausal woman with lymphovascular invasion also has a high rate of local recurrence and should be offered radiotherapy.

Hormone therapy Premenopausal and postmenopausal women, who are oestrogen receptor (ER) positive, should be offered tamoxifen, an oestrogen-receptor blocker. It is possible that the new aromatase inhibitors will be as effective as tamoxifen, and they have fewer side-effects.

Women who are over 80 years of age may be treated with tamoxifen alone. However, if it is possible to perform surgery, it should be done because there is a lower local recurrence rate. These patients may then be treated with tamoxifen, and will have an excellent prognosis.

Chemotherapy Combination chemotherapy, such as anthracycline and cyclophosphamide (AC), or cyclophosphamide, methotrexate and 5-fluorouracil (CMF), reduces the risk of recurrence of breast cancer. This is particularly true in the premenopausal, node-positive patient where a 25% improvement in overall survival has been obtained. For node-negative women, the benefit is less, but there is still a benefit. Recent studies have shown that chemotherapy also has a benefit in node-positive, postmenopausal women.

Table 22.10 Which adjuvant treatment

		Oestrogen Receptor Positive	Oestrogen Receptor Negative
Premenopausal women	Axillary node negative	Combination chemotherapy + Tamoxifen (high risk patients)	Chemotherapy (high risk patients)
		Tamoxifen (low risk patients)	
	Axillary node positive	Chemotherapy + Tamoxifen	Chemotherapy
Post menopausal women	Axillary node negative	Tamoxifen ± chemotherapy	Chemotherapy (high risk patients only)
	Axillary node positive	Chemotherapy ± Tamoxifen	Chemotherapy

Chemotherapy — CMF, cyclophosphamide, methotrexate, FEC, 5-fluorouracil; epirubicin, cyclophosphamide

Combination chemotherapy is more effective than single-agent regimens, and is usually given for four or six cycles. The role of high-dose chemotherapy is still under clinical investigation, where the risk of recurrence is high (i.e. more than four positive axillary nodes). Because high doses of chemotherapy kill haematological cells as well as cancer cells, the stem cells need to be harvested and reinfused after treatment, or protected with granulocyte colony-stimulating factor (GCSF).

Complications of chemotherapy – Alopecia is a feature of all regimens which use doxorubicin or mitozantrone and neutropenia is also common. GCSF can shorten the time that a patient is neutropenic. Nausea and vomiting are also common. $5HT_2$ receptor antagonists (odansetron) has reduced the problem to manageable levels.

Advanced breast cancer (T3/4; N0–2; M+)

Advanced disease may be divided into locally advanced and metastatic disease. In discussing treatment in patients with advanced disease, it is important to bear in mind the quality of life and several recent studies have demonstrated significant improvements in quality of life in patients receiving combination therapy.

Locally advanced disease

These patients may present with a slow-growing tumour, for which the patient has not sought advice until it has become locally fixed or ulcerated, or they may present with fixed axillary nodes, *peau d'orange* or inflammation of the whole breast (inflammatory carcinoma). These patients should all be staged to see if there is metastatic disease, with chest x-ray, ultrasound scan of the liver, and isotope bone scan. If there is no detectable metastatic disease, surgery chemotherapy and radiotherapy may offer prolonged survival.

The patient with locally advanced disease is best treated by radiotherapy and chemotherapy initially, with surgery being kept until the tumour has regressed. Primary surgery has a high rate of local recurrence, and only 30% of patients treated with radiotherapy are free from local recurrence. Chemotherapy and radiotherapy used in combination can increase the local response to 80%. Patients treated in this manner may have significant improvements in quality of life and possibly prolonged survival.

Local recurrence after mastectomy

This occurs in the scar or in the skin flaps, and if diagnosed early is usually amenable to surgery. Unfortunately, it often is followed by systemic relapse. Sometimes the relapse is widespread and is difficult to control. A malodorous infected ulcer on the chest wall may exist for some time in the absence of metastases. Metronidazole creams and charcoal dressings help to relieve the smell and deslough the ulcer.

Metastatic disease

Metastatic breast cancer can run a very variable course. If the cancer is hormone sensitive, the patient may have a good outlook, and may live for several years. However, if the tumour is not hormone sensitive the patient will have a much shorter survival. The average period of survival after the diagnosis of metastatic disease is about 2 years, however there is a wide variation.

Patients with a long disease-free interval survive for longer than patients with a short interval. Patients with metastases in the local lymph nodes or in the bones survive for longer than patients with metastases at other sites such as the liver. Patients with visceral metastases have the poorest survival as they tend to have a short disease-free interval as their cancers are more aggressive.

The treatment of metastatic disease This depends on the site of the metastases and the disease-free interval. If the latter is long and the site is favourable such as bone then hormone treatment may be a reasonable first line. If this fails, then chemotherapy must be considered.

Patients who have poor prognosis disease and a short disease-free interval are best treated with chemotherapy initially (patients with liver metastases). If this fails, then second-line chemotherapy with a non-cross resistant regimen is indicated.

In both groups of patients, the treatment of symptoms is important. Pain needs to be relieved and dyspnoea and nausea should be treated. Radiotherapy is an excellent way of relieving localized bone pain. Steroids have an important place in relieving other symptoms. Bisphosphonates are also effective in treating widespread bone pain.

Pathological fractures

If possible these should be anticipated. They can be recognized by a sharp increase in pain over a few days. Internal fixation followed by radiotherapy will give mobility and can be associated with reasonable survival. If a pathological fracture does occur, it can be managed by the same combination of internal fixation and radiotherapy (Fig. 22.16).

Malignant pleural effusion

Pleural effusion is the second most common effect of metastases from breast cancer. The small ones, which do not cause symptoms, do not require treatment. If the patient complains of significant shortness of breath, then it is better to drain the effusion, rather than aspirate it. Drainage is effective in controlling about one-third of effusions.

However, if tetracycline, inactivated *Corynebacterium parvum* or talc is instilled at the end of the procedure, about 85% of effusions are controlled. This instillation is associated with pain and occasionally pyrexia. The patient should be warned about the pain, and reassured that it is transient.

Hypercalcaemia

This is a major metabolic complication, experienced by women with metastases in the liver and in bone. It is a rare complication in the absence of bone metastases. Some of the breast cancer cells release cytokines, which activate osteoclasts in the bone, and raise the serum calcium. Clinically this is usually non-specific and patients present with fatigue, nausea, constipation, polyuria, and dehydration. There is often considerable bone pain. The high serum calcium can cause cardiac arrhythmias, renal failure, pancreatitis, and psychosis. Bisphosphonates have revolutionized treatment, and should be used as soon as the diagnosis is established.

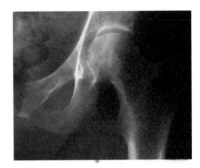

(a)

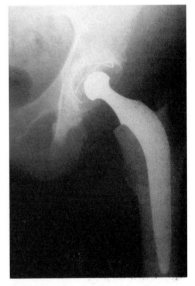

(b)

Fig. 22.16 (a) Radiograph of a pathological fracture. (b) A metastasis in the neck of the femur, with excision and hip replacement.

Table 22.11 The treatment of hypercalcaemia

- Hydration
- Bisphosphonates
- Mobilization
- Orthopaedic treatment before fractures occur
- Treatment of bone pain
  external beam
  analgesics and NSAIDS
  radioactive strontium

The dehydration (if any) should be corrected before administration. Chemotherapy reduces the risk of recurrence, but if the disease is progressive despite this treatment, the bisphosphonates can be administered every 2–4 weeks, intravenously (Table 22.10).

Metastases in the CNS

Any patient who presents with a focal neurological symptom must be investigated with computed tomography (CT) or magnetic resonance imaging (MRI). Isotope brain scanning is unhelpful. If brain metastases are present, the initial treatment is to reduce the oedema with steroids. When the oedema has settled, local treatment with fractionated radiotherapy will stabilize the condition. Unfortunately, the long-term results are disappointing, with most patients dying within 3–4 months. If there is only a solitary metastasis, it can be excised by the neurosurgeons, and long-term survival may occur. CNS metastases are not usually hormone sensitive (Fig. 22.17).

Patients with cord compression caused by spinal bone metastases usually present too late after the onset to be amenable to an emergency laminectomy, but if this cannot be done, dexamethasone and fractionated radiotherapy, given before paraplegia and bladder dysfunction are established, can be very effective.

Infiltration of the brachial plexus is a difficult neurological complication to treat. Palliative radiotherapy may relieve pain, but effective pain relief is often all that can be offered.

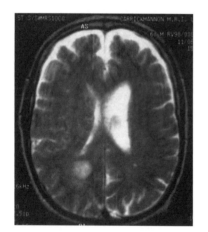

Fig. 22.17 Metastases from breast cancer in the brain, demonstrated by MRI.

Follow-up of the breast cancer patient

As with other cancers, there is no evidence that a follow-up programme detects recurrences. Most recurrences are found by the patient, who draws the attention of their medical attendant to it. However, a regular follow-up programme is a great comfort and support to the patient, and most patients like to be in contact with the breast team at regular intervals. There is another reason for regular follow-up: it gives the breast team an opportunity to evaluate their results. Survival of breast cancer is measured in terms of 5-year survival. All who treat breast cancer ought

---

Box 22.1 *Following up patients treated for breast cancer*

- Follow-up programmes rarely detect recurrences.
- Most recurrences are found by the patient herself.
- Patients find comfort in a regular follow-up programme.
- Follow-up programmes are an opportunity to evaluate results of treatment.
- Clinical follow-up with annual mammography detects recurrence significantly earlier than clinical examination alone.

---

to know what their 5-year survival is, and what percentage of that survival is disease free. It enables comparison of this survival with other units treating breast cancer, and to see how results can be improved.

Breast cancer treated by partial mastectomy has a risk of recurrence, and there is a higher risk of a contralateral tumour developing (unless the patient is on tamoxifen). Annual mammography will pick up these changes before they are apparent clinically, when they can be treated effectively (Box 22.1).

Breast cancer and pregnancy

About 2% of all breast cancers occur in pregnancy, and it is difficult to diagnose because of the difficulty of identifying a discrete mass in an enlarging breast, and so a much higher percentage of women are node positive. Apart from this, there is no evidence that breast cancer occurring in pregnancy is more aggressive than other breast cancer.

Radiotherapy should not be used in pregnancy, and there is a risk that chemotherapy may damage the fetus. So in the first and second trimesters, treatment should be a mastectomy (partial or total) and axillary node clearance. In the third trimester of pregnancy the ideal is to delay treatment until the pregnancy is

---

Box 22.2 *Breast cancer and pregnancy*

- 2 breast cancers occur in every 10 000 pregnancies.
- A high proportion of breast cancers in women under 40 years of age are associated with pregnancy.
- Breast cancers diagnosed in the first and second trimesters of pregnancy should be treated by mastectomy (partial or total) and axillary node clearance.
- Breast cancer diagnosed in the third trimester of pregnancy should be treated by delaying treatment until the patient is 32 weeks and inducing labour. Aggressive chemotherapy, surgery, and radiotherapy can then be used.

---

32 weeks and then deliver the baby. Then aggressive chemotherapy, surgery, and radiotherapy can all be used.

Although there is only limited information, the effect of pregnancy after a breast cancer has been treated does not appear to be deleterious. Because 80% of recurrences occur in the first 2 years, it is usually recommended that the patient should not become pregnant in this time, but pregnancy *per se* does not appear to increase the likelihood of recurrence (Box 22.2).

Breast cancer and the elderly

There are many definitions of elderly, but for this discussion 'elderly' means over the age of 70 years.

The elderly woman should be treated in the same way as her 'younger sister'. A partial mastectomy or even a total mastectomy can be performed under local anaesthesia, and older women can tolerate radiotherapy very well. If the patient is fit for general anaesthesia then the axilla should be cleared, for there is a high risk of axillary recurrence if this is not done. All elderly patients should be offered adjuvant treatment. For those patients who will not tolerate chemotherapy, treated with tomoxifen is recommended

There is a small group of very elderly or unfit patients who cannot be treated surgically. For these women, tamoxifen may be given as a sole treatment, and in the majority it will hold the disease in check for at least 2 years.

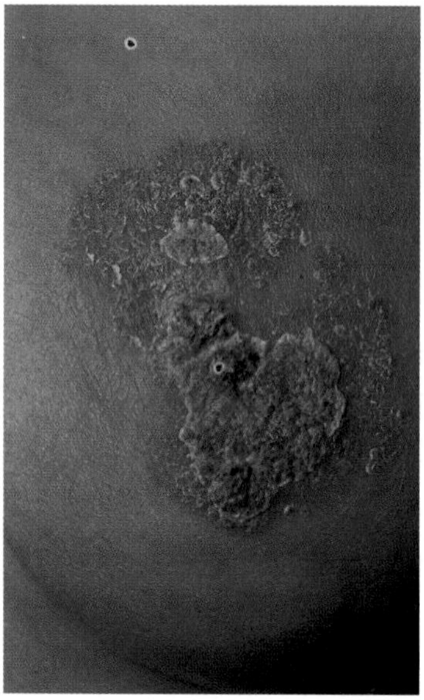

Paget's disease of the nipple

Paget's disease is an eczematous change in the nipple and areola skin, with an underlying breast cancer. The eczematous change is caused by Paget's cells, which are migratory cancer cells invading the epidermis. Clinically, Paget's disease is on the nipple and the areola, whereas eczema is on the areola only. If Paget's disease is suspected, a mammogram should be performed to determine if there is an underlying cancer. If the mammogram is negative, it is worth trying the effect of hydrocortisone cream for 1 week. If this is not effective the lesion must be biopsied (Fig. 22.18).

If Paget's disease is diagnosed histologically, the only treatment that is effective is a total mastectomy. A partial mastectomy would involve the excision of the nipple, and this gives a poor cosmetic result. Adjuvant treatment would depend on ER status, on node status, and on menopausal status (Box 22.3).

Fig. 22.18 Paget's disease of the nipple.

> ### Box 22.3 *Paget's disease of the nipple*
> - Can only definitely be diagnosed by a full thickness skin biopsy
> - Is only associated with 1–2% of breast cancers
> - Occurs on the nipple and areola but eczema is confined to the areola
> - A mammogram may pinpoint the underlying cancer
> - The only effective treatment is a total mastectomy

Support for the breast cancer patient

There is accumulating evidence that psychosocial support influences adjustment to cancer, and clinical observations in various settings suggest that factors ranging from pain control to mortality can be altered by such support. This support can be offered by doctors, medical personnel, specialist breast care nurses, support groups, volunteers, and the families of patients.

Doctors

About 30% of women with breast cancer develop an anxiety state or depressive illness within a year of diagnosis, and few patients mention this to doctors at a breast clinic. Doctors can encourage them to talk about psychological problems by asking questions and clarifying the responses about perceptions a patient has of the nature of their illness and their reactions to it, and about their experience of losing a breast or having radiotherapy or chemotherapy.

By showing sympathy, trying to imagine how the patient is feeling, and summarizing what has been said so far, doctors can encourage patients to talk about their feelings, and to express them.

Getting patients to talk freely is inhibited by closed leading questions, and by giving advice and reassurance. If the psychological concerns are not disclosed despite an open directive style, it is useful to ask about impact of illness on the patient's daily functioning since surgery, relationships with their partner, and their mood (Table 22.11).

Specialist breast care nurses

Breast care nurses are trained to be able to help patients talk about social, emotional, or psychological concerns, and to avoid behaviour that inhibits patients talking about such things. They check the patient's understanding of and reaction

Table 22.12 Symptoms of psychiatric morbidity

Anxiety	Depression
Anxiety, tension and inability to relax. Present for more than 50% of time over 4 weeks	Persistent low mood, which is present for more than 50% of the time over 4 weeks
Cannot be reassured	Cannot be distracted by self or others
Recognized as not normal anxiety	Significantly different from normal mood
Insomnia	Inability to enjoy oneself
Irritability	Diurnal variation of mood
Impaired concentration	Early waking
Intolerance of noise	Impaired concentration
Panic attacks	Feeling hopeless or suicidal
Somatic symptoms	Feelings of guilt, self blame or worthlessness
	Irritability and irrational anger
	Loss of interest
	Retardation or agitation

to the bad news that has been given, and offer further information and practical and emotional support. Breast care nurses need rapid access to a psychiatrist or a clinical psychologist when they uncover severe psychological problems.

There is no firm evidence that helping patients in such a way prevents psychological morbidity, but properly trained nurses can monitor a patient's adjustment and recognize those who need help. This leads to a significant reduction in psychological morbidity. The use of breast care nurses may mean that doctors leave the psychological care to them, but patients' psychological adaptation is determined by what the doctors say about diagnosis and treatment.

Support groups

Breast cancer is frequently associated with difficulty in interpersonal relationships. The presence of someone in the patient's environment, with whom the experience can be shared, lessens the harmful effect. This role is usually filled by a member, or members, of the patient's family, but may be an extended family member or an unrelated friend. The presence of positive social support not only diminishes the psychological distress of breast cancer, but is probably important in modulating survival as well.

The absence of social support, or the loss of a significant person who withdraws during the patient's illness, may be an additional stress and may be more painful than the illness itself.

When these personal forms of support are inadequate, patients will be helped by a support group, but a significant number who elect to join such a group have shared their concerns with their families and friends. People who seek support groups do so because they expect to feel better, and are usually satisfied with what transpires.

The shared goals of all support groups are:

- to provide emotional support
- to maintain the social identity of the member
- to provide education
- to provide tangible environmental support
- to provide a social affiliation.

The groups need a professional facilitator who will help the group to find the information and education relevant to their needs, and who will be able to teach problem solving, stress management, and other coping skills. When the goals are achieved, groups often achieve a high degree of social cohesion, with members visiting one another outside of the group times and having less depression, fatigue, confusion, and maladjusted coping mechanisms.

Volunteers

Patients are often supported by talking to someone who has been through similar experiences as themselves, and there are appropriately trained groups of volunteers throughout the country who can be contacted. Volunteers will often be invaluable to patients who have lost the support of their significant person because of their illness. Volunteers are trained to be able to withdraw gently from this association and to help the patient to find some more permanent support.

Prevention of breast cancer

Because the pathogenesis of breast cancer is unknown, there is very little that can be done to prevent breast cancer. Living a healthy lifestyle, with no smoking and a low alcohol intake may not lower the incidence, and breast-feeding does not appear to make much difference. Women who have lived this lifestyle in the hope that they can avoid breast cancer are often devastated when it strikes them.

Tamoxifen

Women who have breast cancer on one side have an increased chance of developing breast cancer on the contralateral side. However, in those women who are treated with tamoxifen for their breast cancer, the risk of a contralateral breast cancer falls to the same as the risk in the general population. So perhaps tamoxifen will prevent breast cancer in those who are at high risk. Several trials have tried to answer this question, but the results are contradictory. There are ongoing trials that are trying to provide more information and to clarify the situation. All women who are at high risk should be offered one of these trials.

Bilateral subcutaneous mastectomy

Bilateral subcutaneous mastectomy performed at 5 years younger than the youngest family relative to have developed breast cancer might be considered appropriate for women with a strong family history of breast cancer, or who carry mutations of the *BRCA1* or *BRCA2* gene. There is no specific evidence that such individuals will totally avoid breast cancer.

Male breast cancer

Carcinoma of the male breast is an uncommon phenomenon, accounting for less than 1% of all breast cancers. Based on family history, the prognosis and the response to treatment are remarkably similar between the sexes. The age risk is similar to that for females, without the early postmenopausal peak. Relative androgen deficiency may be a cause, and radiation exposure increases risk.

The pathology of male breast cancer is similar to that in females. The vast majority are infiltrating ductal carcinomas, with lobular carcinoma being very rare. Its clinical presentation is the same as in females, with a unilateral painless breast mass.

The treatment is total mastectomy, and axillary node clearance. Radiotherapy is given postoperatively because of the proximity of the pectoralis muscle. As a high percentage of male breast carcinomas are oestrogen-receptor positive they respond well to adjuvant tamoxifen. Survival is good with 80% of the men who are node negative, and 46% of node-positive men still alive at 5 years.

Case histories

Mrs ROD

Mrs ROD was aged 42 when she found a lump in her right breast. She is a married woman with three children. Her first baby was born when she was aged 23 and she had her first period when she was aged 13. She has no family history of breast cancer, and took the oral contraceptive pill from the age of 30 to the age of 40. Her menstrual cycle was regular and normal.

She went to her GP who referred her to the breast clinic. Here it was confirmed that she had a 2×2 cm lump in the upper outer quadrant of the right breast. There was no skin attachment, and no attachment to deep fascia. No glands could be palpated in the axillae or supraclavicular fossa. There was no liver enlargement, no abnormal signs in the chest, and no tenderness over bone prominences.

A mammogram showed that this mass had the characteristics of malignancy, and fine needle aspiration cytology, under ultrasound control to ensure the needle was in the lesion, showed malignant cells.

Diagnostic summary
- Aged 42 (premenopausal)
- No risk factors
- Palpable lump 2×2 cm
- Mammogram – carcinoma (code 5)
- FNAC – malignant (C5)

After discussion with the surgeon and the breast care nurse, Mrs ROD chose to have a partial mastectomy and axillary node clearance. This was performed 1 week after her attendance at the breast clinic, and she was in hospital for 3 days. An axillary drain was left place after the operation, and this was removed after 48 hours. She was mobile and helping to hand out tea in the ward on the morning of discharge. The breast care nurses had taught her exercises to prevent shoulder stiffness, and she felt very well.

At operation a 1.8 cm tumour had been excised, and the margins of excision were 5 mm distant from the nearest tumour edge. The wounds had been closed with subcuticular Vicryl. There were 12 lymph nodes found in level 1, of which four contained metastases, and there were three lymph nodes found in level 2, of which one contained a metastasis. Histologically, the tumour did not show any tubule formation, the nuclei were very pleomorphic, and there were 26 mitoses per high-powered field. Oestrogen and progesterone receptors were negative.

Pathological summary
- Size 1.8 cm
- Grade III (3,3,3)
- Axillary nodes:
  level 1, 4/12
  level 2, 1/3
  total 5/15
- Oestrogen receptors negative, H score = 20
- Progesterone receptors negative

continued

Case histories **continued**

Mrs ROD was referred to the oncologists, who gave her radiotherapy and chemotherapy. The radiotherapy was given to the breast in 25 fractions over 5 weeks, and the chemotherapy was Adriamycin and cyclophosphamide, given every 3 weeks for four courses. Unfortunately, her hair all fell out, but had regrown by the end of the treatment.

She remained well until 2 years and 6 months after her treatment when she began to have nausea. She went to see her GP, who noted that she was jaundiced, and sent her urgently to the oncologist. She was noted to have liver secondaries and started a course of Taxotere, but did not improve. She went downhill rapidly, and died peacefully 2 years and 9 months after the initial diagnosis.

Treatment summary
* Surgery:
  partial mastectomy
  axillary node clearance
* Radiotherapy: 25 fractions
* Chemotherapy:
  Adriamycin
  cyclophosphamide

Mrs CAN

Mrs CAN is aged 62. She was asked by her GP to go to the NHS Breast Screening Centre for a mammogram, and as the mammogram showed an abnormality she was asked to attend an assessment clinic. She had not noticed any abnormality in her breast, and even after the invitation to attend the assessment clinic arrived she still could not find any abnormality.

Mrs CAN has four children. The oldest one was born when she was aged 30, and she had her first period when she was aged 11. When she was aged 52 she experienced the menopause, and was put on hormone replacement therapy. She stopped this therapy 2 years ago. Her mother had breast cancer, treated by a mastectomy when she was aged 58. Her mother subsequently died of a heart attack aged 81.

At the assessment clinic the doctor could not palpate any abnormality, but repeat mammograms showed a spiculated lesion behind the left nipple which was 0.5 cm in diameter. A fine needle aspiration cytology under ultrasound control confirmed that this lesion was malignant.

Diagnostic summary
* Screening mammogram: suspicious
* Assessment mammography: malignant (code 5)
* Ultrasound-guided FNAC: malignant (C5)
* Clinical examination: no lesion discovered

Mrs CAN was advised that a partial mastectomy would give a poor cosmetic result as the lesion was behind the nipple, so she chose a total mastectomy. She was very distressed by the diagnosis and needed the support of the breast care nurse at the assessment clinic, and on two occasions prior to admission, which was 6 days after the

continued

Case histories continued

assessment clinic. When admitted, she was beginning to cope, and said that she had been greatly helped by the breast care nurse being available to listen to her fears and to give her information. She had found the relaxation tape, given by the breast care nurse, particularly useful.

She had a left total mastectomy and axillary node clearance. The level 1 and level 2 nodes were cleared from the axilla. There was a suction drain behind the mastectomy wound and another suction drain in the axilla, when she returned from theatre. These were removed at 48 hours and 72 hours, respectively, and then Mrs CAN went home.

A 0.6 cm tumour was found behind the left nipple. The margins of excision were clear of tumour. Histologically, the tumour showed much tubule formation, the nuclei were very uniform and small in size, and there were only two mitotic figures per high-power field. This is a grade II tumour (1,2,1). There were no metastases in the 16 lymph nodes recovered from the axilla. Oestrogen receptors were positive (H = 250) and so were progesterone receptors (H = 190).

Pathological summary
- Size of the tumour: 0.6 cm
- Grade of the tumour: II (1,2,1)
- Axillary nodes:
  level 1, 0/12
  level 2, 0/4
- Oestrogen receptors positive, H = 250
- Progesterone receptors positive, H = 190

The prognosis for Mrs CAN is therefore good, and her Nottingham Prognostic Index is 3.12. The surgeon and oncologist saw her together and decided she should be treated with tamoxifen, 20 mg daily, and would need no further adjuvant treatment. She was seen by the breast care nurse, who fitted her with a prosthesis to go into the bra. She also attended a support group, and found this a great help.

When seen 5 years after the surgery, there was no evidence of recurrence, and the tamoxifen was discontinued.

Treatment summary
- Surgery:
  total mastectomy
  axillary node clearance
- Radiotherapy: not given
- Chemotherapy: not given

Endocrine therapy: tamoxifen 20 mg daily for 5 years

Further reading

Dixon, J. M. (ed.) (1995) *The ABC of breast diseases*. BMJ. Publishing, London.

Dixon, J. M. and Sainsbury, R. (1999) *Breast cancer*, 2nd edn. Churchill Livingstone, Edinburgh.

Fentiman, I. S. (1998) *The detection and treatment of breast cancer*. Martin Dunitz, London.

Harris, J. R., Leppman, M. E., Morrow, M., and Hellman, S. (1996) *Diseases of the breast*. Lippincott-Raven, Philadelphia.

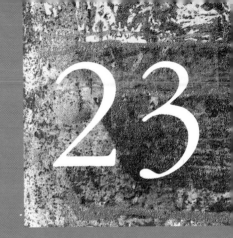

Tumours of the nervous system
Brian Orr

- The space-occupying lesion (SOL)

- Primary brain tumours

- Spinal tumours

- Tumours of the peripheral nervous system (PNS)

Tumours of the nervous system

There are many tumours of the nervous system and there is still controversy over their classification. In 1993, there was a revised classification by the WHO, and this is now used worldwide. Immunostains, electron microscopy, cytogenetics, and, most recently, molecular genetics have helped to bring about a more rational classification as we have learned that some tumours form part of a wider group whereas other tumours are distinct and separate entities.

In the clinical setting, options are rather limited and similar patterns of management occur for different tumours. This chapter attempts to emphasize these themes and state the patient characteristics that also matter in management. These themes can only be approached through a workable tumour classification system and therefore a significant part of this chapter systematically describes this classification but in the most clinically orientated way.

Aetiology of nervous system tumours

A data collection problem has been identified by the International Agency for Research on Cancer (IARC). Brain tumours are not included in a publication of cancer trends because of incomplete and inaccurate data. This has arisen because:

- nervous system tumours are relatively rare;
- there are many different types;
- there are many tumour grades;
- there have been four changes in classification over 70 years.

These factors have made epidemiological studies difficult and as a result there are few certainties in tumour causation. The few certain factors that are known only account for a limited number of tumours. The factors that cause most tumours are therefore likely to be complex. The following is a summary of present knowledge.

Descriptive epidemiology

Person

- Age: tumour incidence peaks in the 65–74 age group.
- Gender: males have higher incidence.
- Race: incidence higher in whites than blacks in USA.
- Social class: incidence higher in upper social classes

Time

- Overall incidence has increased in twentieth century but increase is small.
- The only tumour with substantial increase is primary brain lymphoma.
- A proportion of primary brain lymphoma is AIDS-related.
- A proportion is non-AIDS related and is as yet unexplained.

Place

- International variation is not very striking.
- Tumour cluster studies have failed to provide valid risk factors.

Analytical epidemiology

Observational studies (cohort and case–control studies) have increased our knowledge of causation, especially by ionizing radiation and genetic factors. However, these factors only account for a small proportion of tumours.

Radiation Ionizing radiation can cause nerve sheath tumours, meningiomas, and gliomas. Implicated treatments are:

- radiotherapy to head and neck for benign conditions;
- dental x-rays at an early age;
- *in utero* x-ray exposure.

Reviews investigating dangers of electric power fields have found exposure to be insignificant in causation. There is still controversy surrounding radio-frequency radiation. Reviews of mobile phone exposures are still taking place.

Genetic factors Gene disorders with associated tumour types are shown in Table 23.1.

Diet Nitrosamide exposure in mothers can cause brain tumours in their children. Exposure is complex and includes:

- diet
- smoke
- cosmetics
- some drugs.

Nitrosamide-inhibiting foods (vitamin C and vitamin E) can reduce risks of tumours.

Occupation Increased risks are seen in:

- aircraft pilots
- farm workers (particularly livestock workers);
- health care workers (especially if exposure to formaldehyde).

Infections

Simian virus 40 (SV40) is present in some tumours. So far there is little evidence of a causal role in brain tumours.

Table 23.1 Gene disorders and associated tumour types

Gene disorder	Tumour type
Neurofibromatosis type 1	Astrocytoma, optic gliomas, neurofibroma
Neurofibromatosis type 2	Schwannoma, meningioma
Turcot's syndrome	Glioblastoma, medulloblastoma
Tuberose sclerosis	Subependymal astrocytoma
von Hippel–Lindau syndrome	Haemangioblastoma
Gorlin's syndrome	Medulloblastoma
Sturge–Weber disease	Choroid plexus papilloma

Trauma The best studies indicate an increased risk of meningioma. Most studies have serious confounding features, making results unreliable.

The space-occupying lesion (SOL)

The SOL (Fig. 23.1) is the term used when imaging of the brain gives a radiological diagnosis but as yet a pathological diagnosis has not been made. Imaging using computed tomography (CT) scan or magnetic resonance imaging (MRI) can give the following important information:

- intra- versus extra-axial (within brain substance or without);
- contrast enhancement (how much intravenous contrast is taken up);
- mass effect (how much compression of surrounding brain);
- oedema (how much fluid is accumulated around tumour);
- cysts (presence of abnormal fluid filled cavities);
- hydrocephalus (dilatation of ventricles caused by a block in CSF circulation).

The SOL can be caused by cerebral abscess, cerebral bleed, as well as cerebral tumours. The symptoms at presentation can be similar for all three conditions. The presentation symptoms are:

- raised intracranial pressure (headache and vomiting);
- epilepsy (petit mal, grand mal, temporal lobe type);
- neuropathies (hemiparesis, cranial nerve loss, posterior fossa signs);
- functional loss (personality change, cognitive loss, dysphasia).

The most common brain tumour is a secondary lesion (brain metastasis). This can present as single or multiple lesions and can arise from the following primary sites:

- lung
- breast
- colorectal
- oesophagus or stomach
- skin – melanoma.

The prognosis for brain metastases is dependent on the type of primary cancer, the performance status at presentation, and the response to treatment. The single brain metastasis can be treated with optimal relapse-free duration by a combination of whole brain radiotherapy and radiosurgery. Where radiosurgery is not available, surgery remains first-line treatment but carries with it a certain morbidity, especially so in the older age groups.

Primary brain tumours
Tumours of neuroglial cells or gliomas
Astrocytomas

These account for 80% of gliomas. The astrocyte is a stellate cell. The astrocytomas have a range of cell types, each type similar to a normally differentiated area of brain (Table 23.2).

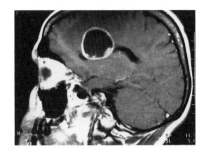

Fig. 23.1 Space-occupying lesion showing rim contrast enhancement.

Table 23.2 Tumour cell types

Tumour cell	Normal area of brain
Protoplasmic	Cortex
Fibrillary	White matter
Pilocytic	Corpus callosum or pyramids
Gemistocytic	Reactive gliosis

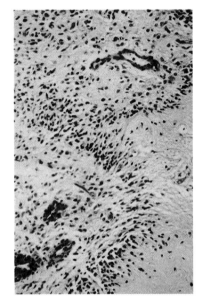

Fig. 23.2 High-grade glioblastoma showing palisading necrosis.

The differences in cell type are due to differing patterns of intracellular intermediate filaments. The grade of the tumour must predict clinical behaviour. The following characteristics are used to assess grade:

• cell pleomorphism

• mitotic activity

• vascular proliferation

• necrosis.

Low-grade astrocytomas are grades I and II, anaplastic astrocytoma is grade III, and glioblastoma is grade IV. Anaplastic astrocytoma and glioblastoma form the high-grade astrocytomas. The radiological appearance of low- and high-grade astrocytoma is very different (Fig. 23.2, Table 23.3).

An exception to this rule is the low-grade pilocytic astrocytoma of the cerebellum or suprasellar area that shows a cystic component and intense enhancement on imaging.

Glioblastoma multiforme accounts for approximately two-thirds of the total number of astrocytomas. Glioblastoma multiforme gives a positive response to glial fibrillary acidic protein (GFAP) staining on immunohistochemistry (IHC) as do the lower grades of astrocytoma. There are a diversity of cell forms in the tumour and characteristically these cells palisade (swirl) around areas of necrosis. The main difference between glioblastoma and anaplastic astrocytoma is the duration of preoperative symptoms and length of postoperative survival.

Treatment of the low-grade astrocytomas is with surgery alone, whereas the treatment of high-grade astrocytomas is with surgery and radiotherapy. It has been concluded that chemotherapy has no significant survival advantage for glio-

Table 23.3 Radiographic appearance of low- and high-grade astrocytomas

Low grade	High grade
Homogeneous tumour	Heterogeneous tumour
Hypodense on CT scan	Mixed density
Little enhancement	Strong enhancement
Little oedema	Significant oedema
No haemorrhage or cysts	Cysts and haemorrhage common

blastoma and therefore it has no role in the primary treatment of this group of tumours. It can be used for relapsed disease when it can palliate symptoms successfully. At present trials are investigating the role of temozolamide (an oral alkylating agent) in primary treatment of high-grade gliomas.

An operation on a high-grade glioma is called a decompression. An internal decompression is the most frequent type and is performed when the infiltrating tumour margins make it impossible to excise the tumour completely. The operation leads to a pathological diagnosis, resolution of pressure symptoms, and improvement in function, allowing more patients to proceed with postoperative radiotherapy. Radiotherapy will prolong the effectiveness of surgery and can increase life expectancy for glioblastoma from 5 to 11 months. Not only can survival be improved, for many there will also be significantly improved quality of life with adequate working abilities. The ideal radiotherapy dose is 60 Gy given during two phases (large fields followed by small fields) but practically this can only be given to patients with good performance status. Brachytherapy (the use of radioactive implants) and radiosurgery (the use of multiple treatment arcs to minimize radiation dose to adjoining normal tissues) can bring further survival advantages but this can only be gained for a superficial tumour and a small tumour (< 3 cm), respectively.

The prognosis for high-grade gliomas depends on tumour grade, the age of the patient, and the performance status of the patient. Some elderly patients with poor performance status will derive little benefit from radiotherapy and the correct decision may be no treatment. The maintenance of quality of life and the steroid-sparing effect of radiotherapy are very important issues and all patients should be carefully assessed by an oncologist.

Oligodendrogliomas

These tumours account for 5% of gliomas. Like astrocytomas, they occur in adult life and in the cerebral hemispheres. Unlike astrocytomas, they have a preponderance for the frontal lobes, are slow growing, and show more calcification. Microscopically, the tumour cell is enlarged and round. The cell would appear to have undergone acute swelling with an empty-looking cytoplasm (in contrast to a fibrillary cytoplasm). The small, round nucleus appears to float and the calcification is confined to the vascular stroma of the tumour. Under electron microscopy it is seen that the cytoplasm is filled with mitochondria instead of glial filaments. There are four tumour grades as in astrocytoma but the most commonly occurring tumour is the anaplastic or grade III tumour.

Oligodendrogliomas are both radio- and chemosensitive. Their slow growth has made it difficult to conclude whether chemotherapy should be given as part of the primary treatment for high-grade (anaplastic) tumours. A recruiting MRC trial is addressing this issue. Surgery and radiotherapy are the accepted treatments for anaplastic tumours. Some treatment centres will report 10-year survival figures above 50% for oligodendrogliomas, showing better survival figures than for astrocytomas.

Ependymomas

These tumours account for 5% of gliomas. They occur in children and young adults; in children they have a tendency to occur in the fourth ventricle, whilst in

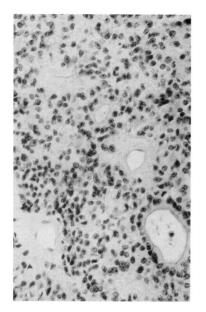

Fig. 23.3 Ependymoma showing ependymal cells arranged around a lumen.

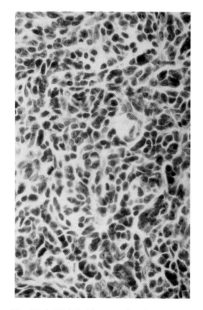

Fig. 23.4 Medulloblastoma showing a Homer Wright rosette.

adults they occur in the spinal cord. The ependymal cell lines the CSF lumen. Ependymomas have prominent endoplasmic reticulum, microvilli on the cell surface, cilia with the 9 + 2 axial complex configuration and basal bodies (blepharoplasts). A diagnostic feature is the ependymal rosette (cells arranged around a lumen), but this is only found in a minority. Perivascular pseudo-rosettes (cells arranged around a blood vessel) are frequent (Fig. 23.3). The ventricular ependymomas can cause hydrocephalus. Supratentorial ependymomas can also occur (not periventricular) and radiologically these are indistinguishable from other gliomas.

The practical classification is low, intermediate, and high grades of tumour. The low-grade tumour is typified by the myxopapillary ependymoma occurring at the cauda equina in the third or fourth decades of life. The tumour cells secrete mucin so the stroma is prominent. Although these tumours are large, they are usually resectable and immediate postoperative radiotherapy is not required. On the other hand, a high-grade ependymoma can recur locally very quickly and the incidence of metastasis to another part of the CNS is approximately 10–15%. The incidence is higher with higher-grade and infratentorial tumours. Staging of these patients should include imaging of the neuroaxis and CSF cytology. Ten or fifteen per cent will have positive cytology and this makes the prognosis worse.

Surgery to decompress the tumour and to correct hydrocephalus is the primary aim. For intermediate- to high-grade tumours, postoperative radiotherapy is required. If there is a significant risk of metastasis, craniospinal radiotherapy is given. Otherwise, involved field radiotherapy is given. Unfortunately, high-grade tumours have a survival similar to glioblastoma, but intermediate-grade tumours can do well. Chemotherapy has been used for relapsed high-grade ependymomas but response duration is short.

Malignant neuronal tumours
Medulloblastoma

By definition this tumour is restricted to the cerebellum. The cell of origin is still not known but it is thought to arise from the external granular layer of the fourth ventricle. This tumour forms 25% of childhood tumours. Maximal incidence occurs at 3–5 years of age. A second peak occurs at age 20–24 years. Seventy per cent of these tumours occur in children; the other 30% occur in young adults. In children the tumour is typically midline; in adults it is typically laterally placed in the cerebellum.

CT appearances are of hyperdense lesions due to the dense cellularity of the tumour. Strong homogeneous enhancement is typical; cysts and haemorrhages are common. Spread of the tumour can be determined by imaging; spread can be by the leptomeningeal route or by drop metastases along cord.

The microscopic appearance is a dense collection of small, round, blue-stained cells. They show scant cytoplasm, round nuclei, and abundant mitoses. A Homer Wright rosette (Fig. 23.4) is a collection of tapering cells with peripheral nuclei. Pseudo-rosettes can also occur; here the cells are arranged around a blood vessel. Positive staining for NSE (an immunostain) is frequently seen.

The optimal treatment is complete resection of tumour followed by craniospinal radiotherapy. Complete resection tends to be more easily accomplished for peripheral tumours. After craniospinal radiotherapy, the posterior fossa is usually boosted to give a total dose of 55 Gy to the tumour bed. Trials are still ongoing to determine the role of chemotherapy in this tumour. Although chemotherapy responses are obtained, they are not durable unless consolidated by radiotherapy. There remains the possibility that chemotherapy may reduce the necessary dose of radiotherapy to achieve cure. This would have enormous potential in very young children with developing nervous systems that may be impaired by radiotherapy at an early age.

The 5-year survival figures for medulloblastoma is 40–45%. Worse prognosis occurs with undifferentiated tumours, incomplete resection, young age, and positive CSF. It is now known that loss of heterozygosity at chromosone 17p13 is associated with poor treatment response.

Other malignant neuronal tumours of CNS

Other malignant neuronal tumours of the CNS are shown in Table 23.4.

The PNET is undifferentiated, showing no neuronal or rosette differentiation. It has a worse prognosis than the medulloblastoma. At the moment, it is considered a separate tumour from the medulloblastoma, but it may be derived from a similar primitive cell in the CNS.

Cerebral lymphoma

The incidence of this tumour is 1 or 2 per million per year. This tumour frequently occurs in AIDS or immunocompromised patients. It frequently is found in elderly patients; however, a significant proportion occurs in middle age.

Primary lymphoma can present as a single lesion in 50% of patients. In these cases it usually involves the fronto-parietal areas of the brain. In the other 50% of patients, the lesions are multiple. A periventricular demarcated pattern can raise suspicions that a tumour is lymphoma. A trial of steroids has also been used in forming a diagnosis; typically a lymphoma may show a response to steroids alone. However, in many patients the diagnosis cannot be made before biopsy or decompression.

CNS lymphoma is a B-cell, high-grade tumour occuring in an extranodal site. Unfortunately, it does not achieve the 45% 2-year survival figures of other high-grade non-Hodgkin's lymphoma tumours. In fact, the median survival of 12–14 months is similar to glioblastoma. Lymphoma is very radio- and chemo-sensitive and recent treatment is combined modality for patients under the age of

Table 23.4 Other malignant neuronal tumours of the CNS

Tumour type	Location
Retinoblastoma	Eye
Pineoblastoma	Pineal gland
Primitive neuroectodermal tumour (PNET)	Cerebral hemispheres

60 years. Prognosis is very dependent on age; those patients over 60 years having a very poor outlook. Recent phase 2 studies combining chemotherapy, containing high-dose methotrexate and cytarabine, followed by whole brain radiotherapy, have seen survival increase to 30–40% at 5 years but this is in a selected young group of patients. Nevertheless, appropriate chemotherapy offers a better hope of cure and should now be considered in fit patients.

The staging of CNS lymphoma should include MRI of the craniospinal axis and CSF cytology. Positive lymphoma cells in the CSF occur in 25% of patients and are an indication for intrathecal methotrexate, usually given along with systemic chemotherapy.

Surgery has a role in obtaining material for histology but has no role in controlling the illness. This is because CNS lymphoma is a generalized disease in a majority of cases (despite radiologically demarcated lesions). When radiotherapy is administered, the posterior orbit and cribriform plate must be included in the fields, otherwise these areas can be sanctuary sites for later disease relapse.

Tumours of the pituitary

Adenomas

A full account of pituitary adenomas is given in Chapter 24 and need not be duplicated here.

When an adenoma is causing an endocrinological problem, medical management is started, using bromocriptine or a suitable alternative. Sometimes inhibition of cortisol biosynthesis is required in Cushing's disease.

When an adenoma causes pressure symptoms or visual field problems despite medical management, then surgery is required. A transphenoidal or transfrontal approach can be made, depending on the extent of tumour in the suprasellar region.

Significant residual tumour and recurrent tumour have both been indications for local radiotherapy. Radiotherapy is most effective following maximal tumour excision and sometimes a second operation should be considered for recurrent tumour, immediately followed by radiotherapy.

It is difficult to talk about evidence-based management for adenomas. Most reported series in the literature have small numbers and the cases are highly selected. However, the evidence would suggest a benefit in treating patients with acromegaly and Cushing's disease with surgery and radiotherapy. These patients frequently develop coincidental morbidity from their endocrine condition because medical management is not fully effective over a whole lifetime. These patients in particular should be considered for radiotherapy early in the natural history of the disease. The improvement in the endocrine state following radiotherapy may take many years to become apparent.

Craniopharyngioma

This is another benign tumour but its management is troublesome because of local recurrence. Strictly this is a tumour of both sella and suprasellar areas. It is thought to arise from Rathké's pouch. Its significance to oncologists arises because it is the most common non-glial tumour in children. It has a peak incidence between 5 and 10 years of age. Approximately 20% arise from the sella; 80% arise from the suprasella area. The symptoms at presentation are typically:

- raised intracranial pressure (headache and vomiting);
- visual dysfunction (visual field defect and blindness);
- endocrine disturbance (polyuria);
- hypothalamic dysfunction (short stature and obesity).

Microscopically, the tumour is composed of anastomosing trabeculae in a connective tissue matrix. Masses of keratin and cholesterol clefts are seen. The tumour undergoes cystic change and the contained fluid has the viscosity of engine oil. There is a characteristically gliotic response in surrounding brain. Complete resection is usually not achieved. Postoperative radiotherapy will lower the risk of relapse by approximately 50%. In patients under 3 years, it is advisable to delay radiotherapy because of morbidity associated with irradiating a developing nervous system.

Tumours of the pineal gland

Germ cell tumours, malignant neuronal tumours, and malignant glial tumours occur in this gland.

Germ cell tumours

The pineal gland is the most common site, followed by the suprasellar region, for CNS germ cell tumours. CNS germ cell tumours comprise 10% of paediatric cranial tumours but only 1% in adults. In reported series, 50–80% of pineal tumours are germ cell. As well as children, there is a significant incidence in young adults with the peak occurring at puberty.

Germinoma – These are more common than teratomas. They have a preponderance in males. On imaging it is common to see a homogeneous mass with strong enhancement and calcification. Hydrocephalus occurs quite commonly. Microscopically, the appearance is similar to gonadal germinomas: lobules of spheroidal cells, showing vacuolated cytoplasm and large nuclei, occurring in vascular connective tissue containing lymphocytes. Immunostains are positive for placental alkaline phosphatase (PLAP) but negative for α-fetoprotein (AFP). Metastases can occur by way of the ventricular system or the meninges. There is a higher incidence in Klinefelter's syndrome and it is associated with isochromosome 12p, but this is not a constant finding. Treatment of choice is radiotherapy. This is a radiosensitive tumour. It is almost mandatory to give craniospinal radiotherapy because the risk of metastases is large.

Teratomas – These tumours have a male preponderance and most occur in the first two decades of life, but on the whole earlier than for germinomas. On imaging they may show calcification but the masses are usually mixed density with cysts. The microscopic appearance can be either mature (features of squamous epithelium or neuroepithelium) or immature (features of neuroblastoma, retinoblastoma, or even rhabdomyosarcoma). Staging involves imaging of the whole CNS axis to look for metastases and determination of tumour markers in serum as well as CSF. Testicular tumour markers, namely AFP and β-human chorionic gonadotropin (β-HCG), are used. A diagnosis of pineal teratoma can be made on radiological grounds with elevated markers in the CSF. Imaging of thorax, abdomen, and pelvis is also performed to rule out involvement at mediastinal or retroperitoneal sites. The treatment of choice has remained systemic chemotherapy as in gonadal teratomas. A standard platinum regimen is chosen. Response can be evaluated by tumour markers as well as imaging. Radiotherapy may also play a role if there is a residual mass after chemotherapy.

Malignant neuronal tumours of pineal gland – pineoblastoma

During development the pineal gland has large, pale-staining cells separated by bands of dense, small cells. In man, the smaller cells disappear so that the parenchymal cells are separated by a connective tissue stroma. These parenchymal cells are neuronal cells containing secretory granules and developing cytoplasmic processes to blood vessels. These cells have similarities to photoreceptor cells, showing positive staining to arrestin and rhodopsin kinase. The sympathetic nerves that serve the pineal gland increase activity of rhodopsin kinase, leading to melatonin release that is thought to synchronize endogenous endocrine rhythms.

Pineoblastoma, a malignancy of the neuronal cell, occurs in children under 10 years of age. The child presents with symptoms of raised intracranial pressure but an additional symptom may be the loss of upward gaze (Parinaud's syndrome). Pineoblastoma has occurred in patients with medulloblastoma and also in patients with retinoblastoma. Imaging usually shows a heterogeneous mass with cysts and necrosis. It shows strong enhancement. Leptomeningeal spread or intraventricular metastases can be detected. Microscopically, the tumour is densely cellular with scanty cytoplasm and round nuclei. Homer Wright rosettes may be present as in medulloblastoma, Flexner–Wintersteiner rosettes may be present as in a retinoblastoma. Treatment follows the pattern of medulloblastoma. Surgical excision should be as extensive as possible. This should be followed by craniospinal radiotherapy as the risk of metastases is very high. The role of chemotherapy has yet to be fully determined. The 5-year survival is approximately 55%, very similar to medulloblastoma.

Malignant glial tumours of the pineal gland

The pineal gland contains fibrillary astrocytes which provide a stroma for the parenchymal cells. A small number of malignant gliomas can occur in the pineal gland.

Meningiomas

These tumours are mainly benign and form 20% of all CNS tumours. They have a predominance in women and occur frequently in middle age. A familial link with von Recklinghausen's disease is known. Aetiological factors are previous radiation and trauma, particularly if it leads to chronic irritation. The sites of occurrence are cerebral convexities, middle third of sagittal sinus, overlying sylvian fissures and base of skull. The radiological appearance is of an extra-axial, well-demarcated, hyperdense lesion showing intense enhancement. Calcification and bone erosion may be seen. The classical types are microscopically grouped as syncytial (syncytial), fibroblastic (spindle cells arranged in whorls) (Fig. 23.5), or transitional (mixed pattern). Surgical excision is usually possible and 80% do not relapse.

Aytpical meningiomas

These tumours microscopically show malignant cell features, malignant morphological features, or invasive features. Malignant cell features are:

- pleomorphism
- multinucleation
- increased mitotic rate.

Malignant morphological features are:

- 'sheeting' (loss of whorls or syncytial growth pattern)
- necrosis.

Invasive features are:

- brain invasion (bad prognostic factor)
- dura or bone invasion (not necessarily poor prognostic indicator).

Complete excision is less likely and earlier recurrences are more frequent. Most of these tumours are treated with postoperative radiotherapy and this decreases the risk of relapse by approximately 50%. Males tend to have a higher risk of relapse; younger patients have also increased relapse rates.

Meningiosarcoma

These tumours are highly malignant, behaving like sarcomas rather than true meningiomas. Despite surgery and radiotherapy, most patients relapse early and die from their disease.

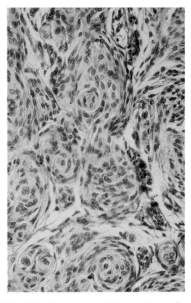

Fig. 23.5 Meningioma with no evidence of mitosis.

Spinal tumours

It is very important that a diagnosis of spinal cord compression (SCC) is made early. The diagnosis should be made on clinical evidence. Patients can complain of loss of balance or co-ordination in their legs, loss of power, which is usually symmetrical but may be uneven, or loss of sensation. Very seldom would a patient volunteer information describing a sensory level on the basis of dermatome innervation but a feeling of numbness and pins and needles are common complaints. The clinician needs the necessary level of suspicion to evaluate these symptoms further by patient examination. It is important to remember also that extradural metastases, which are the commonest cause of spinal cord compression, may cause significant and progressive pain. The patient confined to bed because of poor pain control may also have coincidental SCC, which will be missed if the neurological state is not checked regularly.

Unless the patient has had a previous neurological deficit, the signs are usually easily elicited for SCC. There is decreased:

- co-ordination
- position sense
- power (hip flexion decreased more than extension).

There is increased:

- tone
- reflexes (clonus sometimes demonstrated at knee and ankle).

There is altered:

- plantar reflexes (upgoing)
- pain and temperature sensation.

The sensory level should be demonstrated as accurately as possible. Not only is there the benefit of directing the imaging more efficiently, but there is the opportunity to predict multiple levels of cord compression, which can occur in 20%. A sterile broken tongue depressor is ideal as it provides necessary pain sensation but does not puncture the epidermis. A venepuncture needle is crude as the epidermis is easily traumatized. If a sensory level is demonstrated, the diagnosis is already made.

Imaging for SCC will:

help in determining pathological diagnosis (extradural metastasis or intrinsic tumour);

- determine the extent of lesion (both vertically and laterally);
- determine whether the lesion is single or multiple;
- provide important information on the stability of spinal bodies.

The level of spinal cord compression on imaging will frequently be one or two vertebral bodies above the elicited dermatome level.

If a patient presents with SCC and imaging has suggested a tumour as the cause, the management depends on whether the patient has a known malignancy or not. When there is no previous histological diagnosis, this should now be obtained. In the past some patients have been treated for malignancy when the lesion represented an abscess. The histological diagnosis can be made by CT-guided biopsy or by decompression. There is now a clear role for the use of MRI for spinal tumours. Imaging of the whole spine in different planes can be performed in a short time and this investigation has become the preoperative investigation of choice in these tumours.

Surgical management

- Posterior decompression or laminectomy
- Anterior decompression

An emergency laminectomy is the treatment of choice when the posterior compartment is involved and the spine above and below the lesion is stable. In 50% of patients with SCC, the anterior compartment is the predominant involved site. In this case a posterior decompression, although releasing pressure, has no significant role in improving the functional state. The anterior decompression involves an anterior approach through chest or abdomen and can only be undertaken in fit patients. Again, stability of surrounding spine is required so that stabilizing rods are adequately fixed.

Non-surgical management

Radiotherapy is the primary treatment of SCC when there are multiple bone metastases along the spine in the vicinity of the compression or when there are multiple levels. It is also used following decompression to lower the risk of relapse and maintain the functional state. Treatment is recommended within 12 hours of the definitive imaging. The fractionation used depends on the prognosis. The prognosis is determined by the type of primary tumour and the functional state of the patient. The patient with lung cancer, significant paraparesis and progressing disease at the primary site will have the worse prognosis (median survival 3–6 months). The patient with the haematological malignancy with improving neurological function will have the best prognosis (median survival 2–4 years).

Chemotherapy is used for haematological malignancies causing SCC. The patient with extradural high-grade non-Hodgkin's lymphoma (extranodal site) is usually managed with core biopsy, radiotherapy, and chemotherapy. A standard regimen for non-Hodgkin's lymphoma (cyclophosphamide, Adriamycin, vincristine, and prednisolone) is used. When there is CSF involvement, intrathecal methotrexate and systemic methotrexate regimens are used.

Tumours of the spinal cord and canal

- Astrocytoma (they tend to be high grade and have a poor prognosis).
- Ependymoma (can be the low-grade myxopapillary type or the intermediate-to high-grade tumour of the cervico-thoracic cord in adults).
- Lymphoma (can occur as tumours within cord – intramedullary – or more frequently as tumours compressing cord – extradural).
- Meningioma (resection of these tumours can be difficult and prognosis depends on adequate resection).
- Cordoma (a tumour of notochord remnants occurring in the sacrum, surgery is the treatment of choice; radiotherapy may be required for significant residual disease or relapse).
- Schwannoma (these tumours of the peripheral nervous system can occur on spinal nerve roots and cause SCC).
- Neuroblastoma (this paediatric peripheral nervous system tumour can access the spinal canal, through the intervertebral foramina, causing SCC).

Location of tumours of spinal cord and canal

On imaging the brain, the location of a tumour is either extra- or intra-axial (either outside or inside brain). For the spine the location of tumours are:
- intramedullary (within the cord);
- extramedullary and intradural (within the coverings of cord);
- extradural (outside the cord coverings).

Examples include:
- intramedullary (astrocytoma, ependymoma, and some lymphomas) (Fig. 23.6);
- extramedullary and intradural (meningioma and some schwannomas);
- extradural (metastases, some lymphomas, and some schwannomas).

Tumours of the peripheral nervous system (PNS)

The peripheral nervous system (PNS) contains:
- motor nerves

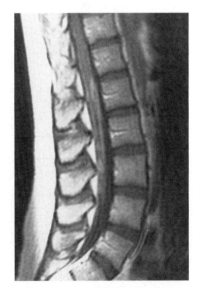

Fig. 23.6 Intramedullary lymphoma involving conus and corda equina.

- sensory nerves
- autonomic nerves.

The autonomic nerves in the PNS are all post-ganglionic neurons. When these neurons develop tumours, they are of two types:
- ganglionic or neuroblastic tumours;
- paraganglionic or neuroendocrine tumours.

Nerve sheath tumours

These tumours are derived from two cell types:
- Schwann cell: this cell is of neural crest origin (neuroectoderm). They are the supportive cells for peripheral neurons and are the equivalent to the oligodendrocyte of the CNS. When it myelinates a neuron, it ensheathes only one axon. There are non-myelinating Schwann cells and some cells perform a macrophage role.
- fibroblast cell: this cell has a mesenchymal origin. It normally inhabits the endoneurium, which is the connective tissue matrix between nerve fibres.

Schwannomas

These benign tumours occur on cranial nerves as well as in the PNS. When multiple, they are usually associated with neurofibromatosis type 2 (a congenital gene disorder with two different genes causing types 1 and 2 syndromes). Microscopically, the appearance is of interwoven bundles of bipolar spindle cells, the alignment of nuclei produces Verocay bodies (seen under the high-power microscope, the body is made up of aligned nuclei of the spindle cells).

In the cranial nerves the most important example is the acoustic nerve schwannoma occupying the cerebellopontine angle. This tumour enlarges the acoustic canal and presents with tinnitus, ataxia, and unilateral deafness. Treatment is with surgery using a joint ENT and neurosurgical approach.

Peripherally, schwannomas can occur on the flexor aspect of the elbow, wrist, or knee. They can also occur on intercostal nerves or in the posterior mediastinum close to spinal nerve roots.

Neurofibromas

These benign tumours likewise occur on cranial nerves as well as in the PNS. When plexiform neurofibromas, occur this is pathognomonic for neurofibromatosis type 1. They are complex tumours having a schwannial (neuroectodermal) component as well as a mesenchymal component. Microscopically, the tumour has a looser texture due to more significant collagen fibres running randomly through it (Fig. 23.7). The cell content is scantier, the cells are bi- or tripolar, and the nuclei are elongated (fusiform).The treatment is surgery and complete resection is very important in reducing the recurrence rate.

Malignant nerve sheath tumours

The distinction between schwannomas and neurofibromas becomes blurred in malignant tumours. Most malignant schwannomas arise in limbs. Microscopically, there is increased cellularity, cell pleomorphism, and the spindle cells form a

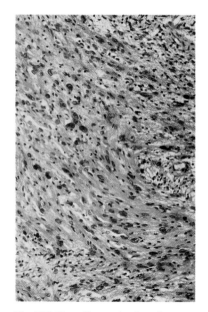

Fig. 23.7 Neurofibroma showing a loose texture and fusiform nuclei.

herring-bone pattern. The tumour shows signs of invasion into neighbouring structures. Malignant neurofibromas arise peripherally in large nerves. The majority are seen in pre-existing plexiform neurofibromas. The mesenchymal element can show metaplasia into cartilage, osteoid, bone, or fat. Surgery is the only effective treatment but clear margins are difficult to achieve.

Peripheral neuroblastic tumours

Neuroblastoma (sympathetic nervous system)

This is a very important paediatric tumour, accounting for approximately 8% of all childhood cancers. It occurs in the adrenal medulla and the organs of Zuckerkandl (present in the neck, mediastinum, and retroperitoneum). This tumour usually presents before 5 years of age, as either an abdominal mass or a paravertebral mass causing cord compression. These tumours produce increased amounts of catecholamines and the metabolites VMA (vanillylmandelic acid) and HVA (homovanillic acid) appear in the urine in 95% of cases.

It is thought that these tumours arise during the development of the sympathetic nervous system. Neural crest cells within this system differentiate into ganglion cells, Schwann cells, and perineurial cells. Three tumour subgroups are possible:

* neuroblastoma (primitive cells without schwannial stroma);
* ganglioneuroblastoma (ganglion cells seen, extensive schwannial stroma);
* ganglioneuroma (mature ganglion cells, mature stroma).

The biologically favourable tumours will have potential for maturation. The cytogenetics of this tumour are well known. There is a deletion of the short arm of chromosome 1. There is gene amplification, usually at the short arm of chromosome 2. MYCN amplification leads to a worse prognosis.

Well-encapsulated tumours are easily resectable, but tumours invading the aorta, liver, or kidney have a poor prognosis. Patients older than 1 year will have a worst prognosis, compared with younger patients. The adrenal gland location has a worst prognosis. Metastases can occur in lymph nodes, bone marrow, liver, and skin and will carry a poor prognosis. Treatment consists of a combination of surgery and radiotherapy and in advanced tumours palliative chemotherapy and radiotherapy are used. Survival figures vary between 20% and 90%, depending on the stage of the tumour.

Peripheral PNET (parasympathetic nervous system)

These tumours are now thought to be derived from primitive neural crest cells that show the morphology or phenotype of the parasympathetic nervous system. The tumours arise in bone, soft tissue, as well as peripheral nerves. These tumours are known as Ewing's sarcoma if location is in bone, or extra-osseous Ewing's sarcoma if location is in soft tissue. If they occur in bone, 50% occur in the central axis skeleton (the other 50% in bony extremities); if they occur in soft tissue, the two most common locations are chest and extremities. Peripheral PNETs present in young and older patients either as a tender mass or with a pathological fracture. Unfortunately, there is no serum or urine marker.

There are distinctive cytogenetics with a chromosomal translocation between chromosomes 11 and 22. This brings about a fusion of a *EWSRI* gene with *ETS* oncogenes. The phenotype of this tumour is characteristically different from neuroblastoma. Although they are composed of densely packed, small, blue cells and can form rosettes, they do not produce neuritic processes. Under electron microscopy there are two types of cells – light and dark cells.

The prognosis does not depend on the age of the patient. Peripheral tumours do better than central tumours. Surgical resection with radiotherapy to the involved site and chemotherapy is the optimal treatment for these tumours. Surgery for central tumours is more difficult. Metastases can occur by the haematogenous route to bone marrow and lung.

Paragangliomas

These neuroendocrine tumours fall into two broad groups.

Chromaffin paraganglia (sympathetic system)

Phaeochromocytomas (adrenal medulla and organs of Zuckerkandl) The majority of these tumours are benign but 5% may be malignant. They occur in children and adult and most are sporadic. Approximately 10% occur within known families as part of multiple endocrine neoplasia (MEN) types 2A or 2B and then they tend to occur early in life. The presenting symptoms are due to excess secretion of catecholamines (not just metabolites) into the serum. Predominant noradrenaline secretion causes sustained hypertension whilst mixed adrenaline/noradrenaline secretion causes fluctuating hypo/hypertension.

These tumours are composed of chief cells, which have variably sized nuclei; some cells are multinucleated. The electron microscope appearance is of dense core granules that are membrane bound and contain catecholamine enzymes. Local invasion can occur even in benign tumours. Treatment is by surgical excision with α-adrenergic blockade. Only about 10% of tumours relapse. The 5-year survival for malignant phaeochromocytomas is only 36%.

Non-chromaffin paraganglia (parasympathetic system)

Chemodectomas The majority of these tumours are benign but 5–10% may be malignant. These tumours are usually non-secreting, but some can secrete noradrenaline. Most occur sporadically, but familial cases occur and the involved gene is on chromosome 11. The primary treatment for these tumours is surgery. The difficulty in location, and the presence of bone destruction, or intracranial involvement, all make radiotherapy an alternative treatment option that may cause less morbidity. Survival figures of 90% at 5 years can be achieved with optimal treatment.

Carotid body tumour This occurs at the bifurcation of the common carotid artery just below the angle of mandible. It can present with hoarseness or Horner's syndrome. Patients are typically between 40 and 60 years old. There is an increased incidence at high altitude. Microscopically, the tumour is composed of chief cells in a highly vascular stroma and electron microscopy shows dense core granules. Bad prognostic features include pleomorphic cells, mitotic figures, and necrosis.

Glomus tympanicum This occurs in the middle ear. The presenting features are of dizziness, tinnitus, and hearing loss.

Glomus jugulare This occurs on the temporal bone at base of skull. Typically presents with loss of cranial nerves IX–XII.

Case histories

Case 1

A 25-year-old chef presented with a 1-month history of weakness and numbness in his left hand. He also described a persistent headache. MRI scan showed a SOL in the right parietal lobe. A stereotactic biopsy showed the presence of a grade III astrocytoma (high-grade glioma). Further surgery would have caused marked morbidity. In the absence of decompression and during radiotherapy planning, the patient received procarbazine, lomustine, and vincristine (PCV) chemotherapy. Following the completion of a 4-week period of radiotherapy (using a three-field plan) he was prescribed a further two courses of PCV chemotherapy

His functional state was unstable during the first course of chemotherapy and during the radiotherapy. He noticed weakness of left leg and increasing spasticity on his left side. He was intolerant to reduction in his steroid dose during this time and during subsequent chemotherapy. His performance status seemed to fall on steroid reduction. He became Cushingoid and the subsequent proximal myopathy was a significant factor in further functional loss. His chemotherapy was stopped, active physiotherapy and rehabilitation was started, and the steroids were correspondingly reduced as efforts were made to reduce spasticity.

Imaging showed a good response to treatment with a smaller involved area in the parietal lobe. The treated area showed high signal but no mass effect, enhancement, or oedema. He has now obtained good functional state without the need for walking aids.

Lessons

- Completion of treatment should always be attempted.
- Loss of functional state can be iatrogenic as well as tumour related.
- Grade III tumours can have significant survival.
- Radiotherapy must be well planned to maximize tumour dose and minimize normal tissue dose.
- Similar results can be obtained with 6 weeks of radiotherapy or 4 weeks of radiotherapy and chemotherapy in grade III gliomas.

Case 2

A 59-year-old man presented with headache, ataxia, and then collapse. CT scan showed a space-occupying lesion in the right parietal lobe of the brain (Fig. 23.8). Decompression was performed and histology showed a high-grade B-cell non-Hodgkin's lymphoma. Staging was by MRI of craniospinal axis (clear), CSF cytology (clear), and CT scan of thorax, abdomen, and pelvis (clear).

His primary treatment was a chemotherapy regimen containing high dose methotrexate and cytarabine. Sodium bicarbonate diuresis was required to facilitate methotrexate clearance. His first course of chemotherapy was complicated by an episode of thrombocytopenia 10 days into his cycle, requiring platelet transfusion. During the second course of chemotherapy, he did not successfully clear the methotrexate in 2–3 days despite optimal diuresis. Renal excretion took a total of 7 days and by this time a haemolytic anaemia had developed, presumably caused by

continued

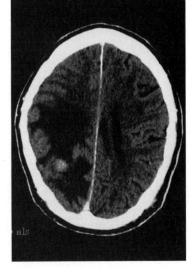

Fig. 23.8 CNS lymphoma in a periventricular location.

Case histories continued

folate deficiency (despite optimal folinic acid rescue). The development of anaemia caused conversion of his controlled atrial fibrillation to uncontrolled atrial fibrillation. Blood transfusion and folic acid supplementation stabilized his condition.

Imaging showed complete response to chemotherapy. He then proceeded to cranial radiotherapy. He received a dose of 30.6 Gy in 17 fractions over 3.5 weeks. The fields included posterior orbit and cribriform plate (sanctuary sites for relapse). He has remained disease free for 1 year.

Lessons
* Lymphoma can appear similar to glioma on imaging.
* High-dose whole brain radiotherapy can cause cognitive function loss.
* Results are excellent for reduced dose radiotherapy, especially if complete response is achieved with chemotherapy.
* Suitable chemotherapy regimens can be very toxic despite optimal precautions.
* Serum methotrexate levels can be measured to determine when adequate clearance has been achieved.
* To avoid a demyelinating condition (encephalopathy), high-dose chemotherapy must be given first in sequence before radiotherapy.

Further reading

Graham, D. I. and Lantos, P. L. (eds) (1997) *Greenfield's neuropathology*, 6th edn, Volumes 1 and 2. Arnold, London.

Bigner, D. D., McLendon, R. E., and Bruner, J. M. (eds) (1998) *Russell and Rubinstein's pathology of tumours of the nervous system*, 6th edn, Volumes 1 and 2. Arnold, London.

Vinken, P. J. and Bruyn, G. W. (eds) (1997) *Handbook of clinical neurology*, Volume 67, Series 23–25, *Neuro-oncology* Parts 1–3. Elsevier, Oxford.

DeVita, V. T., Hellman, S., and Rosenberg, S. A. (eds) (1997) *Cancer: principles and practice of oncology*, 5th edn, Chapter 42, pp. 2013–62. Lippincott-Raven, Philadelphia.

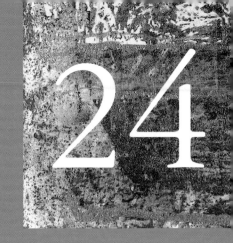

24

Endocrine tumours
Patrick M. Bell and
A. Brew Atkinson

- Pituitary

- Thyroid

- Parathyroid

- Adrenal

- Endocrine tumours of gastrointestinal tract and pancreas

- Multiple endocrine neoplasia (MEN)

- Humoral manifestations of malignancy

Endocrine tumours

Pituitary

Epidemiology, aetiology, and pathology

Pituitary tumours are common, accounting for about 10% of brain tumours coming to surgery. They are almost invariably benign, and present with symptoms either of a mass lesion or hormonal dysfunction (Table 24.1). Annual clinical incidence rates are about 2 per 100 000 population but recently, sophisticated imaging techniques suggest that 20% of the pituitary glands of 'normal' individuals harbour an incidental pituitary abnormality.

Pituitary adenomas are monoclonal in origin and theories of tumour development suggest intrinsic pituitary cell defects. It is likely that the majority of them develop from single transformed cells, which are then further stimulated by a variety of growth factors.

Pituitary adenomas can be classified on the basis of their clinical hormonal manifestations. Tumours are characterized as growth hormone (GH)-producing adenomas associated with acromegaly, prolactin-secreting adenomas and ACTH-producing adenomas causing Cushing's syndrome. Other rare forms include TSH-producing tumours causing thyrotoxicosis. In addition, there is the large group of clinically non-functioning adenomas. Pituitary tumours can also be classified by immunohistochemistry, using highly specific antisera to anterior pituitary hormones.

Presentation

Table 24.1 lists the common presentations. Local symptoms include headache and symptoms secondary to compression of adjacent tissues or nerves, i.e. visual field disturbances (classically bitemporal hemianopia), loss of visual acuity, and ocular palsies.

Symptoms of hormone overproduction (Table 24.2) vary, depending on the particular anterior pituitary hormone being overproduced. Prolactinomas are common. In females they typically cause amenorrhoea and/or galactorrhoea. They are often microadenomas (< 1 cm diameter), whereas in men the adenomas tend to be

Table 24.1 Presentations of pituitary adenoma

1. Local problems
   e.g. field defects, headache

2. Hormone overproduction
   e.g. Cushing's syndrome, acromegaly

3. Hormone underproduction
   e.g. growth failure, hypoadrenalism

4. Mixtures of the above

Table 24.2 Assessment for possible hormone overproduction

1. In many situations a suppression test used. Requires a normal range established in controls without endocrine disease

2. Acromegaly and/or giantism 75 g oral glucose tolerance test with growth hormone levels

3. Cushing's syndrome

    Pituitary origin in 70–80% of cases

    Low dose dexamethasone (synthetic steroid) testing with measurement of serum cortisol to confirm hypercortisolism

    Other tests then required to establish pituitary or other cause of hypercortisolism

4. Hyperprolactinaemia

    Raised prolactin plus clinical features

    No suppression test required

5. TSH induced thyrotoxicosis

    Very rare case of hyperthyroidism

    Always rule out other causes

larger and present with symptoms secondary to tumour compression. Hypogonadism is almost invariable (decreased libido, impotence, and infertility). There is a rough association between tumour size and prolactin production. Before any patient considered to have a non-functioning adenoma is sent to surgery, prolactin should be measured because if it is significantly elevated (> 4000 mU/l), dopamine agonist treatment with cabergoline or bromocriptine can shrink the tumour.

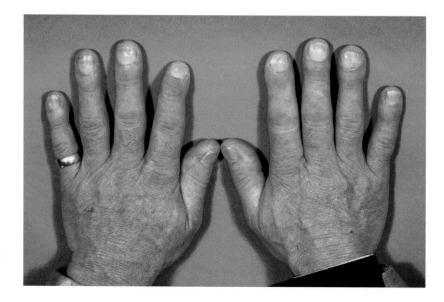

Fig. 24.1 Classical acromegalic hands. Note spatulate fingers and the 'ectopic' wedding ring, which no longer fits the ring finger.

Large tumours with prolactin < 4000 mU/l are, however, unlikely to be pro-lactin-secreting. Hyperprolactinaemia in this situation is caused by the endocrino-logically inactive adenoma compressing the pituitary stalk and preventing hypothalamic dopamine (prolactin-inhibiting factor) from reaching prolactin-secreting cells. It is therefore mandatory to image the pituitary in all cases of mild hyperprolactinaemia before starting drug therapy.

GH-producing adenomas are associated with giantism in children (rare) and acromegaly in adults. Acromegaly is a good example of the different ways pituitary disease can present, with all manifestations in Table 24.1 occurring in some patients. The common results of GH excess are thickening of the skin, classical facial features with thick lips, exaggerated nasolabial folds, and lengthening of the jaw. Hands and feet increase in size, resulting in spade-like digits (Fig. 24.1). Diabetes and hypertension are common. There is increased morbidity and mortality, mainly from respiratory and cardiovascular disease.

Excess adrenocortical function leading to hypercortisolism (Cushing's syndrome) results from a variety of causes. About 70% of cases are due to an ACTH-producing pituitary adenoma. The classical clinical features are weight gain, centripetal obesity, moon face, proximal myopathy, fresh purple striae, thin skin, and easy bruising. Hypertension and diabetes are common. After a diagnosis of hypercortisolism has been made, a very careful investigation is required before pituitary aetiology can be assumed.

Table 24.3 Diagnosis of hypopituitarism

Hormone	Diagnosis	Therapy
TSH, thyroxine	Free thyroxine low, TSH low, normal (inappropriate) or below normal	Thyroxine orally once daily
ACTH, cortisol	Stimulation test (hypoglycaemia as stimulus)	Low-dose hydrocortisone orally, usually twice daily
LH & FSH, testosterone or oestradiol	Low oestradiol or testosterone FSH & LH low normal or below normal	Male: testosterone by IM injection every 2–3 weeks or by daily patch
		Female: oestrogen by cyclical oestrogen/progestogen replacement regimen
		To achieve fertility in women, FSH/LH by daily IM injection with careful monitoring; in men, FSH/LH by IM injection 3 times weekly
Growth hormone	Stimulation test (hypoglycaemia, arginine, or standardized exercise test)	GH daily by SC injections in selected adult cases
Vasopressin	Water deprivation test measuring urinary and plasma osmolality and plasma AVP	Desmopressin intranasally once or twice daily. Tablets also available

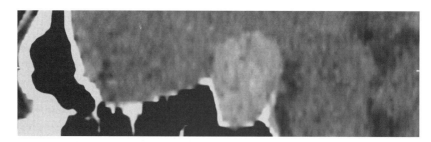

Fig. 24.2 Sagittal CT scan showing extensive pituitary tumour extending into the suprasellar region.

As well as hormonal excess, adenomas can be associated with hormone deficiency, either single or, more commonly, multiple (Table 24.3). The classic sequence of loss of function is, first luteinizing hormone (LH) and follicle-stimulating hormone (FSH), then GH, followed by thyroid-stimulating hormone (TSH), and finally adrenocorticotrophic hormone (ACTH). Posterior pituitary deficiency of vasopressin can occur, leading to diabetes insipidus, but this is a rare preoperative finding with pituitary adenomas. Symptoms of GH deficiency in adults include reduced muscle strength, decreased exercise tolerance and increased body fat. In children, growth velocity is decreased markedly. Gonadotrophin deficiency leads to decreased libido in both sexes, impotence in men and amenorrhoea and infertility in females. TSH deficiency is associated with tiredness, weight gain, and decreased energy. ACTH deficiency causes malaise, loss of energy, poor appetite, weight loss, and postural dizziness. Intercurrent illness can lead to vascular collapse, coma, and, if the condition remains undiagnosed, death.

Examination and investigation

The examination should include visual acuity measurements and visual field estimations by confrontation and by detailed perimetry. Careful checks for signs of overproduction should be made, e.g. classical features of acromegaly or Cushing's syndrome, galactorrhoea, etc. Signs of underproduction may be present, e.g. loss of secondary sexual characteristics (pubic hair, axillary hair, beard growth). Blood pressure may be elevated (acromegaly, Cushing's) or decreased (hypoadrenalism).

Table 24.4 Radiology of the pituitary

CT/MR

- Good at diagnosing or ruling out large tumours
- Not very good with lesion < 1 cm

  Venous sampling from petrosal sinuses

- Indicated in special situations, e.g. possible pituitary aetiology for Cushing's syndrome

  Decisions to operate

- Surgeons often operate on basis of sophisticated endocrinological testing even when CT/MR negative

Table 24.5 Therapy for pituitary adenoma

Transphenoidal pituitary surgery

External pituitary irradiation

Medical therapy

Dopamine agonists, (prolactinoma) bromocriptine, cabergoline

- Somatostatin analogues (acromegaly), octreotide, lanreotide
- Steroid inhibitors (Cushing's), metyrapone, ketoconazole

Supplementary surgery

- Bilateral adrenalectomy (Cushing's)
- Repeat pituitary surgery

Schemes for detection of overproduction (Table 24.2) and underproduction (Table 24.3) are shown. After these tests have been performed, careful radiological imaging of the pituitary by MR or CT is essential (Fig. 24.2). Specialized venous sampling from petrosal sinuses for ACTH gradient is often used in the differential diagnosis of Cushing's syndrome (Table 24.4).

Treatment and prognosis

A variety of treatment options are available (Table 24.5). For prolactinomas the usual initial therapy is medical, using dopamine agonists, either bromocriptine or cabergoline. These shrink over 80% of such tumours. For other types of adenoma, transphenoidal surgery is the therapy of first choice. In acromegaly and Cushing's syndrome, specialized centres report 70–80% remission rates post-operatively. Pre- and perioperative hydrocortisone therapy is given. Patients must be monitored carefully for meningitis and diabetes insipidus. Postoperatively, even though most pituitary adenomas are not entirely removed, the outlook is good. If significant tumour is present at postoperative assessment or if significant regrowth occurs, external pituitary irradiation over 5–6 weeks is very helpful in decreasing morbidity but often causes long-term hypo-pituitarism. If hormone overproduction persists, therapy specific to the particular syndrome should be used, e.g. metyrapone, ketoconazole, or bilateral adrenalectomy in Cushing's syndrome, or somatostatin analogues in acromegaly. Long-term follow-up of pituitary adenomas in a specialist endocrine centre is essential for optimal outcomes.

Thyroid

Thyroid tumours are the commonest endocrine neoplasms. Most present as pain-less lumps in the neck. A major challenge for the clinician is to distinguish malig-nant thyroid tumours from the majority of nodules in the thyroid that are benign.

Classification, aetiology, and pathology (Table 24.6)

By far the commonest thyroid cancers are those arising from follicular epithelial cells. The commonest of these is the papillary type in which the cells form papil-

Key points

Pituitary tumours can present

- tumour compression
- hormone overproduction
- hypopituitarism

Always check prolactin in apparently endocrinologically inactive tumour. Dopamine agonist may shrink prolactinoma.

Transphenoidal surgery indicated for most other tumours.

Table 24.6.   Classification of thyroid carcinoma

Epithelial

- Follicular

  Papillary (70%)

  Follicular (15%)

  Undifferentiated or anaplastic (10%)

- C cells

  Medullary carcinoma (5%)

Non-epithelial

  Lymphoma

Secondaries

Percentages are estimated proportions of commoner types.

lae and have characteristic nuclear changes. Small (< 1 cm diameter) papillary microcarcinomas are a frequent incidental finding at autopsy. The other common epithelial tumour is the follicular type.

Chromosomal abnormalities are a feature of both papillary and follicular types with activation of the *RAS* oncogene. Activation of the *RET* oncogene is relatively specific for papillary carcinoma. External irradiation is a known risk factor for thyroid carcinoma and may influence these genetic changes.

Medullary thyroid carcinoma arising in the C cells is relatively uncommon. In approximately 20% of cases there is a family history and in these, C-cell hyperplasia may precede tumour formation. Familial cases may be associated with multiple endocrine neoplasia (MEN) type 2. In many familial medullary carcinomas a characteristic mutation of the *RET* proto-oncogene is detectable in peripheral blood. This is valuable in screening clinically unaffected family members and has in part replaced screening tests based on tumour calcitonin production.

Lymphomas are rare. They may coexist with Hashimoto's thyroiditis.

Secondaries in the thyroid are a common autopsy finding in widespread malignant disease but are rarely a presenting clinical feature.

Table 24.7 Points in history favouring benign or malignant disease

Benign	Malignant
Abnormal thyroid function (hyper- or hypothyroidism)	Male (though most carcinomas occur in females)
Family history of benign thyroid disease	Family history of thyroid cancer or endocrine neoplasia
Pain (suggesting thyroiditis)	History of external radiation
	Young (< 20 years) or old (> 70 years) at presentation

Clinical features

The usual presentation is of a painless lump in the neck. A careful history may help to distinguish those which harbour thyroid cancers from the majority of thyroid nodules that are benign and harmless (Table 24.7).

On examination of thyroid nodules, features that raise suspicion of malignancy include:

• firm or hard consistency

• irregular shape

• fixity to deep or superficial structures.

Most thyroid carcinomas occur in single nodules and are rare in the presence of a multinodular goitre. However, significant change, or any of the worrying features noted above, in a nodule within a multinodular goitre should raise suspicion of malignancy.

Particular clinical features of the different pathological types are summarized in Table 24.8. Regional lymphadenopathy is relatively common. Signs of local compression such as stridor, hoarseness, or dysphagia are rare except in anaplastic carcinoma where the neck mass may occasionally be painful.

Investigation

Blood tests:

• Free thyroxine, TSH: abnormalities of thyroid function rare in thyroid carcinoma.

• Thyroid autoantibodies: high titre in Hashimoto's thyroiditis where the goitre may occasionally be confused with nodular thyroid disease. Remember that Hashimoto's thyroiditis and carcinoma may coexist.

• Thyroglobulin: produced by follicular epithelial cells and high levels may be present in differentiated carcinoma. There is significant overlap with benign

Table 24.8 Clinical features of different pathological types at presentation

	Sex (M:F)	Age (years)	Findings in the neck	Metastases
Papillary	1:3	30–50	Single nodule, local glands occasionally	Rare
Follicular	1:2	40–60	Single nodule, local glands rare	Bones and lungs
Anaplastic	M<F	60–70	Hard mass, local compression, local glands common	Common, but death from disease in the neck
Medullary	M<F	40–60	Mass, local glands common	Bone, liver, and lung

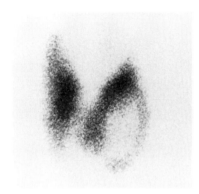

Fig. 24.3 Technetium scan showing 'cold' nodule (reduced isotope uptake) in the left lower lobe.

disease. Thyroglobulin is most useful in monitoring treatment of previously diagnosed epithelial carcinoma.

- Calcitonin: excessive secretion is characteristic of medullary carcinoma.
- *RET* proto-oncogene: present in around 90% of familial cases of medullary carcinoma. In asymptomatic family members a negative result reliably excludes the possibility of developing medullary carcinoma.

Imaging

- Isotope scans: are widely employed to investigate thyroid nodules. Unlike normally functioning thyroid tissue, most thyroid carcinomas do not take up iodine efficiently. Following administration of isotopes such as ^{121}I or technetium (^{99m}Tc), scintigraphic scanning usually shows a 'cold' area (Fig. 24.3). Unfortunately, the majority of benign nodules are also cold and a few carcinomas take up isotope normally. Scans must therefore be interpreted cautiously.
- Ultrasound scanning: a highly sensitive method for detecting thyroid nodules, but of limited value in identifying which are malignant.
- Cytology: samples can be obtained by the technique of fine needle aspiration, which is now the usual investigation of first choice (Fig. 24.4). Provided thyroid cells are adequately represented in the sample, reliable differentiation of malignant from benign lesions can be obtained in the majority of cases. Even after repeated sampling there is uncertainty in a proportion of cases. In this situation surgical resection will allow full histological assessment and provide either reassurance or guide further appropriate treatment.

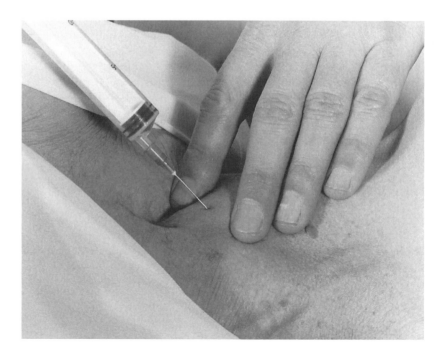

Fig. 24.4 Fine needle aspiration of a thyroid nodule.

Table 24.9 Factors determining less good prognosis in papillary and follicular carcinoma (AGES)

Age (older)
Grade (poorly differentiated)
Extent (local spread or metastases)
Size (of primary lesion)

Staging

Traditionally staging follows a TNM classification. The primary tumour (T) status is defined by the size of the lesion, the nodal (N) status by the presence or absence of regional lymph nodes, and the metastatic (M) status by the presence or absence of distant metastases. In practice, cell type is critical in determining outcome with papillary and follicular having a relatively good prognosis, anaplastic very poor, and medullary carcinoma somewhere in between.

Treatment

Several treatment modalities are available and with the exception of anaplastic carcinoma these have the potential to be highly effective. Given that some lesions, for example, small, well-differentiated papillary carcinomas, follow an indolent course and carry a good prognosis, determining how aggressive treatment should be requires some discretion. Thus decisions about differentiated papillary and follicular lesions will be influenced by several well-defined prognostic indicators (Table 24.9).

Surgery Small differentiated tumours (< 1–2 cm) may be treated by lobectomy. Large lesions usually require near total thyroidectomy with removal of involved lymph nodes where possible. The more radical treatment ensures removal of possible satellite microcarcinoma in the opposite lobe (a feature especially of papillary carcinoma). It also facilitates subsequent treatment of metastases with radioiodine.

Medullary carcinoma is frequently multicentric and is usually treated by total thyroidectomy with removal of involved lymph nodes if possible. In familial cases with mutations in the *RET* proto-oncogene, unaffected members testing positive for the mutation are offered total thyroidectomy at around 5–7 years of age.

Anaplastic lesions are usually inoperable at time of diagnosis.

Thyroxine The rationale for this treatment in thyroid carcinoma is not simply to provide physiological hormone replacement following thyroidectomy. It depends on the evidence that:

- TSH is a promoter of thyroid growth and
- adequate thyroxine will suppress TSH.

The aim is to suppress TSH into the low or undetectable range. This requires larger doses of thyroxine than are needed for the treatment of hypothyroid patients. Therapy is lifelong and should be interrupted only during further investigation or treatment, and then for as short a time as possible.

Radioiodine This treatment is based on the specificity of iodine uptake in differentiated thyroid carcinoma. By administering ^{131}I, radiation can be delivered to the thyroid with little exposure to other parts of the body. Since most thyroid carcinomas are 'cold' compared with normal thyroid tissue, relatively little ^{131}I will be delivered to the tumour in the presence of a largely intact thyroid gland. Radioiodine is therefore used to destroy any remaining thyroid tissue after near total thyroidectomy and this facilitates future use of tracer doses of ^{131}I to detect metastatic disease. Metastases can in turn be treated with larger therapeutic doses of ^{131}I. Before radioiodine treatment commences, thyroxine must be discontinued for several weeks, allowing an increase in TSH, which stimulates iodine uptake.

Small tumours treated by limited surgery generally do not require radioiodine. Medullary and anaplastic carcinomas are not responsive to radioiodine.

Follow-up Treated patients with differentiated thyroid carcinoma should be reviewed after 3 months, then every 6 months for 2 years and if there is no evidence of recurrence annually thereafter. At each visit:

- the neck is palpated;
- free thyroxine and TSH are checked as a guide to thyroxine dosage;
- thyroglobulin is checked. Increased levels suggest presence of tumour tissue and often indicate need for further radioiodine.

Prognosis

Long survival is possible. Prognostic features in well-differentiated thyroid carcinoma have been mentioned (Table 24.9). In a specialized centre overall survival (corrected for deaths not related to thyroid cancer) at 25 years is 94% for papillary, 79% for medullary and 71% for follicular carcinoma. Most recurrences and most mortality are in the first 5–10 years after diagnosis.

Parathyroid

Parathyroid carcinoma is rare, contributing less than 1–2% of all hyperparathyroidism (which is caused by a benign adenoma in over 75% of cases). Carcinoma should be suspected:

- in unusually severe hyperparathyroidism (with very high parathyroid hormone concentrations);
- when hypercalcaemia is associated with a palpable mass in the neck;
- in cases of recurrent hypercalcaemia following parathyroid surgery.

Adrenal

The adrenal gland consists of two parts, the outer cortex and the inner medulla. The cortex produces glucocorticoids (mainly cortisol), mineralocorticoids (mainly aldosterone), and sex steroids. The medulla produces the neurotransmitter hormones adrenaline and noradrenaline. Table 24.10 shows a classification of tumours based on site, hormonal activity, and nature.

Adrenal incidentaloma

Adrenal tumours have always been considered to be relatively uncommon but more recently CT scanning of the abdomen for other conditions has led to a

Table 24.10 Adrenal tumour classifications

Position
- Cortex or medulla

Hormonally active?
- Cortex Hyperaldosteronism, Cushing's syndrome, virilism
- Medulla Phaeochromocytoma

Hormonally inactive?
- Adrenal incidentaloma

Benign or malignant

marked increase in incidentally discovered adrenal tumours often called 'incidentalomas'. They are present in 1–5% of patients imaged with CT. The differential diagnosis includes primary adrenal adenoma or carcinoma, adrenal gland metastasis, and infiltrative disease of the adrenal.

Once discovered, the abnormality must be assessed for hormonal activity (Table 24.11) and for malignancy. Positive results should be followed by more detailed hormonal evaluation in order to make a definite diagnosis. Once hypersecretion is confirmed, therapy is as detailed below for the particular condition.

The size of an incidentaloma is useful in distinguishing between benign and malignant lesions. Those larger than 4 cm have a much greater chance of being malignant and should be either removed or biopsied. In the remainder, CT/MR scanning should be repeated at 6 months and tumours removed if they are growing significantly.

Hypercortisolism

Adrenal adenomas causing Cushing's syndrome are usually associated with a gradual onset whereas carcinomas tend to have a more acute clinical onset often with associated abdominal and back pain. As for all cases of Cushing's syndrome, the diagnosis is made on the basis of increased urinary free cortisol excretion and lack of suppression of serum cortisol after low-dose dexamethasone. ACTH levels are suppressed. Both adenomas and carcinomas are visible on CT or MR scans.

The tumour should be removed surgically if possible (Fig. 24.5). Adenoma patients usually have postoperative suppression of the hypothalamic–pituitary–adrenal axis and require glucocorticoid therapy for many months until the axis has recovered and the remaining adrenal gland is again functioning normally.

Table 24.11 Tests for incidentally found adenomas

- Careful clinical and family history and examination
- 24 hour urinary catecholamines on two occasions
- 0800 hour serum cortisol after 1 mg dexamethasone at 2300 hours
- Uncuffed serum potassium
- Plasma aldosterone and renin activity if hypertensive

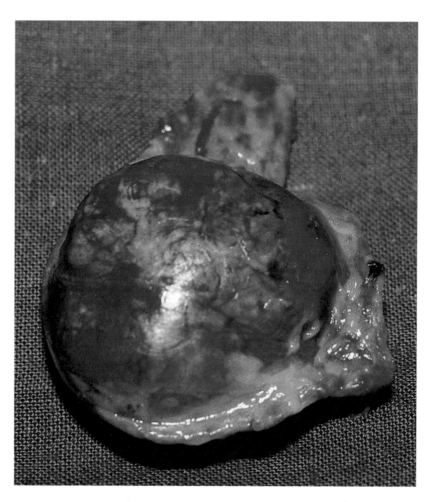

Fig. 24.5 A typical adenoma causing Cushing's syndrome. Note the surrounding rim of normal adrenal tissue.

In adrenal carcinoma, complete resection is unusual. Mitotane (*op*'DDD) is used for non-resectable recurrent disease with mixed results in terms of hormonal and tumour size response. All patients should, however, be treated immediately following the initial operation. Glucocorticoid therapy should be given simultaneously to prevent development of hypoadrenalism. Median survival time is short.

Hyperaldosteronism

This should be suspected in all patients with hypertension and hypokalaemia. The incidence is about 1% of all cases of hypertension. Symptoms can include muscle fatigue and weakness but patients are usually asymptomatic. The disease can be caused by either a unilateral adenoma or bilateral hyperplasia. Aldosterone levels are high and renin levels suppressed. Adrenal carcinoma causing the syndrome is extremely rare.

The diagnosis can be made using a variety of tests including upright aldosterone to renin ratios, overnight supine renin and aldosterone levels and saline suppression tests (infusion of saline normally suppresses aldosterone and this suppression is lost in hyperaldosteronism).

The differential diagnosis between unilateral adenoma and bilateral hyperplasia is important as treatment differs. A careful assessment of both CT scan and the results of adrenal venous sampling is made. Removal of an adrenal adenoma is usually recommended. This restores potassium to normal and may lower blood pressure. Even if it remains raised, treatment options available for reduction of blood pressure are widened. Specific medical therapy with spironolactone, an aldosterone antagonist, or amiloride is used if the diagnosis is bilateral adrenal hyperplasia.

Virilizing adrenal tumours

These are rare. Virilism in females may be a feature of adrenal carcinoma often in association with Cushing's syndrome. Testosterone-secreting adrenal tumours are an unusual cause of hirsutism and virilism. The diagnosis should be suspected when the serum levels of the precursor hormone DHEA-S are very high.

Phaeochromocytoma

These tumours are derived from chromaffin cells and produce catecholamines. They are dangerous because of their ability to release suddenly large amounts of catecholamines with subsequent catastrophic rises in blood pressure and vascular crisis. The diagnosis should be suspected in hypertensive patients with paroxysmal symptoms of headache, sweating, and palpitation (Table 24.12). They may occur in association with medullary carcinoma of the thyroid (MEN type 2) and neurofibromatosis.

About 80% are adrenal, the rest mainly occurring elsewhere in the abdomen. They can be bilateral and about 20% are eventually shown to be malignant so that all require extended follow-up. As with most types of endocrine tumour, it is not easy to distinguish histologically between benign and malignant tumour types, the latter diagnosis being reserved for those cases with metastases or tumour tissue in areas where chromaffin tissue does not occur normally.

The diagnosis of phaeochromocytoma is made by detecting elevated urinary catecholamines (adrenaline and noradrenaline) and/or failure of plasma catecholamines to suppress after administration of clonidine. Tumours are generally sufficiently large to be identified readily by CT and MR scanning.

Table 24.12 Manifestations of phaeochromocytoma

- Paroxysmal attacks
- Tachycardia and sweating
- Headaches
- *Café au lait* spots
- Unusual BP response to surgery, anaesthesia
- Positive family history
- Associated diseases
    Medullary carcinoma thyroid
    Neurofibromatosis
    Hyperparathyroidism

Surgical removal is the definitive treatment option. Careful preoperative medical management is essential using α-receptor blockade to reverse the effects of adrenergic stimulation. β-blockade should never be used until adequate α-blockade has been achieved. A multidisciplinary approach with a team comprising an experienced physician, anaesthetist, and endocrine surgeon, along with intensive care facilities, is essential for good outcomes to be achieved.

When malignancy is evident at first diagnosis, surgical debulking is often helpful. In that situation and where malignancy is diagnosed later, the radiopharmaceutical I meta-iodobenzylguanidine ([131I]MIBG) can be used therapeutically as it is concentrated by chromaffin tissue. Combination chemotherapy with cyclophosphamide, vincristine, and dacarbazine has also been used but with limited success. During treatment chronic medical management with α- and β-blockade is usually needed.

In non-malignant phaeochromocytoma, survival after successful operation approaches normal. Hypertension frequently remains or develops. In malignant phaeochromocytoma there appear to be two subtypes, one with slow and indolent progression and the other with more rapid deterioration. The overall 5-year survival rate is less than 50%.

Endocrine tumours of gastrointestinal tract and pancreas

These rare but fascinating tumours arise from peptide-secreting cells of the gastrointestinal mucosa and pancreatic islets. Because they secrete both hormones and neurotransmitters, and because they were thought to have a common origin from neural crest tissue, they are often called neuroendocrine tumours.

Neuroendocrine cells in fact arise from diverse embryological origin. They have highly differentiated cell function, contain secretory granules, and possess the capacity for Amine Precursor Uptake and Decarboxylation (hence APUD cells) involved in neurotransmitter production. APUD cells are found in many other organs including thyroid, adrenal medulla, and lung. Although a major secretory product dominates any particular tumour syndrome, cells may produce other peptide hormones through enhanced expression of genes normally expressed at a low level.

Neuroendocrine tumours share a number of characteristics:

- symptoms caused by excessive secretion of hormones rather than local tumour growth and invasion;
- secretion of several peptide hormones and neurotransmitters;
- potentially diverse and widespread effects though endocrine (release of hormones into circulation) and paracrine (effects on adjacent cells) effects;
- often slow growing with patients in reasonable health in the presence of metastatic disease;
- may be part of MEN syndromes.

Some of the better recognized clinical syndromes are summarized in Table 24.13.

Investigation

Hormone estimation Diagnosis is suggested by elevated levels of peptide hormone in blood, or of relevant metabolites of neurotransmitters in urine. Abnormal regulation

Table 24.13 Endocrine tumours of the gastrointestinal tract and pancreas

Syndrome or tumour	Cell of origin	Clinical features	Malignant	Hormone product
Carcinoid syndrome	Enterochromaffin	Flushing, diarrhoea, valvular heart disease	100% (with syndrome)	Serotonin (5 HT)
Zollinger–Ellison, gastrinoma	Pancreatic islets duodenal G cell	Peptic ulcers, diarrhoea	70%	Gastrin
Insulinoma	Islet β cell	Hypoglycaemia	10%	Insulin
Watery diarrhoea, hypokalaemia, achlorhydria (or Verner–Morrison) syndrome, VIPoma	Islet cells	Diarrhoea, hypokalaemia, hypochlorhydria	60%	Vasoactive intestinal polypeptide
Glucagonoma	Islet α (A) cells	Diabetes mellitus, rash, diarrhoea	80%	Glucagon
Somato-statinoma	Islet D cells	Diabetes mellitus, diarrhoea, gallstones	70%	Somatostatin

of hormone secretion is the basis of provocative testing, which may be useful for several syndromes, e.g. increased gastrin secretion in response to secretin in gastrinoma.

Imaging A number of techniques are used to identify and define extent of tumours:
- CT and ultrasound scanning for pancreatic lesions and liver metastases;
- barium studies, endoscopy, and ultrasound for mucosal and submucosal lesions;
- for difficult small or multiple lesions angiography and selective venous sampling with hormone estimation.

Treatment

Therapy can be directed against tumour growth and spread or hormone overproduction.

Tumour growth and spread When a localized tumour can be identified, surgery offers the chance of complete cure. However, this is often impossible when a small tumour cannot be found, when tumours are multicentric, and when metastases are already present. Chemotherapy may be effective against the primary tumour, e.g. streptozotocin in insulinoma. Hepatic metastases can occasionally be resected surgically or may be attacked though the hepatic artery by embolization or chemotherapy.

Hormone overproduction The effect of excess hormone production on target organs may be counteracted, e.g. reduction of gastric acid secretion in gastrinoma by proton pump inhibitors or gastric surgery. Alternatively, hormone production may be reduced directly by the synthetic somatostatin analogue octreotide. Somatostatin itself blocks a wide range of peptide hormone secretion but has a very short half-life. The analogues are resistant to peptide degradation and can be administered by regular subcutaneous injection.

Carcinoid syndrome

Carcinoids are the commonest gastrointestinal endocrine tumours. They are slow growing and are a relatively common incidental finding in surgically removed specimens of the appendix. Occasionally gastrointestinal carcinoids present with bleeding or obstruction.

Hormone products of primary gastrointestinal carcinoids pass into the portal circulation and are cleared by the liver. The carcinoid syndrome results from hormone release into the systemic circulation by metastatic liver deposits. Small bowel carcinoids are the most malignant and most likely to be associated with the syndrome. Extra-intestinal carcinoids (e.g. bronchial) may produce the syndrome in the absence of metastases.

The main secretory product is serotonin, which is synthesized by enzymatic modification of tryptophan. Serotonin produces excessive intestinal secretion and hypermotility (responsible for diarrhoea), and stimulates growth of fibroblasts (may contribute to cardiac lesions). The metabolic product of serotonin – 5-hydroxyindoleacetic acid (5-HIAA) – is excreted in the urine and is useful diagnostically. The role of other peptide and monoamine secretions is not yet defined but they may well be responsible for cutaneous flushing.

Clinical features

The classic features of the syndrome are:

- flushing – may be intense, precipitated by food, alcohol, or stress. Flushing is especially prominent with bronchial carcinoids when it may last for days associated with excessive lacrimation;
- diarrhoea;
- valvular heart disease – usually tricuspid and pulmonary (hormone products cleared by the lung spare the left side of the heart except in bronchial carcinoids when there is direct secretion into pulmonary veins).

Less frequent symptoms include:

- wheezing (especially bronchial carcinoid);
- telangiectasia;
- hypotension.

With a very large tumour load, utilization of tryptophan with inadequate conversion to niacin may lead to protein malnutrition and pellagra.

Diagnosis

Confirmation is usually possible by finding increased urinary 5-HIAA. Some food (e.g. bananas) may give false-positive results. Foregut carcinoids (e.g. bronchial) do not produce serotonin from 5 hydroxytryptophan (5-HTP) and no urinary breakdown product is found.

As well as usual imaging procedures, scintigraphic scanning with radiolabelled octreotide is useful for detecting primary and metastatic tumour. Octreotide binds on to somatostatin receptors present on most carcinoid tumours.

Treatment

Surgery rarely cures the syndrome except in isolated bronchial lesions since by definition metastases are present. The burden of tumour may be reduced by surgery, chemotherapy, or hepatic artery embolization. Liver transplant is a possible option.

Control of the syndrome can be achieved in most cases by octreotide. It is useful both in acute life-threatening crises as well as in the longer term.

Prognosis

Prognosis is variable with incidentally discovered appendiceal tumours rarely affecting survival. When liver metastases are present, 5-year survival is about 20%.

Gastrinomas (Zollinger–Ellison syndrome)

About 80% of gastrinomas occur in the pancreas (they are the commonest of the pancreatic islet cell tumours) and most of the others are in the duodenum. The tumours may be multicentric, especially when associated with MEN type 1. Hyperparathyroidism is particularly commonly associated.

Most present with some manifestation of peptic ulcer disease caused by excessive gastric acid secretion. Many also have diarrhoea and this may be the presenting feature. Gastrinoma should be considered in peptic ulcer disease when:

- ulceration is present in unusual sites such as the distal duodenum or jejunum;
- there is associated diarrhoea;
- there is associated hypercalcaemia or pituitary disease in the patient or family.

Formerly the major morbidity and mortality stemmed from complications of peptic ulcer disease (bleeding and perforation). Gastrectomy was a radical but effective way to counteract hypergastrinaemia. Now hyperacidity and peptic ulcer symptoms can be controlled by proton pump inhibitors. There is greater emphasis on localization and resection of primary tumour with potential cure. This remains difficult when tumours are small or multifocal, and impossible if metastatic disease is already present.

Insulinoma

These are the second commonest islet cell tumours. Like gastrinomas, they may be multifocal and are frequently associated with MEN 1.

The presentation is with hypoglycaemia and Whipple's triad should be present:

- symptoms of hypoglycaemia;
- low plasma glucose concentration;
- relief of symptoms after glucose concentration is raised.

Symptoms of hypoglycaemia can be many and varied, as well as confusingly intermittent. They are most often present after fasting, e.g. in the early hours of the morning.

The diagnosis requires demonstration of high insulin concentrations at a time when plasma glucose is low. This will be present if a blood sample can be taken during a hypoglycaemic attack. More often provocative tests, e.g. 72 hour fast under careful in-patient supervision, are required for confirmation. Confusing cases, where hyperinsulinaemia is induced by surreptitious administration of sulphonylurea or insulin, can be ruled out by measurement of sulphonylurea levels and C peptide (a measure of endogenous insulin release).

Surgical treatment is usually possible and highly effective. Even with large metastatic tumours, debulking surgery may relieve hypoglycaemia. For those in whom surgery is not possible there are several medical measures:

- diazoxide: inhibits insulin secretion;
- octreotide: inhibits insulin secretion;
- streptozotocin: chemotherapeutic agent toxic to the β cell, sometimes used to reduce tumour bulk as well as control symptoms.

Multiple endocrine neoplasia (MEN)

Two broad patterns of multiple endocrine neoplasia syndromes have been described, MEN 1 and MEN 2 (Table 24.14). These tumour syndromes share several characteristics:

- cells mostly of APUD type;
- autosomal dominant inheritance;
- progression of multicentric process from hyperplasia to adenoma and occasionally carcinoma.

MEN 1

Formerly patients presented with advanced and frequently diverse manifestations aged 20–40 years. Now many come to light through screening relatives of known cases.

> **Key points**
>
> - Tumours arise from neuroendocrine cells.
> - Symptoms are usually caused by hormone secretion rather than tumour growth and invasion.
> - Other tumours of multiple endocrine neoplasia (MEN) syndrome may be associated.
> - Treatment is directed either against the tumour or towards reducing or counteracting hormone overproduction.

Table 24.14 Multiple endocrine neoplasia (MEN) syndromes

MEN 1	MEN 2A	MEN 2B
Parathyroid hyperplasia (> 95%)	Medullary thyroid carcinoma (90%)	Medullary thyroid carcinoma (> 95%)
Pancreatic islet (80%) Tumour	Phaeochromocytoma (50%)	Phaeochromocytoma (50%)
Most often gastrinoma	Parathyroid hyperplasia (25%)	
Quite often insulinoma		
Pituitary tumour (50%)		With mucosal neuromas
Most often prolactinoma		
Also growth hormone secreting (acromegaly)		

Table 24.15 Screening for MEN 1

- Serum calcium
- Serum prolactin
- ± Serum gastrin
- ± Pituitary imaging

Hyperparathyroidism due to diffuse hyperplasia is almost invariable. Surgical results tend to be less good than in other cases of primary hyperparathyroidism due to a single adenoma. Management of pancreatic islet cell tumours is complicated by the presence of multiple tumours which makes definitive surgery difficult.

Mutations of a tumour suppressor gene (encoding the protein menin) on chromosome 11 seem to be responsible in at least some cases, but in contrast to MEN 2, the diversity of mutations makes reliable genetic screening impossible. Biochemical and radiological tests are undertaken in established cases and family members every 3–5 years from the age of 10 years (Table 24.15).

MEN 2A

Like MEN 1, patients may present with established disease (Table 24.14) with medullary thyroid carcinoma usually being the first manifestation. However, cases are identified increasingly through family screening.

The multicentric nature of medullary thyroid carcinoma makes radical surgery necessary. The potential for phaeochromocytoma to be bilateral should be remembered.

Screening for mutations of the *RET* proto-oncogene, which are present in most cases, should be undertaken at birth or in early childhood. Established cases will usually have had thyroidectomy as a prophylactic or therapeutic procedure. They require regular screening with serum calcium and urinary catecholamines for other components of the syndrome. Measurement of calcitonin (usually after pentagastrin stimulation) helps identify recurrence of medullary thyroid carcinoma.

MEN 2B

This represents only about 5% of all MEN 2 cases. Medullary thyroid carcinoma and phaeochromocytoma are associated with characteristic mucosal neuromas, especially on the distal part of the tongue. Patients are often tall with marfanoid body features. Hyperparathyroidism is an unusual feature.

Screening is along similar lines to MEN 2A.

Humoral manifestations of malignancy

Inappropriate secretion of hormones by tumours of non-endocrine origin is common. The term ectopic (out of place) hormone secretion is often used, although in normal cells in tissues where these tumours originate hormone can be detected in small amounts. Several theories have been proposed to explain inappropriate hormone secretion by non-endocrine tumours. They include a random tumour-related depression of gene control and a dedifferentiation leading to expression of proteins normally seen in fetal or immature cells.

Table 24.16 Common syndromes of inappropriate hormone secretion

Syndrome	Clinical features	Site of tumour	Hormone	Treatment
Hypercalcaemia of malignancy	Dehydration, gastrointestinal symptoms, confusion	Lung, breast	PTHrP (normally a tissue factor). Massive production results in hormonal effects similar to PTH	Rehydration Intravenous diphosphonate pamidronate
Myeloma causes hypercalcaemia by cytokine-induced osteolysis. Lymphoma-associated with increased 1,25-dihydroxyvitamin D.				
Inappropriate antidiuretic hormone release (SIADH)	Water intoxication, hypotonicity	Lung (small cell), brain Note: differentiate from non-tumour causes of inappropriate ADH release	Antidiuretic hormone (ADH)	Water restriction, demeclo-cycline. In severe cases consider hypertonic saline
Ectopic ACTH (corticotrophin)	Cushing's syndrome but compared to usual • more rapid onset • commoner in men • obvious pigmentation • marked hypokalaemia	Lung (small cell) carcinoid (thymus, bronchial)	ACTH, rarely corticotrophin-releasing hormone (CRH)	Surgery for resectable tumour. If inoperable, control hypercor-tisolism by adrenolytic drugs
Hypoglycaemia With non-islet cell tumour	Fasting hypoglycaemia	Large slow-growing sarcomas often abdominal or retroperitoneal	Insulin-like growth factor 2 (IGF-2)	Surgery, curative or debulking. Hypogly-caemia may respond to octreotide, gluco-corticoids or glucagon

Hormone secretion by non-endocrine tumours has several characteristics:

- generally non-suppressible;
- clinical features of hormone excess present only in advanced disease;
- usually involves simple peptide hormones. (Synthesis of glycoproteins, steroids, and thyroxine requires several enzymatic steps with correspondingly more complex gene control. It is less likely that a co-ordinated change in expression will take place to allow excess hormone production);
- related hormone rather than conventionally recognized hormone may be involved, e.g. hypercalcaemia of malignancy usually results from parathyroid hormone-related peptide (PTHrP), which has structural homology with parathyroid hormone (PTH).

Some of the more common syndromes of inappropriately hormone release are summarized in Table 24.16.

Case histories

Case 1

History
A 44-year-old man presented to his GP with headache and a history of bumping his car on two occasions while parking. Further questioning revealed decreased libido and impotence for 2 years.

Examination
He appeared well. Visual acuity was decreased at N10 in the right eye but was normal in the left at N5. There was a bitemporal hemianopia by confrontation. Pubic and axillary hair was sparse and there was poor beard growth.

Investigations
Computerized perimetry confirmed the visual field defect. MR scan showed a large pituitary adenoma extending upwards out of the pituitary fossa and in contact with the optic chiasm.

LH and FSH were low normal and testosterone below normal. Free thyroxine and TSH were normal. Prolactin was 1600 mU/l. GH and cortisol responded normally during an insulin hypoglycaemia test.

Management and explanation
The patient had an urgent transphenoidal hypophysectomy in an attempt to preserve vision. Postoperatively assessment showed the development of other pituitary deficiencies and the patient is now on thyroxine, testosterone, and hydrocortisone. He wears a Medic Alert bracelet and has been instructed to double his dose of hydrocortisone temporarily during episodes of illness and to receive the drug parenterally if there is vomiting or diarrhoea.

The diagnosis is of an endocrinologically silent pituitary adenoma presenting with mass effect and evidence of hypopituitarism. All such patients should have an urgent serum prolactin estimation prior to any surgery. In this case prolactin was raised

continued

Case histories continued

because of compression of the pituitary stalk. If this size of tumour had been pro-lactin-secreting, and therefore amenable to trial of medical therapy, the level would have been over 4000 mU/l. Careful consideration of extended pituitary irradiation is now necessary as it results in lower rates of tumour recurrence.

Case 2

'This thyroid gland of mine is getting larger.'

A 45-year-old lady has had goitre for many years. She points to the left side of the neck, saying that it has become larger in the last few weeks.

On examination there is a bilateral multinodular goitre with a large 5 cm diameter nodule on the upper pole of the left lobe.

Fine needle aspiration reveals 15 ml chocolate-coloured fluid and shrinks the nodule. Cytology reveals no evidence of malignancy.

At review in 3 months there has been no recurrence of the left sided nodule. The rest of the goitre is unchanged.

Thyroid carcinoma in a multinodular goitre is unusual; however, it must be exclud-ed if there is a significant change. In this case it is likely that there has been bleed-ing into a pre-existing cyst or nodule. Aspiration removed cyst fluid and altered blood products. Quite often fluid will re-accumulate in cysts of this type.

Case 3

History and examination

During a routine CT examination for other reasons, a 46-year-old lady was found to have a 2 cm adrenal adenoma. There were no headaches, sweating attacks, or pal-pitation to suggest phaeochromocytoma. BP was 124/82 mmHg. She had no symp-toms or signs of Cushing's syndrome. There was no family history of endocrine disease.

Investigations

Serum potassium was 4.2 mmol/l and supine plasma renin and aldosterone were normal. Two 24 hour urinary catecholamine estimations were normal. An over-night dexamethasone suppression test (1 mg at 2300 hours) was abnormal with incomplete suppression of 0900 hour serum cortisol (200 nmol/l).

Management

Because of abnormality of the pituitary adrenal axis, surgery was recommended. This condition, sometimes known as pre-Cushing's syndrome, with autonomous cortisol production, is often associated with suppression of steroid production by the contralateral gland. Routine hydrocortisone replacement therapy was therefore given for 6 months until demonstration that the axis had recovered.

Explanation

All so-called adrenal incidentalomas should undergo careful clinical assessment followed by simple endocrine screening to rule out early hormonal dysfunction. If abnormalities are found, then surgery is recommended regardless of the size of the adenoma. If the adenoma is non-functioning then observation is recommended if size is less than 4 cm and surgery if more that 4 cm because of the increasing risk of malignancy as size increases.

continued

Case histories continued

Case 4

'Every time I stop omeprazole my tummy pain comes back.'

History

A 31-year-old housewife described presenting to another hospital 4 years earlier with recurrent episodes of slurred speech in the morning. Hypoglycaemia had been demonstrated and she was told she had tumours in the pancreas. Subsequently she underwent surgery, which was successful. She was also told that her calcium level was high due to overactive parathyroid glands and some time later these were removed surgically. Her gastrointestinal symptoms had been present for a year but had not been investigated.

Examination

The only abnormal physical sign was some epigastric tenderness.

Investigation and review of previous treatment

Review of previous medical notes indicated that 4 years ago, helped by CT with contrast enhancement and intraoperative ultrasound scanning, four pancreatic islet cell tumours had been identified and removed by radical distal pancreatectomy. Two of these were confirmed at histology and immunocytochemistry to be insulinomas. A small nodule in the wall of the duodenum was also identified and removed at surgery and this was shown to be a gastrinoma.

At neck exploration a year later enlargement of all four parathyroid glands was noted and a three and one-half gland total parathyroidectomy undertaken. Parathyroid hyperplasia was confirmed at histology. Around this time a non-functioning pituitary adenoma was identified.

Current investigations demonstrated active duodenal ulceration and markedly raised serum gastrin. Serum calcium and pituitary function were normal. CT and octreotide scanning showed no abnormality in the pancreas or elsewhere in the abdomen.

Explanation

This patient has features of MEN 1 with evidence of multiple pancreatic adenomas, a pituitary adenoma, and hyperparathyroidism. It is likely that one or more small gastrinomas are present in the residual pancreas or duodenal wall despite negative imaging procedures. Currently her symptoms are well controlled with full-dose omeprazole. She is being followed up carefully. Arrangements are being made for family screening.

Further reading

Felig, P., Baxter, J. D., and Frohman, L. A. (eds) (1995) *Endocrinology and metabolism*, 3rd edn. McGraw-Hill, New York.

Ganguly, A. (1998) Primary aldosteronism. *N Engl J Med* **339**, 1828–34.

Kulke, M. H. and Mayer, J. (1999) Carcinoid tumours. *N Engl J Med* **340**, 858–68.

Mazzaferri, E. L (1993) Management of a solitary thyroid nodule. *N Engl J Med* **328**, 553–9.

Schlumberger, M. J. (1998) Papillary and follicular thyroid carcinoma. *N Engl J Med* **338**, 297–306.

Service, F. J.(1995) Hypoglycaemic disorders. *N Engl J Med* **332**, 1144–52.

Sheaves, R., Jenkins, P. J., and Wass, J. A. H. (eds) (1997) *Clinical endocrine oncology*. Blackwell, Oxford.

Utiger, D (1997) Treatment and retreatment of Cushing's disease. *N Engl J Med* **336**, 215–17.

Wilson, J. D., Foster, D. W., Kronenberg, H. M., and Larsen, P. R. (eds) (1998) *William's textbook of endocrinology*, 9th edn. W. B. Saunders, Philadelphia.

Working Party from the Endocrinology and Diabetes Committee of the Royal College of Physicians and the Society for Endocrinology in conjunction with the Research Unit of the Royal College of Physicians (1997). Pituitary tumours: recommendations for service provision and guidelines for management of patients. *J R Coll Physicians Lond* **31**, 628–36.

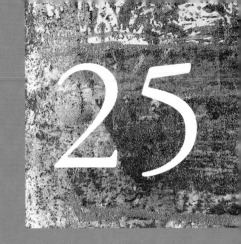

25

Oncological emergencies
Sarah McKenna

- Introduction
- Cancer-related emergencies
- Treatment-related emergencies

Oncological emergencies

Introduction

An oncological emergency is defined as a situation arising in the cancer patient, related either to the cancer itself or its treatment, for which early diagnosis and treatment is necessary to prevent major morbidity or mortality.

Optimal outcomes in these patients rely on recognition of early symptoms and signs, and institution of the appropriate therapy. Avoidance of undue morbidity and mortality is particularly important for patients in whom further treatment may significantly prolong or improve the quality of life.

This chapter deals with the most commonly occurring oncological emergencies. These have been classified as:

- cancer related
- treatment related.

Cancer-related emergencies

Superior vena cava obstruction

Aetiology

The superior vena cava (SVC) lies on the right side of the upper mediastinum, and is closely related to the aorta, right main bronchus, right pulmonary artery, and trachea. It drains the jugular and subclavian veins, which supply the head, neck and arms. It is susceptible to compression because of the low pressure within it, and also because of its location within the relatively rigid bony thorax.

Causes of SVC obstruction may be classified as follows:

- **benign:** e.g. thyroid goitre, mediastinal fibrosis;
- **malignant:** may be due to tumour compressing or invading the SVC;
- **thrombosis:** as a primary event, this is usually related to the presence of an indwelling catheter for venous access. As a secondary event, this is usually due to sluggish blood flow related to obstruction; this may be suspected in the case of SVC obstruction that fails to settle with appropriate management.

The most common aetiology is **malignant disease**, with **bronchogenic carcinoma** being the single most common cause. With the increasing use of indwelling catheters for venous access, however, **thrombosis** as a cause of this syndrome is becoming increasingly common.

Presentation

Obstruction of the SVC leads to engorgement of the internal jugular and subclavian veins. If obstruction occurs over a relatively long time, development of collaterals, particularly with the azygos system, the internal mammary vessels, and the subcutaneous vessels overlying the chest and upper abdomen, may efficiently 'redirect' the obstructed blood. Symptoms and signs may then be minimal. In the

> **Optimal management of oncology emergencies requires:**
> - knowledge of the cancer's natural history;
> - appreciation of the aims of treatment;
> - awareness of the side-effects of the treatment;
> - prompt recognition of the clinical syndrome
> - prompt initiation of appropriate management.

patient with a more acutely developing obstruction, collaterals are not well developed. Pressure in the SVC is thus very high, and symptoms and signs are marked.

Symptoms of SVC obstruction include facial swelling, dyspnoea, headache, nasal stuffiness, hoarseness, and cough. All symptoms tend to be worse in the morning, as lying flat further increases pressure in the SVC.

On examination the patient may have some or all of the following:

- bloated facies
- engorged neck vein (with no evidence of hepatojugular reflux)
- papilloedema
- chemosis
- engorged superficial veins in the neck, arms, and upper chest.

The danger of SVC obstruction is that sluggish blood flow in the cerebral venous circulation may lead to thrombosis or cerebral haemorrhage with catastrophic neurological sequelae. Therefore it is important that this condition is recognized and treated promptly.

Investigation

Patient with a previous diagnosis of cancer Investigation is aimed at confirming the diagnosis of SVC obstruction and identifying the level of obstruction:

- **CXR:** in most cases this reveals a bulky upper right mediastinum. However, it generally gives little information about the aetiology or site of obstruction.
- **Venogram:** useful to confirm the diagnosis of SVC obstruction and confirm its site. It also gives an idea of the degree of collateral formation and is particularly useful if stenting is being considered.
- **Contrast-enhanced CT:** demonstrates the level of obstruction and also helps to determine whether the obstruction is due to thrombus, tumour compression, or invasion.

Patient presenting de novo A diagnosis should be established in the first instance non-invasively. Useful investigations include:

- **Tumour markers:** e.g. elevated α-fetoprotein and/or β-HCG suggest a germ cell tumour;
- **Sputum cytology:** may establish a diagnosis of lung cancer;
- **Biopsy or Fine needle aspiration (FNA)** of an enlarged peripheral node may also be useful.
- **Bronchoscopy:** may also be helpful, although this tends to be technically more difficult in these patients because of the engorged vessels in the upper airways and patients' difficulty in lying flat.

In a minority of cases it is not possible to establish a diagnosis by non-invasive methods. In the past many of these patients would been treated blindly with radiotherapy. Invasive diagnostic measures such as **CT-guided biopsy** or **mediastinoscopy** were believed to be hazardous in these patients due to the risks of haemorrhage. Recent evidence, however, suggests that the risks have been overstated.

Given the increasingly specific anticancer treatments, and the fact that it is often not possible to establish a diagnosis in previously irradiated tissue, almost all patients should have a tissue diagnosis before treatment begins.

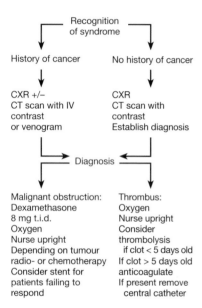

Fig. 25.1 Superior vena cava obstruction.

Treatment

General measures Mildly affected patients require only definitive treatment for their condition. For more severely affected patients, the following measures may improve symptoms:

- bed rest
- oxygen
- high-dose steroids, e.g. dexamethasone 4 mg t.i.d. in patients with a diagnosis of cancer
- avoidance of dehydration as this increases the risk of a complicating thrombus.

Specific measures- The specific treatment depends to a large extent on the underlying aetiology.

- **Malignant aetiology:** very chemosensitive diseases such as small cell lung cancer or lymphoma may be treated with chemotherapy. Less chemosensitive diseases such as non-small cell lung cancer are generally treated with radiotherapy. In both instances an improvement in symptoms should be seen within 72 hours of commencing treatment.

- **Thrombotic aetiology:** in cases where the aetiology is thrombotic, the treatment depends on the length of time for which the patient has had symptoms:
  clot ≤ 5 days old – consider thrombolysis;
  clot > 5 days old **or** thrombolysis contraindicated – anticoagulation with low molecular weight heparin followed by warfarinization is standard treatment.

  Central lines should be removed following initial treatment in these patients if possible.

  In cases where standard therapy is ineffective, or where the syndrome has recurred following treatment, a **stent** may be inserted into the SVC via a brachial or femoral approach. Stents have the advantage of immediately relieving symptoms. Complications, however, include stent migration, infection, and blockage. Nevertheless, their use is increasing, and in some centres they are standard initial treatment for all cases of SVC obstruction. To a certain extent, therefore, the precise treatment of SVC obstruction depends on local expertise.

Prognosis

If symptoms resolve and there have been no neurological consequences, the prognosis is that of the underlying disease.

Pericardial effusion

Aetiology

A pericardial effusion is an abnormal collection of fluid in the pericardial sac. If the collection of fluid is large or develops acutely, the heart cannot relax properly in diastole and so heart filling (particularly on the right side) is reduced. In an attempt to maintain cardiac output, heart rate and myocardial contractility increase. When these compensatory mechanisms are overcome, blood pressure falls. This clinical situation is known as cardiac tamponade.

Malignancy is a common cause of pericardial effusion with bronchogenic carcinoma being the single commonest causative tumour.

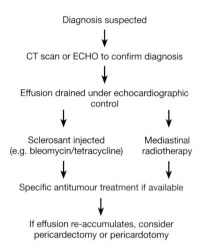

Diagnosis suspected

↓

CT scan or ECHO to confirm diagnosis

↓

Effusion drained under echocardiographic control

↓   ↓

Sclerosant injected   Mediastinal
(e.g. bleomycin/tetracycline) radiotherapy

↓   ↓

Specific antitumour treatment if available

↓

If effusion re-accumulates, consider pericardectomy or pericardotomy

Fig. 25.2 Pericardial effusion.

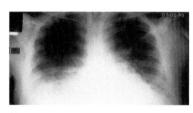

(a)

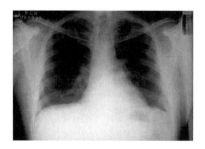

(b)

Fig. 25.3 (a) Chest x-ray showing cardiomegaly in a 56-year-old man with known small cell lung cancer. Note the pericardial catheter inserted to drain the effusion. Bilateral pleural effusions are also present. (b) Repeat chest x-ray 4 months later following radiotherapy and chemotherapy.

Presentation

Common symptoms include dyspnoea and chest pain. Increased pressure in the hepatic and mesenteric veins may cause right upper quadrant pain and nausea.

Signs include tachycardia, pulsus paradoxus (i.e. blood pressure fall of > 10 mmHg on inspiration), an elevated jugular venous pressure, soft heart sounds, hepatomegaly, and ankle oedema.

Similar signs may be seen with cardiac tamponade secondary to pericardial fibrosis. This may complicate mediastinal radiotherapy and usually occurs many years following treatment.

Investigations

- **ECG:** may show small volume complexes.
- **CXR:** may show cardiomegaly with a globular heart. It should be noted that ECG and CXR are often normal.
- **CT scan of thorax:** confirms the diagnosis, and is also useful in determining if there is a fibrotic element.
- **Echocardiography:** the most useful investigation as, in addition to demonstrating the effusion, an assessment of its functional importance can be made.
- **Cytology of the aspirated effusion:** often confirms a diagnosis of malignancy.

Treatment

Asymptomatic effusions Drainage is not generally required, but the patient must be closely monitored for development of symptoms.

Symptomatic effusions General measures include the following:

- oxygen may improve dyspnoea in severely affected patients.
- the patient should be nursed upright.

Specific measures include the following:

- drainage of effusion: this is usually performed via a subxiphisternal approach with echocardiographic guidance. Whilst this provides immediate symptomatic relief, the effusion will almost always re-accumulate without further treatment.
- pericardial sclerosis: instillation of sclerosants (such as tetracycline or bleomycin) into the pericardial sac following drainage may prevent re-accumulation.
- radiotherapy: radiotherapy to the heart following drainage may also prevent re-accumulation.
- pericardectomy or pericardotomy: these procedures may be indicated if the effusion has re-accumulated following radiotherapy or pericardial sclerosis.

The optimal treatment for effusions that recur following drainage is unclear. To a certain extent, therefore, precise treatment will depend on local expertise. For patients with chemosensitive tumours, appropriate chemotherapy will also help prevent re-accumulation of the effusion.

Prognosis

Development of a pericardial effusion usually indicates advanced disease. If the tamponade can be relieved, prognosis depends on efficacy of specific treatment for the disease.

Spinal cord compression

Aetiology

Spinal cord compression occurs when pressure on the cord leads to neurological dysfunction. In most cases the onset is gradual, and damage is believed to be related to disruption of the cord microvasculature. Occasionally, however, the onset may be much more acute and related to occlusion of a major blood vessel such as the anterior spinal artery.

Pressure on the cord commonly results from tumour involving the dural tissues. Most commonly the dura are involved by local tumour spread – either posteriorly from a vertebral body or by paravertebral tumour masses invading via the intervertebral foramen. Less commonly, the dural tissues or medulla of the cord may themselves be the site of blood- or lymphatic-borne deposits.

Metastatic involvement of the vertebral bodies may also lead to bone weakening and subsequent fracture. Bone fragments may be displaced posteriorly and impinge upon the cord. This mechanism is particularly associated with acute occlusion of the anterior spinal artery, and sudden onset of symptoms.

Cancers commonly associated with spinal cord compression include breast, lung, prostate, and myeloma.

Presentation:

Symptoms of cord compression depend on the area of the cord affected:

The thoracic cord is the area most commonly involved. Common symptoms include back pain (typically radicular in distribution); sensory disturbance in the feet; urinary disturbance; and leg weakness. Typically the onset is gradual – initial symptoms may be vague and the diagnosis may be missed. Signs are those of bilateral upper motor neuron lesions in the legs, and a sensory level may be detectable.

The cervical cord is less commonly affected, but its involvement may be suspected if there are neurological symptoms or signs in the arms also.

Malignancy involving the lumbar spine below the level of the cord may lead to compression of the cauda equina. This leads to nerve root pain in the lower back and legs. Urinary disturbance may also be a feature. Signs are those of lower motor neuron lesions in the legs, with commonly also signs of nerve root irritation (ie limited straight leg raising).

Whilst in the late stages a diagnosis of spinal cord compression is obvious, the initial symptoms may be very vague. As outcome is closely related to early treatment, a high index of suspicion must be maintained in order to pick up this complication in the early stages.

Investigation

Patients with a diagnosis of cancer In such patients investigation is focused on confirming

Diagnosis suspected

↓

Diagnosis confirmed CT scan or MRI

↓   ↓

History of cancer   **No history of cancer**
Radiotherapy unless: Establish diagnosis
(1) Chemosensitive   with CT-guided biopsy
    tumour   or combined
(2) Consider surgery   diagnostic/therapeutic
    in good   procedure
    performance
    status patients
    with single site of
    cord compression
    and no systemic
    disease, or if bony
    instability is
    demonstrated

(Patients treated surgically should be followed
up with radiotherapy)

Fig. 25.4 Spinal cord compression.

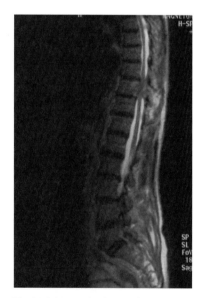

Fig. 25.5 T2-weighted MRI of
thoracolumbar spine. This scan of a
43-year-old woman with known bone
metastases from breast cancer presents with
weakness in both legs. MRI shows a
metastasis in the vertebral body of T10,
spreading posteriorly to block CSF flow and
compress the spinal cord.

the diagnosis of cord compression, and outlining the level at which the cord is compressed.

- **X-Rays of the spine:** may reveal evidence of bony metastatic disease, but gives little information regarding the level of compression.
- **CT Scan:** images the spine by taking 'cuts' through the spine in the coronal plane. Bone is well visualized but disadvantages include:
  - sagittal views to examine the entire spine are not possible – lesions at sites 'between' cuts may be missed;
  - demonstrating obstructed CSF flow necessitates injection of a radiopaque dye into the subarachnoid space (myelography).
- **MRI Scan:** this is the optimal examination in most instances of cord compression:
  - more sensitive and specific than CT scan;
  - better imaging of soft tissue;
  - can visualize the entire spine in the sagittal view;
  - obviates the need for intrathecal contrast.

Patients with no previous diagnosis of cancer In such patients MRI and/or CT myelogram is undertaken to confirm a diagnosis of cord compression. Further investigations, however, are also required to determine the tissue diagnosis. This may be achieved with CT-guided biopsy or at operation where a combined diagnostic and therapeutic procedure may be undertaken.

Treatment

General measures Steroids (e.g. dexamethasone 4 mg t.i.d.) may reduce inflammation associated with the compressive lesion and improve symptoms in the short term.

Specific treatment

- **Radiotherapy:** for patients in whom a cancer diagnosis has been established, most are treated with radiotherapy. Radiotherapy has been shown to have equivalent results to surgery in this instance. It has the added advantages of not requiring a period of convalescence, and also allows several sites of compression to be treated at once. Radiotherapy is also indicated after an operative procedure to reduce the chance of recurrence.
- **Surgery:** surgical candidates include patients in whom cord compression has recurred following a radical dose of radiotherapy, or in whom bony instability or compression of the cord by bone has been demonstrated. Surgery may also be indicated in patients with an unknown diagnosis when biopsy may be combined with an operative procedure. For anteriorly located metastases this usually involves a decompression and stabilization procedure. For the less common, posteriorly located metastases, laminectomy is the procedure of choice.
- **Chemotherapy:** for very chemosensitive tumours such as lymphoma or small cell lung cancer, chemotherapy may be as effective as radiotherapy in relieving symptoms.

Prognosis

Functional outcome depends on:

- ambulatory state at diagnosis: 80% of patients ambulatory at the time of diagnosis will remain so following treatment, whereas < 10% unable to walk at diagnosis will regain mobility. For this reason, early diagnosis and intervention are of the utmost importance.
- tumour type: patients with very radio- or chemosensitive tumours tend to do better than those with less treatment-sensitive tumours.

Brain metastases

Aetiology

Brain metastases result from the spread of cancer from distant sites to the brain, usually via the haematogenous route. Metastases may involve the bony skull, the dural layers, or the leptomenigeal sapce. Most commonly, however, deposits are seen within the brain parenchyma itself.

Tumours which commonly spread to the brain include breast, lung, and melanoma.

Presentation

The presentation of the patient with brain metastases varies according to the site of the lesion. Focal symptoms related to the area involved by the metastases include seizures, mental changes, sensory disturbances, or speech problems. Symptoms may also occur due to increased intracranial pressure. This is most commonly seen with tumours in the posterior fossa due to blockage of CSF flow. Symptoms include headache, which tends to be worse in the morning, nausea, and visual disturbances.

Classically symptoms from brain metastases come on gradually and progress. Atypical presentations may occur, however; a patient may present acutely if there has been haemorrhage into a metastasis, for example.

Early diagnosis of brain metastases is important as untreated brain metastases may cause progressive neurological dysfunction or catastrophic rises in intracranial pressure leading to coma and death. In a patient who is otherwise reasonably well, treatment to control the progression of neurological dysfunction can substantially improve quality of life.

Investigations

The optimal investigation is gadolinium-enhanced MRI. If this is not available, contrast-enhanced CT scan may be used instead, although there is a slightly higher false-negative rate with this investigation.

Treatment

For the majority of patients with cerebral metastases, curative treatment for their cancer is not possible, and the aim of treatment is to reverse neurological symptoms or at least to limit neurological deterioration for the remainder of the patient's life.

Steroids Cerebral oedema may be contributing to symptoms. High-dose steroids (e.g. dexamethasone 8 mg t.i.d.) may lead to a dramatic improvement in symptoms within 24 hours.

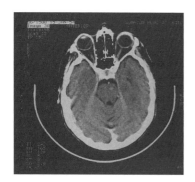

Fig. 25.6 CT scan of brain in a 72-year-old man with lung cancer presents with diplopia. Metastases are poorly demonstrated on this CT scan.

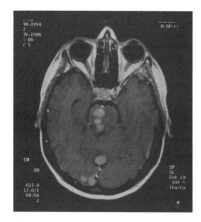

Fig. 25.7 Gadolinium-enhanced T2-weighted MRI of brain in the same patient as in Fig. 25.6. Metastases are much more clearly demonstrated.

Radiotherapy Whole brain radiotherapy is the mainstay of treatment for most patients with cerebral metastases. For patients with good prognostic factors, who may be expected to live beyond 6 months, the long-term problems of whole brain radiotherapy, such as radiation-induced leucoencephalopathy or dementia, may be minimized by prolonging the period over which the treatment is given and reducing treatment fraction size. Patients may initially experience a deterioration in symptoms on commencing radiotherapy due to cerebral oedema. It is important, therefore, that the steroids be continued while the patient is receiving radiotherapy. Steroids can then gradually be reduced – although some patients may require to remain on a small dose of steroids long-term to control symptoms.

Surgery The role of surgery in patients with cerebral metastases is evolving. Its place is most clearly defined in the following circumstances:

- patient presenting acutely with a large bleed into a metastasis may benefit from decompression and drainage of the haematoma;
- patient presenting *de novo* with a cerebral lesion and no primary lesion may undergo surgery to establish a diagnosis;
- selected patients presenting with a solitary brain lesion whose systemic disease is controlled and who have good performance status, may get good long-term disease control (and rarely cure) following metastatectomy. Available trials suggest that survival is further improved by the addition of postoperative radiotherapy.

Chemotherapy

Traditionally chemotherapy has not been used to treat brain metastases, due to the belief that the blood–brain barrier prevented chemotherapy from reaching the brain parenchyma. Recent evidence, however, suggests that this may not be the case, and that for patients with small cell lung and breast cancer, for example, palliative chemotherapy may contribute to the control of cerebral as well as systemic disease.

Prognosis

Whilst in a majority of patients cerebral disease can be controlled for the duration of the patient's lifetime, the outlook for survival is generally poor. Factors adversely affecting survival include:

- multiple brain lesions
- poor performance status
- poor response to steroids
- short disease-free interval between tumour diagnosis and development of metastases
- presence of progressive systemic disease.

Hypercalcaemia
Aetiology

Hypercalcaemia occurs most commonly in the setting of advanced disease. In most cases, hypercalcaemia is a non-metastatic complication of cancer mediated by factors such as parathyroid hormone-like substance.

Tumours particularly associated with hypercalcaemia include lung cancer (especially the squamous subtype), breast cancer, and myeloma.

Presentation

Elevation in serum calcium impairs the reabsorption function of the proximal tubules in the kidney, leading to a salt-losing diuresis and symptoms of polyuria and polydipsia. Other symptoms include abdominal pain, constipation, nausea, and anorexia. On examination, the patient may be dehydrated and changes in mental state may be apparent. These vary from mild confusion to impaired consciousness.

The severity of symptoms associated with hypercalcaemia depends on the absolute level of calcium and also the time over which the hypercalcaemia has developed. Patients with rapidly developing hypercalcaemia tend to be more severely affected than those in whom the hypercalcaemia develops over a longer period of time.

Investigations

Calcium levels should be assayed from an uncuffed venous sample and the value corrected for the albumin level as follows:

Corrected calcium = measured calcium + (40 − albumin) × 0.002 mmol/l

Complications

Prolonged untreated hypercalcaemia leads to dehydration, renal failure and ultimately coma.

Treatment

Symptoms of high calcium are most often seen with a calcium > 3 mmol/l. Elderly patients and those with poor performance status have a reduced tolerance to elevated calcium levels, and a trial of treatment is worthwhile for any degree of hypercalcaemia in these patients.

Rehydration Many of the symptoms of hypercalcaemia are related to dehydration. Rehydration will improve these symptoms and temporarily help to reduce calcium levels. In patients with adequate renal and cardiac function, this replacement may be vigorous (e.g. 3 litres physiological saline over 24 hours). In patients whose renal or cardiac function is compromised, the fluid replacement should be slower, and may be covered with loop diuretics, as these also have a calciuric effect.

Bisphosphonates In order to maintain the normal calcium the patient should be treated with bisphosphonates following rehydration. These interfere with the metabolic activity of osteoclasts, thereby inhibiting release of calcium from the bone. Bisphosphonates reduce serum calcium over a period of 3–6 days, and the effect is maintained for approximately 2–3 weeks. This should be followed by further IV fluids as dictated by the patient's serum urea, electroloytes, and calcium level. Calcium levels should be checked at 2-weekly intervals. Some patients may require regular bisphosphonates to maintain normocalcaemia.

Specific antitumour therapy Where indicated, chemotherapy may help control hypercalcaemia.

Prognosis

The development of hypercalcaemia is usually a late event in the malignant process and is a poor prognostic sign.

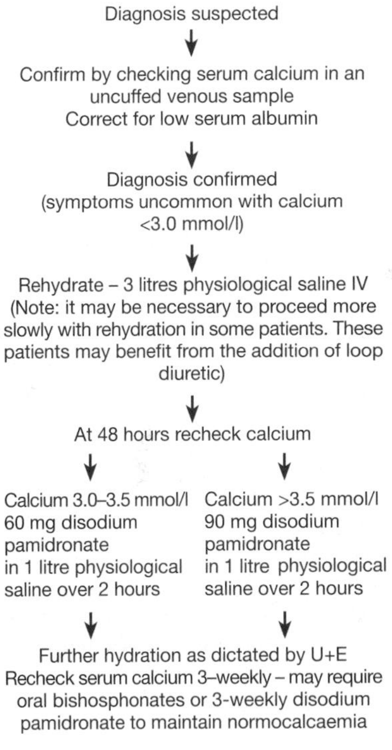

Diagnosis suspected

↓

Confirm by checking serum calcium in an uncuffed venous sample
Correct for low serum albumin

↓

Diagnosis confirmed
(symptoms uncommon with calcium <3.0 mmol/l)

↓

Rehydrate – 3 litres physiological saline IV
(Note: it may be necessary to proceed more slowly with rehydration in some patients. These patients may benefit from the addition of loop diuretic)

↓

At 48 hours recheck calcium

↓   ↓

Calcium 3.0–3.5 mmol/l   Calcium >3.5 mmol/l
60 mg disodium   90 mg disodium
pamidronate   pamidronate
in 1 litre physiological   in 1 litre physiological
saline over 2 hours   saline over 2 hours

↓   ↓

Further hydration as dictated by U+E
Recheck serum calcium 3–weekly – may require oral bishosphonates or 3-weekly disodium pamidronate to maintain normocalcaemia

Fig. 25.8 Hypercalcaemia.

Large airway obstruction

Aetiology

The large airways are comprised of the larynx, trachea, and major bronchi. Obstruction of these airways may result from lesions arising within the lumen of the airways. The most common example of this is bronchogenic carcinoma. Primary laryngeal and tracheal tumours occur much less commonly.

Obstruction may also occur due to lesions compressing or invading the airways from outside. This rarely affects the trachea due to its rigidity, but may involve the large bronchi. Again, the most common cause is bronchogenic carcinoma, but other tumours that may cause this problem include oesophageal cancer, breast cancer, and lymphoma.

Presentation

Obstruction of the large airways leads to dyspnoea and stridor. Symptoms tend to be worse on exertion. More distally located tumours may also cause some atelectasis, with resultant exacerbation of dyspnoea and predisposition to infection.

Investigation

Investigation is aimed at establishing a cause for the obstruction and determining its level.

- **CXR (PA and lateral):** may be suggestive of primary or metastatic lung carcinoma and may show evidence of lung collapse.
- **Bronchoscopy:** will allow visualization and biopsy of tumours in the large airways. Brushings and washings may confirm a diagnosis of lung cancer in more peripherally located lesions.
- **CT scan of thorax:** particularly useful at identifying obstruction arising outside the bronchial walls.

Treatment

General measures

- Bed rest and oxygen for severely affected patients.
- Corticosteroids: these may reduce associated inflammatory changes and improve symptoms temporarily.

Specific measures

- **Radiotherapy:** for the most commonly occurring non-small cell lung cancer, radiotherapy offers the best palliation.
- **Chemotherapy:** for more chemosensitive tumours, such as small cell lung cancer or lymphoma, chemotherapy is the initial treatment of choice.
- **Others:** occasionally symptoms are not relieved with the above measures; referral to the thoracic surgeons should then be considered for consideration of:
  - laser therapy: usually indicated for endobronchial lesions;
  - endobronchial stent insertion: useful for compression due to extrinsic lesions.

Prognosis

Provided the obstruction can be relieved, the prognosis is that of the underlying disease.

Haemoptysis

Presentation

Cancers that arise in or invade the mucosal lining of the major bronchi may cause haemoptysis. Bronchogenic carcinoma is by far the most common cause of this symptom. Metastatic lesions are most commonly located peripherally or sub-pleurally and therefore cause haemoptysis much less commonly.

Commonly, only small amounts of blood are expectorated, but occasionally a large blood vessel may be eroded by the tumour with consequent massive haemoptysis.

Treatment

General measures These include resuscitation with IV fluids, colloids, and packed red cells as required.

Specific measures For the patient that can be stabilized, **radiotherapy** may prevent further episodes. For the patient who continues to have haemoptysis, **intubation** to prevent fatal aspiration may be required.

Further methods to stop haemorrhage include **bronchial artery embolization** or **laser coagulation** of the bleeding site. Occasionally surgery may be appropriate.

Ureteric obstruction

Aetiology

Obstruction of the ureters at any point along their path leads to dilatation of the ureter and back pressure changes in the kidney. Eventually this compromises renal function in the obstructed kidney.

Ureteric obstruction may be classified as causing:

- **Unilateral hydronephrosis:** examples include pelvic tumours (e.g. cervical cancer, rectal cancer) and pelvic or retroperitoneal lymphadenopathy (e.g. due to lymphoma or germ cell tumour). Unless both ureters are affected, the hydronephrosis is unilateral.
- **Bilateral hydronephrosis:** causes include bladder and prostate cancer. The bladder may also be compressed by tumours arising within the pelvis.

Presentation

The presenting symptoms of hydronephrosis depend on whether:

- **obstruction is unilateral or bilateral:** unilateral obstruction may be well tolerated in a patient with a second normally functioning kidney, but renal failure results if both kidneys are obstructed.
- **obstruction is acute or chronic:** renal colic type pain is characteristic of acutely occurring obstruction, whereas chronically developing obstruction are usually painless.

Investigations

- **Serum urea and creatinine:** hyperkalaemia may require urgent treatment.
- **Ultrasound scan:** useful to demonstrate the hydronephrosis and its extent. May also give some clues to aetiology, e.g. demonstrating pelvic lymphadenopathy.

- **Intravenous pyelography:** useful to demonstrate the level of obstruction but is relatively contraindicated in patients with renal failure.
- **CT scan of abdomen and pelvis:** useful for demonstrating 'extrarenal ' causes of obstructive uropathy.
- **Cystourethroscopy:** for patients in whom dilated ureters extend to the bladder, and in whom there is no extrarenal lesion, cystourethroscopy is the investigation of choice.

Treatment

The treatment of this condition must be individualized. For patients in whom obstruction occurs in the setting of advanced disease and for whom no further active treatment is appropriate, no treatment may be indicated. Patients who may require treatment include:

- patients in whom obstructive uropathy occurs as an initial presentation of cancer and for whom active treatment is appropriate. This is particularly true for patients who will receive treatment with nephrotoxic agents such as cisplatin.
- as a palliative measure in patients for whom renal colic type pain is difficult to control.

In general terms, patients with bilateral obstruction require relief of the obstruction on one side only to improve renal function. The kidney chosen is usually that which has the thickest cortex on CT or ultrasound scanning.

Methods for relieving obstruction include:

- **percutaneous nephrostomy tube:** in patients for whom relief of obstruction is required acutely and for whom definitive treatment may well relieve the obstruction (e.g. germ cell tumours, lymphoma), insertion of a percutaneous nephrostomy tube provides a speedy and temporary relief of obstruction.
- **ureteric stent:** in patients for whom the obstruction is predicted to be longer lasting, long-term drainage is best achieved by the endoscopic insertion of ureteric stents (which require replacement every 4–6 months), or formation of a permanent urinary diversion, for example, a urinary conduit.

Complications of both percutaneous and ureteric stents are relatively common and include obstruction, infection, and migration.

In patient with bilateral hydronephrosis due to bladder outlet obstruction, an attempt should be made to pass a **urinary catheter**. If this is not possible a **suprapubic catheter** may relieve obstruction.

Impending bone fracture

Aetiology

Bone is a common site for involvement by metastatic disease. The pattern of disease resulting from the metastases may be sclerotic or lytic, but is most commonly mixed. Common primary tumours include breast, lung, and prostate.

The effect of metastases within bone is to reduce strength and increase the likelihood of fracture. Pathological fractures (particularly in weight-bearing bones) are associated with impaired healing. Orthopaedic intervention is also technically more difficult once the bone has fractured. For these reasons it is important to identify patients at high risk of fracture for consideration of prophylactic orthopaedic intervention.

Presentation

Complaints of bony pain in a patient with cancer should prompt investigations for metastatic disease. This pain is often described as 'boring' in nature. Pain on weight bearing is a particularly sinister symptom.

Investigations

Radiography Plain radiographs will demonstrate bone metastases and give an indication of their extent in a majority of cases. In addition to the area of interest, radiographs of proximal and distal areas should also be obtained. Further lesions may then be treated at the same operation if necessary.

Bone scan This is a more sensitive investigation than plain x-ray. It may identify further unsuspected disease sites.

CT scan This is the optimal investigation to demonstrate mineral content and structurally significant lesions. It may contribute to the decision to proceed with surgery.

Treatment

Ideally, all patients with bony metastases should have intervention before fracture. The decision to proceed to surgery, however, is often difficult for the following reasons:

- in patients with limited life expectancy, predicted duration of convalescence should be taken into account;
- it is impossible to predict with certainty which bony lesions are most likely to cause fracture. However, the following factors have been identified as predicting patients at greatest risk of developing a fracture:
  - site – lesions in weight-bearing bones are at most risk;
  - extent of destruction – destruction of greater than 50% of bony cortex;
  - symptoms – patients complaining of pain, particularly on weight bearing;
  - type of lesion – increased risk in lytic compared to blastic deposits.

The decision to proceed with internal fixation must be individualized and involve consultation with the oncologist and an orthopaedic surgeon experienced in the treatment of oncological problems.

Patients identified as being at high risk of fracture and fit for surgery should undergo internal fixation of the affected bone to prevent fracture. The type of internal fixation device used depends on the site of the lesion and patient performance status. In all cases, internal fixation of the bone should be followed by radiotherapy to control tumour growth and allow healing.

Gastrointestinal obstruction
Aetiology and presentation

Gastrointestinal obstruction in the cancer patient may occur at any point between the oesophagus and the rectum. Causes may be classified as follows:

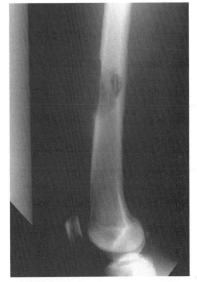

(a)

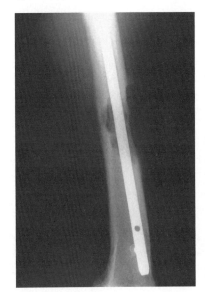

(b)

Fig. 25.9 (a) x-ray left femur in a 60-year-old man with renal cancer, complaining of pain in the left leg, particularly on weight bearing. x-Ray shows a large lytic deposit in the distal left femur. (b) x-ray of the femur following insertion prophylactically of an intramedullary nail.

- tumour related, e.g. ovary, bowel, lymphoma;
- treatment related, e.g. abdominal radiotherapy, drugs such as opioids and anticholinergics.

Symptoms depend on the level of bowel obstructed. Particularly when the obstruction is tumour related, however, multiple sites may be involved, leading to a mixed clinical picture.

Prompt recognition of obstruction in the cancer patient is important for optimal treatment. Those patients for whom medical management has failed, fare best when the decision to proceed to surgery is taken early while their performance status and nutritional status is good.

Investigations

Investigation is aimed at pinpointing the site and cause of obstruction:
- **Plain adominal x-ray:** may reveal dilated bowel loops or fluid levels.
- **Barium studies:** may reveal the level or levels of obstruction.
- **CT scan of abdomen:** the optimal investigation for demonstrating lesions extrinsic to the bowel.

Treatment

Management of the patient with bowel obstruction depends on the tumour type, patient performance status, previous treatments, and the level and degree of obstruction. Patients for whom the aim of care is clearly palliative, and whose performance status is poor, may be managed medically in the majority of cases (see Chapter 12). For patients presenting acutely with a good performance status, more active management is indicated:

Conservative
- Nil orally and IV fluids.
- For small bowel obstruction, passage of a nasogastric tube may considered.
- General measures should include attempts to relieve constipation and the discontinuation of all medications that may be exacerbating the obstruction.

Surgical In selected patients whose symptoms cannot be controlled medically, surgery may relieve symptoms. Surgical procedures include resection of the obstructed bowel, bypass, or stoma formation.

Gut perforation

This may occur secondary to any gastrointestinal malignancy, but is most commonly seen following initial chemotherapy for bulky gastrointestinal non-Hodgkin's lymphoma. Presentation may be atypical due to the fact that many of these patients are on high doses of steroids, and a high index of suspicion should be maintained in this group.

Diagnosis may be confirmed by the presence of air under the diaphragm on x-ray or CT scan. If these investigations are negative, the diagnosis may be confirmed by Gastrografin enema or swallow.

Treatment in all patients who are fit is surgical.

Hyperviscosity syndrome

Aetiology and presentation

In the cancer patient this syndrome occurs when a large number of blast cells or an excessive production of immunoglobulins leads to increased viscosity of the blood and sluggishness in its movement, particularly through small vessels. Symptoms associated with this syndrome include confusion, transient ischaemic attacks, blurred vision, cardiac failure, and bruising due to impaired platelet function.

Treatment

Acutely leucopheresis or plasmapheresis will improve symptoms. Chronically treatment is that of the underlying disease.

Treatment-related emergencies

Neutropenic sepsis

Aetiology

Neutropenia is defined as an absolute neutrophil count of less than 1.5×10^9/L. Causes of neutropenia in the cancer patient include:

- **Chemotherapy:** this is the most common cause. While chemotherapy is toxic to all progenitor cells, granulocyte precursors are particularly sensitive, and neutropenia typically develops 5–7 days following treatment.
- **Radiotherapy** to large areas of marrow containing bone, e.g. mantle radiotherapy for Hodgkin's disease.
- **Involvement** of the bone marrow by tumour: this is most commonly seen in haematological malignancies such as acute myeloid leukaemia.

Neutropenia is associated with an increased risk of serious infection. Gram-negative organisms are the most commonly isolated, although Gram-positive organisms are being seen more frequently in recent years. With prolonged neutropenia, fungal infections become increasingly common. In contrast to immunocompetent patients, most of the pathogens in neutropenic patients are actually part of the patient's own gut or skin flora. Chemotherapy may disrupt the body's natural barriers to bacterial entry, and so further predispose to infection.

The risk of a patient developing an episode of sepsis is related to:

- the absolute neutrophil count: risk increases substantially with a neutrophil count $< 0.5 \times 10^9$/l.
- the duration of neutropenia: risk increases greatly with neutropenia lasting longer than 7 days.
- patient factors: those with mucositis, intercurrent illnesses, and poor performance status are at increased risk.

Presentation

Infection in patients with low neutrophil counts are atypical in their presentation due to the lack of inflammatory response, and signs suggesting a focus for the infection are commonly absent. The only sign of infection initially may be a pyrexia.

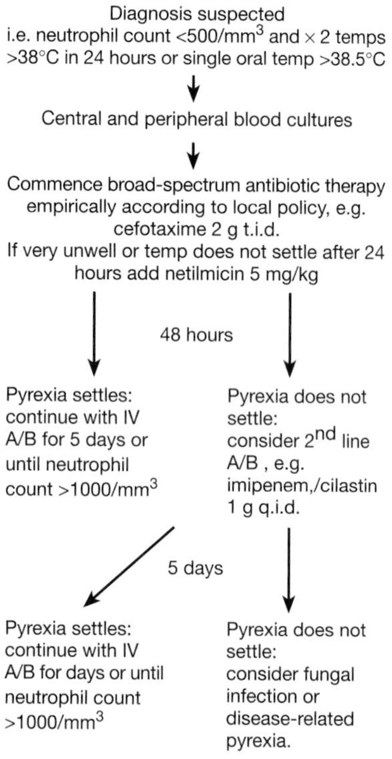

Diagnosis suspected
i.e. neutrophil count <500/mm^3 and × 2 temps
>38°C in 24 hours or single oral temp >38.5°C

↓

Central and peripheral blood cultures

↓

Commence broad-spectrum antibiotic therapy
empirically according to local policy, e.g.
cefotaxime 2 g t.i.d.
If very unwell or temp does not settle after 24
hours add netilmicin 5 mg/kg

48 hours

Pyrexia settles:
continue with IV
A/B for 5 days or
until neutrophil
count >1000/mm^3

Pyrexia does not
settle:
consider 2nd line
A/B , e.g.
imipenem,/cilastin
1 g q.i.d.

5 days

Pyrexia settles:
continue with IV
A/B for days or until
neutrophil count
>1000/mm^3

Pyrexia does not
settle:
consider fungal
infection or
disease-related
pyrexia.

Fig. 25.10 Neutropenic sepsis.

Untreated, the patient may become rapidly unwell. Given the lack of symptoms and signs, a diagnosis of sepsis should be made in any neutropenic patient with:

- two temperatures of greater than 38°C;
- a single temperature of greater than 38°C in a 24-hour period.

It is important to note that, particularly in patients who are very ill or are on steroids, a pyrexia may not be present. In any neutropenic patient, the diagnosis must be suspected and treated empirically in the absence of other obvious diagnosis in an ill patient.

Investigations

- **Blood cultures:** these should be taken from a peripheral vein, and from each lumen of any indwelling vascular device.
- **MSSU.**
- **Throat swabs.**

Other investigations may be indicated according to the clinical situation.

Treatment

General measures Given the high mortality of this condition when treatment is delayed, any discussion of the treatment of neutropenic sepsis should mention measures taken to avoid this complication or facilitate its early diagnosis. These include:

- Patient education: i.e. recognition of symptoms suggestive of sepsis, ready access to medical advice;
- Medical education: i.e. education of all medical staff treating cancer patients. All units with responsibility for treating patients with chemotherapy should have a locally agreed protocol for the treatment of neutropenic sepsis;
- Prevention: good mouth care, avoidance of infected contacts, etc.

Specific measures Initial antibiotic therapy should cover the most common and most virulent organisms. Such antibiotics include broad-spectrum penicillins, and third- or fourth-generation cephalosporins. The following antibiotics may also be added to the initial regimen:

- Aminoglycoside: this may be considered in the shocked patient. Otherwise, studies suggest that it may be safely omitted from the initial regimen and added after 24 hours if the pyrexia fails to settle.
- Metronidazole: considered in the presence of colonic symptoms (such as diarrhoea) or dental problems. These raise the possibility that anaerobic organisms are involved.
- Anti-staphylococcal agent: considered if the patient has an indwelling line.

Failure of fever to settle after 48 hours necessitates a change of antibiotics. Failure of pyrexia to settle after 5 days should prompt suspicion of a fungal infection, and consideration given to the empirical introduction of antifungal agents.

The role of growth factors in this condition is uncertain. They are known to shorten the duration of neutropenia, but the effect on outcome is uncertain.

Prognosis

Factors adversely affecting outcome include:

- delay in commencing treatment;
- prolonged or profound neutropenia;
- underlying disease: patients with haematological malignancies, particularly acute leukaemias, are at very high risk;
- poor patient performance status.

Chemotherapy extravasation

Chemotherapy is commonly administered as an intravenous infusion. Extravasation of certain agents into the surrounding tissues may cause extensive tissue necrosis. Such agents are known as **vesicants**. Importantly, as chemotherapy or its metabolites remain in the tissue for some time, tissue damage may evolve over a period of days or weeks. Such patients must be followed up even when the initial injury seems minor.

Prompt recognition and treatment of extravasation reactions are required to minimize tissue damage.

Examples of commonly used vesicants include:

- Adriamycin
- Epirubicin
- Vincristine
- Vinblastine
- Cisplatin.

Prevention

Guidelines for the administration of chemotherapy help to limit the occurrence of extravasation reactions, and aid prompt diagnosis and treatment when they occur. Chemotherapy should only be administered by trained staff, who are fully aware of the potential problems.

Treatment

Extravasation should be suspected if the patient complains of pain or swelling around the infusion site during infusion of a known vesicant and the following measures taken:

- Discontinue the chemotherapy infusion.
- Leave the venous catheter *in situ* and attempt to aspirate back the instilled chemotherapy.
- Apply ice to the affected area (exception to this is in the case of extravasated vinca alkaloids when a warm pack should be applied).
- Elevate the affected limb.
- Monitor the affected area daily for the first 2 weeks and beyond that if there is continued evidence of inflammation.

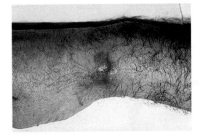

Fig. 25.11 This shows an area of inflammation that developed 3 days following extravasation of Adriamycin. No evidence of inflammation was evident initially. Note that venous catheters should not be positioned over the wrist due to risk of damage to the joint, tendons, and neurovascular structures in the area.

- Consider early plastic surgery referral for any case where signs are progressive. Surgery has the dual effect of removing the offending agent and, secondly, debriding necrotic skin to promote healing.

Specific antidotes have been recommended for some vesicants; evidence supporting the use of these antidotes, however, is limited and often conflicting. There are no standard guidelines, therefore, regarding the use of these agents.

Tumour lysis syndrome
Aetiology:

Chemosensitive tumours with rapid doubling times are associated with large cell kill following treatment. The sudden release of large amounts of intracellular contents into the bloodstream may exceed the kidney's ability to excrete them. This may lead to a number of problems known as tumour lysis syndrome. Features of this syndrome include hyperkalaemia, hyperuricaemia, hyperphosphataemia, and hypocalcaemia. These metabolic disturbances can lead to renal failure, cardiac arrhythmias, and tetany.

Tumours associated with this syndrome include acute leukaemias, high-grade lymphoma, and choriocarcinoma.

Presentation

This syndrome usually presents approximately 24 hours following commencement of chemotherapy. Symptoms include those of acute renal failure, including nausea, confusion, and oliguria or anuria. Patients may also complain of symptoms of hypocalcaemia such as tetany and perioral paraesthesia.

Prevention

- Patient at risk is identified.
- Adequate hydration is ensured – hydration should be commenced 24–48 hours prior to the commencement of chemotherapy and a fluid intake of at least 3 litres daily should be maintained during chemotherapy.
- Allopurinol 300 mg daily is commenced 48 hours prior to commencement of chemotherapy. This should be continued for the duration of the chemotherapy or at least until tumour bulk has significantly reduced.
- Serum electrolytes are monitored throughout treatment.

Treatment

- electrolyte disturbances are treated.
- early dialysis to control metabolic disturbances acutely should be considered.

Thrombocytopenia
Aetiology

Thrombocytopenia is defined as platelet count $< 150 \times 10^9/l$. It occurs most commonly following chemotherapy due to damage to megakaryocyte precursors.

Treatment

In patients who are well, the risk of haemorrhage is significantly raised only at very low platelet counts. Current evidence suggests that the incidence of serious haemorrhage increases markedly only with platelet counts less than $10 \times 10^9/l$. Prophylactic platelet transfusion, therefore, is not recommended until platelet count falls below this level.

In patients who are unwell, due to infection for example, there is an increased risk of haemorrhage. It is recommended that such patients receive prophylactic platelets when the count falls below $30 \times 10^9/l$. Patients receiving platelets prophylactically usually receive platelets from five donors.

Problems with platelet transfusion include transfusion reactions and the development of platelet antibodies, which may limit the efficacy of future transfusions.

Case histories

Case 1

A 52-year-old woman attended her GP. Over the last month she had been complaining of mid-thoracic back pain. Over the last week she had developed some tingling in the feet. On direct questioning by her doctor, she admitted to some urinary hesitancy.

Otherwise she had been feeling very well – in particular she noted no problems with weakness in the arms or legs and her bowels were moving normally.

Her GP noted that she had had a partial mastectomy for node-positive breast cancer 4 years ago. At that time she had been treated with radiotherapy to the breast, chemotherapy, and commenced on tamoxifen, which she was still taking. On review at the breast clinic 2 months ago all appeared to be well with no clinical evidence of disease recurrence.

She had no other significant past medical history.

On examination there was no palpable evidence of disease in either breast, axillae, or supraclavicular fossae. Focal tenderness was noted over the sixth thoracic vertebrae. On neurological examination of the legs, tone was felt to be slightly increased bilaterally, although her doctor felt that this could be due to difficulty in relaxing. Examination was otherwise normal.

What are the possible diagnoses?
The most important diagnosis to be excluded is that of spinal card compression. The most likely reason for this is that the patient has developed vertebral bony metastases which are compressing the cord.

Other possible diagnoses include demyelinating disease, anterior spinal artery thrombosis, or a primary spinal tumour.

continued

Case histories continued

What investigations should be requested?
- X-Ray of spine: mixed lytic/blastic lesions scattered throughout the spine.
- MRI spine: demonstrated a soft tissue lesion extending posteriorly from the sixth and seventh thoracic vertebrae causing compression of the cord and obstruction of CSF flow. Widespread marrow replacement was noted throughout the spine although there were no further areas of cord compression.
- CXR: multiple rib metastases noted but lung fields were clear.
- Ultrasound scan abdomen: no abnormality seen. In particular, the liver appeared clear.

What treatment is indicated?
She was commenced on dexamethasone 4 mg t.i.d. Radiotherapy to the involved spine was commenced.

With commencement of the steroids, the patient noted that the tingling in her feet had resolved. She had no side-effects from the radiotherapy. The steroids were gradually discontinued over the course of radiotherapy treatment.

Given the relatively long disease-free interval, her known oestrogen-receptor positive status at the time of original operation, and the isolated bony nature of the metastases, Tamoxifen was discontinued and second-line hormonal therapy with Arimidex commenced.

She remains alive and well with no recurrence of her symptoms 6 months after this presentation.

Case 2

A 23-year-old man presented to his GP complaining of a 12-hour history of feeling vaguely unwell. He noted that he had had a couple of episodes of 'shaking' but that these had resolved spontaneously.

He had recently been diagnosed as having stage III teratoma and was currently 7 days following his second course of chemotherapy. He had been warned about the risk of infection whilst on this treatment, and to contact the hospital directly should he develop symptoms. Having no more specific signs of infection, however, he was relatively unconcerned but wished to be reassured.

On examination his GP noted that he had a pyrexia of 38.8°C. Examination was otherwise unremarkable.

What is the likely diagnosis and what are the appropriate investigations?
The most likely diagnosis is neutropenic sepsis. Blood cultures were taken from a peripheral vein as well as from each lumen of his Hickman line. An MSSU was also requested. A full blood profile was taken:

- Hb 11 g/dl
- WCC $1.2 \times 10^9/l$
- neutrophil count $0.1 \times 10^9/l$
- platelets $88 \times 10^9/l$.

Case histories continued

What is the appropriate treatment?

A diagnosis of neutropenic sepsis was made, and the patient commenced on the broad-spectrum antibiotics ceftazidime 1.5 g t.i.d. intravenously.

Results of the peripheral blood cultures 2 days later revealed growth of a Gram-negative rod later characterized as *Eschericia coli*. The pyrexia settled over the next 48 hours.

His IV antibiotics were continued for 5 days. By then his neutrophil count had risen to $1.3 \times 10^9/l$.

What are the appropriate precautions to take prior to the next course of chemotherapy?

Given that this is a radical course of treatment, all efforts must be made to continue full chemotherapy doses on schedule. The patient therefore received prophylactic granulocyte colony-stimulating factor (G-CSF) from day 5 following his next course of treatment. He was also given further advice regarding the importance of recognizing the symptoms of neutropenic sepsis early and commencing treatment immediately. He was instructed how to take his temperature at home if he felt unwell and advised to contact the oncology unit directly should symptoms develop.

Further reading

DeVita, V. T., Hellman, S., and Rosenberg, S. A. (1997) *Cancer: principles and practice of oncology*, 5th edn. Lippincott-Raven, Philadelphia.

Peckham, M., Pinedo, H. M., and Veronesi, U. (1995) *Oxford textbook of oncology*. Oxford Medical Publications, London.

Price, P. and Sikora, K. (1995) *Treatment of cancer*, 3rd edn. Chapman and Hall Medical, London.

Souhami, R. and Tobias, J. (1998) *Cancer and its management*, 3rd edn. Blackwell Science, Oxford.

Index

Note: Page numbers in *italics* refer to figures and tables

ABV (Adriamycin, bleomycin, vinblastine) 381
ABVD (Adriamycin, bleomycin, vinblastine, dacarbazine) 336
acanthosis nigrans 57
acinic cell carcinoma 197, 207
acoustic nerve schwannoma 460
acquired immunodeficiency syndrome (AIDS) 24–5, 372, 380–1, *380*, 447, 453
acral lentiginous melanoma (ALM) 180–1, *181*
acromegaly 467, 468, *468*, 470, 471
acupuncture 158, 434
adenocanthoma 175–6
adenocarcinoma 52
  bile duct 243
  endometrial 214
  gall bladder 244
  lung 297–8, *297*, 309
  mucin-secreting 57
  oesophagus 233–4
  ovarian 223–4
  pancreas 238
  prostate 269
  renal 261
  stomach 236
adenoid cystic carcinoma 197
adenoma
  adrenal 477, *478*, 488
  colorectal 45, *45*
  pituitary, *see* pituitary tumours, adenoma
adhesive interactions 56
adjustment styles 100, *100*
adjuvant chemotherapy 121, 378, 433–4
adjuvant psychological therapy 100
adrenal tumours 476–80, *477*
  adenoma 477, *478*, 488
  carcinoma 477, *478*
  case history 488
  hyperaldosteronism 478–9
  hypercortisolism 477–8
  incidentaloma 476–7, *477*, 488
  phaeochromocytoma 462, 479–80, *479*
  virilizing 479
Adriamycin, *see* doxorubicin
adult T-cell leukaemia/lymphoma (ATLL) 24
adult T-lymphoblastic leukaemia 340
aetiology 7, 8, 15–25, *21*
  association or causation 31
  chemical carcinogens 17–20, *17*, *18*

epidemiological evidence 30–5, *32*
  genetic, *see* familial cancer syndromes
  psychological risk factors 95–7
  radiation 20–1
  viruses 21–5, *22*, *23*
  see also specific cancers; carcinogens
aflatoxins 24, 64
AIDS, *see* acquired immunodeficiency syndrome
air pollution 69
AJCC classification
  bone tumours 360, *360*
  soft tissue sarcomas 373, *374*
AJCC staging system, soft tissue sarcomas *374*
alcohol 32, 66
  and breast cancer 66, 420
  and head and neck cancer 67–9, 194
  and tobacco 67–9, 194
alkaline phosphatase 330, 363, 364
alkylating agents 122, 124, 125, *126*, 128, 333
  see also specific drugs
allopurinol 510
alopecia 127, 434
α-fetoprotein (AFP) 12
  in hepatic tumours 241, 402
  in mediastinal germ cell tumours 285–6
  in ovarian cancer 224
  in paediatric germ cell tumours 407–8
  in pineal germ cell tumours 455–6
  in testicular cancer 279, *279*
amiloride 479
aminoglycoside 508
amphibole asbestos 311, 312, *312*
amputation 365, 371
anagrelide 349
anal cancer 253–5
  aetiology 254, *254*
  clinical presentation 254
  epidemiology 253
  investigations 255
  pathology 254
  prognosis 256
  treatment 254, 255–6
analgesics 148, 149–53, *149*, 303
anal melanoma 254
anaplastic large cell lymphoma 340
anaplastic tumours 57
angiography 90–1

angiomyolipoma 263

angiosarcoma 371

Ann Arbor staging system, lymphoma 335, *335*, 339

anorexia/malaise/weakness 156–7

   management 157

anthracyclines 121–2, 127, 327, 432, 433

anti-androgens 274

antibiotics 508

anti-emetics 152, 158–60, *159*

antimetabolites 121–2, 124, 125, *126*

   see also specific drugs

antioxidants 72

anti-staphylococcal agents 508

anxiety disorders 98, *439*

anxiety/restlessness/agitation 164–5

apoptosis 55

APUD cells 480

aromatic compounds 64

asbestos 69, 295–6, 310–12, *311*, *312*

asbestosis 311

ascites 111, 225

L-asparagine 128

Aspergillus flavus 24, 64, 241

aspirin 149, 249

astrocytoma 449–51, *450*, 459, 463

ataxia telangiectasia (AT) 21, 422

atrophic skin lesions 174

atypical ductal hyperplasia 420

atypical hyperplasia 52, 420

axillary node clearance/sampling 429–30, *430*

Bacillus Calmette–Guérin (BCG) 185, 267

barium enema 76, *85*, 86, 237, 251

Barrett's oesophagus 52, 233–5

basal cell carcinoma (BCC) 70, 174, 176, 202, *202*, 206

basement membranes 56

Bayesian approach 34–5

Beckwith–Wiedemann syndrome 392–3, *392*, 402

behavioural factors 95

Bence Jones proteinurea 342, 343

benign tumours 49, 50

benzodiazepines 154, 164–5

3,4–benzpyrene 296

BEP (bleomycin, etoposide, cisplatin) 280

bereavement services, in palliative care 146

ß-carotene 65, 72, 194

ß-human chorionic gonadotrophin (ß-HCG) 224, 279, *279*, 285–6, 402, 407–8, 455–6

betel nut 193

bilateral salpingo-oophorectomy 216

bile duct carcinoma (cholangiocarcinoma) 243–4

   aetiology *241*, 243

   clinical presentation 243

   epidemiology 243

   investigations 243

   pathology 243

   prognosis 244

   treatment 243–4

bile duct obstruction 239

biliary bypass 240

bilobectomy 303

biological response modifiers 128–30

biopsy 58, 91

bisphosphonates 153, 306, 344, 435, 501

bladder cancer 3, 264–8

   diagnosis and staging 264–5, *265*

   invasive 267–8

   pathology 265–6, *266*

   risk factors *264*

   superficial 266–7, *266*

   treatment 266–8

bladder reconstruction 267

blast (primitive) cells 323, 330

bleomycin 125

   in Hodgkin's disease 336

   in Kaposi's sarcoma 381

   in testicular cancer 280

   toxicity 127–8

blood transfusion 113

Bloom and Richardson scale, breast cancer 427

bone fractures 504–5, *505*

   aetiology 504–5

   investigations 505

   in metastatic breast cancer 435, *435*

   in myeloma 343, 344

   presentation 505

   treatment 112, 505

bone marrow plasma cells 341, *341*

bone marrow samples 325–6

bone marrow suppression 127, 352

bone marrow transplantation 352–4, *353*

   in Ewing's sarcoma 368

   in leukaemia 327, 329, 330

   in lymphoma 336, 340

   in neuroblastoma 391

bone pain 153, 435, 505

bone scanning 273, *273*, 505

bone tumours, malignant primary 359–70

   aetiology 359

   case history 382

   classification 360, *360*

   clinical presentation 360

   investigations 360–1

   management *361*, 362

   staging 361, *361*

bowel cancer, *see* gastrointestinal cancer

Bowen's disease 275

brachytherapy 139, 203, *203*, 244, 305, 451

brain tumours

   case histories 463–4

in children *387*, *408*, *410*, 411, 448, 451–3, 455–6
imaging 88–9, 449
metastases 449, 499–500
  aetiology 499
  from breast cancer 436, *436*
  from lung cancer 308
  investigations 499, *500*
  presentation 499
  prognosis 500
  treatment 112, 499–500
  primary 449–57, 467–71
BRCA1 gene *43*, 78, 222, 421, 441
BRCA2 gene *43*, 78, 222, 421–2, 441
breaking bad news 97, *97*, 161
breast cancer 3, *12*, 41, *109*, 371, 415–44
  advanced breast cancer treatment 157, 434–6
    hypercalcaemia 435–6, *436*
    locally advanced disease 434
    local recurrence after mastectomy 434
    malignant pleural effusion 435
    metastatic disease 309–10, 434–5, 436, *436*
    pathological fractures 435, *435*
  case histories 102, 116, 442–4
  diagnosis 59, 422–4
    core biopsy 424
    examination 422, *422*, *423*
    fine needle aspiration cytology 58, *108*, 423–4, *423*, *424*
    history 422, *422*
    mammography 423, *423*
    open biopsy 424, *424*
    ultrasonography 423
  ductal 426–7, *427*, 441
  early breast cancer treatment 429–34
    adjuvant therapy 433–4, *433*
    breast reconstruction, *see* reconstruction after mastectomy (*below*)
    choice of operation 430–1
    histological assessment 432
    primary chemotherapy 432
    primary treatment 429–30, *429*, *430*
  in elderly 438
  follow-up 436–7, *437*
  geographical variation in treatment/survival 5, 6
  history 417–18
  inflammatory carcinoma 431
  lobular 56, 423, 426–7
  male 441
  'no special type' 426
  Paget's disease of nipple 176, 438, *438*
  pathology 426–7
    classification 426, *426*
    extensive *in situ* disease 427
    in situ cancers 426–7, *427*
    lymphovascular invasion 427
    tumour differentiation 427, *427*
  and pregnancy 437–8, *437*

prevention 65, 441
  BRCA1 and *BRCA2* testing 78
  prophylactic surgery 73, 78, 112, 441
  screening 74–5, 424–5, *425*
  tamoxifen 73, 441
psychology 96, 98–9, 101, 102, 439–40, *439*
reconstruction after mastectomy 110, *430*, 431–2
  complications 432
  immediate or delayed 431
  insertion of silicone prosthesis 431
  latissimus dorsi myocutaneous (LD) flap 431
  masking of recurrence 431
  transverse rectus abdominus myocutaneous (TRAM) flap *429*, *430*, 431
risk factors *417*, 418–22
  age 418, *418*
  age at first pregnancy 419
  age at menarche and menopause 418
  alcohol 66, 420
  diet 65, 420
  family history 420–2, *421*
  geographical location 418, *419*
  hormone replacement therapy 420
  lactation 419
  oral contraception 420
  personality 96
  previous benign disease 420
  radiation 420
  sedentary lifestyle 65
  weight 65, 66, 419
'special types' 426
staging 428–9
  oestrogen and progesterone receptors 429
  primary tumour 428
  prognostic index 58, 428–9, *428*
  regional lymph nodes 428
support for patient 439–40
  doctors 439
  groups 440
  specialist breast care nurses 439–40
  volunteers 440
  timing of surgery 110
breast care nurses 439–40
breast self-examination 75
breathlessness, *see* dyspnoea
bronchial artery embolization 503
bronchial carcinoid tumours, *see* carcinoid tumours of lung and bronchus
bronchial obstruction, *see* large airway obstruction
bronchoalveolar carcinoma 298
bronchodilators 154, 156
bronchogenic carcinoma, primary 295–308
  aetiology 295–6, *295*, 311
  chemoprevention 296
  diagnosis 300
  epidemiology 295

bronchogenic carcinoma, primary (*cont.*)
  examination 300
  fitness for radical therapy 302–3
  non-metastatic paraneoplastic syndromes 299–300, *299*
  pathology 296–8, *297*
  presentation 298–300, *299*
  prevention 296
  screening 296
  special situations/emergencies 305–6, 493, 495, 502, 503
  staging 300–2, *300*, *301–2*
  treatment 303–8
bronchoscopy 235, 300, 305, 502
bronchospasm 156, 293
Budd–Chiari syndrome 242
Burkitt's lymphoma 22–3, *23*, 54–5
busulphan 330, 354
BV (bleomycin, vinblastine) 381

CA-19–9 (tumour marker) *12*, 240, 243
CA-125 (tumour marker) 12, *12*, 223, 224
cachexia 57, 156–7
  humoral factors 156–7
  management 157
  metabolic abnormalities 156
caecal carcinoma 56, 114–15, 250–1, *251*
Calman–Hine Report (1995) 6–7
cancer centres 7
cancer-prone/type C personality 96
cancer units 6–7, 59
carboplatin 127, 226, 307
carcinogenesis 17–25, *21*, 50–6
carcinoid syndrome 246, *481*, 482–3
  clinical features 482
  diagnosis 482–3
  prognosis 483
  treatment 483
carcinoid tumours of lung and bronchus 292–4
  aetiology and epidemiology 292
  atypical (AC) 292, 294
  diagnosis 293
  examination 293
  pathology 292–3
  presentation 293, 482
  prognosis 294
  staging 293–4
  treatment 294
  typical (TC) 292, 294
  well-differentiated neuroendocrine carcinoma 292, 294
carcinoma 52, 57
carcinoma in situ *51*, 52
carcinosarcoma 217
cardiac tamponade 114, 310, 495, 496
cardiac transplantation 291–2
cardiac tumours 291–2
  investigation 291

  presentation 291
  treatment and prognosis 291–2
cardiotoxicity, of chemotherapy/radiotherapy 127
caretaker genes 53
carotid body tumour 462
case histories
  brain tumours 463–4
  breast cancer 102, 116, 442–4
  chemotherapy 130–2
  endocrine tumours 487–9
  genitourinary malignancy 281
  gynaecological cancers 227–30
  head and neck cancer 208
  Hodgkin's disease 354
  lung cancer 130–1, 315, *315*, *316*
  nephroblastoma (Wilms' tumour) 412
  neuroblastoma 411–12
  oesophageal cancer 255
  oncological emergencies 511–12
  osteosarcoma 382
  palliative care 166–7
  prostate cancer 141–2, 281
  psychological factors 102
  radiotherapy 141–2
  skin cancer 187–8
  surgery 114–16
  testicular cancer 131–2
CAV (cyclophosphamide, doxorubicin, vincristine) 307
cavernous haemangioma 89
CEA (carcinoembryonic antigen) 12, *12*, 238, 243, 250
cell adhesion molecules 56, 57
cell cycle 55, *55*, 121, *121*, 359
cerebral lymphoma 447, 453–4, 463–4, *463*
cervical cancer 217–21
  aetiology 23, 53, 217–18
  case history 228–9
  diagnosis and staging *219*, 220
  epidemiology 214, 217
  examination 219–20
  pathology 218
  presentation 218–19
  prognosis 221
  screening 75–6, *75*, 217–18
  treatment 220–1
cervical intraepithelial neoplasia (CIN) 76, 217, 221
cervical smear 59, 75–6, 217–18
chemical carcinogens 17–20
  initiation 17–18, *17*, 18–19, *18*, *21*
  promotion 17–18, *17*, 19–20, *21*
  and sarcoma 371
  and skin cancer 175
chemodectoma 197, 462
chemoprevention 72–3, 78, 296
chemotherapy 119–32
  adjuvant therapy 109, 110, 121, 378, 433–4

and bone marrow transplantation 352–3, 354
case histories 130–2
classification of drugs 125–6, *126*
combination therapy 122
cycle-specific agents 121
dose intensity 122
general principles 121–6
-induced toxicities 126–8
  alopecia 127
  bone marrow suppression 127, 352
  cardiotoxicity 127
  extravasation 509–10, *509*
  gonadal damage and sterility 128
  immunosuppression 127, 352
  nausea and vomiting 127, 434
  neurotoxicity 128
  neutropenic sepsis 507
  pulmonary toxicity 127–8
  renal toxicity 127
  tumour lysis syndrome 510
natural products 125, *126*
neoadjuvant therapy 121
new therapeutic approaches 128–30
  biological response modifiers 128–30
  colony-stimulating factors 129
  gene therapy 129–30
  interferons 128
  interleukin-2 and adoptive immunotherapy 128–9
  monoclonal antibodies 129
  tumour vaccines 129
patient performance status 125, *125*
pharmacological aspects
  absorption/distribution/excretion 126
  biotransformation 126
phase-specific agents 121
resistance to 122–5, *123*
  acquired drug resistance 124
  enhanced DNA repair 124
  increased target gene expression 125
  intracellular thiols 124
  intrinsic drug resistance 124
  multidrug resistance (MDR) 124
  transport resistance 124
treatment of
  adult soft tissue sarcomas 378, *378*, 380
  anal cancer 255, 256
  bladder cancer 266–8
  bone tumours 364–5, 367–8
  brain tumours 453–4, 456, 500
  breast cancer 429, 432, 433–4, 435
  cervical cancer 220–1
  colorectal cancer 252–3
  head and neck cancer 203, 205
  hepatoblastoma 403–4
  Kaposi's sarcoma 381

  large airway obstruction 502
  leukaemia 327, 329, 330, 333
  lung cancer 294, 303, 304, 307
  lymphoma 336, 339–40, *339*, 459
  mediastinal tumours 289–90, 291
  melanoma 185–6
  mesothelioma 316
  nephroblastoma 394, 395
  neuroblastoma 391
  ovarian cancer 226
  paediatric germ cell tumours 410–11
  pancreatic cancer 240
  retinoblastoma 401
  rhabdomyosarcoma 398
  spinal cord compression 498
  stomach cancer 238
  testicular cancer 279–80
vascular access 112–13
see also specific drugs
chest radiographs 84–5, *84*
childhood cancers 387, *387*
  acute lymphatic leukaemia 321, 328, 329, 330, 387, *387*
  brain tumours *387*, *408*, *410*, 411, 448, 451–3, 455–6
  mediastinal tumours 285, 289
  solid tumours, non-CNS 385–413
  see also Ewing's sarcoma; osteosarcoma
cholangiocarcinoma, *see* bile duct carcinoma
cholecystectomy 244, 245
chondrosarcoma 359, 369, *369*, *370*
CHOP (cyclophosphamide, Adriamycin (hydroxydaunorubicin), vincristine (Oncovin), prednisone) 333, 339–40
choriocarcinoma 405, 407, 408, 510
chromaffin paraganglia 462
chromosomal abnormalities 321–2, 327, 371
chrysotile (white asbestos) 69, 311, *312*
cigarette smoking, *see* smoking
cirrhosis of liver 241, 404
cisplatin 126, 509
  in anal cancer 256
  in bladder cancer 267–8
  in bone tumours 364, 369
  in cervical cancer 221
  in hepatoblastoma 403–4
  in lung cancer 304
  in mediastinal tumours 291
  in oesophageal cancer 236
  in ovarian cancer 226
  in soft tissue sarcomas 378
  in stomach cancer 238
  in testicular cancer 279, 280
  toxicity 127, 128
cladribine 340
Clark levels 181, *182*
clear cell sarcoma 393, 394, 395

clinical detection
  clinical symptoms or signs 9
  early detection 9
  limits of 121, *121*
Clinical Group staging system, rhabdomyosarcoma 397, 398
clinical psychologists 102
Cloquet's node 213
CNS prophylaxis, haematological malignancy 329, 340
cobalt-60 139
Cochrane Collaboration 34
Codman's triangle 363, *363*
coeliac plexus block 240, 245
cognitive behavioural psychotherapy 100
colectomy 73, 112, 252
colonoscopy 76, 251, 253
colony-stimulating factors (CSFs) 127, 129, 352
colorectal cancer *3*, *4*, *5*, *12*, 247–53
  aetiology 33, 41, 65, 66–7, 248–9, *248*
  and blood transfusion 113
  clinical presentation 250–1, *250*, *251*
  epidemiology 247–8
  hereditary non-polyposis (HNPCC) 44, 53, 249, *249*
  investigations 85, 86, 251–2
  multistep nature 45, *45*, 249–50
  pathology 249–50, *250*
  prevention 65, 72, 73
  prognosis 253
  screening 76, 253
  treatment 109, 252–3, *252*, *253*
colposcopy 76
communication skills 161–2
computerized tomography (CT) 87–9, *88*, 272, 498
confounding 31
congenital mesoblastic nephroma 393
congruence, in doctors 97
coping styles 100, *100*
cordoma 459
core biopsy 58, 91, 424
corticosteroids 157, 333, 502
Corynebacterium parvum 185, 435
cough 155–6, 298, 303
  dry 155–6
  productive 155
cough suppressants 155–6
Courvoisier's sign 239, *239*
cranial nerve palsy 195, 198
craniopharyngioma 454–5
crocidolite (blue asbestos) 69
cruciferous vegetables 66
Cushing's syndrome 454, 467, 469, 470, 471, 477, *478*
cyclizine 158–9
cyclo-oxygenase 2: 72
cyclophosphamide
  and alopecia 127
  and bone marrow transplantation 354

  in bone tumours 367–8
  in breast cancer 433
  in lung cancer 307
  in mediastinal tumours 289
  in nephroblastoma 395
  in non-Hodgkins' lymphoma 339–40
  in ovarian cancer 226
CYP1A1 enzyme 19
cystoscopy 264
cysto-urethrectomy 268
cystourethroscopy 504
cytarabine 127, 327, 454
cytochrome P-450 enzymes 19
cytokines 128–30, 156–7, 342, 435
cytological techniques 58–9

dacarbazine 186, 336, 378
dactinomycin 125, 367–8, 380, 395
daunorubicin 125, 127
day care centres, in palliative care 146
death rattle 165
decompression 451, 452, 458
deep venous thrombosis 113
denial 100
depression 97–8, *439*
desmoid tumours (aggressive fibromatoses) 381–2
desmoplasia 56
detection bias 30
diagnosis 9–10, *10*
  psychological impact 97
  role of surgery 108
  tissue diagnosis 57–9
  see also specific cancers
diamorphine 151
diazepam 154
diazoxide 484
diet 32
  and breast cancer 65, 420
  carcinogens in 24, 63–4, *64*
  and colorectal cancer 65, 249
  fat 65, 249, 420
  fibre 64–5, 249
  fruit and vegetables 65–6
  and head and neck cancer 194, 195
  and nervous system tumours 448
  and prevention 63–7, *66*
  and stomach cancer 236
diethylstilboestrol 420
differentiation, of tumours 50, 57
digital rectal examination (DRE) 77, 271
dihydrofolate reductase 125
dihydropyrimidine dehydrogenase 126
direct-acting carcinogens 18, *18*
DNA 17
  and chemical carcinogens 17, 18, 19

and chemotherapy 124, 125
and radiotherapy 135, 136
DNA excision repair 20, 44
enhanced 124
DNA index (DI) 388
DNA repair genes 43–5
DNA viruses 21–4
dopamine agonists 468, 471
doxorubicin (Adriamycin) 125
in bladder cancer 266, 267–8
in bone tumours 361, 364, 367–8, 369
extravasation 509, 509
in hepatoblastoma 403–4
in hepatoma 242
in Hodgkin's disease 336
in Kaposi's sarcoma 381
in lung cancer 307
in mediastinal tumours 289
in myeloma 343–4
in nephroblastoma 395
in soft tissue sarcomas 378
in stomach cancer 238
toxicity 127
drug resistance, see chemotherapy, resistance to
Dukes system, colorectal cancer 251–2
duodenum 246, 247
dysgerminoma 405, 407, 411
dyskaryosis 75
dysphagia 234, 235, 306
dysplasia 50–2
dyspnoea 154–5
in large airway obstruction 502
in lung cancer 298, 303, 310
in malignant pleural effusion 310
management of daily activities 155
management in terminal phase 155
pharmacological symptom management 154–5

Eaton–Lambert syndrome 57
ECMV (etoposide, cyclophosphamide, methotrexate, vincristine) 306
electromagnetic radiation 137, 137
electron microscopy 57
electrons 136, 137, 139
embryonal carcinoma 405, 407, 408
embryonal tumours 387, 391, 401
emergencies, see oncological emergencies
emotional suppression 96
empathy 97
endocrine tumours 454, 465–90
endoluminal ultrasonography 235
endometrial cancer 214–17, 215
aetiology 65, 66, 214
case history 228
diagnosis 215–16
epidemiology 214

investigation 216
pathology 214–15
presentation 215
prognosis 217
staging 215, 216
treatment 216–17
endometroid adenocarcinoma 223, 224
endoscopic retrograde cholangiopancreatography (ERCP) 111, 240
endoscopy 58, 86, 294
Enneking staging system, primary bone tumours 361, 361
enucleation of eye 401
ependymoma 451–2, 452, 459
epidemiology 3–4, 3, 4, 27–35
and aetiology 30–5, 32
association or causation 31
confounding 31
detection bias 30
evidence synthesis 34–5
exposure bias 31
genetic 33–4
susceptibility bias 30
see also specific cancers
epidermal growth factor (EGF) 40, 312
epidermal growth factor receptor (EGFR) 40
epirubicin 238, 509
Epstein–Barr virus (EBV) 22–3, 33, 194, 334
c-erbB2 oncogene 40–1, 54, 59, 296, 371
erythrocytosis, see polycythaemia vera
erythroplasia of Queyrat 275
essential thrombocythaemia (ET) 348–9, 349
prognosis 349
treatment 349
esthesioneuroblastoma 197
ethics, of surgical oncology 107–8
etoposide 279, 280, 307, 368
Ewing's sarcoma 366–9, 366, 387, 461
extraosseus 366, 461
investigations 366–7
pathology 367, 367
prognosis 368, 369
treatment 367–8, 378
EWS-ERG gene 366, 367
EWS-FLI1 gene 366, 367
excision repair 20, 44, 124
exercise tolerance test 303
exfoliative cytology 59, 296
exocrine pancreas, see pancreatic cancer
exposure bias 31
external auditory meatus 205, 207
extramedullary plasmacytoma 197

faecal occult blood testing 76, 253
familial adenomatous polyposis 72, 248–9, 402
familial cancer syndromes 8, 8, 53–4, 54
and bone and soft tissue sarcomas 359, 371, 396

familial cancer syndromes (*cont.*)
  and breast cancer 78, 420–2
  and colorectal cancer 248–9, *249*
  genetic susceptibility testing 77–8, *78*
  as indicators of tumour suppressor genes 42, *43*
  and nephroblastoma 392–3, *392*
  and nervous system tumours *448*
  see also specific syndromes
fat, dietary 65, 249, 420
fibre, dietary 64–5, 249
fibroblast cells 460
fibrolammellar carcinoma 404
fighting-spirit 100
FIGO staging classification
  cervical cancer *219*, 220
  endometrial cancer *215*
  ovarian cancer 224, *225*
  vulval cancer *212*
fine needle aspiration (FNA) cytology 58, 91
  breast cancer 58, *108*, 423–4, *423*, *424*
  thyroid tumours 474, *474*
finger clubbing 57, 315, *315*
Flexner–Wintersteiner rosettes 399, 456
fludarabine 333
fluid replacement 161, 165, 501, 510
5–fluorouracil (5–FU)
  in anal cancer 255, 256
  biotransformation 126
  in breast cancer 433
  in colorectal cancer 253
  in gallbladder carcinoma 245
  in oesophageal cancer 236
  in pancreatic cancer 240
  in renal cell carcinoma 262–3
  in stomach cancer 238
folinic acid 253
forced expiratory volume in one second (FEV$_1$) 303
formaldehyde 448
fractionation 136
fruit and vegetables 65–6
fulguration 111

gallbladder carcinoma 244–5
  aetiology *241*, 244
  clinical presentation 244
  epidemiology 244
  investigations 245
  pathology 244
  prognosis 245
  treatment 245
gallbladder dilatation 239, *239*
gallbladder polyps 244
gallstones 244
ganglioneuroblastoma 289, 461
ganglioneuroma 289, 461

Gardner's syndrome 249, 371, 381
garlic 66
gastrectomy 237
gastric cancer, *see* stomach cancer
gastrinoma (Zollinger–Ellison syndrome) *481*, 483
gastrointestinal cancer 231–56
  endocrine tumours 480–4, *481*
  imaging 86
gastrointestinal obstruction 505–6
  aetiology and presentation 505–6
  in colorectal cancer 250
  investigations 506
  management 160
  in palliative care 160–1
  treatment 160–1, 506
    surgery 110–11, 114, 161, 506
gastrointestinal symptoms, in palliative care 156–61
gatekeeper genes 53, 54
gemcitabine 240
gene amplification 54
gene therapy 129–30
genetic epidemiology 33–4
genetic susceptibility syndromes, *see* familial cancer syndromes
genetic susceptibility testing 77–8, *78*
genitourinary malignancy 257–82
germ cell tumours
  in children 405–11, 455–6
    clinical presentation 407–8, *408*
    diagnosis 409, *409*
    pathogenesis and epidemiology 405–6
    pathology 406–7, *406*
    prognosis 411
    staging *409*, 410
    therapy 410–11, *410*
  mediastinal 285–6, 290–1, *290*, *409*
  ovarian 222, 224, 226, *406*, *407*, *408*, *408*, *409*, 410
  pineal 455–6
  testicular 277, 278, *278*, 279–80
germinoma 407, 408, 455
germline mutations 42, 53–4, *392*, 399
giant cell tumours 370, *370*
Gleason grading system, prostate cancer 270, 271, *271*
glioblastoma 450–1, *450*
glioma 448, 449–52, 456, 463
glomus jugulare 197, 462
glomus tympanicum 462
glottis 206
glutathione-*S*-transferase 19, 194
Goldie–Coldman hypothesis 124
gonadal damage, and chemotherapy 128
gonadoblastoma 407
G-proteins 41
grading, of tumours 57–8
graft-versus-host disease 353
graft-versus-leukaemia effect 353

granulocyte colony stimulating factor (G-CSF) 352–3, 434
granulocyte-macrophage colony stimulating factor (GM-CSF) 312, 352–3
growth factor receptors 40–1
growth factors 40, 312
growth hormone (GH) deficiency 470
growth hormone (GH)-producing adenoma 467, 469
gut perforation 506
gynaecological cancers 209–30

H19 gene 392–3
haematological and lymphoid tumours 319–55, *319*, 459
   pathogenesis 321–2
haematuria 259, 260, 264
haemoptysis 298, 305, 503
   presentation 503
   treatment 503
hair loss (alopecia) 127, 434
hairy cell leukaemia 128, 340, 345
haloperidol 152, 159, 165
Hashimoto's thyroiditis 472, 473
head and neck cancer 191–208
   aetiology 193–5
   anatomy 195–6, *195*
   case history 208
   diagnosis 198–9
   epidemiology 193
   examination 198, *198*
   genetics 194–5
   pathology 196–7
   pre-malignancy 196
   presentation 197–8
   prevention 72, 195
   prognosis 205–7
   staging 199, *199–200*
   treatment 200–5
   treatment side-effects 205, *205*
health behaviour 95, *95*
hemicolectomy 252
hepatic artery embolization 242
hepaticojejunostomy 240
hepatitis B virus (HBV) 24, 33, 71, 240–1, 242, 404
hepatoblastoma 401–4
   clinical presentation 402
   diagnosis 402, *403*
   epidemiology 401
   genetics 402
   pathology 402
   prognosis 404
   staging 403, *404*
   treatment 403–4
hepatoma (hepatocellular carcinoma (HCC)) 240–2
   aetiology 24, 64, 241, *241*
   in children 404–5
      clinical presentation 405
      diagnosis *403*, 405

      epidemiology 404
      pathology 404
      staging *404*
      treatment and prognosis 405
   clinical presentation 241–2
   epidemiology 240–1
   investigations 242
   pathology 241
   prognosis 242
   treatment 91, 242
hereditary non-polyposis colorectal cancer (HNPCC) 44, 53, 249, *249*
herpes simplex type-2 275
heterogeneity, of tumours 58
heterozygosity, loss of 42, 54
high-fibre diet 64–5
histopathological diagnosis/staging/classification 11–12, 57–8
hMSH2 gene 44, 53
hoarseness 198, 298–9
Hodgkin's disease 333–6, *387*
   aetiology 334
   case history 354
   diagnosis 334
   epidemiology 333
   examination 334
   nodular sclerosing variant 334
   pathology 334, *335*
   presentation 334
   prognosis 336
   quality of life 336
   staging 335–6, *335*
   treatment 336
home care teams, in palliative care 146
Homer Wright rosettes 197, 388–9, 452, *452*, 456
homosexual activity 254, 381
homovanillic acid 285, 390, 461
hormonal therapy
   in bone pain 153
   in breast cancer 433, 435
   in carcinoid tumours of lung and bronchus 294
   in prostate cancer 273–4, *274*
hormone deficiency 469, 470
hormone overproduction 467–9, *468*, 471, 477–9, 480–2
hormone replacement therapy (HRT) 420
hormone secretion, inappropriate, by non-endocrine tumours 485–7, *486*
Horner's syndrome 56, 299, 300, 389
hospices 145–6
human herpes virus 8: 372, 380–1
human immunodeficiency virus (HIV) 24–5, 175, 380–1
human papillomavirus (HPV) 23
   and anal cancer 254
   and cervical cancer 23, 53, 76, 217
   and head and neck cancer 194
   and penile cancer 275
   and vaginal and vulval cancer 211, 221

human T-cell leukaemia virus (HTLV-1) 24, 33
hydration, artificial 161, 165, 501, 510
hydronephrosis 503
5–hydroxyindoleacetic acid (5–HIAA) 482
hydroxyurea 330, 349
hyoscine butylbromide 160
hyoscine hydrobromide 165
hyperaldosteronism 478–9
hypercalcaemia *486*, 500–1, *501*
    aetiology 500–1
    in breast cancer 435–6, *436*
    in bronchogenic carcinoma 306
    complications 501
    investigations 501
    in myeloma 343
    in parathyroid carcinoma 476
    presentation 501
    prognosis 501
    treatment 306, *436*, 501
hypercortisolism 469, 477–8
hyperparathyroidism 476, 483, 485
hyperplasia 52
hypertension 214, 259, 478
hyperviscosity syndrome 343, 507
hypoglycaemia 483–4, *486*
hypopharyngeal tumours 194, 198, 204, 206
hypopituitarism *469*, 470
hysterectomy 216, 220
hysteroscopy 216

ICE (ifosfamide, carboplatin, etoposide) 307
ifosfamide
    in bone and soft tissue sarcomas 368, 369, 378
    in cervical cancer 221
    in lung cancer 304, 307
    toxicity 128
ileum 246, 247
imaging, *see* radiological imaging
immediate early genes 40
immunohistochemistry 57, 59, *374*, 376
immunosuppression
    and chemotherapy 127, 352
    and HIV infection 24
    and skin cancer 175
immunotherapy 128–30
    in bladder cancer 267
    in melanoma 185–6
    in renal cell carcinoma 262–3
indirect-acting carcinogens (procarcinogens) 18, *18*, 19
infectious agents, *see* viruses
inherited predisposition, *see* familial cancer syndromes
initiation 17–18, *17*, 18–19, *18*, 21
insulin-like growth factors (IGFs) 40, 312
insulin-like growth factor type 2 (*IGF2*) gene 392–3
insulinoma *481*, 483–4

interferons 128
    in haematological malignancy 128, 330, 331, 340, 344, 349
    interferon-alpha (IFN-a) 185–6, 262–3, 330
    in Kaposi's sarcoma 381
    in melanoma 185–6
interleukin-1 156–7
interleukin-2 (IL-2) 128–9, 186, 262–3
intermenstrual bleeding 218–19
international comparison, of treatment and outcome 5–7, *5*
International Neuroblastoma Staging System 390, *391*
interstitial brachytherapy 139, 203
intestinal obstruction, *see* gastrointestinal obstruction
intracavity brachytherapy 139
intracellular thiols 124
intracellular transducers 41
intraluminal brachytherapy 305
intravenous fluids 165
intravenous urogram (IVU) 264
invasion 49
ionizing radiation 20–1, *137*
    and bone and soft tissue sarcomas 359
    and breast cancer 420
    and leukaemia *322*, 323
    and nervous system tumours 448
    see also radiotherapy
irinotecan 253
iron-deficiency anaemia 194
isotretinoin (13–*cis*-Retinoic acid) 72

Japan 237–8, 418
jaundice, obstructive 110, 239, 240, 243, 245
jejunum 246, 247

Kaposi's sarcoma 25, 175, 372, 380–1, *380*
kidney, *see* nephroblastoma; renal carcinoma
Krukenberg tumours 236

lactate dehydrogenase (LDH) 278, *279*, 367
laminectomy 458, 498
laparoscopy 108, 111, 237
laparotomy 107–8
large airway obstruction 502
    aetiology 502
    investigation 502
    presentation 502
    prognosis 502
    treatment 114, 305, 502
laryngeal cancer 194, 198, 204, 206
laryngectomy 204
laryngopharyngectomy 204
laryngoscopy, indirect 198, *198*
laser therapy 114, 294, 305, 503
latissimus dorsi myocutaneous (LD) flap 431
leather bottle stomach (linitis plastica) 86, 236, 237
lentigo maligna (melanotic freckle) 179–80

lentigo maligna melanoma (LMM) 181
leukaemia 323–33
    acute 49, 323, *332*
      emergencies 327, 509, 510
      progression to 331, 344, 348, 349, 350, 352
    acute lymphatic (lymphoblastic) (ALL) 323, 324–5, 328–30, *328*
      in children 321, 328, 329, 330, 387, *387*
      prognosis 329, *329*
      quality of life 330
      treatment 329
    acute myeloid *323*, 324, *326*, 327–8
      M_3 (promyelocytic/progranulocytic) variant *326*, 327
      and myeloproliferative disorders *346*
      prognosis 327–8
      quality of life 328
      therapy-related 336
      treatment 327
    aetiology 24, 322, 323
    chronic lymphatic (CLL) 323–4, *323*, 324–5, 331–3, *331*, *332*
      prognosis 333
      quality of life 333
      staging 332, *332*
      treatment 332–3
    chronic myeloid (CML) 323, *323*, 325, 330–1, *332*, *346*
      'blastic transformation' 331
      prognosis 331
      quality of life 331
      treatment 330
    diagnosis 325–6
    examination 324–5
    graft-versus-leukaemia effect 353
    haematological findings *332*
    hairy cell 128, 340, 345
    pathology *322*, 323–4, *323*
    presentation 324, *324*, 325
leukocoria 399, *399*
leukoplakia 72, 196
life events 96
lifestyle factors 33, 95
Li–Fraumeni syndrome 359, 371, 396, 405–6, 422
linear accelerators (Linacs) 137, 139
linear energy transfer (LET) 136
linkage analysis 54
lip cancers 202, *202*, 206
liposarcoma 370, 371
liver cancer
    and alcohol 66
    imaging 88, 89, 108
    secondary, from colorectal cancer 112, 252, *252*, *253*
    see also hepatoblastoma; hepatoma
liver cirrhosis 241, 404
liver transplantion 405
lobectomy, lung 303
locus of control 96
lung cancer *3*, *4*, *5*, 19, 57, 155

carcinoid tumours 292–4
case history 130–1
imaging 84–5, *84*, 87
non-small cell, *see* non-small cell lung cancer (NSCLC)
prevention 67–9, *67*, *68*, 72, 296
primary bronchogenic, *see* bronchogenic carcinoma, primary
secondary 308–10
    from osteosarcoma 365, *365*, 366
    from soft tissue sarcomas 378–9, *378*
    malignant pericardial effusion 310
    malignant pleural effusion 310
    primary/secondary distinction 309
    pulmonary metastasectomy 112, 309–10, *365*, 378–9, *378*
    second primary tumours 309
small cell, *see* small cell lung cancer (SCLC)
luteinizing hormone releasing hormone (LHRH) analogues 274
lymphocyte-activated killer (LAK) cells 186
lymphoedema 371
lymphoepithelioma 197
lymphoma 53, 285, 333–40, 510
    aetiology 33
    cerebral 447, 453–4, 463–4, *463*
    Hodgkin's disease, *see* Hodgkin's disease
    imaging 88
    non-Hodgkin's, *see* non-Hodgkin's lymphoma
    small bowel 246
    spinal 459, *459*
    thyroid 472
lymphosarcoma 371
Lynch I syndrome 249
Lynch II syndrome 249

magnetic resonance imaging (MRI) 89–90, 199, *199*, 272, 498
malignant fibrous histiocytoma 369–70, 371, 372, *372*
malignant melanoma, *see* melanoma
malignant mixed carcinoma 197
malignant pericardial effusion, *see* pericardial effusion
malignant pleural effusion 310, 366, 435
malignant pleural mesothelioma (MPM), *see* mesothelioma
malignant tumours 49–50, *50*
    spread and effects 56–7
mammography
    and breast cancer diagnosis 423, *423*
    and breast cancer follow-up 437
    and breast cancer screening 74–5, 424, *425*
    and hormone replacement therapy 420
    in Paget's disease 438
mantle cell lymphoma 340
mastectomy
    axillary node clearance/sampling 429–30, *430*
    breast reconstruction 110, *430*, 431–2, *431*
    choice of operation 430–1
    in early breast cancer 429–31
    in elderly 438
    history 417–18

mastectomy (*cont.*)
and local recurrence 431, 434
and lymphoedema 371
in men 441
partial 429, *429*, 430–1, 433, 437
and pregnancy 437
prophylactic 73, 78, 112, 441
psychological impact 98–9
total 429, *429*, 430, 432, 438, 441
mediastinal tumours 285–91
diagnosis 89, 285–6
germ cell 285–6, 290–1, *290*, *409*
neurogenic 285, 289–90, *290*
presentation 285
secondary 285
thymic 286–9, *286*
medical dosimetrists 140
medical physicists 141
medical physics 137
medullary thyroid carcinoma *473*
and multiple endocrine neoplasia type 2: 73, 472, 479, 485
prognosis 475, 476
and *RET* proto-oncogene 472, 474, 475
medulloblastoma 452–3, *452*, 456
megestrol acetate 157
melanin 177
melanocytes 177
melanoma 173, 177–87
adjuvant therapy 185–6
anal 254
case history 187–8
clinical presentation 181
diagnosis 181
distant metastases 185, 246, 309–10
genetics 179
head and neck 197
local recurrences 185
management 184–5
prevention 70–1, *71*, 186–7
prognosis 183–4, *183*
risk factors 178–9
spontaneous regression 185
staging 181–2, *182*
treatment 185–6
types 179–81
vulval 211
melphalan 343–4, 354
meningioma 456–7, *457*
aetiology 448, 449
atypical 457
spinal 459
meningiosarcoma 457
mercaptopurine 329
mesorectal excision 252

mesothelioma 310–16
aetiology 69, 310–12, *312*
diagnosis 314
electron microscopy 313
epidemiology 310, *311*
epithelial 313
examination 313
pathology 313
presentation 313
prevention 69, 312–13
prognosis 316
sarcomatous 313
staging 314, *314*
treatment 314–16, *314*
metaplasia 52
metastasis 49, 56–7
methotrexate
in bladder cancer 267–8
in breast cancer 433
in haematological malignancy 329, 340, 454, 459
intrathecal 329, 454, 459
in lung cancer 307
in soft tissue sarcomas 378
in stomach cancer 238
toxicity 126, 127
methotrimeprazine (levomepromazine) 159, 165
metoclopramide 152, 159
metronidazole 508
MIBG (meta-iodobenzylguanidine) scan 390
MIC (Mitomycin C, ifosfamide, cisplatin) 304
microsatellite instability 53, 249
midazolam 154, 164–5
middle ear 205, 207, 462
mismatch repair (MMR) 44–5
Mitomycin C 255, 256, 266, 304
mitotane 478
mitotic inhibitors 126, *126*
see also specific drugs
Moh's micrographic surgery 377
molecular biology 37–46
moles 70–1, 178–9, 181
monoclonal antibodies 129
monoclonal gammopathy of uncertain significance (MGUS) 345
monomorphic adenoma (oncocytoma) 196
MOPP (mustine, Oncovin (vincristine), procarbazine, prednisone) 336
morphine 149–52, *152*
breakthrough pain 151
commencement 150
dose increase 151
dosing frequency 151
forms *151*
side-effects 152
signs of toxicity 152
M-proteins 341–2, *342*, 345, *345*
MTS1 gene 179

mucin-secreting adenocarcinoma 57
mucoepidermoid carcinoma 197, 207
mucosal neuroma 485
mucositis 205, *205*
multidisciplinary teams 13, 59, 107, 140, 145
multidrug resistance (MDR) 124
multiple endocrine neoplasia (MEN) syndromes 292, 371, 484–5
   case history 489
   type 1: 483, 484–5, *484*, 489
   type 2: 73, 472, 479
     A 462, *484*, 485
     B 462, *484*, 485
multistep nature of cancer 45, *45*, 52–3
mustine 336
mutator phenotype 44–5
MVAC (methotrexate, vinblastine, Adriamycin, cisplatin) 267–8
MVP (Mitomycin C, vinblastine, cisplatin) 304
myasthenia gravis 286, 288
c-*myc* oncogene 41, 54–5, 296
mycosis fungoides 175, 340
N-*myc* proto-oncogene 388
myelodysplastic syndromes (myelodysplasia; MDS) 351–2, *351*
   aetiology 352
   pathology *351*, 352
   quality of life 352
   treatment 352
myelofibrosis 349–51, *350*
   aetiology 345–6
   prognosis and quality of life 351
   treatment 350, *350*
myeloma 197, 341–5
   aetiology 341
   diagnosis 343, *343*
   pathology 341–2, *341*, *342*
   presentation 342–3, *342*
   prognosis 344
   quality of life 344
   related conditions 345, *345*
   staging 343, *344*
   treatment 343–4
myeloproliferative disorders 345–51, *346*
   aetiology 345–6
   pathology 346
   presentation 346

naevi (moles) 70–1, 178–9
   congenital melanocytic 178
   dysplastic 178
nasal cavity tumours 205, 207
nasopharyngeal carcinoma (NPC) 195
   aetiology 23, 194–5
   pathology 197
   presentation 198
   prognosis 207
   treatment 205

National Wilms' Tumour Study Group staging system 394, *394*
nausea and vomiting
   assessment of causes 157–8
   and chemotherapy 127, 434
   management 157
   and morphine 152
   in palliative care 157–60, 161
   pathogenesis 158, *158*
   treatment 158–60, *159*
nebulized therapies 154, 156
neck, regions 195–6
neck cancer, *see* head and neck cancer
neck dissection 201, *201*
needle biopsy 58
neoadjuvant chemotherapy 121
neoplasia 49–50
neovascularization 56, 90–1
nephrectomy 262, 263, 394
nephroblastoma (Wilms' tumour) 387, 391–5
   case history 412
   clinical presentation 393, *393*
   diagnosis 393–4
   epidemiology 392, *392*
   genetics and molecular biology 392–3
   pathology 393, *393*
   prognosis 395, *395*
   staging 394, *394*
   treatment 394–5
nephrostomy tube, percutaneous 504
nephro-ureterectomy 268
nerve blocks 148
nerve sheath tumours 290, 448, 460–1
nervous system tumours 445–64
   aetiology 447–9
   analytical epidemiology 448–9
   brain, *see* brain tumours
   descriptive epidemiology 447
   peripheral nervous system 459–62
   space-occupying lesion 449
   spinal 457–9
neurilemmoma 289
neuroblastoma 387–91, *387*, 461
   aetiology/genetics/molecular biology 388
   case history 411–12
   clinical presentation 389, *389*
   diagnosis 390, *390*
   epidemiology 388
   esthesioneuroblastoma 197
   mediastinal 289
   pathology 388–9
   prognosis 391
   spinal 459
   staging 390, *391*
   treatment 391
neuroendocrine tumours 292–4, 462, 480–4

neurofibroma 371, 460, *460*, 461

neurofibromatosis type 1 (von Recklinghausen's disease) 289, 371, 456, 460

neurogenic tumours of mediastinum 285, 289–90, *290*

neuroglial cell tumours 449–52

neuronal tumours of CNS, malignant *453*
    medulloblastoma 452–3
    pineoblastoma 456

neuropathic pain 147, 152–3
    treatment 152–3

neurosurgery 111

neurotoxicity, of chemotherapy 128

neurotransmitters 480

neutropenic sepsis 507–9, *508*
    aetiology 507
    case history 512
    investigations 508
    presentation 507–8
    prognosis 509
    treatment 508

nitrosamide exposure, in mothers 448

N-nitroso compounds 64

nocioceptive pain 147

nodular melanoma 179, *180*, 184

non-chromaffin paraganglia 462

non-Hodgkin's lymphoma (NHL) *3*, 337–40, 387
    aetiology 338, *338*
    B-cell 337–9
    case history 463–4, *463*
    clinical findings 339
    and gut perforation 506
    high-grade 338, 339
    intermediate-grade 338, 339, 340
    low-grade 338, 339, 340
    pathogenesis 338–9
    prognosis 340
    and spinal cord compression 459
    staging 339
    T-cell 337–9, 340
    treatment 339–40, *339*

non-seminomatous germ cell tumours (NSGCT)
    mediastinal 286, 290–1
    testicular 278, *278*, 280, *280*

non-small cell lung cancer (NSCLC)
    aetiology 296
    case history 315, *315*, *316*
    pathology 296–8
    staging 300–2, *300*, *301–2*
    treatment 303–6
        best supportive care 303
        chemotherapy 304
        radiotherapy 304–5
        special situations 305–6, 495
        surgery 303–4
    treatment success rates and prognosis 308

non-soluble fibre 64

non-steroidal anti-inflammatory drugs (NSAIDs) 72, 149, 153, 249

Nottingham Prognostic Index 58, 429, *432*

nuclear hyperchromasia 50, 52

nuclear medicine (radioisotope imaging) 90

nuclear oncogenes (transcription factors) 41

nucleotide excision repair (NER) 20, 44

nutrition
    in palliative care 156, 161
    surgeon's role in management 113
    see also diet

obesity 65, 66–7, 214, 259, 419

occupational carcinogens 33, 69, *70*, 175, 194, 295, 448
    see also specific carcinogens

octreotide 160, 294, 481–2, 483, 484

odansetron 434

oesophageal cancer *3*, 233–6
    aetiology 233–4, *233*
    case history 255
    clinical presentation 234
    epidemiology 233
    investigations 234–5, *234*
    pathology 234
    prognosis 236
    treatment 235–6, *235*

oestrogens 214

oligodendroglioma 451

oncocytoma 196, 263

oncogenes 21, *39*, 40–1, 45, 54–5
    see also specific genes

oncogenic DNA viruses 22–4

oncogenic RNA viruses 24–5

oncological emergencies 491–513
    in acute leukaemia 327, 509, 510
    cancer-related 493–507
    case histories 511–12
    in polycythaemia vera 348
    surgical 114
    treatment-related 507–10

opioids
    in dyspnoea 154
    in pain management 149–52, *150*
    in terminal phase of illness 164

oral cavity cancer 66, 193, 194, 198, 202–3, 206

oral contraceptive 223, 420

Oramorph 150, 151, 154

orchidectomy 274, 279, 410

oropharyngeal cancers 66, 67–9, 198, 203–4, *204*, 206

osteosarcoma 359, 363–6, *363*, 387
    case history 382
    high-grade central 363–4
    intraosseus 364, 365
    investigations 363, *363*
    metastatic 365–6

parosteal 364, 365
pathological classification 363–4, *364*
periosteal 365
presentation 360
prognosis 366
treatment 364–5, 378
ovarian cancer *3, 12,* 222–7
aetiology 222–3
case history 229–30
in children *406,* 407, 408, *408, 409,* 410
examination and diagnosis 224
and intestinal obstruction 160, 246
pathology 223–4
presentation 224
prevention 73, 78, 223
prognosis 226–7
staging 225, *225*
treatment 112, 226
oxygen 154
ozone layer 173, 174

p53 tumour suppressor gene *43, 43,* 55, 296, 359, 421–2
paediatric cancers, *see* childhood cancers
Paget's disease 176
of bone 359, 366, 369
of nipple 176, 438, *438*
pain 147
types 147
pain management 147–53, *153*
aim 147
approaches 148–9
in breast cancer 435
in lung cancer 303
neurosurgery 111
pharmacology 149, *149*
principles 148
in prostate cancer 274
palliative care 143–69
bereavement services 146
case histories 166–7
common symptoms and management 147–61
day care centres 146
defined 145
home care teams 146
hospital units 146
management of terminal phase of illness 162–6
psychosocial and spiritual care 161–2
specialist in-patient units (hospices) 145–6
specialist teams within acute hospital setting 146
palliative medicine 145
palliative radiotherapy 137
palliative surgery 110–11
Pancoast syndrome 299, 300
pancreatic cancer *3,* 238–40
aetiology *239*

clinical presentation 239, *239*
endocrine tumours 480–4, *481,* 485
epidemiology 238
investigations 108, 240
pathology *12,* 238–9
prognosis 240
treatment 240
pancreaticoduodenectomy 240, 243, 244, 247
papillary cystadenoma lymphomatosum (Warthin's tumour) 196
papillomaviruses 23
see also human papillomavirus
paracetamol 149
paraganglioma 462
paraganglionic neurogenic tumours 285, 289
paranasal sinuses 194, 198, 205, 207
paraneoplastic syndromes 57
in lung cancer 299–300, *299*
in neuroblastoma *389*
in renal carcinoma 260, *261*
in thymoma 286, *287,* 288
paraproteins 341–2, *342,* 345, *345*
parasympathetic nervous system 461–2
parathymic syndromes 286, *287,* 288
parathyroid tumours 476
Parinaud's syndrome 456
parity 214, 217, 223, 419
parotid tumours 196
particulate radiation 137, *137*
passive smoking 69
pathological fractures, *see* bone fractures
pathology 47–60
carcinogenesis 50–6
neoplasia 49–50
spread and effects of malignant tumours 56–7
tissue diagnosis 11–12, 57–9
see also specific cancers
patient performance status 125, *125*
PAX gene 380
pegylated liposomal doxorubicin (PLD) 381
pelvic cancer, imaging 89–90
penectomy 277
penile carcinoma 275–7
incidence and aetiology 275, *275*
investigation and treatment 276–7
presentation and pathology 275–6, *275, 276*
prognosis *277*
pentostatin 340
peptic ulcer disease 483
peptide hormones 293, 294, 299, 480–2, 487
pericardial effusion 310, 495–7, *496*
aetiology 495
investigations 496
presentation 496
prognosis 497
treatment 114, 310, 496

pericardial sclerosis 496
pericardiocentesis 114, 310
periorbital ecchymoses 389, *389*
peripheral blood stem cell (PBSC) rescue 336, 340, 344, 353, 368
peripheral nervous system (PNS) tumours 459–62
peripheral neuroblastic tumours 461–2
peripheral neuropathy 128
peritoneal–venous shunt (Denver shunt) 111
personality factors 96–7
phaeochromocytoma 462, 479–80, *479*, 485
Philadelphia chromosome 55, 330
phototherapy 267
pineal gland tumours 455–6
   germ cell 455–6
   glial 456
   pineoblastoma 456
pipe smoking 193
pituitary tumours 467–71
   adenoma 454, 467
      ACTH-producing 467, 469
      case history 487–8
      epidemiology/aetiology/pathology 467
      examination and investigation 470–1, *470*
      growth hormone (GH)-producing 467, 469
      presentation 467–70, *467, 468, 469*
      prolactin-secreting 467–8, 471
      treatment and prognosis 471, *471*
   craniopharyngioma 454–5
placental alkaline phosphatase (PLAP) *279*, 455
plain radiographs 84–6
plasmacytoma 341
platelet apheresis 349
platelet-derived growth factors 349
platelet transfusion 513
platinum analogues 124, 226, 289, 316
   see also specific drugs
pleomorphic adenoma 196, 197
pleomorphism 50, 52
pleural effusion 310, 313, 366, 435
pleural mesothelioma, malignant, *see* mesothelioma
pleurectomy and decortication of lung 314, *314*
Plummer–Vinson's tumour 234
pneumonectomy 303–4, 315
point mutations 55
polycyclic hydrocarbons 19, 194
polycythaemia (rubra) vera 346–8, *347, 348*
   prognosis 348
   quality of life 348
   treatment 347–8
polyembryoma 407
polymerase chain reaction 59
polymorphisms 54
polyposis coli 72, 112, 248–9, 402
positional cloning 54
positron emission tomography (PET) 90

post-cricoid tumours 194, 204
postmenopausal bleeding 215
precursor B/T lymphoblastic lymphoma 340
prednisolone 329
prednisone 329, 336, 339–40, 343
prevention 31, 61–79
   of breast cancer, *see* breast cancer, prevention
   chemoprevention 72–3, 78, 296
   and diet 63–7, *66*
   genetic susceptibility testing 77–8, *78*
   of head and neck cancer 72, 195
   of lung cancer 67–9, *67, 68*, 72, 296
   of mesothelioma 69, 312–13
   and occupational carcinogens 69, *70*
   of ovarian cancer 73, 78
   primary 63–73, *63*
   prophylactic surgery 73, 78, 112, 441
   screening, *see* screening
   secondary 74–8
   of skin cancer 70–1, *71*, 186–7
   surveillance 77
   of viral-related cancer 71, *71*
primitive neuroectodermal tumours (PNET) 366, 367, 453, 461–2
procarbazine 128, 336
progestogens 216–17
progression 53
progressive telomere truncation 55
prolactinoma 467–8, 471
promotion 17–18, *17*, 19–20, *21*
prophylactic cranial irradiation (PCI) 308
prostate cancer *3, 4, 5*, 30, 259, 268–75
   case histories 141–2, 281
   clinical presentation 269, *269*
   diagnosis/staging/grading 270, 271, *271*
   investigations 271–2
   pathology 269–71, *269*
   risk factors 65, *268*
   screening 76–7, 274–5
   treatment options 272–4
prostatic intraductal neoplasia (PIN) 269
prostatic specific antigen (PSA) 12, 77, 271, *272*, 274–5
protein tyrosine kinases (PTK) 40–1
proto-oncogenes 40, *41*
   see also specific genes
psammoma bodies 224
psychology 93–103
   behaviour and cognitions 95, *95, 96*
   and breast cancer 96, 98–9, 101, 102, 439–40, *439*
   case history 102
   personality factors 96–7
   psychological impact 97–9, *97, 98*
   psychological risk factors 95–7
   psychotherapy 99–102
      and psychosocial outcome 99–100, *99*

and survival 100–1, *100*
    treatment provision 101–2
psychoneuroimmunology 100–1
public awareness campaigns *71*, 187
pulmonary haemorrhage 114
pulmonary toxicity, of chemotherapy 127–8
purpura 324
pyrimidine dimers 44

radiation, *see* ionizing radiation; ultraviolet radiation
radiation oncologists 135
radical cystectomy 267
radical hysterectomy 216, 220
radical nephrectomy 262, 263
radical prostatectomy 272–3
radical trachelectomy 221
radical vulvectomy 213
radiobiology 135–7
    '5 Rs' *136*
radiographers 140
radioiodine 476
radiological imaging 10, 81–92
    computerized tomography (CT) 87–9, *88*, 272, 498
    interventional radiology/angiography 90–1, *91*
    magnetic resonance imaging (MRI) 89–90, 199, *199*, 272, 498
    modalities *83*, 84–6
    nuclear medicine (radioisotope imaging) 90
    positron emission tomography (PET) 90
    ultrasound, *see* ultrasound
radiosurgery 451
radiotherapy 133–42
    case histories 141–2
    conformal treatment 138
    external beam 139
    historical perspective 135
    immobilization shell 203, *203*
    -induced malignancy 175, 359, 367, 371, 401, 448
    medical physics 137, *137*
    and neutropenic sepsis 507
    planning process 137–9
        outcome 139
        pre-planning 137
        treatment delivery 138–9
        treatment planning 137–8
    pre-/postoperative 109–10
    radiation oncology department 139–41
    radiobiology 135–7, *136*
    simulation 137–8, 140
    treatment of
        anal cancer 255–6
        bile duct carcinoma 244
        bladder cancer 267
        bone tumours 362, *362*, 365, 367
        brain metastases 308, 500
        brain tumours, primary 411, 451, 452–4, 455, 456

        breast cancer 371, 433
        gynaecological cancers 216, 220, 222
        haemoptysis 503
        head and neck cancer 201, 202, 203, *203*, 204, *204*, 205
        large airway obstruction 502
        leukaemia 329
        lung cancer 294, 304–5, 307–8
        lymphoma 336, 339
        mediastinal tumours 289–90, 291
        mesothelioma 315
        nephroblastoma 394–5
        oesophageal cancer 235
        pericardial effusion 496
        prostate cancer 273
        retinoblastoma 400–1
        rhabdomyosarcoma 398
        skin cancer 177, 185
        soft tissue sarcomas 377
        spinal cord compression 457–8, 498
    raised intracranial pressure 158–9, 449, 455, 499
ras oncogene 41, 55, 472
    K-*ras* oncogene 238, 296
    Ras proteins 41
REAL classification, non-Hodgkin's lymphoma 337, *337*
reciprocal translocation 54–5
reconstructive surgery 110, *430*, 431–2, *431*
rectal cancer, *see* colorectal cancer
red meat 65, 249
Reed–Sternberg cells 334
Reese–Ellsworth staging classification, retinoblastoma *400*
registration systems 29–30
rehydration 161, 165, 501, 510
renal carcinoma 57, 259–63
    aetiology 65, 259–60
    clinical presentation 260, *260*, *261*
    imaging 89
    investigation 261
    pathology 260–1
    treatment 261–3
    see also renal cell carcinoma
renal cell carcinoma (RCC)
    aetiology 259–60
    histopathological grading 261
    immunotherapy 262–3
    incidental detection 259, 260
    nephron-sparing surgery 263
    paraneoplastic effects *261*
    pathology 260–1
    prognosis 263, *263*
    staging *262*
    treatment of localized RCC 261–2
    treatment of metastatic RCC 262
renal toxicity, of chemotherapy 127
respiratory symptoms, in palliative care 153–6
retinoblastoma gene (*RB1*) 399

retinoblastoma (RB) *387*, 398–401, 456
  clinical presentation 399–400, *399*
  diagnosis 400
  epidemiology 398–9
  familial 42, 359, 371, 398–9, 401
  genetics and molecular biology *41*, 42, 53, 399
  pathology 399, *399*
  prognosis 401
  staging *400*
  treatment 400–1
  two-hit theory *41*, 42, 53, 399
retinoids 72, 195, 296
RET proto-oncogene 472, 474, 475, 485
retroviruses 22, *22*, 24–5, 55
rhabdomyosarcoma (RMS) 372, 378, 379–80
  alveolar 379–80, 395–6, *396*
  in children 370, 379, 380, *387*, 395–8
    clinical presentation 396–7, *396*
    diagnosis 397–8, *397*
    epidemiology 395
    pathology and genetics 395–6, *396*
    prognosis 398
    staging *397*, 398
    treatment 380, 398
  embryonal 379, 395, *396*, 398
  pleomorphic 380
RNA viruses 21–2, 24–5, 40
rodent ulcer 176
round cell tumours 367, *367*

sacrococcygeal tumours 407, *409*, 410
salivary gland tumours 196–7, 205, 207
Salmon–Durie staging system, myeloma *344*
sarcoma 53, 57
  bone and soft tissue sarcomas 357–83
SAS gene 371
Schwann cells 460
schwannoma 289, 371, 459, 460–1
sclerosing cholangitis 243
screening 8–9, 74–7
  for breast cancer 74–5, 424–5, *425*
  for cervical cancer 75–6, *75*, 217–18
  for colorectal cancer 76, 253
  for lung cancer 296
  for multiple endocrine neoplasia (MEN) syndrome type 1: 485
  for ovarian cancer 223
  for prostatic cancer 76–7, 274–5
  test requirements *73*, 74, *74*
seborrhoeic keratosis 175
second messengers 41
sedentary lifestyle 33, 65
seminoma
  in children 405, 407
  mediastinal 290–1
  testicular 278, *278*, 279, 407

sentinel node biopsy 184–5
serotonin 293, 482
serous adenocarcinoma 223
Sézary syndrome 340
sigmoid colectomy 252
sigmoidoscopy 76, 251
silicone breast implants 431
simian virus 40 448
c-*sis* gene 312
skin cancer 171–89, *173*
  aetiology 20, 43–4, 174–5, *174*
  benign lesions 175–6
  case history 187–8
  diagnosis 175–6
  head and neck cancers 202, *202*, 206
  malignant lesions 176
  melanoma, *see* melanoma
  pre-malignant lesions 176
  prevention 70–1, *71*, 186–7
  skin metastases 176
  treatment 176–7
skin types 178–9, *178*
small bowel tumours 245–7
  aetiology 245–6
  carcinoids 482
  clinical presentation 246
  epidemiology 245
  investigations 246–7
  pathology 246, *246*
  prognosis 247
  treatment 247
small cell lung cancer (SCLC) 57, 292
  aetiology 41, 296
  pathology 298
  treatment 306–8, *307*, 495
  treatment success rates and prognosis 308
smoked food 64, 236
smoking 8
  and cancer prevention 32, 67–9, *67*, *68*, 96, 296
  and cervical cancer 217
  and head and neck cancer 193, 194
  and lung cancer 19, 67–9, 295–6
  and renal carcinoma 259
soft palate 206
soft tissue sarcomas, adult 370–82
  aetiology 371–2
  clinical presentation 372
  investigations 372–3
  management 376–9
    adjuvant chemotherapy 378
    chemotherapy 378, *378*
    combined radiotherapy and surgery 377, *377*
    pulmonary metastasectomy 378–9, *378*
    radiotherapy 377
    surgery 376–7

pathological classification 373–6, *373, 374*
  prognosis 379, *379*
  staging *375*, 376
solar (actinic/senile) keratosis 176
soluble fibre 65
somatic mutations 42, 53, 392, 399
somatostatin analogues 294, 481–2
space-occupying lesion (SOL) 89, 449, *449*
spinal cord compression (SCC) 457–9, 497–9, *498*
  aetiology 497
  in breast cancer 436
  case history 511–12
  investigation 497–8, *498*
  in lung cancer 306, 459
  presentation 457–8, 497
  prognosis 498–9
  treatment 457–8, 498
spinal tumours 457–9
  imaging 89, 458
  location 459, *459*
  non-surgical management 457–8
  of spinal cord and canal 459
  surgical management 458
spironolactone 479
splenectomy 350
splenic enlargement 325, 330, 349
sputum cytology 296, 300
squamous cell carcinoma (SCC) 52
  cervical *51*, 52, 218
  head and neck 195, 196, 202, 206
  lung 297
  oesophagus 233, 234
  skin 70, 174, 176, 178, 202, 206
  vulva 211
staging 10–12, 58
  surgical 108
  see also specific cancers
sterility, and chemotherapy 128
steroids 155, 453, 495, 498, 499, 500
stilboestrol 221
stomach cancer *3*, 236–8
  aetiology 236
  clinical presentation 237
  early gastric cancer 237, 238
  epidemiology 236
  investigations 237
  pathology 236–7, *237*
  prevention 66
  prognosis 238
  treatment 237–8
streptozotocin 484
stridor 198, 293
subcutaneous administration of drugs 164
subglottis 206
sulindac 72

sunburn 178
sun-ray spiculation 363, *363*
superficial spreading/flat melanoma (SSM) 179, *180*
superior vena cava obstruction 493–5, *494*
  aetiology 493
  in bronchogenic carcinoma 298, 305–6, 493, 495
  investigation 494
  in lymphoma 334
  presentation 493–4
  prognosis 495
  treatment 495
support groups, breast cancer 440
supraglottis 206
surgery 105–17
  anatomy and pathology 109
  avoidance of unnecessary surgery 107–8
  blood transfusion 113
  case histories 114–16
  combined treatment modalities 109–10
  complications of treatment 113
  conservative 110
  diagnostic 108
  emergencies 114
  ethics 107–8
  limb-sparing *361*, 364, 372, 376
  for metastases 112
  minimally invasive 111
  nutrition management 113
  palliative 110–11
  prophylactic 73, 78, 112, 441
  radical 110
  reconstructive 110, *430*, 431–2, *431*
  specialized centres and outcome 6
  and staging 108
  surgeon as part of oncology team 107
  treatment of
    adrenal tumours 477–8, *478*, 480
    adult soft tissue sarcomas 371, 376–7
    bile duct carcinoma 243, 244
    bone tumours *361*, 362, 364, 365, 367, 369, 370
    brain tumours, primary 451, 452–3, 454, 456
    brain tumours, secondary 112, 500
    breast cancer, *see* mastectomy
    cardiac tumours 291–2
    chemotherapy extravasation 510
    colorectal cancer 109, 252, *252*, *253*
    germ cell tumours in children 410
    gynaecological cancer 213, 216, 220, 222, 226
    head and neck cancer 200–1, *201*, 203, 204, 205
    hepatoblastoma 403–4
    hepatoma 242
    impending bone fracture 112, 505
    lung cancer, primary 294, 303–4
    lung cancer, secondary 112, 309–10, *365*, 378–9, *378*
    mesothelioma *314*, 315

surgery (*cont.*)
  treatment of (*cont.*)
    nephroblastoma 394
    oesophageal cancer 235, *235*
    pancreatic cancer 240
    penile cancer 277
    pituitary adenoma 471
    renal carcinoma 261–2, 263
    retinoblastoma 401
    rhabdomyosarcoma 398
    skin cancer 177, 184–5, 202
    small bowel tumours 247
    spinal cord compression 458, 498
    stomach cancer 237–8
    testicular cancer 279
    thymoma 289
    thyroid tumours 475
    urothelial cancer 267, 268
  vascular access 112–13
  see also specific operations
surveillance 77
survival rates 4–6, *5*, 100–1
susceptibility bias 30
sympathetic nervous system 461, 462
synovial sarcoma 370, *371*

talc pleurodesis 310, 315, 435
tamoxifen 73, 214, 420, 433, 438, 441
tat gene 24
taxanes 121–2, 126, 226, 307
Taxol 127
technetium-99m (^{99m}Tc) 90
telomerase 55–6
telomeres 55
temozolamide 451
TENS (transcutaneous electrical nerve stimulation) 148
teratoma
  in children 405, 407, 455–6
  mediastinal 290–1
  ovarian 222, 224, 226
  pineal gland 455–6
  testicular *278*
terminal phase of illness 162–6
  aims of care 163
  approach to symptom management 163–4
  cultural issues and religious practices 165–6
  definition 162–3
  frequency of symptoms *163*
  management of common symptoms 164–5
  role of hydration 165
testicular cancer 277–80
  aetiology 259, *278*
  case history 131–2
  in children 406, 407, *408*, *409*, 410
  classification *278*

clinical presentation 277–8
  investigation *12*, 279, *279*
  pathology 278–9, *278*
  prevention 73
  treatment 279–80
thoracic tumours 283–317
thorotrast 241
thrombocythaemia, essential (ET) 348–9, *349*
thrombocytopenia 510–13
  aetiology 510
  treatment 513
thrombosis
  deep venous 113
  risk in polycythaemia vera 348
  and superior vena cava obstruction 493, 495
thymic carcinoma 288, 289
thymic tumours 286–9, *286*
thymidylate synthase 125
thymoma 286–9
  aetiology and epidemiology 286
  features of presentation 287, 288
  pathology 286–8, *286*
  prognosis 289
  treatment 288–9
thyroglobulin 473–4, 476
thyroidectomy 73, 475
thyroid tumours 471–6
  anaplastic 473, *473*, 475
  blood tests 473–4
  case history 488
  classification/aetiology/pathology 471–2, *472*
  clinical features 472, 473, *473*
  follicular 472, *473*, 475, *475*, 476
  imaging 90, 474, *474*
  investigation 473–4
  medullary, *see* medullary thyroid carcinoma
  papillary 471–2, *473*, 475, *475*, 476
  prognosis *475*, 476
  staging 475
  treatment 475–6
thyroxine 473, 475
tissue diagnosis 57–9
tissue plasminogen activator (TPA) 19
TNM (tumour–node–metastasis) classification 11–12
tobacco, *see* smoking
tongue 195, 198, 206, 485
tonsillar tumours 204, 206
total hysterectomy 216
total pain concept 147
TP53 gene 55
trans-arterial chemo-embolization (TACE) 91
transcription factors 39, 41
transforming growth factor-a (TGF-a) 40
transforming growth factor-beta (TGF-ß) 312
transitional cell carcinoma (TCC) 264

of bladder 266–8, *266*
  of upper urinary tract 268
  of urethra 268, 281
transphenoidal surgery 471
transrectal ultrasound (TRUS) 77, 271–2, *272*
transurethral resection of bladder tumour (TURBT) 264
transverse rectus abdominus myocutaneous (TRAM) flap *430*, 431, *431*
treatment principles 12–13
trephine biopsy 326
trkA gene 388
Troisier's sign 237
tumour boards 140
tumour-infiltrating lymphocytes (TILs) 186
tumour lysis syndrome 510
  aetiology 510
  presentation 510
  prevention 510
  treatment 510
tumour markers 12, *12*
  see also specific markers
tumour necrosis factor 156–7
tumour suppressor genes (TSG) *41*, 42–3, 53–4
  familial cancers as indicators 42
  loss of heterogosity studies 42, *43*
  retinoblastoma paradigm 42
  somatic and microcell genetic studies 42
  see also specific genes
tumour vaccines 129
two-hit theory
  and nephroblastoma 392
  and retinoblastoma *41*, 42, 53, 399
typing, of tumours 57–8

ulceration 56, 174, 184
ulcerative colitis 243, 249
ultrasound 86–7, *86*
  breast cancer diagnosis 423
  endoluminal 235
  intraoperative 108
  transrectal (TRUS) 77, 271–2, *272*
ultraviolet radiation 20, 44, 70–1, 174, 177, 178
umbilical cord blood transplantation 353–4
unconditional positive regard 97
undifferentiated carcinoma 197, 207
ureteric obstruction 503–4
  aetiology 503
  investigations 503–4
  presentation 503
  treatment 114, 504
ureteric stents 504
urethra, transitional cell carcinoma (TCC) 268, 281
urethrectomy 268
urinary diversion 267
urothelial cancer 263–8

clinical presentation 264
diagnosis and staging 264–5
pathology 265–6, *266*
treatment 266–8
uterine cervix, *see* cervical cancer

vaccines 129, 186
vaginal carcinoma 221–2
  aetiology 221
  epidemiology 221
  examination/diagnosis/staging 222
  pathology 221–2
  prognosis 222
  treatment 222
vanillylmandelic acid 285, 390, 461
vegetables and fruit 65–6
venesection 348
venogram 494
venting gastrostomy 161
vesicants 509
VICE (vincristine, ifosfamide, carboplatin, etoposide) 307
vinblastine 126, 509
  in bladder cancer 267–8
  in Hodgkin's disease 336
  in Kaposi's sarcoma 381
  in lung cancer 304
  toxicity 128
vincristine 126, 509
  in bone tumours 367–8
  in leukaemia 329
  in lung cancer 307
  in lymphoma 336, 339–40
  in nephroblastoma 395
  in rhabdomyosarcoma 380
  toxicity 127, 128
virilizing adrenal tumours 479
viruses 33, 55
  and brain tumours 448
  DNA 21–4
  and head and neck cancer 194
  prevention of viral-related cancer 71, *71*
  RNA 21–2, 24–5, 40
  and sarcomas 372
  see also specific viruses
visceral pain 147
vitamins and minerals 65–6, 194, 296
vomiting, *see* nausea and vomiting
vomiting centre 158–9
von Hippel–Lindau (VHL) syndrome 259–60
von Recklinghausen's disease (neurofibromatosis type 1) 289, 371, 456, 460
vulval cancer 211–14, *211*, 221
  adjuvant therapy 213
  aetiology 211
  case history 227

vulvar cancer (*cont.*)
   diagnosis 212
   epidemiology 211
   examination 212
   pathology 211
   presentation 211
   prognosis 213–14
   staging 212–13, *212*
   treatment 213
vulval dystrophy 211
vulval intraepithelial neoplasia (VIN) 211

Waldenström's macroglobulinaemia 345
warts 175

weakness 156–7
Whipple's triad 483
Will Rogers phenomenon 30
Wilms' tumour, *see* nephroblastoma
Wilms' tumour 1 gene (*WT1*) 392
Wilms' tumour 2 gene (*WT2*) 392
workplace carcinogens 33, 69, *70*, 175, 194, 295, 448
   see also specific carcinogens
World Health Organization 3-Step Analgesic Ladder 149, *149*

xeroderma pigmentosum (XP) 20, 43–4, 174, 179
x-rays 135, 137, 139, 448

yolk sac tumour (endodermal sinus tumour) 405, 407, 408

Colon and Other Gastrointestinal Cancers

Cancer
Principles & Practice
of Oncology

10th edition